HANDBOOK OF ADULT RESILIENCE

HANDBOOK OF ADULT RESILIENCE

Edited by
John W. Reich
Alex J. Zautra
John Stuart Hall

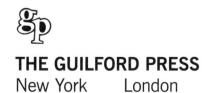

THE GUILFORD PRESS
New York   London

*To Deborah, my wife and continuing role model
for resilient beliefs and actions.*
—J. W. R.

*To Eva, for her tireless support, her ever-present encouragement,
and her enthusiastic embrace of good work
as a key to the good life.*
—A. J. Z.

*To Connie, for her endless contributions
to my resilience, health, and happiness.*
—J. S. H.

©2010 The Guilford Press
A Division of Guilford Publications, Inc.
72 Spring Street, New York, NY 10012
www.guilford.com

Printed in the United States of America

This book is printed on acid-free paper.

Last digit is print number: 9   8   7   6   5   4   3   2   1

Library of Congress Cataloging-in-Publication Data

Handbook of adult resilience / edited by John W. Reich, Alex J. Zautra,
John Stuart Hall.
    p. cm.
  Includes bibliographical references and index.
  ISBN 978-1-60623-488-4 (hardcover)
  1. Resilience (Personality trait). 2. Crisis management. 3. Community
organization. I. Reich, John W., 1937– II. Zautra, Alex. III. Hall,
John Stuart, 1942–
  BF698.35.R47H36 2010
  155.2′4—dc22
                                                    2009023674

About the Editors

John W. Reich, PhD, is Emeritus Professor of Psychology at Arizona State University (ASU). His work has focused on the application of social psychological concepts in understanding societal issues and the development of interventions for improving individuals' well-being. Dr. Reich and the other two coeditors are members of the ASU Resilience Solutions Group, which was the source of the development of this handbook.

Alex J. Zautra, PhD, is Foundation Professor of Clinical Psychology at ASU. His research, clinical work, teaching, and publications explore fundamental mind–body issues such as the role of positive emotion in health and the sources of resilience within the person that restore health and well-being following challenges from stressors at home, at work, and in community life. Dr. Zautra's current research focuses on resilience to chronic pain and resilience as people age.

John Stuart Hall, PhD, is Professor of Public Affairs and Public Service at ASU. A founder and former Director of ASU's School of Public Affairs and its Center for Urban Studies, and Project Director of over 40 large-scale funded and often interdisciplinary urban research projects, Dr. Hall has specialized in linking the University with pressing community public policy and governance issues. His current research interests include building resilience in communities and urban regions, and healthy aging.

Contributors

C. S. Bergeman, PhD, Department of Psychology, University of Notre Dame, Notre Dame, Indiana

Kathrin Boerner, PhD, Jewish Home Lifecare, Research Institute on Aging, Mount Sinai School of Medicine, New York, New York

George A. Bonanno, PhD, Department of Counseling and Clinical Psychology, Teachers College, Columbia University, New York, New York

Allison B. Brenner, MPH, Department of Health Behavior and Health Education, School of Public Health, University of Michigan, Ann Arbor, Michigan

Felipe González Castro, PhD, MSW, Department of Psychology, Arizona State University, Tempe, Tempe, Arizona

Dennis S. Charney, MD, Departments of Psychiatry, Neuroscience, and Pharmacology and Systems Therapeutics, Mount Sinai School of Medicine, New York, New York

Sy-Miin Chow, PhD, Department of Psychology, University of North Carolina at Chapel Hill, Chapel Hill, North Carolina

Jeremy Cummings, MA, Department of Psychology, Bowling Green State University, Bowling Green, Ohio

Mary C. Davis, PhD, Department of Psychology, Arizona State University, Tempe, Tempe, Arizona

Matthew D. Della Porta, MA, Department of Psychology, University of California, Riverside, Riverside, California

Janet Denhardt, DPA, School of Public Affairs, Arizona State University, Phoenix, Phoenix, Arizona

Robert Denhardt, PhD, School of Public Affairs, Arizona State University, Phoenix, Phoenix, Arizona

Michael A. Faber, PhD, Department of Psychology, University of New Hampshire, Durham, New Hampshire

Adriana Feder, MD, Department of Psychiatry, Mount Sinai School of Medicine, New York, New York

Jenna L. Gress, MA, Department of Psychology, Arizona State University, Tempe, Tempe, Arizona

John Stuart Hall, PhD, School of Public Affairs, Arizona State University, Phoenix, Phoenix, Arizona

Vicki S. Helgeson, PhD, Department of Psychology, Carnegie Mellon University, Pittsburgh, Pennsylvania

Atara Hiller, BA, Department of Psychology, Barnard College, New York, New York

Roger A. Hughes, PhD, St. Luke's Health Initiatives, Phoenix, Arizona

Daniela Jopp, PhD, Department of Psychology, Fordham University, Bronx, New York

Paul Karoly, PhD, Department of Psychology, Arizona State University, Tempe, Tempe, Arizona

Martha Kent, PhD, Phoenix VA Health Care System, Phoenix, Arizona

John P. Kretzmann, PhD, Asset-Based Community Development Institute, School of Education and Social Policy, Northwestern University, Evanston, Illinois

Kathryn Lemery-Chalfant, PhD, Department of Psychology, Arizona State University, Tempe, Tempe, Arizona

Lindsey Lopez, MA, Department of Psychology, Carnegie Mellon University, Pittsburgh, Pennsylvania

Linda J. Luecken, PhD, Department of Psychology, Arizona State University, Tempe, Tempe, Arizona

Sonja Lyubomirsky, PhD, Department of Psychology, University of California, Riverside, Riverside, California

Anthony D. Mancini, PhD, Department of Psychology, Pace University, Pleasantville, New York

Ann S. Masten, PhD, Institute of Child Development, University of Minnesota, Minneapolis, Minnesota

John D. Mayer, PhD, Department of Psychology, University of New Hampshire, Durham, New Hampshire

Judith Tedlie Moskowitz, PhD, Osher Center for Integrative Medicine, University of California, San Francisco, San Francisco, California

Kate E. Murray, MA, Department of Psychology, Arizona State University, Tempe, Tempe, Arizona

Eric J. Nestler, MD, PhD, Departments of Neuroscience, Psychiatry, and Pharmacology and Systems Therapeutics, Mount Sinai School of Medicine, New York, New York

Anthony D. Ong, PhD, Department of Human Development, College of Human Ecology, Cornell University, Ithaca, New York

Kenneth I. Pargament, PhD, Department of Psychology, Bowling Green State University, Bowling Green, Ohio

Eshkol Rafaeli, PhD, Department of Psychology, Barnard College, New York, New York

Andrew E. Skodol, MD, Sunbelt Collaborative, Tucson, Arizona, and Department of Psychiatry, University of Arizona College of Medicine, Tucson, Arizona

Maren Westphal, MD, Department of Psychiatry, Mount Sinai School of Medicine, New York, New York

Margaret O'Dougherty Wright, PhD, Department of Psychology, Miami University, Oxford, Ohio

Michael Ungar, PhD, School of Social Work, Dalhousie University, Halifax, Nova Scotia, Canada

Alex J. Zautra, PhD, Department of Psychology, Arizona State University, Tempe, Tempe, Arizona

Marc A. Zimmerman, PhD, Department of Health Behavior and Health Education, School of Public Health, University of Michigan, Ann Arbor, Michigan

Preface

This volume represents an attempt to bring together in one place contemporary scholarship on theory, research, and practice emerging from the newly developing concept of resilience. Although foundational work on this concept initially arose from work on childhood and developmental topics, this handbook fully extends the currency of resilience concepts for the first time from basic biological processes through childhood to the domains of youth and adulthood, to broader societal variables in leadership and community-level processes.

Resilience may well be one of the most heuristic and integrative concepts to appear in 21st-century thinking in the social sciences. Although it has many variations in definitions and characterizations (as will be clear from reading the chapters in this volume), there appear to be two dominant themes in our current thinking that are central to the meaning of this concept: First, as a response to stressful events, resilience focuses on *recovery*, the ability to rebound from stress, a capacity to regain equilibrium quickly and to return to an initial state of health. A second and equally central dimension, *sustainability*, implies the continuation of the recovery trajectory, and even growth and enhancement of function as a result of healthy reactions to the stressful experience. Investigators vary in the degree of focus they place on each of these dimensions, but the themes appear in some version in most contemporary coverage of the concept.

The revolutionary significance of this concept's development perhaps can best be seen in light of the framework described by Thomas Kuhn (1962) in his discussion of the concept of paradigm and, specifically, paradigm shift. Historically, and beginning mainly in the 18th and 19th centuries, as scholars, scientists, and practitioners came to deal with significant individual and societal processes, their main focus was on analysis of, and treatment for, individual and social ills. At the biological level, medical science and practice, such as drug treatment, were applied to physical illness; at the psychological level, Freudian psychotherapy was applied to "mental" illness; and at the broader societal level, public health interventions and government and social welfare programs all arose to reduce or eliminate "sickness," however defined. The same concerns continue to this day.

In Kuhn's framework, the intellectual dominance of paradigms leads participants in these frameworks to adopt a worldview of "normal science," in which there is widespread agreement on the nature of the problem, standardized approaches and procedures to follow in dealing with it, and agreement on what constitutes a "cure." Historically, then, the pervasive acceptance of these various sciences justifies what we can now call the "disease model" as the reigning paradigm of the previous century, and its current manifestations are pervasive even today.

True to Kuhn's model, however, paradigms do not always fit well with the realities of the phenomena under investigation. Initially, these "anomalies" are either ignored or written off as uninteresting error. But over time these anomalies start to bring the normal science paradigm under increasing doubt and scrutiny, and practitioners start to look at nonparadigmatic ways to think about their phenomena. In the face of mounting evidence, the reigning paradigm gets significantly modified or even abandoned, to be replaced by a more acceptable worldview.

That very development characterizes the current shift of focus from the dominant disease model to the current rise of what we call here the resilience model. The standard disease model does not fit well with observations of individual and community responses to stressful experiences. For instance, national surveys in American society have found that nearly 75% of Americans are not now suffering from any diagnoses of emotional or behavioral problems (e.g., Kessler, Chiu, Demler, & Walters, 2005). Children raised in poor socioeconomic circumstances still show healthy developmental processes (Garmezy, 1991). Some groups experiencing high levels of standard risk factors nevertheless show no notable pattern of illness as might be expected from a disease/illness model (Gould, Madan, Qin, & Chavez, 2003). Even the stress in having cancer is followed by a strong sense of growth rather than retreat and withdrawal (Stanton, Bower, & Low, 2006). Community-level analyses provide corroborative evidence. Although communities can be viewed from the perspective of poverty, high school dropout rates, and income equality, newer models focus on social capital: Civic engagement, neighborhood efficacy, social trust, and volunteerism represent resources that can strengthen community health in spite of economic downturns or natural disasters (Putnam, 2000; Vale & Campanella, 2005).

The resilience paradigm suggests that healthy reactions to risk factors are the norm, not the unusual reaction for individuals and communities. A dynamic process of successful adaptation, and not merely an absence of illness, is a key consideration in reactions to stress. The basic parameters of this issue were recognized some time ago in Perry's (1983) review of literature on responses to natural disasters. Healthy and poor outcomes were found to occur, depending on a set of 11 factors that we now call risk and resource factors. An important conclusion is that resilience is a *distinct* process, independent of illness dimensions, and as such it has to be studied in its own right in terms of antecedent, process, and outcome variables.

A review of this volume's table of contents shows that investigators have approached resilience from a number of different angles, but we have categorized them here as moving from the biological, the personal, and up through neighborhood and community levels. We end, in Part IV of the volume, with interventions and applications, with what we see as the most cutting-edge advances as the field moves from basic theoretical and conceptual issues to actual tests of those models in real-world settings. These chapters represent the "payoff" of years of deep conceptual and empirical work to focus this exciting development in actual practice. The aim is not so much to solve problems as to reveal and to strengthen the enabling processes and conditions for actualizing personal and societal well-being.

These chapters approach all levels of resilience from differing perspectives. No single chapter can present everything, but *in toto* they demonstrate the power of the concept's functioning and many uses. We highlight some of the overarching issues at this particular juncture in the development of the resilience paradigm. These themes may suggest to the reader new avenues for thinking about the concept and its implications beyond the specific domains discussed in each chapter. The reader can perhaps apply his or her own structure to these topics, but they are presented here as at least a starting point for applying this new paradigm.

The Role of Stress

If one observes a person or a community functioning well and even growing, this is not *prima facie* evidence that it is a resilient organism or entity. The person may well have high intelligence, good education, or finances, and the community may have a well-functioning system of municipal agencies and available resources, but in contemporary thinking about resilience, as demonstrated in our chapters, these variables are not evidence of resilience per se. The major assumption in these chapters is that resilience has to be studied in the light of either a sudden or an ongoing system stressor. Only when there is a system threat can we be assured that the person or community has exercised the requisite strengths, resources, and capacities that result in shorter- or longer-term resilient adaptation and growth. Successful adaptation is relatively clear-cut and gives a direct report on the role of the various strengths and capacities. Conversely, only under stress are we able to determine that the person or community does not have sufficient amounts or types of resilience resources, whatever they may be, or has them and has failed to deploy them successfully, with poor outcomes. Needless to say, these failures of resilient solutions are quite different in their topographies and suggest distinctly different avenues for recovery of full capacity.

Trait or Process?

Perhaps the easiest explanation (attribution) for a resilient outcome is to say that the person or the community is "resilient," an attribution to a presumably stable entity or indwelling property in the person or community. Of course, as is the case with many such attributions, the logic is circular. But there are standardized measures of this trait version, at least for persons, and these measures are discussed in some of the chapters in this volume.

Other foundational work on resilience explicitly rejected a trait model. For instance, Masten, Best, and Garmezy (1990) wished to avoid thinking in the internal attribution models that would be required for a strict trait approach. They proposed a more open process model in which adaptation to stress is conceived of as a dynamic process involving internal capacities and strengths, and external resources such as a healthy family environment. Of course, traits can refer to stable qualities of social environments, as well as internal processes, but they are rarely used that way in psychological sciences. And the underlying concept of a trait—that it is unchanging—reduces the dynamic capacity of systems to surprise us with their facility to learn new adaptation strategies on the run. The chapters in this volume vary in their treatments of this cause-versus-process issue. There is empirical support for these different approaches, and future investigations will no doubt continue to obtain a broader understanding of them as more evidence is gathered.

Cause versus Outcome?

One of the chief distinctions that must be made early on in studying or applying resilience concepts is where one wants to start in the sequence of events. Does one want to approach the event as existing prior to the stressor, hence as a (pre)existing cause of later reactivity, or does one want to think of it as an outcome of an adjustment process? Thus, is resilience a process that causes positive adaptation, or is it a description of an outcome of preexisting variables or processes?

The chapters in this volume vary in how they approach these concerns. Treating a concern as a cause focuses attention on the states of the person or community prior to a system stressor. A focus on a resilient outcome opens up the additional question about successful shorter- versus longer-term successful adaptation. Each outcome could have differential causal relationships depending on how the original causal model is developed. Even more, though, shifting the focus to the outcome side opens up a new set of questions. How shall we approach the definition, characterization, and certainly the measurement of the behavior of individuals and communities if we want to study their "resilience"? What do we choose for our domain(s) of investigation? These types of issues are raised in the next section, on generalization of our models. For instance, if we choose to study resilience in baby boomers, we have to ask whether older and/or middle-aged adults show the same type of resilient outcomes as younger people. This may depend on the type of stressor and whether types of stressors vary across age levels. The same types of logical and empirical problems arise when considering not age but, for example, different cultural samples. Do Westerners differ from non-Western samples that are considered to have successful resilience outcomes?

Putting the focus on outcomes moves us away from a direct trait/cause model and requires us to conceptualize a more multifaceted approach. This would not, of course, force the abandonment of a simple trait/cause model but would nest it in a larger, more comprehensive approach to the cause–outcome sequence. The chapters in this handbook provide many valuable discussions of the components that have a role in a more integrated, comprehensive picture of resilience thinking.

How General Are Models of Resilience?

This handbook has intentionally recruited authors who devote their attention to the cross-cultural dimensions of resilience. There is little question that the literature to date has been almost totally devoted to Western samples and Western, individualistic thinking. We do not yet know the extent to which our models of resilience are generalizable and which aspects need to be reconceptualized better to fit other cultural prerogatives. Future research is needed to explore that question. The authors here provide comprehensive treatments of the extant literature, limited as it is today, and lay out for us ways we can explore this issue in greater depth across cultures. But to discuss resilience from the perspective of *cross-ethnic* issues should not preclude us from exploring other aspects of our limited sampling: Age, gender, and socioeconomic stratifications of samples, for instance, need to be systematically explored, and *comparative methods* are needed to mark the range and depth of applicability of our findings. Finally, of course, we need to be sure to test the range of applicability of our models to any interventions we design to enhance resilience in diverse populations of interest. The burdens of testing cross-domain generalities of our resilience studies are, of course, no greater than the same issues that arise in other areas of investigation, but those burdens are no less serious for this newly developing body of knowledge.

The issues we have raised here are intended to highlight themes and variations that appear in various forms in the chapters in this volume. Each chapter makes its own outstanding contribution within the framework of the resilience paradigm. The field is too new for Kuhn's (1962) anomalies to be building to the point of crisis, which may someday force a paradigm shift and realignment. Right now, the area is ripe for development and extension in ways we cannot foresee, and the issues we have raised here are intended to help the reader grasp the outlines and deep structure of the concept as it appears in each cutting-edge chapter in this volume. We hope that the reader finds these chapters exciting and brimming with possibilities for applicability of this new paradigm in the social sciences.

References

Garmezy, N. (1991). Resilience and vulnerability to adverse developmental outcomes associated with poverty. *American Behavioral Scientist, 34*, 416–430.

Gould, J. B., Madan, A., Qin, C., & Chavez, G. (2003). Perinatal outcomes in two dissimilar immigrant populations in the United States: A dual epidemiological paradox. *Pediatrics, 111*(6, Pt. 1), 676–682.

Kessler, R. C., Chiu, W. T., Demler, O., & Walters, E. E. (2005). Prevalence, severity, and comorbidity of 12-month DSM-IV disorders in the National Comorbidity Survey Replication. *Archives of General Psychiatry, 62*, 617–627.

Kuhn, T. S. (1962). *The structure of scientific revolutions.* Chicago: University of Chicago Press.

Masten, A. S., Best, K. M., & Garmezy, N. (1990). Resilience and development: Contributions from the study of children who overcome adversity. *Development and Psychopathology, 2*, 425–444.

Perry, R. W. (1983). Environmental hazards and psychopathology: Linking natural disasters with mental health. *Environmental Management, 7*, 543–552.

Putnam, R. D. (2000). *Bowling alone: The collapse and revival of American community.* New York: Simon & Schuster.

Stanton, A. L., Bower, J. E., & Low, C. A. (2006). Posttraumatic growth after cancer. In L. G. Calhoun & R. G. Tedeschi (Eds.), *Handbook of posttraumatic growth: Research and practice* (pp. 138–175). Mahwah, NJ: Erlbaum.

Vale, L. J., & Campanella, T. (2005). *The resilient city.* London: Oxford University Press.

Acknowledgments

This volume arose from ongoing discussions with members of the Arizona State University Resilience Solutions Group (RSG). The scholarly input and personal support of an interdisciplinary team of researchers and educators has been invaluable throughout the activities of the RSG and in the development of this handbook. Some of them have contributed even more by writing chapters for this volume. They are, alphabetically, Leona Aiken, Felipe Castro, Mary Davis, John Stuart Hall, Martha Kent, Richard Knopf, Kathryn Lemery-Chalfant, Linda Luecken, Morris Okun, Maureen Olmsted, John W. Reich, Billie Sandberg, and Alex J. Zautra. The website for RSG is *www.asu.edu/resilience*. Also playing a major role in the activities of the RSG is the support by the St. Luke's Health Initiative and its Director, Dr. Roger Hughes, and by Drs. Jonathan Fink and Rick Shangraw of the Arizona State University Office of the Vice-President of Research and Economic Advancement. The support and encouragement of all of these scholars is hereby gratefully acknowledged.

Contents

IV. INTERVENTIONS FOR ENHANCING RESILIENCE

RESILIENCE AT MANY LEVELS
OF ANALYSIS

1

Resilience

A New Definition of Health for People and Communities

Alex J. Zautra
John Stuart Hall
Kate E. Murray

Beginning with the Framingham Study (Dawber, Meadors, & Moore, 1951), risk factor research has a long and successful history of identifying biological and psychosocial vulnerabilities to chronic, as well as acute, illness. By age 65, most, if not all, Americans will harbor some significant risk for a life-threatening illness. Yet those who live that long may be expected to live an average of 20 more years. In addition, the National Academy of Sciences finds a decrease in disability rates—falling under 20% for the first time in 2000—among elders, citing education, diet, exercise, and medical and public health advances, all leading to a more vigorous and healthy old age (National Research Council, 2001). Even centenarians profess a level of happiness that rivals that of younger groups and laugh at least as often (Jopp & Smith, 2006). How do these people sustain themselves while ill, and how do so many who are ill recover?

The pursuit of knowledge about these capacities is not just about those individuals who beat the odds. There are also considerable anomalies in the community health data (Evans, Barer, & Marmor, 1994)—levels of illness and disablement that cannot be accounted for in the accumulation of risk indices, and surprisingly high levels of functional health in the face of physical illness that cannot be explained by risk factor research. Social status, for example, confers health advantage even after the calculation of multivariate risk ratios between risk and poor health (Marmot & Fuhrer, 2004). Furthermore, there are apparent paradoxes in the findings for some groups that cut against the social gradient (Heidrich & Ryff, 1993). The best known among them is the Hispanic paradox. Even at high risk on the standard indicators, those with strong attachment to their Hispanic heritage appear healthier as a group than their social status would warrant (Fuentes-Afflick, Hessol, & Perez-Stable, 1999; Gould, Madan, Qin, & Chavez, 2003).

These anomalies may be due to a matrix of factors woven within the fabric of the lives of people and their communities that confer resilience. Indices of this capacity for resilience may be found within the person, his or her primary network of kith and kin, and the sociocultural profiles of the neighborhood and community settings. In this chapter we offer resilience as an integrative construct that provides an approach to understanding how people and their communities achieve and sustain health and well-being in the face of adversity. Our aim is to define resilience based on current thinking in biopsychosocial disciplines, to outline key research methods employed to study resilience, and to suggest how this approach may further the development of public health and other intervention programs designed to promote health and well-being.

What Is Resilience?

We begin with definitions of the term. The need for clarity here is made all the more important by its popularity in everyday discourse, becoming what Rutter (1999) has called the "millennium Rorschach." Until recently, scholarly work on resilience was the sole province of developmental psychology (Luthar, 2006). In that arena, resilience has been studied as a dynamic process of successful adaptation to adversity revealed through the lens of developmental psychopathology. Across research and practice, there has been considerable debate over the definition and operationalization of resilience (Luthar, Cicchetti, & Becker, 2000). Is resilience best categorized as a process, an individual trait, a dynamic developmental process, an outcome, or all of the above? In addition, where does one draw the line at successful and resilient adaptation versus nonresilient responses?

In our view, *resilience* is best defined as an outcome of successful adaptation to adversity. Characteristics of the person and situation may identify resilient processes, but only if they lead to healthier outcomes following stressful circumstances. Two fundamental questions need to be asked when inquiring about resilience. First is *recovery*, or how well people bounce back and recover fully from challenge (Masten, 2001; Rutter, 1987). People who are resilient display a greater capacity to quickly regain equilibrium physiologically, psychologically, and in social relations following stressful events. Second, and equally important, is *sustainability*, or the capacity to continue forward in the face of adversity (Bonanno, 2004). To address this aspect of resilience we ask how well people sustain health and psychological well-being in a dynamic and challenging environment.

Definition 1. Recovery: From Risk to Resilience

One of the problems we have in understanding the processes of recovery from stressful events is that most models of physical and mental health have not developed an adequate understanding of the meaning of recovery. This problem is made even more apparent by the frequency with which people and communities actually recover from adversity. Masten (2001), in referring to the many children who survive difficult even abusive home environments, called it "ordinary magic." It is most consistent with resilience we observe in human communities: a natural capacity to recover and at times even further one's adaptive capacities. In fact, the modal response to calamity in our community studies has been not to despair but "to see the silver lining." People report they "discovered what really mattered in life," "found out how much others cared," and "uncovered hidden strengths within (or hidden capacities for generosity in others)" (Zautra, 2003). Researchers who have focused narrowly on developmental risks often see resilience in response to adversity as the exception rather than the rule (Luthar, 2006). However, people are extraordinary, and it is common, not rare, to observe these feats of resilience in children (Garmezy, 1991) and across the lifespan (Bonanno, 2004; Greve & Staudinger, 2006). Some initial psychological distress following stressful experiences is expected and may even be potentially beneficial to adaptation. From a resilience perspective, speed and thoroughness of recovery from harm are the key outcomes to observe. A resilient "recovery" may not be without some remaining emotional "scars," but the return to health is often well beyond what our models of psychopathology would have predicted. A broader and more differentiated view of physical and mental health would be a place to start to capture these resilience experiences.

Though the resilience response may be nearly universal, it is unlikely that we are all the same in this capacity, and that the environmental forces that strengthen or weaken resilience to stress are distributed equally in the population. People differ in their inner strength, flexibility, and "reserve capacity" (Gallo, Bogart, Vranceanu, & Matthews, 2005) just as communities differ in resources and overall resilience capacities. Furthermore, the responsiveness of the social and physical environment differs from one family to another, and from one community to the next (Garmezy, 1991). Some resilience researchers have focused on personality features (e.g., Friborg, Barlaug, Martinussen, Rosenvinge, & Hjemdal, 2005), and have given relatively short shrift to the social-environmental determinants of response capacities of individuals. Yet without attention to social, as well as psychological, capital within our communities, models of resilience may have limited applicability. A social and community psychology of resilience is needed if we are to understand why many of us are not always able to preserve well-being and sustain our progress toward the goals we have set for ourselves and for those about whom we care (Cowen, 1994). In addition, attention to the social and contextual factors may provide greater insights into differences in resilient processes across cultures, an area that requires greater theoretical and empirical interrogation.

We often fail to recognize that communities recover as well, albeit in potentially different ways across cultures and countries.

In fact, recovery from horrific devastation is one of the most important themes of the history of cities. As chronicled in *The Resilient City* (Vale & Campanella, 2005) cities have been destroyed throughout history. Only 42 cities worldwide were permanently abandoned (Chandler & Fox, 1974), and all others have recovered, rising like the mythical phoenix. As Kelly (1970) has reminded us, adaptation principles apply as much to human communities as they do to other ecosystems. It is frequently observed that in the process of recovery from devastation, most members of affected communities demonstrate unusually high levels of cooperation and bonding. Alas, these changes in behavior may not last. Whether it be dramatic examples, such as New York City following 9/11, or more frequent natural disasters, such as floods or hurricanes, people often tend to return to business as usual once the sandbags are removed, the debris is cleared, the insurance claims are filed, and so forth. For many communities, "community resilience" ends with immediate recovery. "Social resilience" may partially result from crises, but lasting sustainable resilience capacities seem to require purposeful intervention in multiple aspects of community, and there are unique approaches to recovery enacted by different systems of governance around the globe. Communities clearly recover; how they do so, and with what implications for future resilience capacity, deserve our attention.

Definition 2. Sustaining Pursuit of the Positive

The second major definition of resilience is adopted from the field of ecology and linked directly to the concept of reserve capacity. Holling, Schindler, Walker, and Roughgarden (1995) define the *resilience* of an ecosystem as its capacity to absorb perturbations/disturbances before fundamental changes occur in the state of that system. By changes in state, Holling and colleagues and others (e.g., Adger, 2000) do not mean a change in the level of a given profile of interactions, but a dynamic, nonlinear change in the nature of the relationships among constituent parts of the system. When people reach and go beyond their capacities to cope with events, we observe not simply a change in levels of cognition, affect, and behavior but also a change in the nature of relationships among these core elements of the human response.

The study of chronic pain patients provides one illustration. During episodes of pain and stress, there are changes in not only the level of negative emotion but also the relation between positive and negative states, revealing a reduction in the complexity of a person's affective experiences (Zautra, 2003; Zautra, Fasman, et al., 2005). Based on these findings, it seems that heightened stress and pain lower the capacity of the person to distinguish between positive emotion and the absence of negative emotion, lowering the sustainability of positive affective engagement.

Kelly (1955) was among the first to point out that the constructs we use to understand ourselves are oriented to the prediction and control of future events. We follow his lead in proposing that the natural course of one's life has a forward lean toward engagement, purpose, and perseverance. Mind–body homeostasis is sustained not by emotional neutrality but by ongoing, purposeful, affective engagement. From this perspective, resilience is expected to extend beyond the boundaries of a person's capacity to stave off pathological states, or a community's ability to recover from a disaster; thus, it includes sustaining pursuits of the positive. In this sense, *individual resilience* may be defined by the amount of stress that a person can endure without a fundamental change in capacity to pursue aims that give life meaning. The greater a person's capacity to stay on a satisfying life course, the greater his or her resilience. Whereas resilient *recovery* focuses on aspects of healing of wounds, *sustainability* calls attention to outcomes relevant to preserving valuable engagements in life's tasks at work, in play, and in social relations.

Behavioral scientists, as well as clinicians, who are unaware of the shortcomings of their conceptual models of health and mental health have difficulty understanding the discontinuities between a person's level of suffering and capacity for psychological growth. Attributes of the positive, such as "satisfying life course," are often left undefined, or are defined on the basis of the absence of some negative attribute. Yet we all know people and communities that appear perfectly adjusted to their circumstances but do not have the capacity to plan for them. Their ship is still in the harbor. We know of people who carry full diagnoses of illness, even mental illness, yet show spark, wit, and perseverance that is remarkable for even the healthiest of us. The absence of illness and pain is no guarantee of a good life. Some paradigms within the clinical sciences that have focused on revealing hidden pathologies within us have often appeared blind to the natural capacities of people, even those who are ill, to resolve problems, bounce back from adversity, and find and sustain energy in the pursuit of life's goals.

There are parallels in the study of communities. We often define the *quality of life* within a community by the absence of crime, the safe streets, the convenience to stores selling everyday commodities, and a relatively unfettered path from home to work and back again. If this were all that attracted us to community, though, no one would bother with Manhattan, San Francisco, or Los Angeles. These very diverse, vibrant places prosper because they attend to the basics, as well as provide high levels of stimulation and opportunity, even though they may introduce more hazards into everyday life (Florida, 2004). People need the structure of a coherently organized physical environment that affords them basic goods. They also benefit from communities that support their needs for social connection and psychological growth. Resilient community structures build on peoples' hopes, as well as provide a means of circling the wagons to provide a "defensible space." We need definitions that go beyond the absence of problems: not just risk, but also capacity, thoughtfulness, planning, and a forward-leaning orientation that includes attainable goals and a realistic vision for the community as a whole.

How does our focus on sustainability of the positive as resilient compare in saliency to recovery? The capacity to mount effective responses to stress and to resist illness is a fundamental imperative. But survival is not enough for resilience. A fulfilling life is also fundamental to well-being, so changes that affect our plans and goals for ourselves, our families, and our communities need attention as well.

The Role of Awareness in Resilient Lives

Recovery and sustainability are different in one critical respect. For recovery, homeostasis is the fundamental principle: a return to a former, more balanced, state. Sustainability, on the other hand, is not based on push-and-pull mechanisms of action and reaction. This condition depends on unique human capacities for appraisal, planning, and intentional action. Whereas automaticity characterizes homeostatic processes, awareness and choice characterize the development of sustainable human values and purposes.

The implications of this distinction are profound. First, it seems possible, even likely, that many people recover from adversity without giving the experience much thought at all. Physiological systems are built to bounce back. One's blood pressure rises under stress, even "boils" when one is angry, but returns to resting levels without any special work on the person's part. Psychological levels of well-being and distress, and social perceptions, such as interpersonal trust, show changes in response to adversity only within a range of values, returning to preadversity levels except under the most extraordinary circumstances. Loss naturally leads to sorrow. For some the grief is remarkably understated, but for others the grief seems so strong as to be frightening. At the time we are faced with grief at its peak levels, it may appear that we will never recover. But just as

we say that to ourselves, a light appears at the end of the tunnel, and we begin to move toward it.

There are cultural differences in how people rebound from adversity. David Brooks (2008) noted how little trauma and grief there was among the survivors of an earthquake that struck China's Sichuan Province in 2008, killing 70,000 people. Instead of sorrow, he observed a pragmatic mentality: "Move on, don't dwell, look to the positive, fix what needs fixing, and work together." But even in Western nations, quick recovery is the rule. Bonnano (2004) found that a high proportion of those who lost a close family member showed no grief reaction, and another significant proportion showed rapid recovery following the death.

Individuals may differ in the extent to which they are able to rebound fully and rapidly. McEwen (1998) introduced the idea of *allostatic load* to describe elevations in physiological indicators that appear to defy homeostatic principles: cortisol levels and blood pressure that do not go lower during the day, for example. Depression and anxiety may be added to the list of indicators of load that, once elevated, does not fall back to normal levels for some people. But these are exceptions to the principle of recovery. The science and practice of psychosomatic medicine arose to address just these kinds of abnormal "heterostatic" patterns.

The normal course of human response is to return to baseline. Interventions are not needed to coax most people back to health, unless there are other problems. A physiological propensity toward autoimmunity, for example, might lead to rheumatoid arthritis for those suffering from episodes of major depression. Some people have great difficulty admitting that they suffer, and they deny painful experiences even to themselves. In psychoanalytic frameworks, denial can turn ordinary experiences into nightmares, a dynamic that influences our emotional lives in unpredictable ways, sometimes leaving us more troubled than we were by the original experience.

The young are without the means to comprehend fully a highly threatening experience. Often unprepared to cope with implications of highly stressful events, a youth's emotional wounds may be left unhealed. Abuse and early trauma can invade awareness years later, disrupting homeostatic processes and chronically elevating central psychological and physiological processes in homeostatic regulation (e.g., Luecken & Appelhans, 2006; Luecken, Appelhans, Kraft, & Brown, 2006). Researchers in behavioral medicine have verified these kinds of costs of early trauma, but even here, not every child is distressed. If we look, we see plenty of the "ordinary magic" of resilience (Masten, 2001) throughout development.

Sustainability and Awareness

Sustainability of purpose invites more consideration of existential questions than does recovery. How do we want to live? What do we wish to accomplish? Which voice within do we listen to most fervently? This is the world of choice and value, and it is surprising how little time most of us spend in this world. Nevertheless, sustainability is a moot point unless we are aware enough to have pursuits that give our lives meaning beyond recovery and survival (Ryff & Singer, 1998). Without a sense of purpose, there is no purpose to sustain, and without a sense of value, no meaning can lengthen the life of the emotions that accompany a positive experience. We are willows in the wind, without a direction of our own.

Awareness is a prerequisite to these higher-order processes, and it is only logical to extend this discussion to include levels of awareness. Some forms of consciousness are more likely than others to yield a rich bounty of meaning and value. Tolle (2005) and others talk about differences in types of awareness. Here it is possible to introduce a range of possible definitions of the quality of the conscious experience. Different cultures have different ways to order the quality of conscious experiences

as well (e.g., Diener & Suh, 2000). Western and Eastern philosophies, for example, offer contrasting views on the nature of conscious experience most likely to sustain well-being. Western views focus on choice and mastery over the environment, whereas Eastern philosophies emphasize full awareness and acceptance of experience, however painful, to gain an enlightened and "joyous" view of the world. These cultural differences underscore that there is more than one way to be resilient, and that greater understanding of resilience processes across cultures is needed.

When thinking of a community's resilience, this distinction between recovery and sustainability is all the more apparent. However, "awareness" is not a property typically ascribed to communities, so, at first glance, it would appear irrelevant. For many, an effectively managed community is one that operates like clockwork. The trains run on time regardless of what is happening, and people shuffle forward as expected, undeterred by calamity. Indeed, an effective future plan for recovery in a community following a natural disaster is one that arranges resources in such a way that the response is as swift and automatic as possible. Emergency deployments are thoughtfully planned before the fact. During the disaster, members of the community hope that everyone knows what he or she is to do without question. They may be guided to safety by set programs, modified in process from the top by only a select few engineers with authority. Yet, from experience, we know that a substantial transfusion of cooperation as a result of disaster can sometimes be the key ingredient in community recovery. Two key research questions remain:

1. Why is it that increased cooperation and bonding occurs in some communities but not in others, despite similarity of the event?
2. Why is it that immediate cooperative responses often dissipate and do not lead to continued collaboration after immediate recovery?

Sustainability of community life requires a different kind of thinking and planning, one that relies on raising awareness and participation of the whole, not just investment in the skills of a few. Fundamental to elevation of awareness to purposeful collective action are processes that promote awareness, social cohesion, and connectedness, and participation by all in the functioning of a healthy community system. Here is where the Sarason (1974) concept "sense of community" is most applicable. Without a shared sense of purpose within the community, there may not be much of a community to sustain anyway. There may be "bricks and mortar" to be sure, but for purposes not defined by those who live and work there. Just as there are levels of awareness and conscious engagement within individuals, communities vary in the quality of citizen awareness, contribution, and commitment to goals. We believe the sustainability of a community's future is in direct proportion to the quality and extent of collective awareness, and direction for growth and development.

What contributes to these capacities, and how to foster these processes within people and their communities, are the key questions that need to be addressed by resilience researchers. New innovative programs focused on resilience are under way and would benefit from paradigm guidance and a better articulated and integrative set of methodologies. Next, we examine measures and methods that may be useful in the study of resilience within people and across communities. We propose one important distinction to keep in mind: Resilience is an outcome of successful adaptation to adversity, and is revealed by sustainability, recovery, or both. Resilience processes are those that have garnered empirical support as variables that increase the likelihood of those outcomes. For the field to advance it is essential to keep the processes and outcomes distinct. Doing so allows us to develop ways to examine the evidence for resilience processes, without confusing independent and dependent variables (see also Greve & Staudinger, 2006).

Identifying Indicators of Resilience Processes

At this stage of resilience research, social scientists have advanced the field with propositions regarding the key biopsychosocial processes that further recovery and sustainability (e.g., Hawkley et al., 2005; Ong, Bergeman, & Bisconti, 2004). Reliable measures of core aspects of positive mental health (Ryff & Keyes, 1995), personal agency, emotional maturity, and subjective well-being (Vaillant, 2003) have provided substantive means of evaluating those propositions. Furthermore, Charney (2004) and Curtis and Cicchetti (2003) have reviewed potential neurohormonal and genetic processes that may yield physiological markers of resilience. Greater specificity in reliable measurement is increasingly available across the levels of inquiry.

A key question for resilience research is how new indicators of resourcefulness differ from established ones of vulnerability. Table 1.1 illustrates how such indices of resilient processes compare to more conventional indices of risk across different levels of analysis. On the left side are examples of risk factors culled from studies of health risk, beginning with the Framingham Study (Dawber et al., 1951). These "usual suspects" are well-established markers of high risk for a number of health problems as people age. On the right side of the graph is a contrasting set of variables that identify biopsychosocial and community resources. Many of these indices have been associated with better psychological and physiological functioning, but for fewer studies have been conducted on the positive side of the ledger.

Resilience Processes as a Separate Dimension

The evidence to date indicates that resilience resources illustrated in Table 1.1 are not qualities found at the positive end of a single continuum of risk but are a separable factor of well-being altogether that confers unique physical and mental health advantages not

TABLE 1.1. Risk and Resilience Resource Indices

Risk factor index	Resilience resource index
Biological	
• Blood pressure: diastolic > 90, systolic > 140	• Heart rate variability
• Cholesterol > 240 mg, resting glucose > 124, body mass index > 25	• Regular physical exercise
• Genetic factors associated with anxiety	• Genetic factors associated with stress resilience
• High C-reactive protein and/or other elevations in inflammatory processes	• Immune responsivity and regulation
Individual	
• History of mental illness	• Positive emotional resources
• Depression/helplessness	• Hope/optimism/agency
• Traumatic brain injury	• High cognitive functioning, learning/memory and executive functioning
Interpersonal/family	
• History of childhood trauma/adult abuse	• Secure kith/kin relations
• Chronic social stress	• Close social ties
Community/organizational	
• Presence of environmental hazards	• Green space and engaging in the natural environment through community gardening
• Violent crime rates	• Volunteerism
• Stressful work environment	• Satisfying work life

accounted for by assessments of relative risk (e.g., Steptoe, Wardle, & Marmot, 2005). To characterize the nature of risk and resilience we need models that contain at least two separate factors: One that estimates vulnerabilities and another that estimates strengths (Zautra, 2003). Resilience depends as much on keeping separate that which is different as on integrating parts that fit together to make a congruent whole. A psychological economy that equates the positive with the absence of the negative is a model for simplicity within the mind, not growth.

One reason we need to distinguish factors is that they address two fundamentally different motivational processes: the need to protect and defend against harm, and the need to move forward and to extend one's reach toward positive aims (Bernston, Caccioppo, & Gardner, 1999). These processes infuse a two-factor meaning structure into emotion, cognition, and behavioral intention. Indeed, neurophysiological responses, including both electroencephalographic (EEG) and functional magnetic resonance imaging (fMRI) data, support distinct neural structures for the regulation of positive as opposed to negative emotive responses (Canli et al., 2001; Watson, Wiese, Vaidya, & Tellegen, 1999). Underlying cognitions of personal control and mastery show two factors (Reich & Zautra, 1991): one of agency, optimism, and hope, and another of helplessness, pessimism, and despair. Social relations have similar differentiated structures. The extent of negative social ties does not predict the extent of positive social ties (Finch, Okun, Barrera, Zautra, & Reich, 1989). Even within intimate spousal relations the extent of negative social interaction does not account for the extent of positive exchanges between partners (Stone & Neale, 1982).

When investigators have constructed separate indices of positive and negative aspects of the person and/or social relations, they have uncovered surprising currency for positive aspects in prediction of health and illness that is not accounted for in measures of negative affective factors (Cohen, Doyle, Turner, Alper, & Skoner, 2003; Moskowitz,

2003; Pressman & Cohen, 2005; Russek & Schwartz, 1997; Seeman et al., 1995). Laughter, positive affect, and optimism; emotional range, as well as maturity (Vaillant & Mukamal, 2001); and the capacity for empathy and support for others all may infuse people with potentially life-sustaining resources even in the face of considerable distress (Zautra, Johnson, & Davis, 2005). It is important not to overstate the amount of psychological muscle it might take to be resilient. Resilient actions often start just with a smile or a moment for reflection that welcomes a broader perspective and encourages a thoughtful optimism about events.

In collaboration with other investigators, we have conducted three studies of risk and resilience with patients challenged by chronic pain disorders (Furlong, Zautra, Puente, López, & Valero, 2008; Johnson-Wright, Zautra, & Going, 2008; Smith & Zautra, 2008). Each of these studies examined whether measures of resilience resources formed separate factors and predicted health outcomes over and above risk factors in patients with rheumatic conditions, including rheumatoid arthritis, osteoarthritis, and fibromyalgia. Although each study relied on somewhat different predictors and different health outcomes, each found evidence of separate but inversely correlated factors of resilience and risk, and in each case the resilience factors predicted key health outcomes after researchers controlled for risk. The Smith and Zautra study of patients with rheumatoid arthritis, for example, identified a resilience factor that comprised measures of active coping, acceptance, positive reinterpretation and growth, purpose in life, and optimism that had a modest negative correlation ($r = -.31$) with a vulnerability factor containing scales measuring anxiety, depression, interpersonal sensitivity, and pessimism. Scores on vulnerability (but not resilience) predicted daily fluctuations in negative affect, including elevations in negative emotion on days of elevated pain. Those participants with high resilience reported more everyday positive interpersonal events,

more positive emotion, and greater responsivity to daily positive interpersonal events. Vulnerability scores were unrelated to those positive affective outcomes.

Indicators of Individual Resilience: Resources and Outcomes

At the level of the individual, resilience concepts have led researchers to develop indices of *positive adaptation*, with items such as "I tend to bounce back quickly after hard times" (e.g., Smith et al., in press). They constitute self-report measures of resilient outcomes. In child development, this research has focused on competence and adaptation, stating that adaptation is identified by children successfully meeting developmental criteria (Luthar, 2006). For adults and older adults, preservation of health and well-being in the face of adversity provides key resilience outcomes. Here we urge further work to distinguish between the resilience outcomes of recovery and sustainability. Speed with which a person regains physiological homeostasis following inflammation in an autoimmune flare-up is one example of *recovery* aspects of resilience. The length of time to return to prestress levels of depression is an example of recovery in mental health. In contrast, *sustainability* in mental health is revealed by the preservation of energy and commitment to purposeful engagements in work and family life under the adaptation challenges imposed by psychosocial distress. For example, resilience may be examined through estimates of sustainability of daily physical functioning under the stress of an episode of chronic pain. In a recent public health study, retention of 20 or more teeth was used as the primary index of resilience to urban poverty (Sanders, Lim, & Sohn, 2008).

To assess resilience resources, the researcher needs to be guided by theoretical models of how people adapt successfully to stressful events. To date, emphasis has been placed on variables linked by theory and/or data to greater endurance. Investigators have begun to examine several key variables of this capacity, including measures of coping, flexibility, and personal agency; sense of purpose; positive emotional engagement in daily life at home, work, and at play; emotion regulation; and indicators of physiological buoyancy, such as heart rate variability (Connor & Davidson, 2003; Keyes, 2004; Masten & Powell, 2003; Ryff & Singer, 1998; Seligman & Csikszentmihalyi, 2000). Theoretical models, research, and interventions must also take into account cultural values, beliefs, and norms to increase understanding of resilience resources in the experiences of individuals around the globe.

Public health researchers have studied related processes for some time as antidotes to stress and vulnerability. Two examples of this emphasis are the study of social support (Berkman & Glass, 2000) and personal control (Pearlin & Schooler, 1978; Reich & Zautra, 1990; Schulz, 1976), both seen as resources that promote adaptation to stressful situations. Indeed, concepts of personal mastery and social support are among the most thoroughly conceptualized, researched, and applied concepts in all the social sciences (Coyne & Downey, 1991; Skinner, 1996). The perception that one can achieve desirable goals and retain a sense of mastery when life events threaten one's personal control beliefs defines the resilient individual. Furthermore, the person's social world provides the meaning structures and supportive resources that enable him or her to meet adaptation challenges. A science of resilience utilizes the best of these approaches in the development of indices that promote recovery and/or sustainability.

Some Candidate Indicators of Community Resilience

Work with communities should also take into account a two-factor model of resilience in developing indicators. As with individual research, examination of community-level variables has grown out of a risk-based tra-

dition. There are numerous assessments that focus on community risk, such as crowded housing, poverty, high school dropout rates, and income inequality promoted by the urban Hardship Index, now in its third edition (Montiel, Nathan, & Wright, 2004). Other indices and models that focus on community and neighborhood stress, such as the Community Stress Index (CSI; Ewart & Suchday, 2002) and measures of neighborhood problems (Steptoe & Feldman, 2001), have also been developed to examine psychosocial effects of environmental stress. Links between neighborhood stress and deprivation, and individual mortality and illness constitute an important field of inquiry in public health (e.g., Tonne et al., 2005).

As Beck (1992) has noted, we tend to focus on living in a "risk society," where our public policies, social services, nonprofit and other organizations work to identify problems and areas of weakness in our communities, and in turn attempt to alleviate those symptoms. In fact, studies of neighborhood crime and safety; poverty alleviation; welfare reform; economic development of poor, inner-city neighborhoods; and so forth represent a virtual subfield of urban inquiry. Even former Senator Daniel Patrick Moynihan, remembered in part for his famous critique of the poverty industry–complex, accepted the risk society model. Such attitudes and beliefs trickle down from policies and community leaders to color the way people construe their life experiences and their motivations.

However, the last two decades have given way to an outcropping of research on community resources that foster resilience. At the forefront of this research, extensive examinations of *social capital* have underscored the importance of social trust, reciprocity, neighborhood efficacy, and civic engagement in many aspects of community life (Coleman, 1990; Portes, 2000; Putnam, 2000; Putnam, Felstein, & Cohen, 2003; Putnam, Leonardi, & Nanetti, 1993). Not surprisingly, given the importance of social support and personal mastery as resources that promote adaptation to the most stressful situations, social connectedness and cohesion have been shown to be linked to greater vitality and stability in communities (Langdon, 1997). Studies probing the link between different indicators of social capital and health outcomes (Kawachi, Kennedy, Lochner, & Prothrow-Stith, 1997; Veenstra et al., 2005), and empirical research examining the "mosaic" of community risk and protective factors continue to highlight the critical influence of place on individuals (Fitzpatrick & LaGory, 2003). These studies help us understand the complex and variable matrix of capacities that communities rely on to enhance the physical, mental, and financial outcomes of their constituents and the individual consequences of developing greater social and human capital.

Just as some individuals appear more resilient than others, similar variation in resilience capacity has been found among communities (Chaskin, Brown, Venkatesh, & Vidal, 2001; Pelling, 2003; Vale & Campanella, 2005), with some communities better able to maintain healthy growth and development, and to respond to stressors such as economic downturns or natural disasters. This general finding raises profoundly important questions about the nature of the relationship between individual and community resilience, and the community role in crafting deeper wells of resilience. To what extent do communities teach, or instill, resilience in people as opposed to either nurturing or blunting resilience tendencies that people bring to a situation? How much of the variation in community resilience can be manipulated by community programs, resources, and activities versus variance that is more predetermined, ranging from genetic determinants to some social, economic, and educational factors that are difficult to change?

Previous researchers have developed several hypotheses and potential advances in identifying key factors of community resilience capacity but less hard data with which to discern how best to conceptualize and assess these qualities (Flower, 1994; National Civic League, 1999). These questions call for thorough empirical study grounded in theory and guided by advanced methods of inquiry that rely on a multilevel framework for conceptualizing and evaluating the relationships between indices of social, community, and personal capacity. We suggest that attention to distinctions between recovery and sustainability may add clarity to research linking social worlds to health outcomes. Wen, Browning, and Cagney (2007), for example, studied neighborhood correlates of physical exercise, a good indicator of sustainability of health. Other researchers may attend to neighborhood rates of recovery following illness. Different community factors may be responsible for sustainability versus recovery outcomes.[1]

A working hypothesis that guides current research on community resilience is that communities, like people, can be taught to be resilient. But we are learning that this is not an endeavor of quick and easy fixes. Communities must also nurture and build resilience from existing natural relationships and among existing institutions. For communities, as well as individuals, sustainable resilience capacities are built over time, require a focus (often a refocus) on strengths not weaknesses, and rest on improved self-organization, self-control (mastery), and social connection.

The bridge from culture to health is built across neighborhoods and communities that connect individuals who share common space, as well as common ground, to support a collective hope and efficacy (Duncan, Duncan, Okut, Strycker, & Hix-Small, 2003). Research on racial segregation and health disparities has shown how neighborhood resources can profoundly influence individual health outcomes (e.g., St. Luke's Health Initiatives, 2003). These research efforts indicate that communities vary dramatically in their capacity to promote and sustain health and healthy communities (Kretzmann & McKnight, 1993). Yet studies that have examined the relations between community-level factors such as social capital and person-level variables (e.g., health behaviors) have had mixed results (Carpiano, 2006; Portes, 2000; Ziersch, Baum, Macdougall, & Putland, 2005), suggesting we have only begun to understand the boundaries of influence of the social domain on individuals.

Inconsistencies are not surprising given that different variables have been used in each study to describe community capacity, resilience, health, and well-being. In addition, many questions remain in community research, such as how to define communities and isolate their effects beyond that of individual variables. Communities are complex, as are the few partial theories explored by analyses of these variables (Bourdieu, 1986; Coleman, 1990; O'Campo, 2003; Portes, 2000; Szreter & Woolcock, 2004). Broad descriptive analyses of communities that range from socioeconomic to environmental factors, from crime statistics to educational outcomes, are now available, but they lack integrative focus. Research papers are brimming with hypotheses identifying key factors of community capacity but contain little hard data with which to discern how best to conceptualize and assess these qualities (Flower, 1994; Hall, 2002; National Civic League, 1999). Both individual and community inquiry would benefit from integrative theory and multilevel approaches to this research.

In Table 1.2 we illustrate how measures of resilience resources may be paired with the resilience outcomes of recovery and sustainability across three levels of inquiry: individual, family, and community. These pairs represent hypothesized relationships between resilience resources and outcomes, and may serve as a guide to building a science of resilience over the next decade of research. For example, under individual resources we list "efficacy expectations" and pair that resource with prevention of chronic disablement following injury or illness. There is evidence of this relationship already in the literature (Bodenheimer, Lorig, Holman, & Grumbach, 2002), but we do not know the full extent of that relationship, nor do we

TABLE 1.2. Illustrations of Resilience Resources and Hypothesized Resilient Outcomes

Resources	Hypothesized outcomes
Individual recovery	
• Heart rate variability	• Physiological recovery following stress
• Supportiveness of social network	• Low depression and anxiety following loss
• Coping capacity/efficacy expectations	• Prevention of disablement following injury
• T-helper cell type 1 and 2 (Th1/Th2) balance of immune response	• Rapid immune response to acute illness/injury
Individual sustainability	
• Sense of purpose	• Sustained elevations in positive emotion and hope
• Emotional awareness and clarity	• High levels of emotion differentiation/complexity
• Social connection/affiliation	• Social meaning and value sustained under stress
Family/community recovery	
• Empathetic concern for family/neighborhood/ community	• Rapid return to normal pace of community life following disaster
• Rapid response crisis training	• Absence of collateral damage during recovery
• Fairness in allocation of local resources	• Minimal "place" clustering of chronic illness
Family/community sustainability	
• Leadership fostering citizen participation	• Vitality/enthusiasm for living shared by members
• Culture of democratic decision making	• Lasting trust in governance of community resources
• Reciprocity and mutual respect in community relations	• High levels of well-being shared by those in the family/community

know for whom this connection is more or less likely. The resilience outcomes for sustainability are different than those designated as "recovery." These outcomes fall within the realm of positive mental health (Ryff & Singer, 1998; Zautra, 2003), identifying the growth and maturation of some of the best qualities of the human experience.

In family/community levels we propose links between attributes of group relations and outcomes favorable to community resilience, such as rapid recovery following a natural disaster and trust. We include these kinds of hypotheses to encourage greater attention to the broader social context and the role of "community" in sustaining well-being for populations. Often researchers only study characteristics of the person and his or her "perceived" social world to test predictions of individual well-being. The role of social relations is too fundamental to sustaining health and recovery from illness to be ignored any longer by research.

Methods of Inquiry and Resilience Outcomes

Longitudinal Design

To develop the appropriate technologies for the study of resilience we need to follow a few basic principles. First, we need to study resilience over time. People develop themes in their lives that offer them hope, optimism, purpose, emotional clarity, and a wisdom built on a complex and accepting view of their social relationships. But they do not do so all at once. Resilience, as we see it, takes time to unfold. Furthermore, there are many bumps along the way, periods of life in which many people look anything but resilient. If we fail to keep the cameras rolling past the point of an illness episode, we then miss capturing the evidence we seek. A focus on the presence or absence of the episode leads us to see people as healthy only until they exhibit signs of illness; then they are sick. This way of thinking places enormous constraints on the development of constructs that can inform our understanding of adaptation

across the lifespan. For example, a person may be nourished by awareness of complex and at times painful emotions, a benefit that is not always immediately apparent. Only through longitudinal observation and carefully conducted birth cohort studies (e.g., Silva & Stanton, 1996) peppered with qualitative evidence from life-changing narratives do we discover how the person has been and can yet be resilient (McAdams, 2006).

Developmental tasks are natural challenges to resilience across the lifespan that identify problems, as well as reveal hidden capacities within. People who look resilient in youth may not retain their resilient capacities in later life, though we suspect that the qualities that make one resilient do tend to generalize to other situations and continue to support successful adaptation and recovery later in life. The degree of cross-situational consistency and stability of resilience over time is important to develop further in future studies. Both the development of these capacities and their sustainability requires us to understand the trajectories of the resilient mind and body over the life course.

Several longitudinal studies within developmental psychology provide a starting point for such inquiry. A seminal study by Werner and Smith (2001) followed children on the island of Kauai from infancy through adulthood, with the initial sample targeting all pregnancies on the island in a given year. Through data collection and analysis spanning 40 years, this research has been able to identify key risk and protective factors that influence outcomes across child development and into adulthood. Findings have emphasized several key factors influencing resilience outcomes, including (1) individual characteristics, such as self-esteem and purpose in life; (2) characteristics of families, such as maternal caregiving and extended family support; and (3) the larger social context, especially having adult role models who provide additional support (Luthar et al., 2000; Werner & Smith, 2001). This study, along with other major longitudinal studies within child development (see Luthar, 2006, for a review), provides a framework for tracking resilience development among children and adolescents over time and in their transitions into adulthood. Although resilience research in child development provides a critical foundation, longitudinal inquiries of health and well-being across adulthood introduce unique challenges (Ong, Bergeman, Bisconti, & Wallace, 2006). The specific risk and protective factors, and their salience to the desired goals for competence and adaptation, vary across the lifespan and are influenced by culture and context.

Resilience research with adults must also address physical health, a domain diminished in the child literature due to difficulty in detection of physiological processes in the early years of life that increase risk for illness later. To fully understand resilience in adults, we advocate a mind–body approach that incorporates both physical and mental health, and the interactions between the two. The Framingham Study (Dawber et al., 1951) has identified many critical risk factors for illness and pathology over the course of adulthood, such as the role of cigarette smoking and unhealthy diet on physical health outcomes. The next question then is, what are the predictors of continued good health and functioning throughout life? Antonovsky (1987) identifies *generalized resistance resources* as the attributes and resources that help individuals to maintain homeostasis and optimal health. Others (Evans & Stoddart, 1990; Singer & Ryff, 2001) also have recognized the need to examine not only trajectories of illness but also trajectories of health. Resilience theories that provide coherent and integrative biopsychosocial models of adaptation would provide this type of inquiry.

Multilevel Analysis

We define the content of inquiries into resilience as (1) the study of the processes of recovery from adversity, and (2) the processes underlying sustainability of purpose.

The best methods to advance these inquiries are multilevel: the examination of resilience capacities at the levels of the biological, psychological, social, and organization–community. Though any single study may focus on core manifestations of resilience at one or two levels, a full understanding of resilience requires methods that can examine how levels interact in the prediction of resilience in the face of adversity.

The examination of resilience at the level of community poses formidable challenges to researchers. Yet communities of location (Black & Hughes, 2001) provide the context in which all individuals (spanning life cycles, income brackets, and cultural heritage) work, love, and live. The complexity of communities provides considerable methodological challenges, demanding multilevel analyses that examine the richness of individual experiences, as well as the cumulative effects of environmental variables. The bidirectional influences of environmental and individual characteristics raise questions of causality, highlighting the importance of feedback loops, cascading effects, and the endless interaction between levels of analysis. Researchers across fields recognize the challenges of understanding, measuring, and evaluating the interplay between individuals and communities (Macintyre, Ellaway, & Cummins, 2002; Rappaport & Seidman, 2000; Sampson, Morenoff, & Gannon-Rowley, 2002; Subramanian, 2004; Subramanian, Jones, & Duncan, 2003).

The "place effects" that were once considered a black box (Macintyre et al., 2002) may now be more clearly delineated, with advances in analysis methods that do justice to the many layers of influence on individual lives. Statistical analyses are now better able to tease apart the differences between and within individuals and communities, allowing us to examine the diversity within our samples rather than look solely at aggregated data (Subramanian, 2004). The obtained increases in predictive power permit an understanding of the richness of individuals and communities, and tests of the independent impact of risk and resilience factors (Zautra, Hall, & Murray, 2009).

Knowledge of core ingredients of resilience within the person shapes the agenda for insights at the community level, but awareness of ecological forces at work changes and extends the metaphor of recovery and sustainability to include relational constructs such as leadership, reciprocity, and culture. With this greater understanding comes the "opportunity for simultaneous pursuit of new knowledge and more effective practice" (Price & Behrens, 2003, p. 219). The use of multilevel modeling permits us to estimate better the influence of community-level variables and to examine variability both within and across communities, allowing us to inquire, for example, about the determinants and influence of the average level of "trust" within a neighborhood, over and above the influence of the individual (Subramanian, Lochner, & Kawachi, 2003). Improved research design and analysis can aid in identifying the short- and long-term effects, from behaviors and attitudes to the accumulated stress and environmental impact of a neighborhood on individual outcomes (Ellen, Mijanovich, & Dillman, 2001). These analyses provide the rich opportunity to look at different layers of effects over time and have been recognized by community researchers as an essential tool in carrying out macro-level research.

However, different levels of analysis often require attention to ecological influences, raising fundamental questions about the resilience process under study as well. The study of trust is a case in point (see Table 1.3). Trust is best understood at the level of the person and his or her social interactions. However, it can also be examined at a biological level as a "safety response," with physiological markers of parasympathetic activation, and with neurohormones such as oxytocin, which has been associated with trusting others with personal resources (Kosfeld, Heinrichs, Zak, Fischbacher, & Fehr, 2005). Mutuality and cohesiveness characterize trusting family networks. At the level of community, this quality may be best characterized as collaborative ties and fairness in the distribution of resources, measured through indicators that can detect evidence of reciprocity in institutional relationships, neighborhoods, and municipalities. Personal income is a valuable resource for resilience, but at the community level, high levels of income disparity among groups within the community (Wilkinson, 1996) may undermine processes of reciprocity and cooperation that permit the expression of trust in interactions among members of those groups, thereby weakening the psychological sense of community (Brodsky, O'Campo, & Aronson, 1999). Resilience researchers need to be mindful of the shifts in meaning of constructs such as trust across levels of analysis. Measurement properties of the variable, and how that variable is related to other key aspects of adaptation, may change dramatically from the level of the person to that of the community.

TABLE 1.3. The Study of Trust across Multiple Levels of Analysis

Level of analysis	Sample constructs	Research approaches
Biological basis	Oxytocin	Experimental designs, lab assessments
Individuals	Interpersonal trust	Cross-sectional studies, daily diary studies
Families	Family cohesion, mutuality, and trust	Cross-sectional, family, and genetic studies
Communities	Collaborative ties, reciprocity, and fairness	Epidemiological/community samples, social indicator research

Studying Resilience in Action

Resilience scholars shift the focus of research on health and well-being through their emphasis on processes that aid in the restoration of well-being following stressful experiences. Stress reactivity research has correctly emphasized the need to examine responses close in time to the occurrence of the stressor (Linden, Rutledge, & Con, 1998; Lovallo & Gerin, 2003; Treiber et al., 2003). Only when the organism is challenged are its capacities fully tested and its vulnerabilities revealed (Light et al., 1999; Matthews, Woodall, & Allen, 1993). An important area of research concerns the identification of genes that promote resilience under stress. Caspi and colleagues (2003) reported that a functional polymorphism in the promoter region of the serotonin transporter gene protects individuals from depression following stressful life events. Young adults who were homozygous for the long allele had fewer depressive symptoms, diagnoses of depression, and suicidality than individuals with one or two copies of the short allele. Some researchers ask whether we can identify genetic factors in neural plasticity that can shape development of resilience (Curtis & Cicchetti, 2003), and whether we can identify factors that slow the effects of age on the decay of resilience (Hawkley et al., 2005).

A stress–diathesis approach that focuses solely on amplitude of the stress response is not sufficient, however. To estimate fully success of psychophysiological adaptation to stress, researchers need to assess both initial reaction and recovery (McEwen, 1998; Sapolsky, 1998). Frankenhauser (1983) has shown that heart rate increases during the workday at all occupational levels but downregulates more rapidly afterward for those in higher-status occupations. A focus on resilience calls attention to the effect of time in the restoration of homeostasis. The failure to down-regulate following a stress response and to restore homeostasis both physiologically and psychologically is the central contributor to allostatic load (McEwen, 1998;

Seeman, Singer, Ryff, Dienberg Love, & Levy-Storms, 2002). To study resilience properly, we need to identify the critical factors within the person and his or her social situation that preserve health and well-being by promoting restoration of homeostasis.

Advanced field methods offer ways to study resilience processes as they unfold in everyday life. Electronic diaries may be used to monitor affects, cognitions, and behaviors thought to be sources of resilience, as well as those thought to place the person at risk. These methods can be used to record resilient responses and also failures of resilience day-to-day or even minute-to-minute, or hour-to-hour, if one wants to be this precise. Ambulatory recording devices permit within days examination of physiological processes that may underlie recovery following stress as well (Almeida, 2005).

The resilience capacities of individuals and their families may be further tested through longitudinal research following major life crises. Bonanno (2005), for example, has developed a model of resilience built upon observations of how people respond to the loss of a loved one. Chronic burdens in family life pose special challenges to adaptive capacities. Most people have suffered through at least one highly stressful circumstance, and to understand resilience requires a careful assessment of the variables that contributed to emotional, cognitive, and behavioral changes that facilitated their recoveries.

The interpersonal contributions to resilient outcomes are likely substantial. Most stressors are shared: Family and friends are involved, directly and indirectly, in the paths to recovery for people in crisis. Homelessness, divorce, and chronic mental and physical illnesses are examples of situations that recruit whole families into them. To understand resilience requires us to advance our methods, as well as our concepts, to evaluate the capacities of families to rebound when faced with stressful circumstances. At the level of the individual, we may focus on a person's capacity for optimism, but at the family level, emotional leadership and a climate of acceptance may be the critical features that hold families together during a crisis. Family interaction research can be used to characterize the behavior of resilient families, and social climate measures can add an emotional profile.

Advances in neuroscience have permitted investigations of how family members exchange biological goods as well as social ones. Reacting to and sharing experiences are revealed in changes in neurohormones, the heart and gut, as well as behavior (Charney, 2004; Craig, 2009). Anxiety, hope, trust, and attachment are shared qualities of families that are observable, in principle at least, at the level of genes, neurophysiology, behavior, cognition, and emotion. The dynamic changes in these family qualities in response to stress across levels and over time would be needed to capture resilience processes under way at home.

Communities also respond to a broad range of stressful events; some are acute disruptions, whereas others are chronic. Some of these stressors, such as discrimination based on income and race, lack of affordable housing, and/or jobs for residents, are deeply significant yet often partially hidden or denied. Others are relatively straightforward: a road closure, salmonella poisoning at the local elementary school, an acute shortage of gasoline. There can also be catastrophic threats to public health, such as a terrorist threat aimed at the water supply, or the sustained failure of the electric power grid during the hot summer months. The survival and well-being of individuals and their families depends on not only the resourcefulness of the people themselves but also the responsiveness of the community. Community responsiveness in turn can be impacted by deep and unresolved fissures of the types mentioned earlier.

As columnist Neal Peirce (2005) noted in his article about intergovernmental response to Hurricane Katrina, spending billions on recovery can be viewed as an enormous opportunity, if the best minds are brought to the table to develop scenarios for public de-

bate, if desirable community goals and visions are derived from this process, and if long-term, effective communitywide investments are made. These natural experiments may lead us to uncover the best ways to assess and strengthen community capacity.

Examining Sustainability

Our second definition of resilience shifts our attention to those factors that preserve ongoing goal-related and highly-valued activities that are keys sources of psychological and community well-being. Ecologists remind us that time is a central factor in sustainability. Some systems and societies survive well in the short term only to collapse later (Diamond, 2005). So too do some people appear unaffected by stressors, only to develop illness and emotional disturbance later. Most research examining the person's affective responses to stress focus on the extent of negative affects provoked. However, other outcomes may be more central to preservation of long-term functioning: the degree to which positive engagements continue uninterrupted, the maintenance of broad affective range, and evidence of clear purposeful steps forward, unimpeded by stress, even if taken only one at a time (Ong et al., 2004). However, with some notable exceptions (e.g., Bonanno, 2004; Bonanno et al., 2002; Ong et al., 2004, 2006), studies of sustainability are rare when compared to the rich literature on stress and recovery.

The adoption of a *two-factor approach* allows us the conceptual space needed to develop methods of inquiry into the processes of sustainability of goals, purpose, and life satisfaction independent of the study of the negative affective reactions to stressful change. Although stressors may increase psychological distress, they may have little or no effect on how much hope the person sustains for the future, personal efficacy expectations, and trust in social relationships. Similarly, hope, efficacy, and trust are also central to community health and at least partially independent of collective stress. In fact, the role of crisis and disaster in forging positive public policy for the future is a frequent theme of the public policy literature (Vale & Campanella, 2005). A prominent American historian Kevin Rozario (2005) writes:

> Dominant colonial traditions encouraged a remarkably constructive approach to calamity, leading settlers on a constant search for silver linings. Disaster narratives became self-fulfilling prophecies, inspiring a faith in betterment, and generating the energy, will and capital commitment that made reconstruction viable—ultimately turning calamities into opportunities and thereby ... making progress. (p. 34)

Communities have recently developed additional tools to build resilience while enhancing the quality of community life. Substantial progress in collaborative leadership, and efforts to develop communitywide goals and indicators of progress toward those goals in a range of community domains can be observed in projects across the United States. The best of these projects are inclusive longitudinal efforts that rest on the contributions of a diverse array of community stakeholders, institutions, and sectors (e.g., Sustainable Seattle Regional Indicator Program; *http://www.sustainableseattle.org*). These community efforts typically aim to enhance some combination of community social, educational, economic, physical, environmental, health, and quality-of-life domains. As such, these projects are inherently geared to build connections among people across central areas of community life, and promote interdisciplinary and cross-sector collaboration. An interdisciplinary focus on resilience offers additional insight when examined at the level of neighborhood and community.

Fostering Individual Resilience

When applying themes of resilience in the design of interventions, we sharpen the saw of current approaches and also encourage new frameworks that take as their principal aim the development of personal and community resources. For individuals there are many useful prevention programs, and many valuable therapies, but few interventions that have articulated a focus on resilience per se. Nevertheless, the skills and ingenuity of consulting and clinical practitioners have led to many methods that are likely to be proven highly successful in boosting individual capacity to recover from difficult times and sustain positive engagements.

One change is apparent with a focus on resilience: a shift away from exclusive attention on therapeutic methods and the endorsement of a broader scope of interactions designed to further strengthen existing talents. Alongside psychotherapy is a host of other potentially valuable interventions, including "coaching" (Hart, Blattner, & Leipsic, 2001), life course review (Viney, 1993), exercise, and mindful meditation, to name a few. Snyder (2002) advocated workshops to encourage pathways that strengthen the person's capacity for hope. With a resilience framework, the targets for lifting demoralization are made more explicit. From a two-factor framework, we know, for instance, that restoring hope does not demand exclusive attention to alleviation of psychological distress. A person can be hopeful even when still anxious. Optimism can be urged even for those who cannot (or will not) give up their fundamentally pessimistic outlooks. Attention to emotion regulation that includes embracing the positive extends the metaphor of the therapeutic beyond that of coping and adjustment to include encouragement of feelings of joy, pleasure, and exhilaration that come from pursuits of core values.

Reich (2006) identified three core principles to follow in developing resilience interventions following catastrophic events: sense of control, coherence, and connectedness. There is broad applicability of these "three C's," to which we might add a fourth: culture. Both social context and the interior of the mind shape what constitutes a positive experience and distinguish it from that which is negative. We assert that resilience can be a universal outcome, with multiple methods and interventions that may be more or less effective depending on the challenges faced and individual, family, community, and cultural influences. Many of the interventions proposed and tested to date emphasize Western theories and values, and further development of interventions to foster resilience across cultures is needed.

A number of interventions within the positive psychology framework have been proposed in the last decade (see Snyder & Lopez, 2002). These interventions have focused specifically on fostering positive engagement, with attention to constructs such as "flourishing" rather than psychopathology and the alleviation of distress (e.g., Keyes & Haidt, 2002). Another approach has been to encourage methods of "forgiveness," thereby releasing restraints on the positive feelings that family members with a history of conflict still may have toward one another (e.g., McCullough, Pargament, & Thoresen, 2000). In a large Internet-based study of positive psychology interventions, Seligman, Steen, Park, and Peterson (2005) found that when individuals wrote about three good things that happened each day and used their identified signature strengths in new ways each week, they reported higher ratings of happiness and lower ratings of depression up to 6 months postintervention. These techniques are not new. Effective interventions for depression have often included positive activity "homework" for those with major depression (Lewinsohn & Graf, 1973). What is new is the paradigm: attention to the positive for the explicit purpose of enhancing well-being and not as medicine for troubled states of mind. When seen with a two-factor lens, this approach is not simply compensatory or even rehabilitative in nature, but a means to further human development along independent trajectories. Thus, the key to resilience is not only the capacity for calm but also the development of greater self-awareness, resulting in the attainment of personal hopes and social purposes.

Fostering Community Resilience

Resilience themes can be applied to the development of social and community interventions as well. Here, the focus is on furthering the expansion of social capital and strengthening connectivity by the reorganization of social exchange. Individual capacity to learn, achieve, and excel at work is strengthened by organizational reforms that shift responsibility (and accountability) for complex tasks downward. Programs in job enrichment (Herzberg, 1966), built upon an understanding of personal needs for mastery and growth on the job, can be highly beneficial to the company profits as well, building greater collective capacity and furthering the firm's social capital. These efforts are examples of effective resilience solutions in which personal development and organizational capacity are threaded together as a long-term investment strategy for a healthy and energetic organization.

A broad systemic view of intervention often is not taken. For a host of reasons, interventions often "morselize" (Lane, 1962) instead. They focus on narrow dimensions of "the problem" and immediate achievable measures of outcomes, such as quarterly profits or election validations, rather than building systemwide capacity for the long term. This is particularly evident in the proliferation of community activities designed to help people cope with problems in living. Marginal tinkering with programs and minor investments in neighborhoods are unlikely to foster resilient communities. In fact, many limited and targeted grant efforts do just the opposite, reinforcing separation and segregation, and in some cases even destroying communities (Chaskin et al., 2001; Churchill, 2003; Peirce, 2005).

Wildavsky (1988) explores the public policy implications of the fact that risk (danger) and safety are inextricably intertwined and should be viewed in a systems context. Wildavsky points to the danger of thinking in terms of "all good" and "all bad," and counsels a search for safety and development of the whole, which involves reduction but not elimination of risk overall. In advocating resilience over resistance as a central organizing theme for city planning and management, Churchill (2003) advises "conserving and investing in the human, social, intellectual and physical capital which constitutes its *protective factors*, rather than expending a large part of the energy of its leadership in short-term efforts" (p. 357, emphasis added).

Innovative resilience programs can change the structure of social exchange within our communities. The Experience Corps (Fried et al., 2004) is one example. This program engages retired senior citizens to advance the chances of young children within inner-city schools. The seniors are provided a way to participate meaningfully in bettering the lives of children in their community. In turn, the children have a surrogate, caring grandparent, who watches over them during part of the school day. Success is measured by markers of well-being among the seniors, as well as retention rates of the children in high school.

Saint Luke's Health Initiatives (2008), a public foundation in Phoenix, Arizona, has launched a 5-year, multimillion-dollar program that blends the authors' resilience model with strength-based community development as a key to resilience (Kretzmann & McKnight, 1993). Called Health in a New Key (HNK), this intervention awards community organizations that develop new partnerships to implement resilience-based interventions that focus on assets, not deficits. The effort is defined as "a way of identifying, framing and responding to issues that focuses first on existing strengths and assets ... and avoids the pervasive culture and model of deficits and needs" (St. Luke's

Health Initiatives, 2003, p. 22). This initiative marks an important step in providing funds to move beyond threat and response paradigms to funding resilience and assets-based research and interventions that can be sustained within communities.

HNK is based on a redefinition of health and measures of progress in that domain. According to the designers of HNK, in the traditional definition of *health* (health in the standard key), "health proceeds through diagnosis and treatment based on science, evidence and best practices. Illness, pathology, needs and deficiencies are identified. Treatment and services are provided. Patients and communities are restored to health" (St. Luke's Health Initiatives, 2003, p. 5). Juxtaposed to this definition is HNK: "Health is the harmonious integration of mind, body and spirit within a responsive community. Diagnosis and treatment, yes, but the focus shifts to strengths and assets first, not just deficits" (p. 6). By providing financial support in the form of nine 5-year partnership grants to collaborations of public and private nonprofit organizations throughout the vast Phoenix metropolitan area, Saint Luke's Health Initiatives hopes to promote resilience and better community health by nurturing exciting organizations, instilling a new approach to health in the region (St. Luke's Health Initiatives, 2008).

Examples from current funded partnerships include collaborative efforts designed to foster broad goals of community building and resilience, while meeting the following important targeted objectives:

1. Develop sustainable asset mobilization that improves community response to health challenges.
2. Increase the number of Phoenix Hispanic families that are willing and able to provide foster and/or adoptive homes for Hispanic children.
3. Identify *promotoras* to serve as leaders addressing community health priorities to improve measurably maternal and infant outcomes in South Phoenix and

Maryvale (Phoenix communities with large poverty populations) (St. Luke's Health Initiatives, 2008).

Other examples include the Healthy Communities Initiatives by the World Health Organization (WHO; 1997), as well as the National Civic League's All-American Cities awards and its development of the Civic Index (National Civic League, 1999). The Resilience Alliance is an international network of institutions and agencies that focuses on social-ecological systems, promoting adaptability and sustainability surrounding developmental policy and practice. The Community Resilience Project based in British Columbia has developed manuals and guides to enhance the capacity of individuals and communities in responding to change. These programs, and many more, represent a new era of public policy and programming that attend to both the needs and the deficits within our communities. Future efforts must strive to continue to unify theory and integrate social activism, with models of health and well-being built upon a solid empirical foundation.

Resilience: More Than a Metaphor

Resilience has become a powerful metaphor for human endurance in a wide array of literature, ranging from scholarly articles about ecology and urban affairs to the financial and sports pages of the daily newspaper. We hope we have shown that there is now substantial, if not universal, evidence of its paradigm-building strength among social scientists interested in models of health and well-being across the lifespan. As metaphor, resilience exerts a powerful influence on how we think about physical health, psychological well-being, and community functioning. In this chapter, our aim has been to develop resilience as more than a metaphor by providing guidance to scientific inquiry. We have advocated measurement methods, multilevel designs, and a two-factor approach to

modeling health and well-being for individuals and their communities. In our view, only by gathering longitudinal data in studies of the turning points in the trajectory of an individual or a community, along with contemporaneous assessments of everyday life, and conducting controlled laboratory studies that provoke challenges to adaptation will we begin to specify the mechanisms that underlie resilience. By establishing urban observatories to mark progress along dimensions of resilience for collectivities, and testing the efficacy of interventions that seek to strengthen resilience for people and their social worlds, we may arrive at the point to declare, as Edward Jenner (1801) did with the smallpox vaccine, that the evidence favoring this approach to health was "too manifest to admit of controversy" (p. 75). Meanwhile, there will be plenty of criticism of resilience concepts, and much healthy debate about measures and methods of change. In science, this is as it should be.

Acknowledgments

Alex J. Zautra and John Stuart Hall contributed equally to this work. We wish to thank Billie Sandberg and members of the Resilience Solutions Group (RSG). The members of the RSG in addition to the authors of this chapter are, in alphabetical order, Leona Aiken, Felipe Castro, Mary Davis, Roger Hughes, Martha Kent, Rick Knopf, Kathy Lemery-Chalfant, Linda Luecken, Morris Okun, and John Reich. This work is supported in part by a grant from the National Institute on Aging (No. R01 AG 026006), Alex J. Zautra, Principal Investigator, John Stuart Hall, Co-Principal Investigator. In addition, we are grateful to St. Luke's Charitable Trust and the Arizona State University Office of the Vice President for Research for invaluable support of the RSG.

Note

1. To develop specific answers to these questions, the RSG of Arizona State University (*www.asu.edu/resilience*) has begun a comprehensive, 5-year study of residents of 40 diverse

"social worlds" in greater Phoenix, Arizona. Results from that study and related research may provide empirical evidence to support a community resilience index and a menu of most effective options for building resilience in communities.

References

Adger, W. N. (2000). Social and ecological resilience: Are they related? *Progress in Human Geography, 24,* 347–364.

Almeida, D. M. (2005). Resilience and vulnerability to daily stressors assessed via diary methods. *Current Directions in Psychological Science, 14,* 64–68.

Antonovsky, A. (1987). *Unraveling the mystery of health: How people manage stress and stay well.* San Francisco: Jossey-Bass.

Beck, U. (1992). *Risk society: Towards a new modernity* (M. Ritter, Trans.). London: Sage.

Berkman, L. F., & Glass, T. A. (2000). Social integration, social networks, social support, and health. In L. F. Berkman & I. Kawachi (Eds.), *Social epidemiology* (pp. 137–173). New York: Oxford University Press.

Bernston, G. C., Caccioppo, J. T., & Gardner, W. L. (1999). The affect system has parallel and integrative processing components: Form follows function. *Journal of Personality and Social Psychology, 76,* 839–855.

Black, A., & Hughes, P. (2001). *The identification and analysis of community strengths and outcomes* (No. ISSN 1444-965n). Canberra: Commonwealth of Australia.

Bodenheimer, T., Lorig, K., Holman, H., & Grumbach, K. (2002). Patient self-management of chronic disease in primary care. *Journal of the American Medical Association, 288,* 2469–2475.

Bonanno, G. A. (2004). Loss, trauma, and human resilience: Have we underestimated the human capacity to thrive after extremely aversive events? *American Psychologist, 59,* 20–28.

Bonanno, G. A. (2005). Resilience in the face of potential trauma. *Current Directions in Psychological Science, 14,* 135–138.

Bonanno, G. A., Wortman, C. B., Lehman, D. R., Tweed, R. G., Haring, M., Sonnega, J., et al. (2002). Resilience to loss and chronic grief: A prospective study from preloss to 18-months postloss. *Journal of Personality and Social Psychology, 83,* 1150–1164.

Bourdieu, P. (1986). The forms of capital. In J. Richardson (Ed.), *Handbook of theory and research for the sociology of education* (pp. 241–258). Westport, CT: Greenwood Press.

Brodsky, A. E., O'Campo, P. J., & Aronson, R. E. (1999). PSOC in community context: Multi-level correlates of a measure of psychological sense of community in low-income, urban neighborhoods. *Journal of Community Psychology, 27,* 659–679.

Brooks, D. (2008). Where's the trauma and the grief? *New York Times,* p. A19.

Canli, T., Zhao, Z., Desmond, J. E., Kang, E., Gross, J., & Gabrieli, J. D. (2001). An fMRI study of personality influences on brain reactivity to emotional stimuli. *Behavioral Neuroscience, 115,* 33–42.

Carpiano, R. M. (2006). Toward a neighborhood resource-based theory of social capital for health: Can Bourdieu and sociology help? *Social Science and Medicine, 62,* 165–175.

Caspi, A., Sugden, K., Moffitt, T. E., Taylor, A., Craig, I. W., Harrington, H., et al. (2003). Influence of life stress on depression: Moderation by a polymorphism in the 5-HTT gene. *Science, 301,* 386–389.

Chandler, T., & Fox, G. (1974). *3000 years of urban growth.* New York: Academic Press.

Charney, D. S. (2004). Psychobiological mechanisms of resilience and vulnerability: Implications for successful adaptation to extreme stress. *American Journal of Psychiatry, 161,* 195–216.

Chaskin, R. J., Brown, P., Venkatesh, S., & Vidal, A. (2001). *Building community capacity.* New York: Aldine De Gruyter.

Churchill, S. (2003). Resilience, not resistance. *City, 7,* 349–360.

Cohen, S., Doyle, W. J., Turner, R. B., Alper, C. M., & Skoner, D. P. (2003). Emotional style and susceptibility to the common cold. *Psychosomatic Medicine, 65,* 652–657.

Coleman, J. (1990). *Foundations of social theory.* Cambridge, MA: Harvard University Press.

Connor, K. M., & Davidson, J. R. T. (2003). Development of a new resilience scale: The Connor–Davidson Resilience Scale (CD-RISC). *Depression and Anxiety, 18,* 76–82.

Cowen, E. L. (1994). The enhancement of psychological wellness: Challenges and opportunities. *American Journal of Community Psychology, 22,* 149–179.

Coyne, J. C., & Downey, G. (1991). Social factors in psychopathology: Stress, social support, and coping processes. *Annual Review of Psychology, 42*, 401–425.

Craig, A. D. (2009). How do you feel—now?: The anterior insula and human awareness. *Nature Reviews Neuroscience, 10*, 59–70.

Curtis, W. J., & Cicchetti, D. (2003). Moving research on resilience into the 21st century: Theoretical and methodological considerations in examining the biological contributors to resilience. *Development and Psychopathology, 15*, 773–810.

Dawber, T. R., Meadors, G. F., & Moore, F. E. J. (1951). Epidemiological approaches to heart disease: The Framingham Study. *American Journal of Public Health, 41*, 279–286.

Diamond, J. (2005). *Collapse: How societies choose to fail or succeed*. New York: Viking.

Diener, E., & Suh, E. M. (2000). *Culture and subjective well-being*. Cambridge, MA: MIT Press.

Duncan, T. E., Duncan, S. C., Okut, H., Strycker, L. A., & Hix-Small, H. (2003). A multilevel contextual model of neighborhood collective efficacy. *American Journal of Community Psychology, 32*, 245–252.

Ellen, I. G., Mijanovich, T., & Dillman, K. (2001). Neighborhood effects on health: Exploring the links and assessing the evidence. *Journal of Urban Affairs, 23*, 391–408.

Evans, R. G., & Stoddart, G. L. (1990). Producing health, consuming health care. *Social Sciences and Medicine, 31*, 1347–1363.

Evens, R. G., Barer, M. L., & Marmor, T. S. (Eds.). (1994). *Why some people get sick and others don't*. New York: Aldine.

Ewart, C. K., & Suchday, S. (2002). Discovering how urban poverty and violence affect health: Development and validation of a Neighborhood Stress Index. *Health Psychology, 21*, 254–262.

Finch, J. F., Okun, M. A., Barrera, M., Jr., Zautra, A. J., & Reich, J. W. (1989). Positive and negative social ties among older adults: Measurement models and the prediction of psychological distress and well-being. *American Journal of Community Psychology, 17*, 585–605.

Fitzpatrick, K. M., & LaGory, M. (2003). "Placing" health in an urban sociology: Cities as mosaics of risk and protection. *City and Community, 2*, 33–46.

Florida, R. (2004). *The rise of the creative class*. New York: Basic Books.

Flower, J. (1994). *Measuring what's working: Alternative community assessment* (Healthy Communities Action Kits, Module 3). San Francisco: Healthcare Forum.

Frankenhauser, M. (1983). The sympathetic–adrenal and pituitary–adrenal response to challenge. In T. Dembroski, T. Schmidt, & G. Blumchen (Eds.), *Biobehavioral basis of coronary heart disease* (pp. 91–105). Basel, Switzerland: Karger.

Friborg, O., Barlaug, D., Martinussen, M., Rosenvinge, J. H., & Hjemdal, O. (2005). Resilience in relation to personality and intelligence. *International Journal of Methods in Psychiatric Research, 14*, 29–40.

Fried, L. P., Carlson, M. C., Freedman, M., Frick, K. D., Glass, T. A., Hill, J., et al. (2004). A social model for health promotion for an aging population: Initial evidence on the Experience Corps model. *Journal of Urban Health, 81*, 64–78.

Fuentes-Afflick, E., Hessol, N. A., & Perez-Stable, E. J. (1999). Testing the epidemiologic paradox of low birth weight in Latinos. *Archives of Pediatrics and Adolescent Medicine, 153*, 147–153.

Furlong, L. V., Zautra, A. J., Puente, C. P., López, P., & Valero, P. B. (2008). Cognitive–affective assets and vulnerabilities: Two factors influencing adaptation to fibromyalgia. *Psychology and Health*, pp. 1–16.

Gallo, L. C., Bogart, L. M., Vranceanu, A. M., & Matthews, K. A. (2005). Socioeconomic status, resources, psychological experiences, and emotional responses: A test of the reserve capacity model. *Journal of Personality and Social Psychology, 88*, 386–399.

Garmezy, N. (1991). Resiliency and vulnerability to adverse developmental outcomes associated with poverty. *American Behavioral Scientist, 34*, 416–430.

Gould, J. B., Madan, A., Qin, C., & Chavez, G. (2003). Perinatal outcomes in two dissimilar immigrant populations in the United States: A dual epidemiologic paradox. *Pediatrics, 111*, e676–e682.

Greve, W., & Staudinger, U. M. (2006). Resilience in later adulthood and old age: Resources and potentials for successful aging. In D. Cicchetti & D. J. Cohen (Eds.), *Developmental psychopathology: Risk, disorder, and adaptation* (2nd ed., pp. 796–840). New York: Wiley.

Hall, J. S. (2002). Reconsidering the connection between capacity and governance. *Public Organization Review, 2*, 23–43.

Hart, V., Blattner, J., & Leipsic, S. (2001). Coaching versus therapy: A perspective. *Consulting Psychology Journal, 53*, 229–237.

Hawkley, L. C., Berntson, G. G., Engeland, C. G., Marucha, P. T., Masi, C. M., & Cacioppo, J. T. (2005). Stress, aging, and resilience: Can accrued wear and tear be slowed? *Canadian Psychology, 46*, 115–125.

Heidrich, S., & Ryff, C. D. (1993). Physical and mental health in later life: The self-system as mediator. *Psychology and Aging, 8*, 327–338.

Herzberg, F. (1966). *Work and the nature of man.* New York: Crowell.

Holling, C. S., Schindler, D. W., Walker, B. W., & Roughgarden, J. (1995). Biodiversity in the functioning of ecosystems: An ecological synthesis. In C. Perrings, K. G. Maler, C. Folke, C. S. Holling, & B. O. Jansson (Eds.), *Biodiversity and loss: Economic and ecological issues* (pp. 44–83). Cambridge, UK: Cambridge University Press.

Jenner, E. (1801). *An inquiry into the causes and effects of the variolae vaccinae, a disease discovered in some of the western counties of England, particularly Gloucestershire, and known by the name of the cow pox.* (3rd ed.). London: Sampson Low.

Johnson-Wright, L., Zautra, A. J., & Going, S. (2008). Adaptation to early knee osteoarthritis: The role of risk, resilience, and disease severity on pain and physical functioning. *Journal of Behavioral Medicine, 36*, 70–80.

Jopp, D., & Smith, J. (2006). Resources and life-management strategies as determinants of successful aging: On the protective effect of selection, optimization, and compensation. *Psychology and Aging, 21*, 253–265.

Kawachi, I., Kennedy, B. P., Lochner, K., & Prothrow-Stith, D. (1997). Social capital, income inequality, and mortality. *American Journal of Public Health, 87*, 1491–1498.

Kelly, G. A. (1955). *The psychology of personal constructs.* New York: Norton.

Kelly, J. G. (1970). Antidotes for arrogance: Training for community psychology. *American Psychologist, 25*, 524–531.

Keyes, C. L. (2004). Risk and resilience in human development: An introduction. *Research in Human Development, 1*, 223–227.

Keyes, C. L., & Haidt, J. (2002). *Flourishing: Positive psychology and the life well-lived.* Washington, DC: American Psychological Association.

Kosfeld, M., Heinrichs, M., Zak, P. J., Fischbacher, U., & Fehr, E. (2005). Oxytocin increases trust in humans. *Nature, 435*, 673–676.

Kretzmann, J. P., & McKnight, J. L. (1993). *Building communities from the inside out: A path toward finding and mobilizing a community's assets.* Chicago: ACTA Publications.

Lane, R. E. (1962). *Political ideology: Why the American common man believes what he does.* New York: Free Press of Glencoe.

Langdon, P. (1997). *A better place to live: Reshaping the American suburb.* Amherst: University of Massachusetts Press.

Lewinsohn, P. M., & Graf, M. (1973). Pleasant activities and depression. *Journal of Consulting and Clinical Psychology, 41*, 261–268.

Light, K. C., Girdler, S. S., Sherwood, A., Bragdon, E. E., Brownley, K. A., West, S. G., et al. (1999). High stress responsivity predicts later blood pressure only in combination with positive family history and high life stress. *Hypertension, 33*, 1458–1464.

Linden, W., Rutledge, T., & Con, A. (1998). A case for the usefulness of laboratory social stressors. *Annals of Behavioral Medicine, 20*, 310–316.

Lovallo, W. R., & Gerin, W. (2003). Psychophysiological reactivity: Mechanisms and pathways to cardiovascular disease. *Psychosomatic Medicine, 65*, 36–45.

Luecken, L. J., & Appelhans, B. M. (2006). Early parental loss and cortisol stress responses in young adulthood: The moderating role of family environment. *Development and Psychopathology, 18*, 295–308.

Luecken, L. J., Appelhans, B. M., Kraft, A., & Brown, A. (2006). Never far from home: A cognitive-affective model of the impact of early-life family relationships on physiological stress responses in adulthood. *Journal of Social and Personal Relationships, 23*, 189–203.

Luthar, S. (2006). Resilience in development: A synthesis of research across five decades. In D. Cicchetti & D. J. Cohen (Eds.), *Developmental psychopathology: Risk, disorder, and adaptation* (2nd ed., pp. 739–795). New York: Wiley.

Luthar, S. S., Cicchetti, D., & Becker, B. (2000). The construct of resilience: A critical evaluation and guidelines for future work. *Child Development, 71*, 543–562.

Macintyre, S., Ellaway, A., & Cummins, S. (2002). Place effects on health: How can we conceptualize, operationalize and measure them? *Social Science and Medicine, 55,* 125–139.

Marmot, M. G., & Fuhrer, R. (2004). Socioeconomic position and health across midlife. In O. G. Brim, C. D. Ryff, & R. C. Kessler (Eds.), *How healthy are we?: A national study of well-being at mid-life* (pp. 64–89). Chicago: University of Chicago Press.

Masten, A. S. (2001). Ordinary magic: Resilience processes in development. *American Psychologist, 56,* 227–238.

Masten, A. S., & Powell, J. L. (2003). A resilience framework for research, policy and practice. In S. S. Luthar (Ed.), *Resilience and vulnerability: Adaptation in the context of childhood adversities* (pp. 1–25). Cambridge, UK: Cambridge University Press.

Matthews, K. A., Woodall, K. L., & Allen, M. T. (1993). Cardiovascular reactivity to stress predicts future blood pressure status. *Hypertension, 22,* 479–485.

McAdams, D. (2006). *The redemptive self: Stories Americans live by.* New York: Oxford University Press.

McCullough, M. E., Pargament, K. I., & Thoresen, C. E. (2000). *Forgiveness: Theory, research, and practice.* New York: Guilford Press.

McEwen, B. S. (1998). Protective and damaging effects of stress mediators. *New England Journal of Medicine, 338,* 171–179.

Montiel, L., Nathan, R., & Wright, D. (2004). *An update on urban hardship.* Albany, NY: Rockefeller Institute of Government.

Moskowitz, J. T. (2003). Positive affect predicts lower risk of AIDS mortality. *Psychosomatic Medicine, 65,* 620–626.

National Civic League. (1999). *The Civic Index: Measuring your community's civic health.* Denver: Author.

National Research Council. (2001). *Preparing for an aging world: The case for cross-national research.* Washington, DC: National Academy Press.

O'Campo, P. (2003). Invited commentary: Advancing theory and methods for multilevel models of residential neighborhoods and health. *American Journal of Epidemiology, 157,* 9–13.

Ong, A. D., Bergeman, C. S., & Bisconti, T. L. (2004). The role of daily positive emotions during conjugal bereavement. *Journals of Ger-*

ontology B: Psychological Sciences and Social Sciences, 59, 168–176.

Ong, A. D., Bergeman, C. S., Bisconti, T. L., & Wallace, K. A. (2006). Psychological resilience, positive emotions, and successful adaptation to stress in later life. *Journal of Personality and Social Psychology, 91,* 730–749.

Pearlin, L. I., & Schooler, C. (1978). The structure of coping. *Journal of Health and Social Behavior, 19,* 2–21.

Peirce, N. (2005). Katrina's opportunity—a new new federalism. Retrieved August 15, 2006, from *www.stateline.org/live/details/story?contentId=55197.*

Pelling, M. (2003). *The vulnerability of cities: Natural disasters and social resilience.* London: Earthscan.

Portes, A. (2000). The two meanings of social capital. *Sociological Forum, 15,* 127–137.

Pressman, S. D., & Cohen, S. (2005). Does positive affect influence health? *Psychological Bulletin, 131*(6), 925–971.

Price, R. H., & Behrens, T. (2003). Working Pasteur's quadrant: Harnessing science and action for community change. *American Journal of Community Psychology, 31,* 219–223.

Putnam, R. D. (2000). *Bowling alone: The collapse and revival of American community.* New York: Simon & Schuster.

Putnam, R. D., Felstein, L. M., & Cohen, D. (2003). *Better together: Restoring the American community.* New York: Simon & Schuster.

Putnam, R. D., Leonardi, R., & Nanetti, R. Y. (1993). *Making democracy work: Civic traditions in modern Italy.* Princeton, NJ: Princeton University Press.

Rappaport, J., & Seidman, E. (Eds.). (2000). *Handbook of community psychology.* New York: Klunem Academic/Plenum Press.

Reich, J. W. (2006). Three psychological principles of resilience in natural disasters. *Disaster Prevention and Management: An International Journal, 15,* 793–798.

Reich, J. W., & Zautra, A. J. (1990). Dispositional control beliefs and the consequences of a control-enhancing intervention. *Journal of Gerontology, 45,* 46–51.

Reich, J. W., & Zautra, A. J. (1991). Experimental and measurement approaches to internal control in older adults. *Journal of Social Issues, 47,* 143–188.

Rozario, K. (2005). Making progress: Disaster

narratives and the art of optimism in modern America. In L. J. Vale & T. J. Campanella (Eds.), *The resilient city* (pp. 27–54). London: Oxford University Press.

Russek, L. G., & Schwartz, G. E. (1997). Perceptions of parental caring predict health status in midlife: A 35-year follow-up of the Harvard Mastery of Stress Study. *Psychosomatic Medicine, 59,* 144–149.

Rutter, M. (1987). Psychosocial resilience and protective mechanisms. *American Journal of Orthopsychiatry, 57,* 316–331.

Rutter, M. (1999). Resilience as the millennium Rorschach: Response to Smith and Gorrell Barnes. *Journal of Family Therapy, 21,* 159–160.

Ryff, C. D., & Keyes, C. L. (1995). The structure of psychological well-being revisited. *Journal of Personality and Social Psychology, 69,* 719–727.

Ryff, C. D., & Singer, B. (1998). The contours of positive human health. *Psychological Inquiry, 9,* 1–28.

Saint Luke's Health Initiatives. (2003). Resilience: Health in a new key. Phoenix, AZ: Author. Available at *www.slhi.org/publications/issue_briefs/pdfs/ib-03fall.pdf.*

Saint Luke's Health Initiatives. (2008). Health in a new key. Phoenix, AZ: Author. Available at *www.slhi.org/new_key/index.shtml.*

Sampson, R. J., Morenoff, J. D., & Gannon-Rowley, T. (2002). Assessing "neighborhood effects": Social processes and new directions in research. *Annual Review of Sociology, 28,* 443–478.

Sanders, A. E., Lim, S., & Sohn, W. (2008). Resilience to urban poverty: Theoretical and empirical considerations for population health. *American Journal of Public Health, 98,* 1101–1106.

Sapolsky, R. M. (1998). *Why zebras don't get ulcers: A guide to stress, stress-related disease, and coping* (3rd ed.). New York: Freeman.

Sarason, S. (1974). *The psychological sense of community: Prospects for a community psychology.* San Francisco: Jossey-Bass.

Schulz, R. (1976). Effects of control and predictability on the physical and psychological well-being of the institutionalized aged. *Journal of Personality and Social Psychology, 33,* 563–573.

Seeman, T. E., Berkman, L. F., Charpentier, P. A., Blazer, D. G., Albert, M. S., & Tinetti, M. E. (1995). Behavioral and psychosocial predictors of physical performance: MacArthur Studies of Successful Aging. *Journals of Gerontology A: Biological Sciences and Medical Sciences, 50,* 177–183.

Seeman, T. E., Singer, B. H., Ryff, C. D., Dienberg Love, G., & Levy-Storms, L. (2002). Social relationships, gender, and allostatic load across two age cohorts. *Psychosomatic Medicine, 64,* 395–406.

Seligman, M. E. P., & Csikszentmihalyi, M. (2000). Positive psychology: An introduction. *American Psychologist, 55,* 5–14.

Seligman, M. E. P., Steen, T. A., Park, N., & Peterson, C. (2005). Positive psychology progress: Empirical validation of interventions. *American Psychologist, 60,* 410–421.

Silva, P. A., & Stanton, W. R. (1996). *From child to adult: The Dunedin Multidisciplinary Health and Development Study.* New York: Oxford University Press.

Singer, B., & Ryff, C. D. (2001). *New horizons in health: An integrative approach.* Washington, DC: National Academy Press.

Skinner, E. (1996). A guide to constructs of control. *Journal of Personality and Social Psychology, 71,* 549–570.

Smith, B., & Zautra, A. J. (2008). Vulnerability and resilience in women with arthritis: Test of a two factor model. *Journal of Consulting and Clinical Psychology, 76,* 799–810.

Smith, B. W., Dalen, J., Wiggins, K., Tooley, E., Christopher, P., & Bernard, J. (in press). The Brief Resilience Scale: Assessing the ability to bounce back. *International Journal of Behavioral Medicine.*

Snyder, C. R. (2002). Hope theory: Rainbows in the mind. *Psychological Inquiry, 13,* 249–275.

Snyder, C. R., & Lopez, S. (2002). *Handbook of positive psychology.* Oxford, UK: Oxford University Press.

Steptoe, A., & Feldman, P. J. (2001). Neighborhood problems as sources of chronic stress: Development of a measure of neighborhood problems, and associations with socioeconomic status and health. *Annals of Behavioral Medicine, 23,* 177–185.

Steptoe, A., Wardle, J., & Marmot, M. (2005). Positive affect and health-related neuroendocrine, cardiovascular, and inflammatory processes. *Proceedings of the National Academy of Sciences USA, 102,* 6508–6512.

Stone, A. A., & Neale, J. M. (1982). Development of a methodology for assessing daily experiences. In A. Baum & J. Singer (Eds.), *Advances in environmental psychology: Environment and health* (Vol. 4, pp. 49–83). Hillsdale, NJ: Erlbaum.

Subramanian, S. V. (2004). The relevance of multilevel statistical methods for identifying causal neighborhood effects. *Social Science and Medicine, 58*, 1961–1967.

Subramanian, S. V., Jones, K., & Duncan, C. (2003). Multilevel methods for public health research. In I. Kawachi & L. F. Berkman (Eds.), *Neighborhoods and health* (pp. 65–111). New York: Oxford University Press.

Subramanian, S. V., Lochner, K. A., & Kawachi, I. (2003). Neighborhood differences in social capital: A compositional artifact or a contextual construct? *Health and Place, 9*, 33–44.

Szreter, S., & Woolcock, M. (2004). Health by association?: Social capital, social theory and the political economy of public health. *International Journal of Epidemiology, 33*, 650–667.

Tolle, E. (2005). *A new Earth: Awakening to your life's purpose.* New York: Penguin Books.

Tonne, C., Schartz, J., Mittleman, M., Melly, S., Suh, H., & Golgberg, R. (2005). Long-term survival after acute myocardial infarction is lower in more deprived neighborhoods. *Circulation, 111*, 3063–3070.

Treiber, F. A., Kamarck, T., Schneiderman, N., Sheffield, D., Kapuku, G., & Taylor, T. (2003). Cardiovascular reactivity and development of preclinical and clinical disease states. *Psychosomatic Medicine, 65*, 46–62.

Vaillant, G. E. (2003). Mental health. *American Journal of Psychiatry, 160*, 1373–1384.

Vaillant, G. E., & Mukamal, K. (2001). Successful aging. *American Journal of Psychiatry, 158*, 839–847.

Vale, L. J., & Campanella, T. (2005). *The resilient city.* London: Oxford University Press.

Veenstra, G., Luginaah, I., Wakefield, S., Birch, S., Eyles, J., & Elliott, S. (2005). Who you know, where you live: Social capital, neighbourhood and health. *Social Science and Medicine, 60*, 2799–2818.

Viney, L. L. (1993). *Life stories: Personal construct therapy with the elderly.* New York: Wiley.

Watson, D., Wiese, D., Vaidya, J., & Tellegen, A. (1999). The two general activation systems of affect: Structural findings, evolutionary considerations, and psychobiological evidence. *Journal of Personality and Social Psychology, 76*, 820–838.

Wen, M., Browning, C. R., & Cagney, K. A. (2007). Neighbourhood deprivation, social capital and regular exercise during adulthood: A multilevel study in Chicago. *Urban Studies, 44*, 2651–2671.

Werner, E. E., & Smith, R. S. (2001). *Journeys from childhood to midlife: Risk, resilience, and recovery.* Ithaca, NY: Cornell University Press.

Wildavsky, A. (1988). *Searching for safety.* New Brunswick, NJ: Transaction Books.

Wilkinson, R. (1996). *Unhealthy societies: The afflictions of inequality.* London: Routledge.

World Health Organization (WHO). (1997). *Twenty steps for developing a healthy cities project* (3rd ed.). Copenhagen: WHO Regional Office for Europe.

Zautra, A. J. (2003). *Stress, emotions and health.* New York: Oxford University Press.

Zautra, A. J., Fasman, R., Reich, J. W., Harakas, P., Johnson, L. M., Olmsted, M. E., et al. (2005). Fibromyalgia: Evidence for deficits in positive affect regulation. *Psychosomatic Medicine, 67*, 147–155.

Zautra, A. J., Hall, J. S., & Murray, K. E. (in press). Community development and community resilience: An integrative approach. *Community Development: Journal of the Community Development Society.*

Zautra, A. J., Johnson, L. M., & Davis, M. C. (2005). Positive affect as a source of resilience for women in chronic pain. *Journal of Consulting and Clinical Psychology, 73*, 212–220.

Ziersch, A. M., Baum, F. E., Macdougall, C., & Putland, C. (2005). Neighbourhood life and social capital: The implications for health. *Social Science and Medicine, 60*, 71–86.

II

BASIC DIMENSIONS OF RESILIENCE

A

Biological Dimensions of Resilience

2

Psychobiological Mechanisms of Resilience to Stress

Adriana Feder
Eric J. Nestler
Maren Westphal
Dennis S. Charney

Most people are exposed to one or more traumatic events during their lifetime, and many must endure stressful conditions that persist over time. Although historically most research has focused on the negative impact of stressful life events, the past several years have witnessed a surge of new information on the psychological and neurobiological mechanisms involved in promoting resilient responses to stress. The construct of *resilience* refers to the ability of individuals to adapt successfully in the face of acute stress, trauma, or chronic adversity, maintaining or rapidly regaining psychological well-being and physiological homeostasis (Charney, 2004). Resilience is not just the absence of psychopathology; adaptive responses to stress can be promoted by strengthening potential protective factors. Recent studies suggest that genetic influences on biological processes are larger than influences on complex behavioral responses, and thus easier to identify and to study (Hasler, Drevets, Manji,

& Charney, 2004; Zhou et al., 2008). An integrative model of resilience incorporating information from multiple phenotypic levels, including the behavioral and psychological, is likely to yield a range of preventive and treatment strategies for stress-related disorders (Charney, 2004; Zhou et al., 2008). This chapter reviews current perspectives on psychosocial, developmental, neurochemical, genetic, and neural factors associated with resilient responses to stress. We conclude with a review of promising preventive and therapeutic strategies.

Psychosocial Factors Associated with Resilience

Studies have identified a range of psychosocial factors that promote successful adaptation to stress, including active coping strategies, positive emotionality, cognitive reappraisal, the presence of social supports, and a sense of purpose in life, among others.

Active Coping and Facing Fears

Active coping strategies, such as planning and problem solving, have been linked to a higher degree of well-being and capacity to handle stress, trauma, and medical illness (Southwick, Vythilingam, & Charney, 2005). Active coping involves facing one's fears. Resilient individuals are more likely to utilize fear as a guide to appraise threat and direct appropriate action. By contrast, maladaptive strategies involving escape/avoidance of stressful situations—such as denial and behavioral disengagement—have been linked to higher distress levels (Carver, 1997; Folkman & Moskowitz, 2004; Southwick et al., 2005). Individuals with posttraumatic stress disorder (PTSD) avoid facing reminders of the trauma, which might contribute to maintenance of conditioned fear.

Positive Emotions and Optimism

An increasing number of studies have provided evidence for the key role of dispositional optimism and positive emotions in enhancing psychological resilience (Ong, Bergeman, Bisconti, & Wallace, 2006; Tugade & Fredrickson, 2004). Positive emotions frequently co-occur with negative emotions in the face of highly stressful personal situations (Ong et al., 2006). According to the broaden-and-build model (Fredrickson, 2001), positive emotions provide a buffer against the adverse consequences of stress by decreasing the autonomic arousal produced by negative emotions, and by increasing flexibility of thinking and problem solving. In fact, studies have shown that positive emotions are associated with faster cardiovascular recovery from negative emotional arousal and decreased stress reactivity (Tugade & Fredrickson, 2004).

Cognitive Reappraisal

The capacity for cognitive reappraisal allows individuals to reevaluate or reframe adverse experiences in a more positive light. Meaning-making processes open multiple alternative avenues to well-being, further discussed below (Seligman, 2005). The ability of resilient individuals to infuse stressful life events with positive meaning, as well as the use of humor, might help to regulate negative emotions (Folkman & Moskowitz, 2000).

Social Support

A large number of studies have documented the importance of social support as a protective variable in stress-related disorders such as PTSD (Charuvastra & Cloitre, 2008). Research has shown that affiliative behaviors in animals and humans alleviate the effects of stress, injury, and infection (DeVries, Glasper, & Detillion, 2003; Robles & Kiecolt-Glaser, 2003). Secure attachment relationships help to reduce negative affect and physical arousal in stressful situations (Bowlby, 1982; Charuvastra & Cloitre, 2008; Mikulincer, Shaver, & Pereg, 2003).

Purpose in Life, Moral Compass, and Spirituality

A sense of purpose in life and the presence of an internal set of beliefs about right and wrong have been linked to resilience. Traumatic events may deeply affect a person's beliefs and sense of meaning (Janoff-Bulman, 1992). Regaining a sense of purpose might be central for the process of recovery. In a recent cross-sectional study of African American individuals exposed to severe trauma, a sense of purpose in life was significantly associated with psychological resilience, as well as recovery from psychiatric disorders (Alim et al., 2008). Counseling sessions focused on meaning making with cancer patients were found to decrease depression and increase life satisfaction in another study (Lee, Cohen, Edgar, Laizner, & Gagnon, 2004). For many individuals, religious or spiritual beliefs and practices provide a framework that facilitates recovery and finding meaning after traumatic or highly stressful experiences (Pargament, Smith, Koenig, & Perez, 1998).

Resilience and Early Life Environment

Adverse early life experiences are known to increase risk for depression and PTSD in adulthood by producing long-lasting hormonal, neurotransmitter, and central nervous system changes that may affect resistance to later stress (Heim & Nemeroff, 2001; Vythilingam et al., 2002). Similarly, animal studies have shown enduring effects of early, prolonged maternal separation (Heim & Nemeroff, 2001). In contrast, there are many examples of resilient development despite early exposure to severe stress, as exemplified by studies of Romanian children adopted away from institutional orphanages into stable homes (Masten, 2001; Rutter, 1998), and by animal studies showing that exposure to an enriched environment can make rodents less vulnerable to stress and to drugs of abuse (Green, Gehrke, & Bardo, 2002), and can reverse some of the behavioral impairments induced by early maternal separation (Francis, Diorio, Plotsky, & Meaney, 2002).

A key factor identified in children who are able to overcome adversity is a close relationship with a caring adult (Luthar, Sawyer, & Brown, 2006; Masten, Best, & Garmezy, 1991). For example, the quality of caregiving that children receive after the loss of a parent can mitigate risk for depression. Children are also able to adapt better in the context of war or disasters when they are not separated from their parents (Masten et al., 1991). Conversely, problematic parental bonding characterized by affectionless control has been identified as a risk factor for depression in adulthood (Parker, 1983). Of note, this important risk predictor has shown robust intergenerational transmission in women, thus providing an opportunity for early intervention (Miller, Kramer, Warner, Wickramaratne, & Weissman, 1997). Rodent studies have shown that early positive maternal care in the form of high levels of licking/grooming and arched-back nursing produces offspring who are less fearful as adults and show attenuated hormonal responses to stress (Weaver et al., 2004). Cross-fostering experiments have demonstrated that these effects are transmitted behaviorally, and recent research has suggested an epigenetic basis of this phenomenon (see below; McGowan et al., 2009; Meaney & Szyf, 2005; Weaver et al., 2004). Other factors associated with resilience during development include social competence and agreeableness, positive emotionality, and the capacity for self-regulation (Masten & Coatsworth, 1998).

Less well researched is the finding that prior exposure to mild or "manageable" stress during development might actually promote more adaptive responses to stress in the future. For example, some studies suggest that adults cope better with a range of stressors, including work-related stressors, spousal loss, or accidents, if they previously have experienced and coped successfully with stressors as children or adolescents (Lyons & Parker, 2007). Lyons and colleagues (Parker, Buckmaster, Schatzberg, & Lyons, 2004) have examined this phenomenon of *stress inoculation* in young squirrel monkeys. Exposure of young squirrel monkeys to short-term isolation from other monkeys induces better social and emotional functioning upon later exposure to mild stressors. Similarly, brief maternal separation of rat pups reduces behavioral and hormonal responses to stress later in life (Meaney & Szyf, 2005) . Importantly, the degree of behavioral control an animal has over stress is a key determinant of whether an individual's response is adaptive or maladaptive: the more control, the more resilient the individual (Maier, Amat, Baratta, Paul, & Watkins, 2006).

Neurochemical Stress Responses Associated with Resilience

The term *allostasis*, coined by Sterling and Eyer (1988), denotes the dynamic process through which the body adapts to daily stressors and maintains homeostasis. When faced with unexpected, sudden stressful events, the brain responds by releasing catecholamines and other stress hormones that prepare the organism to cope with the situation and avert harm to the organism. Interindividual variability in stress resilience depends on differences in the coordinated function of numerous hormones, neurotransmitters and neuropeptides involved in the stress response.

Hypothalamic–Pituitary–Adrenal Axis

Secreted by the hypothalamus in response to stress, the corticotropin-releasing hormone (CRH) activates the release of the adrenocorticotropic hormone (ACTH) from the anterior pituitary gland, which in turn stimulates the synthesis and secretion of cortisol by the adrenal cortex. Cortisol inhibits the release of CRH and ACTH through a complex negative feedback system that keeps in check stress-induced increases in cortisol (de Kloet, DeRijk, & Meijer, 2007). Elevation in hypothalamic–pituitary–adrenal (HPA) axis activity in response to stress sets off a cascade of hormonal processes that facilitate cognitive, metabolic, immunological, and behavioral adaptations to environmental demands (Sapolsky, Romero, & Munck, 2000; Weiner, 1992). The same chemical mediators that promote survival, however, may produce negative health consequences when the stressors become chronic or are perceived as overwhelming, resulting in *allostatic overload* (McEwen & Wingfield, 2003). In the brain, excessive cortisol is associated with complex structural effects in the hippocampus and amygdala in humans and animals, including atropic effects in certain neuronal cell types (McEwen & Milner, 2007). Studies have shown that early life stress is associated with chronic elevation of CRH levels lasting into adulthood (Heim & Nemeroff, 2001). Disturbances in HPA axis function seem to differ between psychiatric disorders. For example, whereas patients with major depressive disorder have elevated cerebrospinal fluid CRH and plasma corti-

sol levels, patients with PTSD have elevated CRH but reduced cortisol levels (de Kloet, Joels, & Holsboer, 2005). Resilience is associated with the rapid activation and efficient termination of the stress response, and is thought to involve an optimal balance of glucocorticoid and mineralocorticoid receptor function (Charney, 2004; de Kloet et al., 2005, 2007).

Dehydroepiandrosterone (DHEA), an adrenal steroid released concurrently with cortisol in response to stress, may increase stress resistance by protecting against neural damage resulting from prolonged HPA axis activity. DHEA and its metabolites counteract corticosteroid-induced neurotoxicity in the hippocampus (Morfin & Starka, 2001). In studies of patients with PTSD, higher plasma DHEA and DHEA-sulfate levels, and higher capacity for adrenal release of DHEA, have been linked to reduced illness severity and greater symptom improvement (Rasmusson et al., 2004; Yehuda, Brand, Golier, & Yang, 2006). Higher DHEA-sulfate–cortisol ratios during stress might be protective in healthy individuals; in a group of soldiers participating in military survival school, higher DHEA-sulfate–cortisol ratios were associated with fewer dissociative symptoms and better performance under stress (Morgan et al., 2004).

The Locus Ceruleus–Norepinephrine System

Another neural system that affects sympathetic nervous system functioning and HPA axis responses to stress is the locus ceruleus–norepinephrine (LC-NE) system. The LC serves a general alarm function within the body, responding to potential threats by triggering the release of NE within the amygdala, nucleus accumbens, prefrontal cortex (PFC), and hippocampus. Activation of the LC also inhibits neurovegetative functions, such as sleep and feeding behavior. A chronically hyperresponsive LC-NE is thought to predispose the organism to heightened anxiety by inhibiting PFC function, thus interfering with more complex cognitive, emotion regulation processes, and leading to cardio-vascular problems (Charney, 2003, 2004). Blockade of beta-adrenergic receptors in the amygdala can oppose the development of aversive memories in animals and humans (Charney, 2003; McGaugh, 2004). Collectively, these findings suggest that resilience might be associated with reduced responsiveness of the LC-NE system.

The Serotonergic System

Serotonin (5-HT) neurons project widely in the brain. Acute stress is associated with increased 5-HT turnover in several brain regions, including the amygdala, the nucleus accumbens, and the PFC. 5-HT has neuromodulatory effects on other neurotransmitter systems that are implicated in mood and anxiety. Depending on the forebrain region involved and which receptor subtype is activated, the release of 5-HT may have anxiogenic or anxiolytic effects (Charney, 2004). Early life stress may lead to diminished stress tolerance in later life by increasing CRH and cortisol levels, which in turn lower 5-HT_{1A} receptor activity. Levels of 5-HT_{1A} receptor during early postnatal development, particularly in frontal cortex and hippocampal regions, may influence anxiety thresholds in adulthood (Lanzenberger et al., 2007). Research using a transgenic mice model suggests that 5-HT_{1A} receptor expression may shape development of anxiety during critical developmental periods (Gross & Hen, 2004).

The Dopaminergic System

Dopamine neurons are activated by rewarding stimuli and inhibited by aversive stimuli. Stress activates dopamine release in the medial PFC (mPFC) and inhibits its release in the nucleus accumbens, a key component of the reward circuitry. Animal and human studies have provided evidence that balance between mesocortical and mesoaccumbens dopamine responses to stress might be crucial in protecting against the negative impact of stress on mood and physical well-being (Cabib, Ventura, & Puglisi-Allegra, 2002). Excessive mesocortical dopamine release after stressful events might be associated with increased vulnerability (Cabib et al., 2002). Dopamine signaling facilitates fear extinction, but its role in resilience per se is unclear.

Neuropeptide Y

There is increasing evidence that neuropeptide Y (NPY), a neuropeptide that is widely distributed in the brain, might have a stabilizing effect on neural circuits that are implicated in the regulation of emotional and behavioral responses to stress. NPY is thought to reduce anxiety by counteracting the anxiogenic effects of CRH in the amygdala, hippocampus, hypothalamus, and LC (Britton, Akwa, Spina, & Koob, 2000; Heilig, Koob, Ekman, & Britton, 1994). Balance between NPY and CRH neurotransmission appears to be crucial to maintaining emotional homeostasis under stress (Sajdyk, Shekhar, & Gehlert, 2004), and might thus be related to resilience.

Studies of combat veterans have revealed an association between low NPY levels and PTSD (Rasmusson et al., 2000; Yehuda, Brand, & Yang, 2006). Findings from a study of Special Forces soldiers undergoing rigorous military training suggest that elevated NPY levels might be associated with better performance under stressful conditions (Morgan et al., 2000). These findings are consistent with those of animal studies, showing that direct injection of NPY into the central nucleus of the amygdala in rats inhibits fear conditioning, results in increased efforts to initiate contact with a stranger, and promotes resilient responses to stress (Sajdyk et al., 2008).

Brain-Derived Neurotrophic Factor

Brain-derived neurotrophic factor (BDNF), an important nerve growth factor, is expressed at high levels in the brain. Although animal and human postmortem studies have shown that BDNF exerts a protective function in the hippocampus, it has very different effects in other brain regions. For example, whereas stress decreases BDNF expression in the hippocampus (Duman & Monteggia, 2006), it increases BDNF levels in the nucleus accumbens in rodents, and this increase is associated with depression-like effects (Berton et al., 2006; Eisch et al., 2003). Resilient animals, however, show no increase in BDNF levels in this latter brain region (Krishnan et al., 2007). These findings are consistent with human studies of depressed patients, who also show increased BDNF in the nucleus accumbens (Krishnan et al., 2007). Less is known about the effects of stress in other brain regions.

Galanin

Another abundant neuropeptide, galanin, is coreleased with NE in response to stress (Barrera et al., 2006). It has been shown to be involved in a variety of physiological and behavioral functions, including regulation of food intake, metabolism, anxiety, and stress. Starting in the LC, the dense galanin fiber system innervates multiple structures in the forebrain and midbrain that form part of the emotional circuitry, including the hippocampus, hypothalamus, amygdala, and PFC (Perez, Wynick, Steiner, & Mufson, 2001). Galanin coexists and functionally interacts with several neurotransmitter systems that are involved in the pathophysiology of mood and anxiety disorders, including NE and 5-HT (Holmes, Yang, & Crawley, 2002). Galanin recruitment might help to downregulate negative emotional states that may result from stress-induced noradrenergic hyperactivation (Karlsson & Holmes, 2006). In a recent rodent study, low behavioral disruption upon exposure to predator scent stress was associated with upregulation of galanin messenger RNA (mRNA) in the hippocampus (Kozlovsky, Matar, Kaplan, Zohar, & Cohen, 2009).

Genetic, Epigenetic, and Transcriptional Mechanisms Associated with Resilience

Genetic susceptibility to most psychiatric disorders involves allelic variations or polymorphisms that are common in the general population. Each allelic variation, however, is associated with a small increase in disorder risk (Rutter, Moffitt, & Caspi, 2006). Thus, each gene might contribute to the causal pathway of psychiatric disorders in combination with other genes, and with environmental influences (Rutter et al., 2006). Recent scientific and technological advances have made it possible to examine genetic influences on not only complex behavioral responses but also underlying biological processes, such as endocrine responses to stress or neural responses to affective stimuli measured with brain imaging.

Gene–environment interactions seem to play a crucial role in determining the degree of adaptability of stress response systems to acute or chronic stressors, both during development and in adulthood (McEwen, 1998). Certain alleles might be associated with hypersensitivity to stress (DeRijk et al., 2006) and might eventually increase risk for developing psychiatric disorders such as PTSD or depression in the wake of stressful life events. The best-known example of gene–environment interaction involves a polymorphism in the serotonin transporter gene promoter region (5-HTTLPR) in humans. This polymorphism has been linked to differential risk for major depression upon exposure to stressful life events in some (Caspi et al., 2003; Kendler, Kuhn, Vittum, Prescott, & Riley, 2005) but not all studies (Gillespie, Whitfield, Williams, Heath, & Martin, 2005; Munafo, Durrant, Lewis, & Flint, 2009; Risch et al., 2009), and to differential amygdala reactivity (Hariri et al., 2005; Munafo, Brown, & Hariri, 2008) and amygdala–cingulate connectivity (Pezawas et al., 2005) in healthy volunteers. Recent studies have begun to identify several polymorphisms in other genes of relevance for resilience, including genes affecting HPA axis function, and the genes coding for catechol-O-methyltransferase (COMT), BDNF, and NPY, among others. In these studies, genetic polymorphisms have been linked to differences in anxiety responses, endocrine function, and differential activation of brain regions to negative stimuli, as summarized in Table 2.1. In addition, studies have identified gene × gene interactions modifying the function of stress response systems, summarized in Table 2.2.

Epigenetics refers to stable changes in chromatin structure that underlie long-

TABLE 2.1. Genetic Polymorphisms Affecting Stress Response Systems

Gene	Examples of studies	Finding
5-HTTLPR	Caspi et al. (2003) Kendler et al. (2005)	Short allele carriers have increased risk for depression upon exposure to stressful life events.
	Hariri et al. (2005)	Short allele carriers show increased amygdala reactivity to threat-related facial expressions.
	Pezawas et al. (2005)	Short allele carriers show decreased amygdala–perigenual cingulate connectivity.
	Kaufman et al. (2004)	Social support mitigates effect of short allele on risk for depression.
	Munafo et al. (2008, 2009) Risch et al. (2009)	Recent meta-analyses.
CRH type 1 receptor	Bradley et al. (2008)	Certain alleles and haplotypes moderate the influence of childhood abuse on depressive symptoms during adulthood.
MR and GR	DeRijk & de Kloet (2008)	Carriers of the N363S variant of the GR gene exhibit higher cortisol responses to the Trier Social Stress Test.
FKBP5	Binder et al. (2008)	Four SNPs of this gene coding for a "chaperone" protein that regulates GR receptor sensitivity interact with childhood abuse severity in predicting PTSD symptoms in adults.
COMT	Heinz & Smolka (2006)	Low-functioning Met 158 allele is associated with higher circulating levels of dopamine and norepinephrine, higher anxiety levels, and increased limbic reactivity to unpleasant stimuli.
	Schmack et al. (2008)	Val158Met polymorphism is associated with interindividual variability in neural responses to reward anticipation.
BDNF	Chen et al. (2006)	Val66Met polymorphism alters anxiety-related behaviors.
	Egan et al. (2003)	Val66Met polymorphism affects human episodic memory and hippocampal function.
	Krishnan et al. (2007)	In mice, the Met BDNF allele is associated with reduced BDNF function, greater anxiety-like behavior, and impaired hippocampal-dependent learning, but increased resilience to chronic stress.
NPY	Zhou et al. (2008)	Low expression diplotype is associated with increased trait anxiety and increased amygdala reactivity to threat-related facial expressions.

Note. 5-HTTLPR, serotonin transporter promoter polymorphism; CRH, corticotropin-releasing hormone; MR, mineralocorticoid receptor; GR, glucocorticoid receptor; FKBP5, FK506 binding protein 5; COMT, catechol-O-methyltransferase; BDNF, brain-derived neurotrophic factor; NPY, neuropeptide Y.

TABLE 2.2. Gene–Gene Interactions Affecting Stress Response Systems

Interaction	Study	Finding
MAO$_A$ by COMT	Jabbi et al. (2007)	Affects endocrine responses to psychological challenge task
5-HTTLPR by COMT by stressful life events	Mandelli et al. (2007)	Affects risk for depression
COMT by 5-HTTLPR	Smolka et al. (2007)	Affects limbic reactivity to unpleasant stimuli in healthy individuals
5-HTTLPR by BDNF Val66Met by stressful life events	Kaufman et al. (2006)	Predicts risk for depression in children
	Kim et al. (2007)	Predicts risk for depression in older adults

Note. MAO$_A$, monoamine oxidase A; COMT, catechol-*O*-methyltransferase; 5-HTTLPR, serotonin transporter promoter polymorphism; BDNF, brain-derived neurotrophic factor.

lasting alterations in gene expression without altering the deoxyribonucleic acid (DNA) sequence (Tsankova, Renthal, Kumar, & Nestler, 2007). Histones constitute the main protein components of chromatin and can be visualized as spheres around which the DNA is wound. Epigenetic mechanisms involve the differential acetylation or methylation of histones by a variety of chromatin-modifying enzymes, as well as differential DNA methylation. The resulting changes in nucleosome properties make the DNA more or less accessible for transcription, thereby mediating the impact of environmental stimuli on gene expression. For example, animal models have shown that drugs of addiction and chronic stress can gradually reduce the activity of histone deacetylase 5 (HDAC5) in the nucleus accumbens, a key brain reward region, leading to increased transcription of genes associated with heightened vulnerability to stress (Renthal et al., 2007). Studies performed in genetically identical mice raised in strictly defined environments demonstrate wide variability in stress responses and degree of resilience. This finding points to the role of chromatin remodeling events, such as histone acetylation or methylation (Krishnan et al., 2007). As mentioned earlier, epigenetic changes can also occur during development and are capable of mediating differential sensitivity to stress, as demonstrated by a series of studies conducted by Meaney and Szyf (2005).

Animal studies are beginning to elucidate the molecular mechanisms associated with resilience. A series of studies focusing on the ventral tegmental area (VTA)–nucleus accumbens reward circuitry demonstrate that resilience is not just the absence of vulnerability, but is associated with a unique set of adaptive changes. C57Bl/6 mice were subjected to social defeat by being placed in the home cage of a larger CD1 mouse daily for 10 days. A subset of mice demonstrated resilient responses, characterized only by anxiety-like symptoms, but no social avoidance, anhedonia, or metabolic disturbances (demonstrated by vulnerable mice). Resilient mice not only lacked the changes in gene expression observed in the VTA–nucleus accumbens of vulnerable mice but they also showed induction of distinct changes in gene expression present only in this subset of mice (Krishnan et al., 2007). These changes included, among many others, the induction of several K$^+$ channel subunits in VTA dopamine neurons, which prevents changes seen in vulnerable mice in response to stress, including increased VTA excitability and associated release of BDNF into the nucleus accumbens. A related study showed that individual variability in the development of learned helplessness in mice was related to the induction of delta-FosB transcription factor in the midbrain, which ultimately resulted in reduced substance P transmission to the nucleus accumbens, associated with resilience (Berton et al., 2007). Many other molecular and transcriptional changes like these are being elucidated in subsets of resilient animals, and may ultimately lead to the development of new treatments for stress-related disorders.

Neural Circuits and Resilience

Animal studies and human neuroimaging studies have begun to identify a number of interconnected brain circuits that mediate different aspects of mood and emotion under normal circumstances and in various pathological conditions that are indicative of low resilience. The field has identified several limbic regions in the forebrain that are highly interconnected and function as a series of integrated parallel circuits that regulate emotional states. Each of these regions is heavily innervated by the brain's monoaminergic systems (norepinephrine, dopamine, and 5-HT), which are thought to modulate their activity. The amygdala, located in the temporal lobe, is particularly important for conditioned aspects of learning and memory, for example, establishing associations between environmental cues and emotional stimuli. While it is best understood for its role in fear conditioning and aversive learning, it has an analogous function with respect to reward-related learning (Davis & Whalen, 2001; Everitt, Cardinal, Parkinson, & Robbins, 2003). The nucleus accumbens, part of the ventral striatum, is best understood as a key reward region of the brain that regulates an individual's responses to natural rewards (e.g., food, sex, social interaction), and that mediates the addicting actions of drugs of abuse. It is thought to function as a key link between motivation for rewarding stimuli and the motor responses needed to obtain rewards (Hyman, Malenka, & Nestler, 2006). More recent research has demonstrated that

it serves an analogous function in avoiding aversive stimuli (Nestler & Carlezon, 2006). The hippocampus, in the temporal lobe, is best characterized for its crucial role in *declarative memory*—the memory of persons, places, and things in time. However, it likely functions more broadly in regulating emotional behavior (Bast, 2007), although the specifics are poorly understood. The hypothalamus is responsible for coordinating the body's peripheral hormonal and metabolic responses with the environment. Its control over the HPA axis and numerous other factors is thought to exert pervasive effects on mood (Nestler & Carlezon, 2006). Probably the most important, but least understood, are regions of PFC, such as medial PFC, anterior cingulate cortex (ACC), and orbitofrontal cortex, among others, which mediate working memory, and provide executive control over planning and execution of all activities. In the sections that follow, we review how these various regions, and several others, integrate to mediate distinct emotional behaviors related to resilience.

Neural Circuitry of Fear

The neural circuitry of fear involves primarily the amygdala, the hippocampus, and the ventromedial PFC (vmPFC). The amygdala is a key structure in mediating fear conditioning, the process by which a previously neutral stimulus, such as a tone, becomes fear inducing or "conditioned" after being paired with a naturally aversive or "unconditioned" stimulus, such as a foot shock (Delgado, Olsson, & Phelps, 2006). The hippocampus mediates the contextual and temporal aspects of fear conditioning (Bast, 2007). Fear conditioning is thought to occur via long-term potentiation of synapses in the lateral amygdala and hippocampus. Over time, existing memories may become reactivated and strengthened by reconsolidation, or weakened by extinction. Both the amygdala and vmPFC are involved in successful extinction, a process that involves new memory formation (Delgado et al., 2006).

The pathophysiology of PTSD might involve abnormal fear learning and underlying dysfunction of fear circuits (Liberzon & Sripada, 2008; Rauch, Shin, & Phelps, 2006; Yehuda & LeDoux, 2007). Individuals with PTSD tend to overgeneralize from specific conditioned stimuli to other stimuli in their environment, which also become associated with their original trauma and are thus fear inducing. Resilience might involve the capacity of avoid overgeneralization of fear cues, as reflected in differential functioning of fear conditioning and extinction processes. For example, enhanced inhibition of the amygdala by the vmPFC may enable more controlled responses to acute stressors (Liberzon & Sripada, 2008). In a recent functional magnetic resonance imaging (fMRI) study of healthy volunteers, the vmPFC became active as fear responses shifted when initially threatening stimuli became safe during the experiment (Schiller, Levy, Niv, LeDoux, & Phelps, 2008). Preliminary findings from a study in patients with PTSD suggest that exposure therapy might work at least in part by increasing rostral ACC and reducing amygdala activation during fear processing (Felmingham et al., 2007). Although fear circuitry function is important in resilience, it has not been carefully studied in resilient individuals. A recent study in healthy individuals suggests that the lateral PFC, activated by cognitive regulation of emotions, might act through vmPFC connections to the amygdala to diminish fear responses (Delgado, Nearing, LeDoux, & Phelps, 2008).

Neural Circuitry of Reward

The nucleus accumbens, part of the ventral striatum, regulates an individual's responses to natural rewards and also mediates addictive behaviors. The mesolimbic dopamine system, the best understood reward circuit, has been increasingly studied in animal models. This system comprises dopaminergic neurons in the VTA, located in the midbrain, that project to the nucleus accumbens and other limbic regions. A recent study using the social defeat stress model in mice showed a relationship between resilience and the ability of some animals to up-regulate potassium channels in the VTA, preventing a stress-induced increase in neuronal excitability and resulting BDNF release in this region, both associated with vulnerability to stress (Krishnan et al., 2007, 2008).

Human fMRI studies have found evidence of reward system dysfunction in both psychiatric and trauma-exposed populations (Dillon et al., 2009; Drevets, Price, & Furey, 2008). Altered neural reward processing has been reported in patients with major depression (Forbes et al., 2009) and PTSD (Sailer et al., 2008), and in young adults with a history of childhood maltreatment (Dillon et al., 2009). In a study using a monetary reward task, healthy adolescents showed greater striatal reactivity during reward anticipation and outcome than did depressed adolescents (Forbes et al., 2009). Furthermore, degree of striatal activation was correlated with level of positive affect measured in naturalistic settings with the Positive and Negative Affect Scale (PANAS), demonstrating a link between positive emotions and reward system function (Forbes et al., 2009).

As mentioned earlier, positive emotionality and optimism have been linked to resilience. In a recent fMRI study, Sharot, Riccardi, Raio, and Phelps (2007) demonstrated increased amygdala and rostral ACC activation while participants were imagining future autobiographical positive events (compared with negative events). Of note, degree of rostral ACC activation was positively correlated with dispositional optimism, measured with the Life Orientation Test—Revised (LOT-R). These results suggest a mechanism through which resilient individuals might be better able to maintain an optimistic outlook even while facing stressful situations. Little is known about reward system function in resilient individuals. A preliminary study in Special Forces soldiers, however, showed differential reactivity of reward-processing regions, including the nucleus accumbens and subgenual PFC, in these highly resilient individuals compared to civilian healthy controls (Vythilingam et al., 2009).

Neural Circuitry of Emotion Regulation

Stress resilience has been related to a greater capacity for emotion regulation (Masten & Coatsworth, 1998), whereas psychopathology might be associated with abnormalities in emotion regulation systems (Johnstone, van Reekum, Urry, Kalin, & Davidson, 2007; Masten & Coatsworth, 1998). Phillips, Drevets, Rauch, and Lane (2003a) have described a neural model of emotion regulation that comprises a ventral system (including the amygdala, insula, ventral striatum, and ventral ACC and PFC) and a dorsal system (including the hippocampus and dorsal ACC and PFC). The ventral system is important for identification of emotional stimuli and production of an appropriate emotional response, whereas the dorsal system is important for effortful regulation of emotional responses (Phillips et al., 2003a). Distinct patterns of abnormalities in these systems are associated with different psychiatric disorders (Phillips, Drevets, Rauch, & Lane, 2003b). Studies in mood and anxiety disorders have most consistently identified abnormalities in amygdala, hippocampus, subgenual ACC, and PFC function (Ressler & Mayberg, 2007).

Imaging genomic studies suggest that differential amygdala reactivity to negative stimuli might represent an intermediate phenotype associated with differential vulnerability to anxiety and depressive disorders (Smolka et al., 2007). For example, studies in healthy individuals have identified a link between polymorphisms in the 5-HT transporter and the *COMT* genes, and increased vulnerability to anxiety and negative moods, as well as increased amygdala reactivity to negative stimuli, and differential coupling between amygdala and cortical regulatory regions (Drabant et al., 2006; Hariri et al., 2005; Pezawas et al., 2005).

As discussed earlier, *cognitive reappraisal* is a mechanism through which resilient individuals may successfully reduce or control emotional responses to stressful situations. Cognitive reappraisal has received increased attention in recent fMRI studies. Findings from studies instructing participants to reappraise the meaning of negative images point to the involvement of the lateral and medial PFC in regulating emotional responses through top-down regulation of amygdala activation during cognitive reappraisal (Goldin, McRae, Ramel, & Gross, 2008; Ochsner et al., 2004). A recent study suggests that the PFC may act on both the amygdala and the nucleus accumbens, with differential effects on reappraisal success (Wager, Davidson, Hughes, Lindquist, & Ochsner, 2008). Greater use of reappraisal in everyday life has also been linked to greater PFC and lower amygdala activation to negative stimuli (Drabant, McRae, Manuck, Hariri, & Gross, 2009), suggesting a possible neural mechanism through which reappraisal might increase stress resistance. Limited information is available on central emotion regulation systems in trauma-exposed resilient individuals. In a recent fMRI study of resilient women with a history of sexual assault but absence of psychopathology, resilience was associated with an increased capacity for cognitive enhancement of emotional responses to negative pictures, a finding that merits further study (New et al., in press).

Additional Neural Circuitry Relevant to Social Behavior

Research suggests that oxytocin and arginine vasopressin, neuropeptides implicated in prosocial behaviors and neuroendocrine responses to stress in animals, might mediate some of the protective and anxiety-reducing effects of affiliative behaviors (Kosfeld, Heinrichs, Zak, Fischbacher, & Fehr, 2005; Young & Wang, 2004). Receptors for these two neuropeptides are spread across a network of cortical and subcortical neural systems related to emotion in monogamous nonhuman mammals (Insel, 1997). Supportive intimate gestures, such as handholding and other types of soothing physical contact, produce an increase in endogeneous opioid activity by triggering the release of oxytocin from the paraventricular nuclei of the hypothalamus (Uvnas-Moberg, 1998). In an fMRI study of married women, handholding with their husband attenuated neural responses to the threat of receiving a shock (Coan, Schaefer, & Davidson, 2006).

Animal studies have shown that intravenous administration of oxytocin attenuates stress responses in the central nervous system (Izzo et al., 1999). In humans, it appears that the combination of social support and oxytocin is most effective in reducing anxiety and HPA reactivity in response to psychosocial stress. Thus, in an experimental study by Heinrichs, Baumgartner, Kirschbaum, and Ehlert (2003) participants who received both social support and oxytocin had lower levels of cortisol, and reported greater calmness and lower anxiety during the Trier Social Stress Test than the placebo group, with and without social support, and the oxytocin-only group.

Oxytocin might also facilitate an individual's ability to infer the mental states of others (Domes, Heinrichs, Michel, Berger, & Herpertz, 2007). The capacity for empathy might be related to social competence, a characteristic of resilient individuals (Iarocci, Yager, & Elfers, 2007; Schulte-Ruther, Markowitsch, Fink, & Piefke, 2007). *Mirror neurons* are a group of cortical neurons that become activated both when an animal performs an action and when it observes the action performed by another animal of the same species (Rizzolatti & Craighero, 2004). The mirror neuron system might play a role in understanding others' emotions and intentions, working together with limbic brain regions, as suggested by preliminary findings from a study of children instructed to imitate emotional faces (Pfeifer, Iacoboni, Mazziotta, & Dapretto, 2008). As discussed earlier, social competence and use of social supports have been linked with increased re-

silience to adversity. Further study is needed to clarify the relationship between the capacity for empathy and resilience to stress, and to elucidate further the underlying neural mechanisms mediating the protective effects of social support on stress responses.

Resilience Interventions

More information is available about treatment interventions with clinical populations than about interventions that might foster resilience and prevent the development of psychopathology upon exposure to stress or trauma. Structured psychological treatments for PTSD, such as prolonged exposure therapy, cognitive-behavioral therapy, and interpersonal psychotherapy, have been shown to be effective in helping patients practice cognitive reappraisal and other coping strategies to confront memories of traumatic events and associated emotions (Butler, Chapman, Forman, & Beck, 2006). Psychotherapeutic approaches with trauma survivors include establishing safety, gradually facing fears in a safe environment, memory consolidation, making meaning, helping patients establish social supports that may have been disrupted or lost in the aftermath of the trauma, and supporting a gradual shift from helplessness to personal agency.

Prolonged exposure therapy, a form of cognitive-behavior therapy based on principles of learning theory (habituation and extinction), was developed specifically for PTSD and has shown the most efficacy for this disorder (Foa et al., 1999; Schnurr et al., 2007). This form of therapy includes imaginal exposure to traumatic memories and *in vivo* exposure to previously avoided situations. More general cognitive-behavioral techniques include addressing previously distorted cognitions and maladaptive behaviors, and focusing on increasing positive social supports and improving problem-solving abilities. Interpersonal psychotherapy focuses on restructuring negative interpersonal relationships and promoting positive social interactions to decrease negative affect and cognitions (Bleiberg & Markowitz, 2005). Regular physical exercise has also been shown to have positive effects on physical hardiness, mood, and self-esteem, and has been linked to neurobiological effects that promote resilience (Cotman & Berchtold, 2002).

Mindfulness-based approaches to stress reduction may help individuals become more emotionally aware, and have been shown to be effective in reducing anxiety and dysphoria in both healthy (Astin, 1997; Shapiro, Schwartz, & Bonner, 1998) and clinical populations (Speca, Carlson, Goodey, & Angen, 2000; Teasdale, Williams, Ridgeway, Soulsby, & Lau, 2000). Davidson and colleagues (2003) found that healthy individuals who participated in an 8-week mindfulness meditation program showed increased left-sided anterior activation (which is associated with positive affect), measured with electroencephalography, and increased antibody titers to influenza vaccine from baseline, compared to subjects in a waiting-list control group. Approaches based on positive psychology are also promising in promoting psychological resilience (Seligman & Csikszentmihalyi, 2000).

Neuroimaging studies have demonstrated that participation in psychotherapy for mood and anxiety disorders can result in measurable changes in brain activity in neural areas implicated in emotion regulation and positive reappraisal (Beauregard, 2007; Roffman, Marci, Glick, Dougherty, & Rauch, 2005). Further research is needed to examine whether treatment-related changes in neural functioning can also reduce the likelihood of developing psychopathology in response to future stressors.

Progress in understanding the neurobiological underpinnings of resilience and vulnerability to stress-related illnesses will also broaden pharmacological treatment approaches. Medications can target responsiveness to reward, hypervigilance to threat, and dysregulated physiological responses. Drug trials currently under way are evaluat-

ing a range of compounds, including NPY enhancers, substance P antagonists, N-methyl-D-aspartic acid (NMDA) antagonists, antiadrenergics, and compounds that downregulate glucocorticoid receptors (Friedman, 2000). Recent data suggest that D-cycloserine, an NMDA receptor partial agonist, can facilitate fear extinction when used in conjunction with exposure therapy (Norberg, Krystal, & Tolin, 2008). Although beta-adrenergic antagonists have been tested in trauma-exposed patients, studies have yielded mixed results (Stein, Kerridge, Dimsdale, & Hoyt, 2007).

Stress resilience reflects an individual's capacity for successful adaptation in the face of acute stress, trauma, or more chronic forms of adversity. Resilience is an active process—not just the absence of pathology—that can be promoted by enhancing potentially protective factors. Novel intervention modalities may become possible with increased understanding of psychological predictors of resilience and the associated underlying genetic, neural, and neurochemical influences that shape these observable psychological strengths.

References

Alim, T. N., Feder, A., Graves, R. E., Wang, Y., Weaver, J., Westphal, M., et al. (2008). Trauma, resilience, and recovery in a high-risk African-American population. *American Journal of Psychiatry, 165,* 1566–1575.

Astin, J. (1997). Stress reduction through mindfulness meditation: Effects on psychological symptomatology, sense of control, and spiritual experiences. *Psychotherapy and Psychosomatics, 66,* 97–106.

Barrera, G., Hernandez, A., Poulin, J. F., Laforest, S., Drolet, G., & Morilak, D. A. (2006). Galanin-mediated anxiolytic effect in rat central amygdala is not a result of corelease from noradrenergic terminals. *Synapse, 59,* 27–40.

Bast, T. (2007). Toward an integrative perspective on hippocampal function: From the rapid encoding of experience to adaptive behavior. *Reviews in the Neurosciences, 18,* 253–281.

Beauregard, M. (2007). Mind does really matter: Evidence from neuroimaging studies of emotional self-regulation, psychotherapy, and placebo effect. *Progress in Neurobiology, 81,* 218–236.

Berton, O., Covington, H. E., III, Ebner, K., Tsankova, N. M., Carle, T. L., Ulery, P., et al. (2007). Induction of deltaFosB in the periaqueductal gray by stress promotes active coping responses. *Neuron, 55,* 289–300.

Berton, O., McClung, C. A., Dileone, R. J., Krishnan, V., Renthal, W., Russo, S. J., et al. (2006). Essential role of BDNF in the mesolimbic dopamine pathway in social defeat stress. *Science, 311,* 864–868.

Binder, E. B., Bradley, R. G., Liu, W., Epstein, M. P., Deveau, T. C., Mercer, K. B., et al. (2008). Association of FKBP5 polymorphisms and childhood abuse with risk of posttraumatic stress disorder symptoms in adults. *Journal of the American Medical Association, 299,* 1291–1305.

Bleiberg, K. L., & Markowitz, J. C. (2005). A pilot study of interpersonal psychotherapy for posttraumatic stress disorder. *American Journal of Psychiatry, 162,* 181–183.

Bowlby, J. (1982). *Attachment and loss* (Vol. 1, 2nd ed.). New York: Basic Books.

Bradley, R. G., Binder, E. B., Epstein, M. P., Tang, Y., Nair, H. P., Liu, W., et al. (2008). Influence of child abuse on adult depression: Moderation by the corticotropin-releasing hormone receptor gene. *Archives of General Psychiatry, 65,* 190–200.

Britton, K. T., Akwa, Y., Spina, M. G., & Koob, G. F. (2000). Neuropeptide Y blocks anxiogenic-like behavioral action of corticotropin-releasing factor in an operant conflict test and elevated plus maze. *Peptides, 21,* 37–44.

Butler, A. C., Chapman, J. E., Forman, E. M., & Beck, A. T. (2006). The empirical status of cognitive-behavioral therapy: A review of meta-analyses. *Clinical Psychology Review, 26,* 17–31.

Cabib, S., Ventura, R., & Puglisi-Allegra, S. (2002). Opposite imbalances between mesocortical and mesoaccumbens dopamine responses to stress by the same genotype depending on living conditions. *Behavioural Brain Research, 129,* 179–185.

Carver, C. S. (1997). You want to measure coping but your protocol's too long: Consider the brief COPE. *International Journal of Behavioral Medicine, 4,* 92–100.

Caspi, A., Sugden, K., Moffitt, T. E., Taylor, A., Craig, I. W., Harrington, H., et al. (2003). Influence of life stress on depression: Moderation by a polymorphism in the 5-HTT gene. *Science, 301,* 386–389.

Charney, D. S. (2003). Neuroanatomical circuits modulating fear and anxiety behaviors. *Acta Psychiatrica Scandinavica, 108*(S417), 38–50.

Charney, D. S. (2004). Psychobiological mechanisms of resilience and vulnerability: Implications for successful adaptation to extreme stress. *American Journal of Psychiatry, 161,* 195–216.

Charuvastra, A., & Cloitre, M. (2008). Social bonds and posttraumatic stress disorder. *Annual Review of Psychology, 59,* 301–328.

Chen, Z. Y., Jing, D., Bath, K. G., Ieraci, A., Khan, T., Siao, C. J., et al. (2006). Genetic variant BDNF (Val66Met) polymorphism alters anxiety-related behavior. *Science, 314,* 140–143.

Coan, J. A., Schaefer, H. S., & Davidson, R. J. (2006). Lending a hand: Social regulation of the neural response to threat. *Psychological Science, 17,* 1032–1039.

Cotman, C. W., & Berchtold, N. C. (2002). Exercise: A behavioral intervention to enhance brain health and plasticity. *Trends in Neuroscience, 25,* 295–301.

Davidson, R. J., Kabat-Zinn, J., Schumacher, J., Rosenkranz, M., Muller, D., Santorelli, S. F., et al. (2003). Alterations in brain and immune function produced by mindfulness meditation. *Psychosomatic Medicine, 65,* 564–570.

Davis, M., & Whalen, P. J. (2001). The amygdala: Vigilance and emotion. *Molecular Psychiatry, 6,* 13–34.

de Kloet, E. R., DeRijk, R. H., & Meijer, O. C. (2007). Therapy Insight: Is there an imbalanced response of mineralocorticoid and glucocorticoid receptors in depression? *Nature Clinical Practice Endocrinology and Metabolism, 3,* 168–179.

de Kloet, E. R., Joels, M., & Holsboer, F. (2005). Stress and the brain: From adaptation to disease. *Nature Reviews Neuroscience, 6,* 463–475.

Delgado, M. R., Nearing, K. I., LeDoux, J. E., & Phelps, E. A. (2008). Neural circuitry underlying the regulation of conditioned fear and its relation to extinction. *Neuron, 59,* 829–838.

Delgado, M. R., Olsson, A., & Phelps, E. A. (2006). Extending animal models of fear conditioning to humans. *Biological Psychology, 73*, 39–48.

DeRijk, R. H., & de Kloet, E. R. (2008). Corticosteroid receptor polymorphisms: Determinants of vulnerability and resilience. *European Journal of Pharmacology, 583*, 303–311.

DeRijk, R. H., Wust, S., Meijer, O. C., Zennaro, M. C., Federenko, I. S., Hellhammer, D. H., et al. (2006). A common polymorphism in the mineralocorticoid receptor modulates stress responsiveness. *Journal of Clinical Endocrinology and Metabolism, 91*, 5083–5089.

DeVries, A. C., Glasper, E. R., & Detillion, C. E. (2003). Social modulation of stress responses. *Physiology and Behavior, 79*, 399–407.

Dillon, D. G., Holmes, A. J., Birk, J. L., Brooks, N., Lyons-Ruth, K., & Pizzagalli, D. A. (2009). Childhood adversity is associated with left basal ganglia dysfunction during reward anticipation in adulthood. *Biological Psychiatry, 66*(3), 206–213.

Domes, G., Heinrichs, M., Michel, A., Berger, C., & Herpertz, S. C. (2007). Oxytocin improves "mind-reading" in humans. *Biological Psychiatry, 61*, 731–733.

Drabant, E. M., Hariri, A. R., Meyer-Lindenberg, A., Munoz, K. E., Mattay, V. S., Kolachana, B. S., et al. (2006). Catechol-O-methyltransferase val158met genotype and neural mechanisms related to affective arousal and regulation. *Archives of General Psychiatry, 63*, 1396–1406.

Drabant, E. M., McRae, K., Manuck, S. B., Hariri, A. R., & Gross, J. J. (2009). Individual differences in typical reappraisal use predict amygdala and prefrontal responses. *Biological Psychiatry, 65*, 367–373.

Drevets, W. C., Price, J. L., & Furey, M. L. (2008). Brain structural and functional abnormalities in mood disorders: Implications for neurocircuitry models of depression. *Brain Structure and Function, 213*, 93–118.

Duman, R. S., & Monteggia, L. M. (2006). A neurotrophic model for stress-related mood disorders. *Biological Psychiatry, 59*, 1116–1127.

Egan, M. F., Kojima, M., Callicott, J. H., Goldberg, T. E., Kolachana, B. S., Bertolino, A., et al. (2003). The BDNF val66met polymorphism affects activity-dependent secretion of BDNF and human memory and hippocampal function. *Cell, 112*, 257–269.

Eisch, A. J., Bolanos, C. A., de Wit, J., Simonak, R. D., Pudiak, C. M., Barrot, M., et al. (2003).

Brain-derived neurotrophic factor in the ventral midbrain–nucleus accumbens pathway: A role in depression. *Biological Psychiatry, 54*, 994–1005.

Everitt, B. J., Cardinal, R. N., Parkinson, J. A., & Robbins, T. W. (2003). Appetitive behavior: Impact of amygdala-dependent mechanisms of emotional learning. *Annals of the New York Academy of Sciences, 985*, 233–250.

Felmingham, K., Kemp, A., Williams, L., Das, P., Hughes, G., Peduto, A., et al. (2007). Changes in anterior cingulate and amygdala after cognitive behavior therapy of posttraumatic stress disorder. *Psychological Science, 18*, 127–129.

Foa, E. B., Dancu, C. V., Hembree, E. A., Jaycox, L. H., Meadows, E. A., & Street, G. P. (1999). A comparison of exposure therapy, stress inoculation training, and their combination for reducing posttraumatic stress disorder in female assault victims. *Journal of Consulting and Clinical Psychology, 67*, 194–200.

Folkman, S., & Moskowitz, J. T. (2000). Positive affect and the other side of coping. *American Psychologist, 55*, 647–654.

Folkman, S., & Moskowitz, J. T. (2004). Coping: Pitfalls and promise. *Annual Review of Psychology, 55*, 745–774.

Forbes, E. E., Hariri, A. R., Martin, S. L., Silk, J. S., Moyles, D. L., Fisher, P. M., et al. (2009). Altered striatal activation predicting real-world positive affect in adolescent major depressive disorder. *American Journal of Psychiatry, 166*, 64–73.

Francis, D. D., Diorio, J., Plotsky, P. M., & Meaney, M. J. (2002). Environmental enrichment reverses the effects of maternal separation on stress reactivity. *Journal of Neuroscience, 22*, 7840–7843.

Fredrickson, B. L. (2001). The role of positive emotions in positive psychology: The broaden-and-build theory of positive emotions. *American Psychologist, 56*, 218–226.

Friedman, M. J. (2000). What might the psychobiology of posttraumatic stress disorder teach us about future approaches to pharmacotherapy? *Journal of Clinical Psychiatry, 61*(Suppl. 7), 44–51.

Gillespie, N. A., Whitfield, J. B., Williams, B., Heath, A. C., & Martin, N. G. (2005). The relationship between stressful life events, the serotonin transporter (5-HTTLPR) genotype and major depression. *Psychological Medicine, 35*, 101–111.

Goldin, P. R., McRae, K., Ramel, W., & Gross, J. J. (2008). The neural bases of emotion regulation: Reappraisal and suppression of negative emotion. *Biological Psychiatry, 63,* 577–586.

Green, T. A., Gehrke, B. J., & Bardo, M. T. (2002). Environmental enrichment decreases intravenous amphetamine self-administration in rats: Dose–response functions for fixed- and progressive-ratio schedules. *Psychopharmacology (Berlin), 162,* 373–378.

Gross, C., & Hen, R. (2004). The developmental origins of anxiety. *Nature Reviews Neuroscience, 5,* 545–552.

Hariri, A. R., Drabant, E. M., Munoz, K. E., Kolachana, B. S., Mattay, V. S., Egan, M. F., et al. (2005). A susceptibility gene for affective disorders and the response of the human amygdala. *Archives of General Psychiatry, 62,* 146–152.

Hasler, G., Drevets, W. C., Manji, H. K., & Charney, D. S. (2004). Discovering endophenotypes for major depression. *Neuropsychopharmacology, 29,* 1765–1781.

Heilig, M., Koob, G. F., Ekman, R., & Britton, K. T. (1994). Corticotropin-releasing factor and neuropeptide Y role in emotional integration. *Trends in Neurosciences, 17,* 80–85.

Heim, C., & Nemeroff, C. B. (2001). The role of childhood trauma in the neurobiology of mood and anxiety disorders: Preclinical and clinical studies. *Biological Psychiatry, 49,* 1023–1039.

Heinrichs, M., Baumgartner, T., Kirschbaum, C., & Ehlert, U. (2003). Social support and oxytocin interact to suppress cortisol and subjective responses to psychosocial stress. *Biological Psychiatry, 54,* 1389–1398.

Heinz, A., & Smolka, M. N. (2006). The effects of catechol-O-methyltransferase genotype on brain activation elicited by affective stimuli and cognitive tasks. *Reviews in the Neurosciences, 17,* 359–367.

Holmes, A., Yang, R. J., & Crawley, J. N. (2002). Evaluation of an anxiety-related phenotype in galanin overexpressing transgenic mice. *Journal of Molecular Neuroscience, 18,* 151–165.

Hyman, S. E., Malenka, R. C., & Nestler, E. J. (2006). Neural mechanisms of addiction: The role of reward-related learning and memory. *Annual Review of Neuroscience, 29,* 565–598.

Iarocci, G., Yager, J., & Elfers, T. (2007). What gene–environment interactions can tell us about social competence in typical and atypical populations. *Brain and Cognition, 65,* 112–127.

Insel, T. R. (1997). A neurobiological basis of social attachment. *American Journal of Psychiatry, 154,* 726–735.

Izzo, A., Rotondi, M., Perone, C., Lauro, C., Manzo, E., Casilli, B., et al. (1999). Inhibitory effect of exogenous oxytocin on ACTH and cortisol secretion during labour. *Clinical and Experimental Obstetrics and Gynecology, 26,* 221–224.

Jabbi, M., Korf, J., Kema, I. P., Hartman, C., van der Pompe, G., Minderaa, R. B., et al. (2007). Convergent genetic modulation of the endocrine stress response involves polymorphic variations of 5-HTT, COMT and MAOA. *Molecular Psychiatry, 12,* 483–490.

Janoff-Bulman, R. (1992). *Shattered assumptions: Towards a new psychology of trauma.* New York: Free Press.

Johnstone, T., van Reekum, C. M., Urry, H. L., Kalin, N. H., & Davidson, R. J. (2007). Failure to regulate: Counterproductive recruitment of top-down prefrontal–subcortical circuitry in major depression. *Journal of Neuroscience, 27,* 8877–8884.

Karlsson, R. M., & Holmes, A. (2006). Galanin as a modulator of anxiety and depression and a therapeutic target for affective disease. *Amino Acids, 31,* 231–239.

Kaufman, J., Yang, B. Z., Douglas-Palumberi, H., Grasso, D., Lipschitz, D., Houshyar, S., et al. (2006). Brain-derived neurotrophic factor–5-HTTLPR gene interactions and environmental modifiers of depression in children. *Biological Psychiatry, 59,* 673–680.

Kaufman, J., Yang, B. Z., Douglas-Palumberi, H., Houshyar, S., Lipschitz, D., Krystal, J. H., et al. (2004). Social supports and serotonin transporter gene moderate depression in maltreated children. *Proceedings of the National Academy of Sciences USA, 101,* 17316–17321.

Kendler, K. S., Kuhn, J. W., Vittum, J., Prescott, C. A., & Riley, B. (2005). The interaction of stressful life events and a serotonin transporter polymorphism in the prediction of episodes of major depression: A replication. *Archives of General Psychiatry, 62,* 529–535.

Kim, J. M., Stewart, R., Kim, S. W., Yang, S. J., Shin, I. S., Kim, Y. H., et al. (2007). Interactions between life stressors and susceptibility genes (5-HTTLPR and BDNF) on depression in Korean elders. *Biological Psychiatry, 62,* 423–428.

Kosfeld, M., Heinrichs, M., Zak, P. J., Fischbacher, U., & Fehr, E. (2005). Oxytocin increases trust in humans. *Nature, 435,* 673–676.

Kozlovsky, N., Matar, M. A., Kaplan, Z., Zohar, J., & Cohen, H. (2009). The role of the galaninergic system in modulating stress-related responses in an animal model of posttraumatic stress disorder. *Biological Psychiatry, 65,* 383–391.

Krishnan, V., Han, M. H., Graham, D. L., Berton, O., Renthal, W., Russo, S. J., et al. (2007). Molecular adaptations underlying susceptibility and resistance to social defeat in brain reward regions. *Cell, 131,* 391–404.

Krishnan, V., Han, M. H., Mazei-Robison, M., Iniguez, S. D., Ables, J. L., Vialou, V., et al. (2008). AKT signaling within the ventral tegmental area regulates cellular and behavioral responses to stressful stimuli. *Biological Psychiatry, 64,* 691–700.

Lanzenberger, R. R., Mitterhauser, M., Spindelegger, C., Wadsak, W., Klein, N., Mien, L. K., et al. (2007). Reduced serotonin-1A receptor binding in social anxiety disorder. *Biological Psychiatry, 61,* 1081–1089.

Lee, V., Cohen, S. R., Edgar, L., Laizner, A. M., & Gagnon, A. J. (2004). Clarifying "meaning" in the context of cancer research: A systematic literature review. *Palliative and Supportive Care, 2,* 291–303.

Liberzon, I., & Sripada, C. S. (2008). The functional neuroanatomy of PTSD: A critical review. *Progress in Brain Research, 167,* 151–169.

Luthar, S. S., Sawyer, J. A., & Brown, P. J. (2006). Conceptual issues in studies of resilience: Past, present, and future research. *Annals of the New York Academy of Sciences, 1094,* 105–115.

Lyons, D. M., & Parker, K. J. (2007). Stress inoculation–induced indications of resilience in monkeys. *Journal of Traumatic Stress, 20,* 423–433.

Maier, S. F., Amat, J., Baratta, M. V., Paul, E., & Watkins, L. R. (2006). Behavioral control, the medial prefrontal cortex, and resilience. *Dialogues in Clinical Neuroscience, 8,* 397–406.

Mandelli, L., Serretti, A., Marino, E., Pirovano, A., Calati, R., & Colombo, C. (2007). Interaction between serotonin transporter gene, catechol-O-methyltransferase gene and stressful life events in mood disorders. *International Journal of Neuropsychopharmacology, 10,* 437–447.

Masten, A. S. (2001). Ordinary magic: Resilience processes in development. *American Psychologist, 56,* 227–238.

Masten, A. S., Best, K. M., & Garmezy, N. (1991). Resilience and development: Contributions from the study of children who overcome adversity. *Development and Psychopathology, 2,* 425–444.

Masten, A. S., & Coatsworth, J. D. (1998). The development of competence in favorable and unfavorable environments: Lessons from research on successful children. *American Psychologist, 53,* 205–220.

McEwen, B. S. (1998). Protective and damaging effects of stress mediators. *New England Journal of Medicine, 338,* 171–179.

McEwen, B. S., & Milner, T. A. (2007). Hippocampal formation: Shedding light on the influence of sex and stress on the brain. *Brain Research Reviews, 55,* 343–355.

McEwen, B. S., & Wingfield, J. C. (2003). The concept of allostasis in biology and biomedicine. *Hormones and Behavior, 43*(1), 2–15.

McGaugh, J. L. (2004). The amygdala modulates the consolidation of memories of emotionally arousing experiences. *Annual Review of Neuroscience, 27,* 1–28.

McGowan, P. O., Sasaki, A., D'Alessio, A. C., Dymov, S., Labonte, B., Szyf, M., et al. (2009). Epigenetic regulation of the glucocorticoid receptor in human brain associates with childhood abuse. *Nature Neuroscience, 12,* 342–348.

Meaney, M. J., & Szyf, M. (2005). Environmental programming of stress responses through DNA methylation: Life at the interface between a dynamic environment and a fixed genome. *Dialogues in Clinical Neuroscience, 7,* 103–123.

Mikulincer, M., Shaver, P. R., & Pereg, D. (2003). Attachment theory and affect regulation: The dynamics, development, and cognitive consequences of attachment-related strategies. *Motivation and Emotion, 27,* 77–102.

Miller, L., Kramer, R., Warner, V., Wickramaratne, P., & Weissman, M. (1997). Intergenerational transmission of parental bonding among women. *Journal of the American*

Academy of Child and Adolescent Psychiatry, 36, 1134–1139.

Morfin, R., & Starka, L. (2001). Neurosteroid 7-hydroxylation products in the brain. *International Review of Neurobiology, 46,* 79–95.

Morgan, C. A., Southwick, S., Hazlett, G., Rasmusson, A., Hoyt, G., Zimolo, Z., et al. (2004). Relationships among plasma dehydroepiandrosterone sulfate and cortisol levels, symptoms of dissociation, and objective performance in humans exposed to acute stress. *Archives of General Psychiatry, 61,* 819–825.

Morgan, C. A., Wang, S., Mason, J., Southwick, S. M., Fox, P., Hazlett, G., et al. (2000). Hormone profiles in humans experiencing military survival training. *Biological Psychiatry, 47,* 891–901.

Munafo, M. R., Brown, S. M., & Hariri, A. R. (2008). Serotonin transporter (5-HTTLPR) genotype and amygdala activation: A meta-analysis. *Biological Psychiatry, 63,* 852–857.

Munafo, M. R., Durrant, C., Lewis, G., & Flint, J. (2009). Gene × environment interactions at the serotonin transporter locus. *Biological Psychiatry, 65,* 211–219.

Nestler, E. J., & Carlezon, W. A., Jr. (2006). The mesolimbic dopamine reward circuit in depression. *Biological Psychiatry, 59,* 1151–1159.

New, A. S., Fan, J., Murrough, J. W., Liu, X., Liebman, R. E., Guise, K. G., et al. (in press). A functional magnetic resonance imaging study of deliberate emotion regulation in resilience and posttraumatic stress disorder. *Biological Psychiatry.*

Norberg, M. M., Krystal, J. H., & Tolin, D. F. (2008). A meta-analysis of D-cycloserine and the facilitation of fear extinction and exposure therapy. *Biological Psychiatry, 63,* 1118–1126.

Ochsner, K. N., Ray, R. D., Cooper, J. C., Robertson, E. R., Chopra, S., Gabrieli, J. D., et al. (2004). For better or for worse: Neural systems supporting the cognitive down- and upregulation of negative emotion. *NeuroImage, 23,* 483–499.

Ong, A. D., Bergeman, C. S., Bisconti, T. L., & Wallace, K. A. (2006). Psychological resilience, positive emotions, and successful adaptation to stress in later life. *Journal of Personality and Social Psychology, 91,* 730–749.

Pargament, K. I., Smith, B. W., Koenig, H. G., & Perez, L. (1998). Patterns of positive and negative religious coping with major life stressors. *Journal for the Scientific Study of Religion, 37,* 710–724.

Parker, G. (1983). Parental "affectionless control" as an antecedent to adult depression. A risk factor delineated. *Archives of General Psychiatry, 40,* 956–960.

Parker, K. J., Buckmaster, C. L., Schatzberg, A. F., & Lyons, D. M. (2004). Prospective investigation of stress inoculation in young monkeys. *Archives of General Psychiatry, 61,* 933–941.

Perez, S. E., Wynick, D., Steiner, R. A., & Mufson, E. J. (2001). Distribution of galaninergic immunoreactivity in the brain of the mouse. *Journal of Comparative Neurology, 434,* 158–185.

Pezawas, L., Meyer-Lindenberg, A., Drabant, E. M., Verchinski, B. A., Munoz, K. E., Kolachana, B. S., et al. (2005). 5-HTTLPR polymorphism impacts human cingulate-amygdala interactions: A genetic susceptibility mechanism for depression. *Nature Neuroscience, 8,* 828–834.

Pfeifer, J. H., Iacoboni, M., Mazziotta, J. C., & Dapretto, M. (2008). Mirroring others' emotions relates to empathy and interpersonal competence in children. *NeuroImage, 39,* 2076–2085.

Phillips, M. L., Drevets, W. C., Rauch, S. L., & Lane, R. (2003a). Neurobiology of emotion perception I: The neural basis of normal emotion perception. *Biological Psychiatry, 54,* 504–514.

Phillips, M. L., Drevets, W. C., Rauch, S. L., & Lane, R. (2003b). Neurobiology of emotion perception II: Implications for major psychiatric disorders. *Biological Psychiatry, 54,* 515–528.

Rasmusson, A. M., Hauger, R. L., Morgan, C. A., Bremner, J. D., Charney, D. S., & Southwick, S. M. (2000). Low baseline and yohimbine-stimulated plasma neuropeptide Y (NPY) levels in combat-related PTSD. *Biological Psychiatry, 47,* 526–539.

Rasmusson, A. M., Vasek, J., Lipschitz, D. S., Vojvodal, D., Mustone, M. E., Shi, Q. H., et al. (2004). An increased capacity for adrenal DHEA release is associated with decreased avoidance and negative mood symptoms in women with PTSD. *Neuropsychopharmacology, 29,* 1546–1557.

Rauch, S. L., Shin, L. M., & Phelps, E. A. (2006). Neurocircuitry models of posttraumatic stress disorder and extinction: Human neuroimaging research—past, present, and future. *Biological Psychiatry, 60,* 376–382.

Renthal, W., Maze, I., Krishnan, V., Covington, H. E., III, Xiao, G., Kumar, A., et al. (2007). Histone deacetylase 5 epigenetically controls behavioral adaptations to chronic emotional stimuli. *Neuron, 56,* 517–529.

Ressler, K. J., & Mayberg, H. S. (2007). Targeting abnormal neural circuits in mood and anxiety disorders: From the laboratory to the clinic. *Nature Neuroscience, 10,* 1116–1124.

Risch, N., Herrell, R., Lehner, T., Liang, K.-Y., Eaves, L., Hoh, J., et al. (2009). Interaction between the serotonin transporter gene (5-HTTLPR), stressful life events, and risk of depression. *Journal of the American Medical Association, 301,* 2462–2471.

Rizzolatti, G., & Craighero, L. (2004). The mirror-neuron system. *Annual Review of Neuroscience, 27,* 169–192.

Robles, T. F., & Kiecolt-Glaser, J. K. (2003). The physiology of marriage: Pathways to health. *Physiology and Behavior, 79,* 409–416.

Roffman, J. L., Marci, C. D., Glick, D. M., Dougherty, D. D., & Rauch, S. L. (2005). Neuroimaging and the functional neuroanatomy of psychotherapy. *Psychological Medicine, 35,* 1385–1398.

Rutter, M. (1998). Developmental catch-up, and deficit, following adoption after severe global early privation: English and Romanian Adoptees (ERA) Study Team. *Journal of Child Psychology and Psychiatry, 39,* 465–476.

Rutter, M., Moffitt, T. E., & Caspi, A. (2006). Gene–environment interplay and psychopathology: Multiple varieties but real effects. *Journal of Child Psychology and Psychiatry, 47,* 226–261.

Sailer, U., Robinson, S., Fischmeister, F. P., Konig, D., Oppenauer, C., Lueger-Schuster, B., et al. (2008). Altered reward processing in the nucleus accumbens and mesial prefrontal cortex of patients with posttraumatic stress disorder. *Neuropsychologia, 46,* 2836–2844.

Sajdyk, T. J., Johnson, P. L., Leitermann, R. J., Fitz, S. D., Dietrich, A., Morin, M., et al. (2008). Neuropeptide Y in the amygdala induces long-term resilience to stress-induced reductions in social responses but not hypothalamic–adrenal–pituitary axis activity or hyperthermia. *Journal of Neuroscience, 28,* 893–903.

Sajdyk, T. J., Shekhar, A., & Gehlert, D. R. (2004). Interactions between NPY and CRF in the amygdala to regulate emotionality. *Neuropeptides, 38,* 225–234.

Sapolsky, R. M., Romero, L. M., & Munck, A. U. (2000). How do glucocorticoids influence stress responses?: Integrating permissive, suppressive, stimulatory, and preparative actions. *Endocrine Reviews, 21,* 55–89.

Schiller, D., Levy, I., Niv, Y., LeDoux, J. E., & Phelps, E. A. (2008). From fear to safety and back: Reversal of fear in the human brain. *Journal of Neuroscience, 28,* 11517–11525.

Schmack, K., Schlagenhauf, F., Sterzer, P., Wrase, J., Beck, A., Dembler, T., et al. (2008). Catechol-O-methyltransferase val158met genotype influences neural processing of reward anticipation. *NeuroImage, 42,* 1631–1638.

Schnurr, P. P., Friedman, M. J., Engel, C. C., Foa, E. B., Shea, M. T., Chow, B. K., et al. (2007). Cognitive behavioral therapy for posttraumatic stress disorder in women: A randomized controlled trial. *Journal of the American Medical Association, 297,* 820–830.

Schulte-Ruther, M., Markowitsch, H. J., Fink, G. R., & Piefke, M. (2007). Mirror neuron and theory of mind mechanisms involved in face-to-face interactions: A functional magnetic resonance imaging approach to empathy. *Journal of Cognitive Neuroscience, 19,* 1354–1372.

Seligman, M. (2005). *Handbook of positive psychology.* New York: Oxford University Press.

Seligman, M. E., & Csikszentmihalyi, M. (2000). Positive psychology: An introduction. *American Psychologist, 55,* 5–14.

Shapiro, S. L., Schwartz, G. E., & Bonner, G. (1998). Effects of mindfulness-based stress reduction on medical and premedical students. *Journal of Behavioral Medicine, 21,* 581–599.

Sharot, T., Riccardi, A. M., Raio, C. M., & Phelps, E. A. (2007). Neural mechanisms mediating optimism bias. *Nature, 450,* 102–105.

Smolka, M. N., Buhler, M., Schumann, G., Klein, S., Hu, X. Z., Moayer, M., et al. (2007). Gene-gene effects on central processing of aversive stimuli. *Molecular Psychiatry, 12,* 307–317.

Southwick, S. M., Vythilingam, M., & Charney, D. S. (2005). The psychobiology of depression and resilience to stress: Implications for prevention and treatment. *Annual Review of Clinical Psychology, 1,* 255–291.

Speca, M., Carlson, L., Goodey, E., & Angen, M. A. (2000). A randomized wait-list controlled trial: The effects of a mindfulness meditation-based stress reduction program on mood and symptoms of stress in cancer outpatients. *Psychosomatic Medicine, 62,* 613–622.

Stein, M. B., Kerridge, C., Dimsdale, J. E., & Hoyt, D. B. (2007). Pharmacotherapy to prevent PTSD: Results from a randomized controlled proof-of-concept trial in physically injured patients. *Journal of Traumatic Stress, 20,* 923–932.

Sterling, P., & Eyer, J. (1988). Allostasis, a new paradigm to explain arousal pathology. In S. Fisher & J. Reason (Eds.), *Handbook of life stress, cognition and health* (pp. 629–649). New York: Wiley.

Teasdale, J. D., Segal, V. Z., Williams, J. M. G., Ridgeway, V. A., Soulsby, J. M., & Lau, M. A. (2000). Prevention of relapse/recurrence in major depression by mindfulness-based cognitive therapy. *Journal of Consulting and Clinical Psychology, 68,* 615–625.

Tsankova, N., Renthal, W., Kumar, A., & Nestler, E. J. (2007). Epigenetic regulation in psychiatric disorders. *Nature Reviews Neuroscience, 8,* 355–367.

Tugade, M. M., & Fredrickson, B. L. (2004). Resilient individuals use positive emotions to bounce back from negative emotional experiences. *Journal of Personality and Social Psychology, 86,* 320–333.

Uvnas-Moberg, K. (1998). Oxytocin may mediate the benefits of positive social interaction and emotions. *Psychoneuroendocrinology, 23,* 819–835.

Vythilingam, M., Heim, C., Newport, J., Miller, A. H., Anderson, E., Bronen, R., et al. (2002). Childhood trauma associated with smaller hippocampal volume in women with major depression. *American Journal of Psychiatry, 159,* 2072–2080.

Vythilingam, M., Nelson, E. E., Scaramozza, M., Waldeck, T., Hazlett, G., Southwick, S. M., et al. (2009). Reward circuitry in resilience to severe trauma: An fMRI investigation of resilient special forces soldiers. *Psychiatry Research, 172,* 75–77.

Wager, T. D., Davidson, M. L., Hughes, B. L., Lindquist, M. A., & Ochsner, K. N. (2008). Prefrontal–subcortical pathways mediating successful emotion regulation. *Neuron, 59,* 1037–1050.

Weaver, I. C., Cervoni, N., Champagne, F. A., D'Alessio, A. C., Sharma, S., Seckl, J. R., et al. (2004). Epigenetic programming by maternal behavior. *Nature Neuroscience, 7,* 847–854.

Weiner, H. (1992). *Pertrubing the organism: The biology of stressful experience.* Chicago: University of Chicago Press.

Yehuda, R., Brand, S. R., Golier, J. A., & Yang, R. K. (2006). Clinical correlates of DHEA associated with post-traumatic stress disorder. *Acta Psychiatrica Scandinavica, 114,* 187–193.

Yehuda, R., Brand, S., & Yang, R. K. (2006). Plasma neuropeptide Y concentrations in combat exposed veterans: Relationship to trauma exposure, recovery from PTSD, and coping. *Biological Psychiatry, 59,* 660–663.

Yehuda, R., & LeDoux, J. (2007). Response variation following trauma: A translational neuroscience approach to understanding PTSD. *Neuron, 56,* 19–32.

Young, L. J., & Wang, Z. X. (2004). The neurobiology of pair bonding. *Nature Neuroscience, 7,* 1048–1054.

Zhou, Z., Zhu, G., Hariri, A. R., Enoch, M. A., Scott, D., Sinha, R., et al. (2008). Genetic variation in human NPY expression affects stress response and emotion. *Nature, 452,* 997–1001.

3

Genes and Environments
How They Work Together to Promote Resilience

Kathryn Lemery-Chalfant

Resilience is a dynamic developmental process that involves many influences. Personal characteristics and social environments have received most of the research attention, but advances in genetics and brain imaging now permit closer study of the biological underpinnings of resilience, well-being, and flourishing in life. Contrary to previous notions, the genome is not a passive blueprint guiding development; rather, gene expression is highly responsive to the environment, and variations in the environment, throughout life.

At the species level, genetic variation is the key to survival across a wide range of changing environments. Natural selection has maintained genes with adaptive effects, with the qualification that these processes operate purely on differential probabilities relating to survival and reproduction, and may be blind to present-day definitions of resilience and well-being. Each person comes into this world with predispositions, potentials, and biases, and this diversity has ensured the

survival of the species over time. Because of this diversity, the same environment can elicit different responses from individuals and has wide-ranging effects on resilience.

Science has advanced beyond the nature versus nurture debate, or the relative importance of genes and environments for developing a person, with the current focus moving toward understanding of gene–environment (GE) interplay. Over the past two decades the human genome has been mapped, and scientists are beginning to understand how different *genetic alleles* (or various forms of a gene) impact our biology, behavior, and overall health and well-being. Humans have approximately 25,000 protein coding genes, most of which are shared with other species, with individuals differing from one another on only about 1.0 to 1.5% of their genes. This small percentage suggests that there are limits to the main effects of genes on behavior, just as there are limits to the main effects of environments. Each of us has two copies of each gene, one inherited from our mother, and one from our father. Many genes only have one form, or *allele*; heredity focuses on genes that have different alleles that may influence individual variation in the observed trait, or *phenotype*. A *dominant* allele can dominate the expression of the other, *recessive* allele, or alleles can be additive, with each contributing to the phenotype.

Research has uncovered examples of inherited diseases that originate from a *genetic mutation*, or a change in a section of deoxyribonucleic acid (DNA) that makes up a gene, such as red–green color blindness and Huntington's disease. However, diseases caused by inherited genetic mutations are relatively rare, and complex psychological traits, such as intelligence and personality, are influenced by many genes, as well as by many environments. Resemblance of family members on intelligence, for example, depends on how many genes they share in common. Plomin, DeFries, McClearn, and Rutter (1997) reported that identical twins were correlated .85 on intelligence, whereas fraternal twins were correlated .60, full siblings ($r = .45$), half siblings ($r = .30$), cousins ($r = .15$), and two individuals selected at random ($r = .00$). Thus, intelligence is heritable, with similarity between individuals depending on how many genes they share in common. *Polygenic traits* are influenced by multiple genes that typically impact rank-ordering on quantitative dimensions.

Multifactorial causation, the idea that multiple genes and multiple environments are involved in the process of resilience, ensures that genes have probabilistic rather than deterministic effects. In fact, it seems that each gene carries only a very small effect on traits or disorders, with odds ratios usually substantially less than two for psychiatric disorders (Kendler, 2005), for example. However, effect sizes increase as one studies *intermediate phenotypes*, or characteristics that are closer to the direct physiological effects of genes. Further evidence of the probabilistic role of genes stems from the finding that genetic variations that increase susceptibility to disease or disorder are quite common in the population. Evidence from twin, family, and adoption studies suggests that genetic predispositions vary across individuals and typically explain 25–60% of the observed phenotypic variance. A particular allele constitutes neither necessary nor sufficient cause of disorder or well-being, but is inherited along with other influential alleles in the environmental context. Therefore, genetic predispositions are now conceptualized as acting nonspecifically, by increasing or decreasing an individual's sensitivity to environmental contexts and challenges.

It is important to emphasize that the influence of genes on disorder or well-being is indirect. The terminology *genes for* is quite misleading, with the rare exception of a few genetic mutations that cause genetic disorders. Specifically, a *gene* is an inherited segment of DNA that directs the synthesis of messenger ribonucleic acid (mRNA), then specifies the synthesis of polypeptides, which then form a particular protein. It is these proteins that make up our bodies, skeletal systems, muscular systems, and also our nervous systems. However, other segments of DNA, called *transcription factors*, influence the transcription and expression of the gene (Rutter, Moffitt, & Caspi, 2006). These are nonprotein-coding DNA elements or genes, such as promoters, enhancers, or silencers. *Transcription*, or the process by which DNA specifies the synthesis of mRNA, is influenced by other genetic and environmental factors. Importantly, most gene regulation is not hardwired in the genes; rather, gene activity depends on the internal and external environments and experience. A change in the environment signals particular genes to turn on and off; pumping iron signals genes to turn on processes to build muscle mass.

The relations between genes and the brain, or genes and behavior, or genes and social relationships, are all complex, incorporating genetic and environmental influences. The influence of genes is probabilistic, with social information altering gene expression, physiology, and behavior.

There are many levels of neural and neuroendocrine regulation that lie between the genome and a social behavior, including transcription, translation, posttranslational modifications, epigenetic changes, brain metabolism, neural (electrochemical) activity, and neuromodulation. Moreover, this regulation occurs in complex and dispersed temporal and spatial patterns within the brain, over physiological time, developmental time, and throughout an individual's life. (Robinson, Fernald, & Clayton, 2008, p. 899)

Identifying genes that play a role in resilience is only a first step because the process by which genes are associated with resilience and well-being also need to be elucidated. As outlined in the National Research Council report, science must extend *From Neurons to Neighborhoods* (Shonkoff & Phillips, 2000) to elucidate GE interplay and the underpinnings of resilience.

The focus of this chapter is how genes and environments work together to promote resilience. To this end, the chapter embeds relevant empirical findings within methodological descriptions of genetically informative designs. There are two main approaches: quantitative genetic designs and molecular genetic designs. *Quantitative genetic designs* use resemblance of relatives (e.g., in twin, family, adoption studies) to determine the relative importance of genetic and environmental influences for phenotype variances and covariances, whereas *molecular genetic designs* incorporate measured genes or DNA variants into study designs, determining the covariation between these variants and the phenotype of interest. Three main types of GE interplay are discussed, including GE correlations, GE interactions, and epigenetics. Two overarching themes are emphasized and supported with empirical findings. First is the idea that genetic influences on resilience cannot be discussed without intimate knowledge of the environment. It makes no sense to classify alleles as "good" or "bad," or even as "protective" or "risk," without also specifying the environmental circumstance. Genetic predispositions are now typically conceptualized as increasing or decreasing sensitivity to adverse or supportive environments. The second theme is that we ultimately advance our understanding of how genes and environments work together to promote resilience, using a systems perspective that can elucidate pathways from genes to resilience and well-being.

Defining Resilience

Generally, *resilience* is a process of successful adaptation to adversity (Zautra, Hall, & Murray, 2008). *Successful adaptation* is defined somewhat differently, depending on whether the adversity is acute or chronic. *Recovery* is the extent to which one recovers fully from an acute adverse event, whereas *sustainability* is the extent to which one continues forward in the face of chronic adversity (Bonanno, 2004). "Whereas resilience 'recovery' focuses on aspects of healing of wounds, 'sustainability' calls attention to outcomes relevant to preserving valuable engagements in life's tasks at work, play and in social relations" (Zautra et al., 2008, p. 44). Resilience leads to measureable, positive outcomes that are not restricted to initial states (Luthar, Cicchetti, & Becker, 2000).

Resilience involves intrinsic and extrinsic processes of successful adaptation, and genetic variations contribute to individual differences in these capacities. Genetic variations can be classified as *risk factors*, or factors that increase the likelihood of, but do not determine, poor adaptation or disease (Rutter, 2006). Smoking, for example, is a well-known risk factor for lung cancer. It increases the likelihood of getting lung cancer, but many individuals smoke and do not get cancer, and many individuals get lung cancer who do not smoke. Genetic variations can also be classified as *protective factors*, which may be the opposite of risk factors; low cholesterol may provide protection from coronary artery disease, and high cholesterol may increase risk, for example (Rutter,

2006). Protective factors can also buffer the influence of adversity or risk factors. Thus, their protective impact is not felt unless one is exposed to adversity. Immunizations are protective in that they help one to resist harmful viruses. Similarly, the effects of a genetic or neurobehavioral vulnerability to depression may be buffered by growing up in a low-stress caregiving environment (Eley et al., 2004).

Risk and protective processes can operate at genetic, neurobiological, individual, and social levels. They can also interact across these levels. "What is clear is that we need to consider both risk and protective processes in relation to genetic, as well as environmental, effects" (Rutter, 2006, p. 21).

Resilience can be influenced by an individual's development over time. With a new phase in life (i.e., marriage, parenthood, an empty nest, grandparenting, entering a retirement home), established protective factors can be challenged in the face of new risk factors. What was effective before may not work in a new environment. Resilience is dynamic; adaptive systems reorganize to create new resilience in new environments. The dynamic development process of resilience, then, may differ in different phases of life. One valuable approach for understanding the dynamics of resilience is the use of family resemblance designs.

Quantitative Genetic Designs for Studying Genetic Influences on Resilience

Quantitative genetic designs, such as twin and adoption studies, do not identify specific resilience genes; rather, they focus on the phenotypic or behavioral expression of the entire genotype. Genetic and environmental influences are directly estimated from the resemblance of relatives. The basic linear model of quantitative genetics parses the phenotypic variance into that due to genetic and environmental influences. Symbolically, $V_P = V_G + V_E + 2\text{Cov}(G)(E) + V_{G \times E}$, where V_P is the phenotypic variance (the sum of the individuals' squared deviations from the mean, divided by the number of individuals), V_G is the genetic (G) variance, V_E is the environmental (E) variance, $2\text{Cov}(G)(E)$ is the covariance between G and E, and $V_{G \times E}$ represents nonadditive effects of G and E. If relatives are more similar to each other than individuals picked randomly from the population on a particular trait, then there is phenotypic covariation for that trait, which is then parsed into genetic and environmental components.

The twin study is one example of a quantitative genetic design. The classic twins-reared-together design includes both identical, monozygotic (MZ) twins, who share 100% of their genes, and fraternal, dizygotic (DZ) twins, who share on average 50% of their segregating genes. MZ twins are more similar to each other than DZ twins for a heritable trait. If an identical twin is schizophrenic, the chances are 45% that the cotwin is also schizophrenic, however, if a fraternal twin is schizophrenic, the chances are 17% that the other one is also affected (Plomin, DeFries, McClearn, & Rutter, 1997). Similarly, if an identical twin is autistic, the chances are 60% that the cotwin is also autistic; however, the concordance between fraternal twins is only 17%. Thus, twin studies can establish whether heritability is important for a particular trait in a given environmental context.

Even more powerfully, multivariate designs allow a decomposition of the covariance between two or more traits. For example, the same genetic factor influenced the age when teens started smoking and drinking (genetic $r = 1.0$), but once these behaviors were initiated, the genetic influences on frequency of smoking and drinking were substance specific (genetic $r = .25$) (Dick, Rose, Viken, & Kaprio, 2000). Multivariate designs are very useful when one studies development, such that a phenotype may be highly heritable at both early and later ages, but different genetic factors may be at work at different ages. In this case, the genetic contribution to continuity would be low. Thus, one can make significant progress in understanding influences on development.

Defining Heritability

Heritability is the proportion of the phenotypic variance due to genetic variance among individuals in a population. Because heritability is a proportion, estimates of heritability will differ in different environments. It is a descriptive statistic that describes the group currently; changes in genetic influences due to migration, or in environmental influences due to educational intervention, may change heritability statistics. If trait-relevant environments for most individuals in a sample are equal, this yields high heritability estimates, with individual differences due primarily to genetic differences. Systematic environmental factors may play a larger role in societies where between-family disparity in socioeconomic status is substantial, for example. Heritability decreases when the relevant environment varies a lot from individual to individual, and heritability increases if the environment is nearly the same for all individuals. Conversely, heritability is greater if the population has greater variability in the relevant genes, and it decreases if the population shares nearly all genes that affect a particular phenotype. Thus, a heritability estimate is specific to the population studied and can be generalized only to groups that share a distribution of relevant genes and environments.

Because heritability may change if environmental circumstances alter, it is imperative that researchers study environments that are representative of the population of interest. This is less of an issue with representative national surveys; however, it may be a big issue with studies of animals kept in artificial contexts. Unless resilience is studied in natural contexts, with the full range of behaviors and environments represented, generalization is difficult, if not impossible.

As a final note, it is useful to consider what heritability is not. The heritability statistic is often misinterpreted, or overinterpreted. Based on twin and adoption study results, the heritability of well-being is thought to range from 50% (Braungart, Plomin, De-Fries, & Fulker, 1992; Tellegen et al., 1988) to 80% (Lykken & Tellegen, 1996). Lyubomirsky, Sheldon, and Schkade (2005) interpreted this moderate to high heritability as providing a "genetically determined set point (or set range) for happiness. ... Its large magnitude suggests that for each person there is indeed a chronic or characteristic level of happiness" (pp. 112–113). Genetic influences do not operate in isolation from environmental influences; thus, high heritability does not imply immutability, and there is no reason to assume that the higher the heritability, the less modifiable the trait is through environmental intervention. Adult height is highly heritable, for example, yet mean height has increased substantially over the past 50 years.

In conclusion, heritability should increase if opportunities for the expression of a trait become greater (Rutter et al., 2006). Heritability, as a descriptive statistic, is also intimately related to environmental influences.

Defining Categories of Environmental Influence

Environment includes all influences other than genetic influences in genetically informative designs, including nongenetic biological and prenatal events, as well as parenting, chaotic home environments, accidents, and illnesses. Environmental influences are parsed into *shared environmental influences* that create similarities among individuals, and *nonshared environmental influences* that create differences among individuals. Evidence for shared environmental effects exist for some traits, such as positive emotionality and personality, yet the majority of environmental influences are nonshared.

Without the use of genetically informative designs, it is difficult to determine the influence of the environment on resilience. Many commonly used "environmental" measures are genetically influenced (see review, below). A full understanding of heritability and environmental influences comes with variations in empirical findings across adverse environments, social environments, cohorts, and age.

Moderators of Heritability

Adverse Moderators of Heritability

The importance of genetic factors for individual differences in resilience is expected to be lower in subsections of the population exposed to adversities that impact the behavior or trait being studied (e.g., posttraumatic stress disorder in war veterans). The heritability of psychopathology was significantly lower in children with very low birthweight compared to children with a normal birthweight in relation to gestational age (Wichers et al., 2002). Similarly, extreme premature birth predicted low intelligence, which was environmentally mediated, whereas genetic factors accounted for a quarter of the variance in intelligence for children who were born after 34 weeks of gestation (Koeppen-Schomerus, Eley, Wolke, Gringras, & Plomin, 2000). In addition, the heritability of antisocial behavior in youth was much greater in the absence of family dysfunction than in the presence of dysfunction (Button, Scourfield, Martin, Purcell, & McGuffin, 2005).

Social Moderators of Heritability

Social factors, such as marriage and religion, have also been found to impact heritability estimates. The heritability of alcohol consumption was lower in married than in unmarried women (Heath, Jardine, & Martin, 1989; Koopmans, Slutske, van Baal, & Boomsma, 1999), whereas individual differences in the personality trait disinhibition (characterized by partying, drinking, and multiple sex partners) were not heritable for those with a religious upbringing (Boomsma, de Geus, van Baal, & Koopmans, 1999).

Cohort Moderators of Heritability

Because heritability changes with environmental circumstance, we might expect differences by cohort. In fact, when there was an overall mean increase in height attributed to improved nutrition from 1928 to 1957 in Finland, there was a corresponding increase in the heritability of height (Silventoinen, Kaprio, Lahelma, & Koskenvuo, 2000). Interestingly, the heritability of smoking in females rose over time as it became more socially acceptable, with no change in men (Kendler, Thornton, & Pedersen, 2000). Furthermore, low heritability of age at first sexual intercourse in women and men who reached adolescence during an era of high social controls inhibiting sex contrasted with high heritability for those reaching adolescence in an era of greater sexual tolerance (Dunne et al., 1997). Thus, lower social controls allow for the expression of heritable individual differences.

Changes in Heritability across the Lifespan

Twin study results suggest that heritability also changes across the lifespan. For example, the variation in neonatal temperament (e.g., irritability, activity) is due to the environment (Riese, 1990), whereas temperamental variation later in infancy is heritable (Goldsmith, Lemery, Buss, & Campos, 1999). The heritability of intelligence increases with age (Boomsma, 1993; Pedersen, Plomin, Nesselroade, & McClearn, 1992), whereas the environment begins to have a larger impact on antisocial behavior after the transition to adolescence. Genetic factors were not as important in predicting antisocial behavior in adolescence because it becomes normative for adolescents to engage in antisocial acts, and many more individuals begin to express these behaviors for sociocultural reasons (Moffitt, 1993). Although new genetic influences emerge in toddlerhood and adolescence (Plomin et al., 1993; Reiss, Neiderhiser, Hetherington, & Plomin, 2000), broad spans of adult life are more quiescent (Johnson, McGue, & Krueger, 2005; Kendler, Neale, Kessler, Heath, & Eaves, 1993; McGue & Christensen, 2003; Pedersen & Reynolds, 1998; Plomin, Pedersen, Lichtenstein, & McClearn, 1994).

Studies stemming from moderational designs bring us closer to understanding the process of GE interplay. Three main types of GE interplay are now considered: GE correlations, GE interactions, and epigenetics.

GE Correlations as One Type of GE Interplay

GE correlations occur when genetic predispositions influence environment selection. For example, genes affect lifestyle selection, dietary preferences, and exercise habits, which in turn influence obesity and body mass, which are associated with poor health outcomes. The literature identifies three types of GE covariance: passive, evocative, and active (Plomin, DeFries, & Loehlin, 1977). *Passive GE correlations* arise because an individual's genotype is correlated with the environment of his or her parents and siblings (who have similar genotypes). Child maltreatment, for example, is more common in families with antisocial parents. Because antisocial behavior is moderately heritable, it is possible that the maltreatment is a marker for genetic risk, and is linked to children's conduct problems for genetic reasons.

Evocative GE correlations occur when others react to particular individuals on the basis of some of their inherited characteristics. The environment becomes correlated with genetic differences when inattentive children, for example, are taught less material in a less effective manner in school. *Active GE correlations* are present when individuals seek out environments that are conducive to developing further their genetic tendencies. Those with antisocial personality disorder, for example, may seek to associate with peers who are also easily frustrated and prone to attribute hostile intent to benign actions of others.

Thus, classic psychosocial study designs that treat measures of the "environment" as causal are sometimes confounded by heritable traits. These traits influence exposure to environments, as well as health outcomes.

Heritable Measures of the "Environment"

Genetic factors account for a significant proportion of the variance in "environmental" measures commonly used in the social and behavioral sciences. Heritable characteristics influence social behavior and interactions, as well as exposure to environmental adversities. Specifically, research has documented genetic influences on styles of parenting (Deater-Deckard, Fulker, & Plomin, 1999; Perusse, Neale, Heath, & Eaves, 1994; Wade & Kendler, 2000), adolescent peer groups (Iervolino et al., 2002; Manke, McGuire, Reiss, Hetherington, & Plomin, 1995), propensity to marry (Johnson, McGue, Krueger, & Bouchard, 2004), marital adversity and divorce (Jockin, McGue, & Lykken, 1996; Kendler et al., 1993; McGue & Lykken, 1992; Spotts et al., 2004), educational and occupational social strata (Lichtenstein & Pedersen, 1997), and social support (Bergeman, Plomin, Pedersen, McClearn, & Nesselroade, 1990; Kessler, Kendler, Heath, Neale, & Eaves, 1992; Spotts et al., 2005). Major life stresses are moderately heritable, with higher heritability for controllable events (in adolescents: Billig, Hershberger, Iacono, & McGue, 1986; in adults: Bolinskey, Neale, Jacobson, Prescott, & Kendler, 2004; Kendler et al., 1993; Plomin, Lichtenstein, Pedersen, & McClearn, 1990). In contrast, stresses that are uncontrollable (e.g., earthquakes, death of relative or friend) are not heritable.

Genetically influenced differences in personality seem to account for many of these effects. Specifically, genetic influences on neuroticism, extraversion, and openness accounted for all of the genetic influences on stressful life events in older adults (Saudino, Pedersen, Lichtenstein, McClearn, & Plomin, 1997). Similarly, genetic influences on cognitive abilities accounted for a significant portion of the genetic influence on education and occupational status (Lichtenstein & Pedersen, 1997).

In addition, genetic factors account for significant covariation between putative measures of the environment and adjustment. For example, the correlation between negative relationships between mothers and their adolescents was .59, with genetic factors explaining 69% of this covariation (Reiss et al., 2000). Genetic factors also explained the covariance of family structure (two parents vs. mother only) and adolescent problem behavior (Cleveland, Wiebe, van den Oord, & Rowe, 2000; Jacobson & Rowe, 1999). Shared genetic liability explained part of the co-occurrence of negative life events and depression as well (in adults: Kendler & Karkowski-Shuman, 1997; in adolescents: Thapar, Harold, & McGuffin, 1998). Thus, genetics plays a central role in these types of associations reported in the literature.

Although many of the "environmental" risk factors identified in the psychological and sociological literatures contain some genetic variance, this does not preclude an environmental influence on the trait (Waldman, 2007). Marital stability, corporal punishment, and physical maltreatment all have environmental influences on children's externalizing problems, when researchers control for the genetic association (D'Onofrio et al., 2005; Jaffee, Caspi, Moffitt, & Taylor, 2004).

Whereas GE correlations reflect genetic differences in exposure to environments, GE interactions refer to genetic differences in susceptibility to environments.

GE Interactions as a Second Type of GE Interplay

GE interactions refer to the same environment leading to different outcomes depending on individual genotypes. Genetic inheritance thus influences susceptibility to environments, with particular alleles supporting resilience by acting as buffers against the negative effects of environmental adversity. In the absence of adversity, however, the allele does not always have a main effect on the phenotype. GE interactions are pervasive. In agriculture, for example, some plants grow better in dry versus wet soil, low versus high elevation, or clay versus sandy soil. Furthermore, plants of the same genotype may be short and bushy at high elevation, and long and slender at lower elevations. Intuitively, GE interactions make sense with psychological traits as well. Individuals who score high on neuroticism (which is a genetically influ-

enced personality trait) react differently to novel environments than do individuals who score high on extraversion.

Adoption designs are conducive to testing for GE interactions if good measures of birth parents are used. The biological parents' phenotypes (e.g., diagnosis) are taken as estimates of offspring genotype depending on the heritability of the trait or disorder. The adoptive parents' phenotypes can then be taken as estimates of environmental influence. Main effects represent independent effects of genotype or environment, and statistical interactions are measures of GE interaction. An increasingly common approach to identifying GE interactions is the *molecular genetic approach*, or including measured genes into study designs. Molecular genetic approaches are described in more detail later in the chapter.

Designs to test GE interaction should include appropriate controls. Each assessment of the environment likely includes some genetic influence. Thus, investigators should account for the association between the measure of the environment and the target gene before considering GE interaction, to determine whether "environmental" effects are genetically or environmentally mediated. Silberg and colleagues (1999) reported that a combination of GE correlation and interaction brought about a greater exposure to (GE correlation), and sensitivity to (GE interaction), stressful life events in adolescence than in childhood. Designs that consider the main effects of genes on a sample of individuals exposed to relevant environments (e.g., child maltreatment, social support) are problematic because they do not simultaneously account for GE correlation. Additionally, investigators must be cognizant of the fact that spurious GE interaction can occur because of scaling artifacts (Eaves, 2006). Spurious interactions may be especially likely with assessments of abnormal behaviors, which typically are not normally distributed across the sample.

To date, molecular genetic approaches to identifying GE interaction have primarily focused on negative effects of particular genetic alleles being manifest if an individual had an adverse childrearing environment or is currently exposed to stress. Luecken and Lemery (2004) reviewed studies that underscore the role of stressful early environments in altering brain neurotransmitter systems, changes that appear stable into adulthood and dispose individuals to stress hypersensitivity. Interestingly, the early environment had a different effect on individuals, depending on their genotype. In a study with rhesus monkeys, the effect of early maternal deprivation was reduced for monkeys with the long allele of the serotonin transporter gene promoter (Suomi, 2000). In humans, men who had been maltreated as children showed more antisocial behavior as young adults, but not as much in those with an active X-linked *monoamine oxidase A (MAO-A)* gene (Caspi et al., 2002). Considering risk for Alzheimer's disease, low paternal socioeconomic status increased the likelihood of disease only for those with the apolipoprotein E (APOE) e4 allele (Moceri, Kukull, Emanuel, van Belle, & Larson, 2000). Similarly, head injury increased the likelihood of Alzheimer's disease, especially for those with APOE e4, with disease risk increasing 10-fold with this combination, exceeding the additive effect of each risk factor (Mayeux et al., 1995).

These examples illustrate that genes operate both as protective and as risk factors in the context of adversity. What has been less studied is how positive, supportive environments may interact with genes to influence resilience, health, and well-being. In the face of low socioeconomic status and maltreatment, children with two versions of the short risk allele of the serotonin transporter promoter showed more symptoms of depression than abused children with two long alleles and nonabused children (Kaufman et al., 2004). Importantly, these genetically at-risk children were more likely to benefit from social support, with support ameliorating the effect of abuse and the high-risk genotype. Thus, genetic inheritance influences susceptibility to both adverse and protective environments.

Relevant environments are not limited to the social environment, and the field of epigenetics focuses on a third type of GE interplay involving the microenvironment.

Epigenetics as a Third Type of GE Interplay

The study of epigenetics is an emerging frontier of science. *Epigenetics* refers to changes in the regulation of gene activity and expression due to the microenvironment that result in changes in the phenotype. The Greek prefix *epi-* in *epigenetics* implies features that are "on top of" or "in addition to" genetics; thus, *epigenetic* traits exist on top of, or in addition to, the organism's underlying DNA sequence. These changes are stable between cell divisions and sometimes can be passed on to the next generation. Epigenetic mechanisms are cell specific and are involved in directing normal development, differentiation, organogenesis, tissue formation, and aging. Whereas epigenetics refers to the study of single genes or sets of genes, *epigenomics* refers to more global analyses of epigenetic changes across the entire genome.

Epigenetic mechanisms are linked to gene activation, gene silencing, and chromosomal instability, but little is known about most of the molecular mechanisms underlying these associations. Specific epigenetic processes include chromatin remodeling and higher-order chromatin structural alterations; post-translational modifications, which include methylation, acetylation, ubiquitination, and phosphorylation of histone tail domains; and gene regulation through noncoding RNAs.

Because epigenetic changes can sometimes be passed on to the next generation, epigenetics is an exciting breakthrough in understanding evolution and short-term adaptation of species. Epigenetic modifications allow organisms to switch between phenotypes that express and repress a particular gene on a multigenerational timescale, without altering the gene.

Some investigators believe epigenetic processes hold the key to understanding human psychopathology:

> It is unlikely that psychopathology results from ancient genetic mechanisms not previously eliminated through the operation of natural selection. It is more likely that the various ways in which the process of gene expression contributes to psychopathology are the result of mechanisms developed by natural selection to facilitate adaptation to the social and physical environment. (Kramer, 2004, p. 26)

The best example to date of the role of epigenetics in resilience was conducted by Weaver and colleagues (2004), with a cross-fostering design in rats. The offspring of mothers with high pup licking, grooming, and arched-back nursing were less fearful as adults and had more modest hypothalamic–pituitary–adrenocortical (HPA) axis responses to stress than offspring of mothers low in these behaviors. Cross-fostering the offspring of high and low licking and grooming, and arched-back nursing mothers led to adult rats with the stress response patterns of their rearing mother. Increased glucocorticoid receptor (GR) mRNA in the offspring of high licking and grooming mothers suggested altered gene expression in the HPA axis. Specifically, the chromatin structure of a GR gene promoter was changed in the hippocampus. DNA methylation is associated with stable variations in gene expression, and the offspring of the high licking and grooming mothers had lower C-methylation of the exon 17 GR promoter sequence. Cross-fostering produced C-methylation changes consistent with the maternal behavior of the foster mother. The behavioral changes persisted into adulthood, and were potentially reversible by the infusion of a histone deacetylase inhibitor. Thus, the early maternal environment influences expression of offspring DNA to adapt best to the environment.

In conclusion, integrating the study of epigenetics with other methods of GE interplay holds great promise for elucidating mechanisms of normal development, resilience, and complex diseases. Environmental exposures can alter gene expression, and these changes are stable and can persist even across generations. It is important to note that the presence of epigenesis does not negate findings from quantitative genetic designs, such as twin and adoption studies, although epigenetic processes may contribute to dynamic resilience processes and well-being.

Next, estimates of heritability from empirical studies using quantitative genetic methodology are given for components of resilience and well-being.

Heritability of Resilience Characteristics

The ability to be happy with life appears to be the central factor in resilience and well-being (Diener, 1984; Lyubomirsky et al., 2005). Happy people live longer lives (Danner, Snowdon, & Friesen, 2001; Ostir, Markides, Black, & Goodwin, 2000), have stronger immune systems (Dillon, Minchoff, & Baker, 1985; Stone et al., 1994), and show greater self-regulation, self-control, and coping (Aspinwall, 1998; Fredrickson & Joiner, 2002; Keltner & Bonanno, 1997). Classic studies of psychosocial resilience conducted by Garmezy, Masten, and Tellegen (1984), Luthar and Cicchetti (2000), Masten and Coatsworth (1998), and Werner and Smith (1992) further cluster characteristics that facilitate and enhance the dynamic developmental process of resilience across the lifespan. These interrelated characteristics were summarized by Southwick, Vythilingam, and Charney (2005) and include (1) positive emotions (including optimism and humor), (2) cognitive flexibility (including positive explanatory style, positive reappraisal, and acceptance), (3) active coping style (including exercise and training), (4) meaning (including religion, spirituality, and altruism), and (5) social support (including role models). We next turn to representative findings from quantitative genetic studies that elucidate the role of heritability in accounting for individual differences in these characteristics.

Heritability of Positive Emotions and Resilience

Across adulthood (25–74 years of age), positive affect was moderately heritable (.60, in men, .59 in women; Boardman, Blalock, & Button, 2008). Recognizing the importance of adversities in resilience, these investigators then operationalized resilience as the residual in positive affect after controlling for social and interpersonal stressors. The heritability of residual positive affect was .52 in men, whereas it was .38 in women, a significant sex difference. Self-acceptance accounted for much of the heritable variance in resilience among men and women. Men also were more influenced by environmental mastery than women. One interpretation is that men have a greater opportunity to express resilience due to gender socialization in this society. "In other words, gender socialization may interact with genetic factors to either diminish resilience for women, or help men to actualize some genetic potential that confers resilience" (Boardman et al., 2008, p. 17).

Heritability of Humor

With a sample from the United Kingdom, genetic and nonshared environment factors accounted for variation in self-reported affiliative and self-enhancing humor, as well as aggressive and self-defeating humor (Vernon, Martin, Schermer, Cherkas, & Spector, 2008). With use of the same questionnaire with a U.S. sample, affiliative and self-enhancing humor was heritable, whereas aggressive and self-defeating humor was attributed to the shared and nonshared environment. Across samples, the tendency to enjoy particular types of humorous stimuli developed as a consequence of experience and was not heritable (Cherkas, Hochberg, MacGregor, Snieder, & Spector, 2000).

Heritability of Mental Toughness

Mental toughness was operationalized as the four traits of control over life, commitment, confidence, and the ability to face new challenges (Vernon, Martin, Schermer, & Mackie, 2008). It was positively correlated with extraversion, and negatively correlated with neuroticism. Heritability was .52 for mental toughness in a Canadian sample.

Heritability of Social Support and Marital Satisfaction

Social support is protective against chronic physical diseases, such as coronary heart disease, hypertension, and stroke, as well as mental illnesses and general functional ability (Seeman et al., 1995). Marital quality is similarly associated with both physical and mental health (Kiecolt-Glaser & Newton, 2001). Previous research has reported moderate heritability of social support (Bergeman et al., 1990; Kessler et al., 1992; Spotts et al., 2005), and marital quality (Spotts et al., 2004, 2005). In Chinese subjects, subjective social support and utilization of support were heritable and also influenced by the shared environment, whereas objective social support was not heritable (Ji et al., 2008).

Heritability of Psychological Well-Being

Kessler, Gilman, Thornton, and Kendler (2004) reported heritabilities ranging from .11 to .43 for six aspects of psychological well-being, including purpose in life, self-acceptance, autonomy, mastery, personal growth, and positive social relationships. Well-being scales included on large personality inventories, such as the Multidimensional Personality Inventory, ranged from .50 to .80 (Bergeman, Plomin, Pedersen, & McClearn, 1991; Braungart et al., 1992; Finkel & McGue, 1997; Lykken & Tellegen, 1996; Spotts et al., 2005; Tellegen et al., 1988). However, well-being measured by the Center for Epidemiologic Studies Depression

Scale was minimally heritable (Gatz, Pedersen, Plomin, & Nesselroade, 1992). Stability and change in heritability of well-being was considered in Norway (Nes, Roysamb, Tambs, Harris, & Reichborn-Kjennerud, 2006). The genetic influences on well-being were largely stable, with cross-time correlations for genetic effects of .85 for males and .78 for females. Nonshared environmental influences, on the other hand, were largely time specific.

Heritability of Religiosity

Several studies have reported modest to moderate heritability of religiosity, with a heritability of .28 reported in Martin and colleagues (1986). Religious attendance yielded heritability estimates from .25 to .42, depending on sex (Maes, Neale, Martin, Heath, & Eaves, 1999; Truett et al., 1994). Personal devotion yielded a similar heritability estimate of .29, whereas the estimate was .12 for institutional conservatism, which was based on religious affiliation (Kendler, Gardner, & Prescott, 1997).

There is some evidence that heritability of religiosity is moderated by age and race. With a large sample of Dutch adolescent and young adult twins, Boomsma and colleagues (1999) reported little to no genetic influence on religious upbringing, religious affiliation, and participation in religious activities. Similarly, with a sample of Finnish adolescents, Winter, Kaprio, Viken, Karvonen, and Rose (1999) reported heritabilities of .11 and .22 for girls and boys, respectively, for religious fundamentalism. Thus, genetic influences on religiosity appear to be attenuated with younger samples. However, higher heritability estimates were obtained with African American (AA) versus European American/ other ancestry (EA) adolescent girls, suggesting that race may also moderate the heritability of religiosity (Heath et al., 1999). Specifically, girls' heritability was estimated at .78 in AA versus .15 in EA for religious involvement, .56 in AA versus .33 in EA for reliance on religious teachings, .74 in AA versus .09 in EA for belief in God, .70 in AA versus .06 in EA for guidance by religious beliefs, and .81 in AA versus .24 in EA for turning to prayer.

Thus, heritability of components of resilience is also subject to moderation by age, race, cohort, and culture, with individual differences within subgroups in the population more or less heritable. These components of resilience are also interdependent, such that the relation between religiosity and well-being is largely mediated through multiple other factors, such as positive emotions, optimism, purpose and meaning in life, rest and rejuvenation, a healthy lifestyle, greater access to resources, and social support (Southwick et al., 2005). The next section introduces molecular genetic techniques that do not rely on traditional family resemblance methods to estimate genetic influences.

Molecular Genetic Techniques for Studying Genetic Influences on Resilience

Phenotypes that are shown to be heritable through quantitative genetic methods can now be explored further, and actual genes may be identified. Specific information about genotypes can be incorporated into behavior genetic or pedigree models to test the importance of individual genes on behavior, or the effect of genes may be associated with behavior in samples of unrelated individuals. Once a gene is identified, we can track how variations in the gene affect protein expression and resulting phenotypes.

The most common study design in this area, the *association study*, examines whether there is a statistical association between particular genetic variants and phenotypes, such as dimensions of personality. A significant association could mean that the gene confers risk or protection for the behavior of interest. However, it could also mean that the gene does not play a causal role but is, for example, located near an important gene on the same chromosome. An association could also arise as an artifact of mixed ethnicity, in that frequencies of particular alleles can vary substantially among populations. Careful control for population stratification is needed when using these designs.

The availability of the entire human genome sequence and hundreds of thousands of genetic variants called *single-nucleotide polymorphisms* (SNPs) has greatly facilitated this area of research, and the field is quickly moving toward models incorporating a large number of measured genetic variants simultaneously. *Haplotype mapping*, which tracks the distribution of clusters of SNPs that segregate as a group, has also aided in the selection of appropriate, somewhat orthogonal genetic variants. Important interactions among genetic variants likely also play a large role in resilience processes and can be modeled when multiple genetic variants are measured.

Simultaneous testing of association with large numbers of genetic variants inevitably leads to false-positive associations. One way to handle this is to take a systems approach and measure intermediate *endophenotypes*, which exist along the pathway from genotype to phenotype, and may be endocrinological, biochemical, neurophysiological, neuroanatomical, neuropsychological, or cognitive (Gottesman & Gould, 2003). To be useful, endophenotypes should be genetically influenced, as well as associated with one or more candidate genes and the phenotype. Incorporating endophenotypes into our models can elucidate pathways from genes to behavior. For example, nonaffected siblings of children with attention-deficit/hyperactivity disorder (ADHD) had deficits in response inhibition similar to that of their affected siblings, although their behavior was similar to that of controls (Slaats-Willemse, Swaab-Barneveld, deSonneville, van der Meulen, & Buitelaar, 2003), suggesting that response inhibition is a putative endophenotype for ADHD.

Geneticists and psychologists easily slip into using shorthand language of "gene for … " and even "risk allele" and "protec-

tive allele." These labels mean little without also specifying the environmental circumstance, with some variations more successful in particular environments. An allele may confer risk in one context and be protective in another, increasing risk of antisocial behavior but predisposing to scientific creativity, for example. It is also often the case that the so-called "risk" allele is the most common version of the gene in the population, again emphasizing that the influence of genes is probabilistic rather than deterministic. Studies that incorporate a large number of measured SNPs or genes generally indicate the presence of mechanisms that both increase and decrease expression of the phenotype, and no single genetic variant is necessary or sufficient for the phenotype. Thus, in most cases, there are costs and benefits to each allele.

A review of associations between a functional polymorphism in the catechol-O-methyltransferase gene and cognitive and emotional phenotypes is descriptive of this fundamental point. One allele is associated with enhanced cognitive processing but exaggerated stress reactivity, whereas the other allele is a risk factor for cognitive dysfunctions but a protective factor in stressful environments.

Risk or Resilience?: Variations in the Catechol-*O*-Methyltransferase Gene

Catechol-O-methyltransferase (COMT) is a key enzyme in the breakdown of dopamine in the prefrontal cortex (Boulton & Eisenhofer, 1998). Dopamine is critical for modulating cognitive functioning, which impacts behavior, thoughts, and emotions. The association is U-shaped, with too little or too much dopamine having deleterious effects on cognitive functioning (Papaleo et al., 2009). The COMT gene has a common functional diallelic polymorphism (*Val158Met*, *rs4680 G/A*) with codominant alleles, such that individuals with the Val/Val genotype have the highest activity of COMT, those with the

Met/Met genotype have the lowest activity of COMT, and heterozygous individuals are intermediate.

Low-activity COMT (Met rather than Val) is related to elevated dopamine in the prefrontal cortex and denser nerve connections. These endophenotypes lead not only to better concentration and executive functioning overall (Sheldrick et al., 2008) but also to more behavioral rigidity, reduced ability to shift attention, and higher personality disorganization. Thus, individuals with low-activity COMT have enhanced cognitive function but may ruminate on stressful thoughts, leading to anxiety. Specifically, the COMT-Met allele has been associated with increased levels of anxiety (Domschke et al., 2004; Drabant et al., 2006; Enoch, Xu, Ferro, Harris, & Goldman, 2003; McGrath et al., 2004; Montag et al., 2008; Olsson et al., 2005, 2007; Woo et al., 2004), obsessive–compulsive disorder (Pooley, Fineberg, & Harrison, 2007), panic disorder, alcoholism, high neuroticism, low sensation seeking, extraversion, reward dependence, and pain sensitivity (Diatchenko et al., 2005; Drabant et al., 2006; Heinz & Smolka, 2006; Lang, Bajbouj, Sander, & Gallinat, 2007; Nackley et al., 2007; Reuter & Hennig, 2005; Stein, Fallin, Schork, & Gelernter, 2005; Zubieta, Heitzeg, et al., 2003; Zubieta, Ketter, et al., 2003).

In contrast, high-activity COMT (Val substitution) leads to less dopamine in the synapses and has been associated with poorer cognitive functioning (Sheldrick et al., 2008), specifically, poorer performance on prefrontally mediated tasks (Barnett, Jones, Robbins, & Muller, 2007; Goldberg et al., 2003; Joober et al., 2002; Malhotra et al., 2002) and prefrontal inefficiency during working memory and cognitive control tasks measured by electroencephalography (Winterer, Musso, et al., 2006) and neuroimaging (Blasi et al., 2005; Egan et al., 2001; Winterer, Egan, et al., 2006).

These human association findings are supported by research using an animal model. Papaleo and colleagues (2009) studied three types of mice: (1) genetically engineered mice lacking a functional COMT (2) a new transgenic mouse overexpressing the human COMT-Val allele, and (3) normal wild-type mice. This genetic manipulation affected specific cognitive and stress reactivity measures analogous to those used with humans. Increased COMT activity was associated with cognitive disadvantage, but a stress and pain sensitivity advantage, whereas decreased COMT activity improved memory but was associated with exaggerated emotional responsivity.

A GE interaction study with the COMT gene supports the notion that one mechanism by which genes influence resilience is by exacerbating susceptibility to relevant environments. Using an experimental design, Jabbi and colleagues (2007) reported that the Val–Met polymorphism moderated subjects' neuroendocrine and subjective responses to acute social stress in the laboratory (i.e., speech preparation, speech, and mental arithmetic conducted in front of a small audience and videotaped). Specifically, healthy participants with the Met–Met alleles had higher endocrine and subjective reports of stress under these conditions.

Taken together, increased COMT activity is a protective factor in stressful situations, but a risk factor for cognitive dysfunctions more generally. COMT reduction enhances working memory processes but is also associated with exaggerated stress reactivity. Each allele has an environmentally specific selective advantage, and both alleles are maintained at high levels in populations worldwide. This apparent evolutionary trade-off between cognitive efficiency and emotional resilience lead to the formation of the "warrior–worrier" model (Goldman, Oroszi, & Ducci, 2005). Importantly, the COMT example underscores the role of environmental selection in resilience processes and moves us away from categorizing alleles as either "risk" or "protective," without specifying contexts and outcomes. In the next section, recent findings associating genetic variants with resilience are reviewed.

A Selective Review of Measured Genes Associated with Resilience Characteristics

We next turn to illustrative findings from molecular genetic studies that elucidate associations between measured candidate genes and individual differences in responses to stress, trait resilience, and social attachments.

Neuropeptide Y (*NPY*) is abundantly expressed in regions of the limbic system and regulates diverse functions, including appetite, weight, and the assignment of emotional valences to stimuli and memories. An SNP (*rs16147*) located in the promoter region of the *NPY* gene alters expression *in vitro* and seems to account for more than half of the variation in expression *in vivo* (Zhou et al., 2008). Higher gene-controlled *NPY* expression was associated with reduced amygdala activation, reduced trait anxiety, and increased resilient responding to moderate levels of sustained muscular pain. Those with genetic variants supporting higher *NPY* released more opioid neurotransmitter in response to the stress challenge, and also had attenuated emotional responses to the pain. *NPY*, then, is a promising candidate resilience gene, playing an important role in neurobiological systems implicated in emotion regulation and resilience to stress.

Brain-derived neurotrophic factor (*BDNF*) is a key regulator of the mesolimbic dopamine pathway, which identifies and responds to emotionally salient stimuli. Research has largely focused on the *Val66Met* SNP (*rs6265*), with the *Met*-allele attenuating secretion of *BDNF* (Egan et al., 2003). The *BDNF Val*-allele carriers have larger amygdalar, hippocampal, and prefrontal cortical volumes compared to the homozygous *Met*-allele carriers (Frodl, Moller, & Meisenzahl, 2008; Pezawas et al., 2004; Sublette et al., 2008), higher levels of self-reported social support and social interactions (Taylor et al., 2008), and higher trait resilience overall. Specifically, Surtees and colleagues (2007) operationalized resilience as sense of coherence, made up of compre-

hensibility, manageability, and meaningfulness to life. A dose–response pattern was observed with *Val* carriers displaying the most resilience. *BDNF* is a candidate resilience gene, with the *Val* allele associated with the ability to be adaptable and to cope flexibly with stress, as well as endophenotypes, such as larger hippocampal volume.

Vasopressin is an important hormone for attachment to offspring and mates. Humans have polymorphisms in three repeat sequences in the 5′ flanking region of the arginine vasopressin receptor 1a (*AVPR1a*) gene. A longer variant of the DNA preceding the gene (i.e., allele 334) was associated with men's marital status, partner bonding, and marital quality perceived by spouses (Walum et al., 2008). This same variant was also associated with altruism (Knafo et al., 2007). This gene shows promise as a candidate for supporting marital success, perhaps by increasing the reward for giving and loving.

The genes reviewed earlier are only the tip of the iceberg in terms of candidate genes for resilience. A number of additional genes have been implicated in attention and affective processing (e.g., *tryptophan hydroxylase 2* gene: Canli, Congdon, Constable, & Lesch, 2008; Reuter et al., 2008), and behavioral resilience to stress exposure (e.g., *activity-regulated cytoskeletal-associated protein* gene: Kozlovsky et al., 2007; *Bcl-2-associated athanogene*: Maeng et al., 2008). Next year, next month, or even tomorrow there will be even more candidates from which to choose. Importantly, this field will advance by incorporating measures of endophenotypes and intermediate phenotypes using a systems perspective to elucidate pathways from genes to behavior, and ultimately to resilience and flourishing in life.

Conclusion

From this chapter I hope the reader can appreciate that it is impossible to discuss the genetics of resilience without intimate knowledge of the environment. Genetic influences are probabilistic, and we should guard against explaining health, well-being, and flourishing in life in a reductionistic "genetic engineering" manner. With quantitative genetic designs, we see variations in heritability estimates depending on cohort, gender, age, marital status, and other risk and protective processes present in the environment. Sociocultural norms impact heritability, with smoking in females becoming more heritable as it became more socially acceptable (Kendler et al., 2000). Thus, lower social controls allow for the expression of heritable individual differences, and heritability should increase with greater opportunities for the expression of a trait (Rutter et al., 2006).

Following from this logic, it makes no sense to classify genes or alleles as "good" or "bad," or even as "protective" or "risk," without also specifying the environmental circumstance. Whether a particular allele is good or bad depends on the environment for polygenic phenotypes, such that the *COMT-Met* allele is associated with cognitive capacity and stress reactivity, whereas the *Val-* allele is protective in stressful environments but confers risk for cognitive dysfunctions. A central concept of evolution is that individual differences are adaptive; there is no single prototype that is ideal for all conditions. Some variations are more successful than others depending on the environment. This argument can be expanded to refer to change across the lifespan: Some variations support resilience at one life stage, whereas other variations may support resilience later in life. Thus, it is largely diversity, rather than good genes or bad genes, that matters.

This chapter introduces three main types of GE interplay: GE correlation, GE interaction, and epigenetics. Whereas GE correlations reflect genetic differences in exposure to environments, GE interactions refer to genetic differences in susceptibility to environments, with genes increasing or decreasing an individual's sensitivity to both risk and protective aspects of the environment.

Epigenetic studies focus on how microenvironments alter gene expression, with relatively stable changes across the lifespan, and sometimes passed from one generation to the next.

GE correlations are often ignored in the psychosocial literature, with genetic influences on early maltreatment, stressful life events, social support, and marital quality, for example, not considered when studying environmental risk and protection. To date, molecular genetic approaches to identifying GE interaction have almost exclusively focused on putative risk alleles and adverse environments, leaving unstudied the role of gene × protective environment interactions. GE interaction studies have, however, elucidated process, with the risk of depression after a stressful event elevated among individuals with one version of the serotonin transporter gene, for example, and diminished among those with the other (Caspi et al., 2003). Furthermore, variations in the serotonin transporter and the monoamine oxidase genes are associated with specific differences in neuroregulation, which are linked to dimensions of temperament that place individuals at risk for psychopathology (Bertolino et al., 2005; Hariri et al., 2005; Pezawas et al., 2005). Recent epigenetic studies, controlling for genetic associations, have underscored the causal role of early parenting in resilient responding to stress (Weaver et al., 2004). As we learn more about GE interplay, we can match environments to genetic propensities to maximize potentials and support resilience through prevention and intervention.

Because genetic influences do not operate in isolation from environmental influences, and high heritability does not imply immutability, genetically influenced polygenic behaviors and traits are largely modifiable through environmental intervention. Disease risk, for example, may be determined by environmental exposure, which then mediates the association between genotype and disease. The classic example is that of *phenylketonuria* (PKU), a single gene disorder characterized by the inability to metabolize the amino acid phenylalanine. A buildup of phenylalanine in the brain and body leads to mental retardation; however, the detrimental effects can be greatly minimized by a diet low in proteins containing phenylalanine. Furthermore, the existence of significant GE interaction suggests that interventions may be most effective in genetic subpopulations. From a resilience perspective, even though genes are not typically modifiable, positive experiences within the social environment can compensate for and buffer individuals against the negative effects of genetic risk. For example, favorable environments may exert effective social control over youth with a heritable risk for using illicit drugs and sexual promiscuity (Shanahan & Hofer, 2005). In this way, findings from GE interplay studies guide the development of social resilience interventions to reduce the burden of disorder and disease on individuals, communities, and countries.

In conclusion, resilience involves intrinsic and extrinsic processes of successful adaptation to adversity, and genetic variations contribute to individual differences in these capacities, with adaptation and positive outcomes not limited to initial states. Resilience is dynamic; adaptive systems reorganize to create new resilience in new environments, and may be different in difference phases of life. Risk and protective processes operate at genetic, neurobiological, individual, and social levels, and do not act in isolation. The understanding of how genes and environments work together to promote resilience will advance by incorporating measures of endophenotypes and intermediate phenotypes using a systems perspective to elucidate pathways from genes to flourishing in life.

References

Aspinwall, L. G. (1998). Rethinking the role of positive affect in self-regulation. *Motivation and Emotion*, 22, 1–32.

Barnett, J. H., Jones, P. B., Robbins, T. W., & Muller, U. (2007). Effects of the catechol-O-methyltransferase Val158Met polymorphism on executive function: A meta-analysis of the Wisconsin Card Sort Test in schizophrenia and healthy controls. *Molecular Psychiatry*, 12, 502–509.

Bergeman, C. S., Plomin, R., Pedersen, N. L., & McClearn, G. E. (1991). Genetic mediation of the relationship between social support and psychological well-being. *Psychology and Aging*, 6, 640–646.

Bergeman, C. S., Plomin, R., Pedersen, N. L., McClearn, G. E., & Nesselroade, J. R. (1990). Genetic and environmental influences on social support: The Swedish adoption/twin study of aging: SATSA. *Journal of Gerontology: Psychological Science*, 45, 101–106.

Bertolino, A., Arciero, G., Rubino, V., Latorre, V., DeCandia, M., Mazzola, V., et al. (2005). Variation of human amygdala response during threatening stimuli as a function of 5'HTTL-PR genotype and personality style. *Biological Psychiatry*, 57, 1517–1525.

Billig, J. P., Hershberger, S. L., Iacono, W. G., & McGue, M. (1986). Life events and personality in late adolescence: Genetic and environmental relations. *Behavior Genetics*, 26, 543–554.

Blasi, G., Mattay, V. S., Bertolino, A., Elvevag, B., Callicott, J. H., Das, S., et al. (2005). Effect of catechol-O-methyltransferase val158met genotype on attentional control. *Journal of Neuroscience*, 25, 5038–5045.

Boardman, J. D., Blalock, C. L., & Button, T. M. M. (2008). Sex differences in the heritability of resilience. *Twin Research and Human Genetics*, 11, 12–27.

Bolinskey, P. K., Neale, M. C., Jacobson, K. C., Prescott, C. A., & Kendler, K. S. (2004). Sources of individual differences in stressful life event exposure in male and female twins. *Twin Research*, 7, 33–38.

Bonanno, G. A. (2004). Loss, trauma, and human resilience: Have we underestimated the human capacity to thrive after extremely aversive events? *American Psychologist*, 59, 20–28.

Boomsma, D. I. (1993). Current status and future prospects in twin studies of the development of cognitive abilities: Infancy to old age. In T. J. Bouchard & P. Propping (Eds.), *Twins as a tool of behavioral genetics* (Life Sciences Research Report No. 53) (pp. 67–82). Oxford, UK: Wiley.

Boomsma, D. I., de Geus, E. J. C., van Baal, G. C. M., & Koopmans, J. R. (1999). A religious upbringing reduces the influence of genetic factors on disinhibition: Evidence for interaction between genotype and environment on personality. *Twin Research, 2,* 115–125.

Boulton, A. A., & Eisenhofer, G. (1998). Catecholamine metabolism: From molecular understanding to clinical diagnosis and treatment: Overview. *Advanced Pharmacology, 42,* 273–292.

Braungart, J. M., Plomin, R., DeFries, J. C., & Fulker, D. W. (1992). Genetic influence on tester-rated infant temperament as assessed by Bayley's Infant Behavior Record: Nonadoptive and adoptive siblings and twins. *Developmental Psychology, 28,* 40–47.

Button, T. M. M., Scourfield, J., Martin, N., Purcell, S., & McGuffin, P. (2005). Family dysfunction interacts with genes in the causation of antisocial symptoms. *Behavior Genetics, 35,* 115–120.

Canli, T., Congdon, E., Constable, R. T., & Lesch, K. P. (2008). Additive effects of serotonin transporter and tryptophan hydroxylase-2 gene variation on neural correlates of affective processing. *Biological Psychology, 79,* 118–125.

Caspi, A., McClay, J., Moffitt, T. E., Mill, J., Martin, J., Craig I. W., et al. (2002). Role of genotype in the cycle of violence in maltreated children. *Science, 297,* 851–854.

Caspi, A., Sugden, K., Moffitt, T., Taylor, A., Craig, I. W., et al. (2003). Influence of life stress on depression: Moderation by a polymorphism in the 5-HTT gene. *Science, 301,* 386–389.

Cherkas, L., Hochberg, F., MacGregor, A. J., Snieder, H., & Spector, T. D. (2000). Happy families: A twin study of humour. *Twin Research, 3,* 17–22.

Cleveland, H. H., Wiebe, R. P., van den Oord, E. J., & Rowe, D. C. (2000). Behavior problems among children from different family structures: The influence of genetic self-selection. *Child Development, 71,* 733–751.

Danner, D. D., Snowdon, D. A., & Friesen, W. V. (2001). Positive emotions in early life and longevity: Findings from the Nun Study. *Journal of Personality and Social Psychology, 80,* 804–813.

Deater-Deckard, K., Fulker, D. W., & Plomin, R. (1999). A genetic study of the family environment in the transition to early adolescence. *Journal of Child Psychology and Psychiatry, 40,* 769–775.

Diatchenko, L., Slade, G. D., Nackley, A. G., Bhalang, K., Sigurdsson, A., Belfer, I., et al. (2005). Genetic basis for individual variations in pain perception and the development of a chronic pain condition. *Human Molecular Genetics, 14,* 135–143.

Dick, D. M., Rose, R. J., Viken, R. J., & Kaprio, J. (2000). Pubertal timing and substance use: Associations between and within families across late adolescence. *Developmental Psychology, 36,* 180–189.

Diener, E. (1984). Subjective well-being. *Psychological Bulletin, 95,* 542–575.

Dillon, K. M., Minchoff, B., & Baker, K. H. (1985). Positive emotional states and enhancement of the immune system. *International Journal of Psychiatry in Medicine, 15,* 13–18.

Domschke, K., Freitag, C. M., Kuhlenbaumer, G., Schirmacher, A., Sand, P., Nyhuis, P., et al. (2004). Association of the functional V158M catechol-O-methyl-transferase polymorphism with panic disorder in women. *International Journal of Neuropsychopharmacology, 7,* 183–188.

D'Onofrio, B. M., Turkheimer, E., Emery, R. E., Slutske, W. S., Heath, A. C., Madden, P. A., et al. (2005). A genetically informed study of marital instability and its association with offspring psychopathology. *Journal of Abnormal Psychology, 114,* 570–586.

Drabant, E. M., Hariri, A. R., Meyer-Lindenberg, A., Munoz, K. E., Mattay, V. S., Kolachana, B. S., et al. (2006). Catechol-O-methyltransferase val158met genotype and neural mechanisms related to affective arousal and regulation. *Archives of General Psychiatry, 63,* 1396–1406.

Dunne, M. P., Martin, N. G., Statham, D. J., Slutske, W. S., Dinwiddie, S. H., Bucholz, K. K., et al. (1997). Genetic and environmental contributions to variance in age at first sexual intercourse. *Psychological Science, 8,* 211–216.

Eaves, L. (2006). Genotype × environment interaction in psychopathology: Fact or artifact. *Twin Research and Human Genetics, 9,* 1–8.

Egan, M. F., Goldberg, T. E., Kolachana, B. S., Callicott, J. H., Mazzanti, C. M., Straub, R. E., et al. (2001). Effect of COMT Val108/158 Met genotype on frontal lobe function and risk for schizophrenia. *Proceedings of the*

National Academy of Sciences of the United States of America, 98, 6917–6922.

Egan, M. F., Kojima, M., Callicott, J. H., Goldberg, T. E., Kolachana, B. S., Bertolino, A., et al. (2003). The BDNF val66met polymorphism affects activity-dependent secretion of BDNF and human memory and hippocampal function. Cell, 112, 257–269.

Eley, T. C., Liang, H., Plomin, R., Sham, P., Sterne, A., Williamson, R., et al. (2004). Parental familial vulnerability, family environment, and their interactions as predictors of depressive symptoms in adolescents. Journal of the American Academy of Child and Adolescent Psychiatry, 43, 298–306.

Enoch, M. A., Xu, K., Ferro, E., Harris, C. R., & Goldman, D. (2003). Genetic origins of anxiety in women: A role for a functional catechol-O-methyltransferase polymorphism. Psychiatric Genetics, 13, 33–41.

Finkel, D., & McGue, M. (1997). Sex differences and nonadditivity in heritability of the Multidimensional Personality Questionnaire scales. Journal of Personality and Social Psychology, 72, 929–938.

Fredrickson, B. L., & Joiner, T. (2002). Positive emotions trigger upward spirals toward emotional well-being. Psychological Science, 13, 172–175.

Frodl, T., Moller, H. J., & Meisenzahl, E. (2008). Neuroimaging genetics: New perspectives in research on major depression. Acta Psychiatrica Scandinavica, 118, 363–372.

Garmezy, N., Masten, A. S., & Tellegen, A. (1984). The study of stress and competence in children: A building block for developmental psychopathology. Child Development, 55, 97–111.

Gatz, M., Pedersen, N. L., Plomin, R., & Nesselroade, J. R. (1992). Importance of shared genes and shared environments for symptoms of depression in older adults. Journal of Abnormal Psychology, 101, 701–708.

Goldberg, T. E., Egan, M. F., Gscheidle, T., Coppola, R., Weickert, T., Kolachana, B. S., et al. (2003). Executive subprocesses in working memory: Relationship to catechol-O-methyltransferase Val158Met genotype and schizophrenia. Archives of General Psychiatry, 60, 889–896.

Goldman, D., Oroszi, G., & Ducci, F. (2005). The genetics of addictions: Uncovering the genes. Nature Review Genetics, 6, 521–532.

Goldsmith, H. H., Lemery, K. S., Buss, K. A., & Campos, J. (1999). Genetic analyses of focal aspects of infant temperament. Developmental Psychology, 35, 972–985.

Gottesman, I. I., & Gould, T. D. (2003). The endophenotype concept in psychiatry: Etymology and strategic intentions. American Journal of Psychiatry, 160, 636–645.

Hariri, A., Drabant, E., Munoz, K., Kolachana, B., Venkata, S., Egan, M., et al. (2005). A susceptibility gene for affective disorders and the response of the human amygdala. Archives of General Psychiatry, 62, 146–152.

Heath, A. C., Jardine, R., & Martin, N. G. (1989). Interactive effects on genotype and social environment on alcohol consumption in female twins. Journal of Studies on Alcohol, 50, 38–48.

Heath, A. C., Madden, P. A. F., Grant, J. D., McLaughlin, T. L., Todoroy, A. A., & Bucholz, K. K. (1999). Resiliency factors protecting against teenage alcohol use and smoking: Influences of religion, religious involvement and values, and ethnicity in the Missouri Adolescent Female Twin Study. Twin Research, 2, 145–155.

Heinz, A., & Smolka, M. N. (2006). The effects of catechol-O-methyltransferase genotype on brain activation elicited by affective stimuli and cognitive tasks. Reviews in the Neurosciences, 17, 359–367.

Iervolino, A. C., Pike, A., Manke, B., Reiss, D., Hetherington, E. M., & Plomin, R. (2002). Genetic and environmental influences in adolescent peer socialization: Evidence from two genetically sensitive designs. Child Development, 73, 162–174.

Jabbi, M., Kema, I. P., van der Pompe, G., te Meerman, G. J., Ormel, J., & den Boer, J. A. (2007). Catechol-O-methyltransferase polymorphism and susceptibility to major depressive disorder modulates psychological stress response. Psychiatric Genetics, 17, 183–193.

Jacobson, K. C., & Rowe, D. C. (1999). Genetic and environmental influences on the relationships between family connectedness, school connectedness, and adolescent depressed mood: Sex differences. Developmental Psychology, 35, 926–939.

Jaffee, S. R., Caspi, A., Moffitt, T. E., & Taylor, A. (2004). Physical maltreatment victim to antisocial child: Evidence of an environmentally mediated process. *Journal of Abnormal Psychology, 113,* 44–55.

Ji, W., Hu, Y., Huang, Y., Cao, W., Lu, J., Qin, Y., et al. (2008). A genetic epidemiologic study of social support in a Chinese sample. *Twin Research and Human Genetics, 11,* 55–62.

Jockin, V., McGue, M., & Lykken, D. T. (1996). Personality and divorce: A genetic analysis. *Journal of Personality and Social Psychology, 71,* 288–299.

Johnson, W., McGue, M., & Krueger, R. F. (2005). Personality stability in late adulthood: A behavioral genetic analysis. *Journal of Personality, 73,* 523–551.

Johnson, W., McGue, M., Krueger, R. F., & Bouchard, T. J. (2004). Marriage and personality: A genetic analysis. *Journal of Personality and Social Psychology, 86,* 285–294.

Joober, R., Gauthier, J., Lal, S., Bloom, D., Lalonde, P., Rouleau, G., et al. (2002). Catechol-O-methyltransferase Val-108/158-Met gene variants associated with performance on the Wisconsin Card Sorting Test. *Archives of General Psychiatry, 59,* 662–663.

Kaufman, J., Yang, B. Z., Douglas-Palumberi, H., Houshyar, S., Lipschitz, D., Krystal, J. H., et al. (2004). Social support and serotonin transporter gene moderate depression in maltreated children. *Proceedings of the National Academy of Sciences USA, 101,* 17316–17321.

Keltner, D., & Bonanno, G. A. (1997). A study of laughter and dissociation: Distinct correlates of laughter and smiling during bereavement. *Journal of Personality and Social Psychology, 73,* 687–702.

Kendler, K. S. (2005). "A gene for … ": The nature of gene action in psychiatric disorders. *American Journal of Psychiatry, 162,* 1243–1252.

Kendler, K. S., Gardner, C. O., & Prescott, C. A. (1997). Religion, psychopathology, and substance use and abuse: A multimeasure, genetic epidemiologic study. *American Journal of Psychiatry, 154,* 322–329.

Kendler, K. S., & Karkowski-Shuman, L. (1997). Stressful life events and genetic liability to major depression: Genetic control of exposure to the environment? *Psychological Medicine, 27,* 539–547.

Kendler, K. S., Neale, M. C., Kessler, R., Heath, A., & Eaves, L. (1993). A twin study of recent life events and difficulties. *Archives of General Psychiatry, 50,* 789–796.

Kendler, K. S., Thornton, L. M., & Pedersen, N. L. (2000). Tobacco consumption in Swedish twins reared apart and reared together. *Archives of General Psychiatry, 57,* 886–892.

Kessler, R. C., Gilman, S. E., Thornton, L. M., & Kendler, K. S. (2004). Health, well-being, and social responsibility in the MIDUS twin and sibling subsamples. In O. G. Brim, C. D. Ryff, & R. C. Kessler (Eds.), *How healthy are we?: A national study of well-being at midlife* (pp. 124–152). Chicago: University of Chicago Press.

Kessler, R. C., Kendler, K. S., Heath, A. C., Neale, M. C., & Eaves, L. J. (1992). Social support, depressed mood, and adjustment to stress: A genetic epidemiologic investigation. *Journal of Personality and Social Psychology, 62,* 257–272.

Kiecolt-Glaser, J., & Newton, T. L. (2001). Marriage and health: His and hers. *Psychological Bulletin, 127,* 472–503.

Knafo, A., Israel, S., Darvasi, A., Bachner-Melman, R., Uzefovsky, F., Cohen, L., et al. (2007). Individual differences in allocation of funds in the dictator game associated with length of the arginine vasopressin 1a receptor RS3 promoter region and correlation between RS3 length and hippocampal mRNA. *Genes, Brain and Behavior, 7,* 266–275.

Koeppen-Schomerus, G., Eley, T. C., Wolke, D., Gringras, P., & Plomin, R. (2000). The interaction of prematurity with genetic and environmental influences on cognitive development in twins. *Journal of Pediatrics, 137,* 527–533.

Koopmans, J. R., Slutske, W. S., van Baal, G. C. M., & Boomsma, D. I. (1999). The influence of religion on alcohol use initiation: Evidence for genotype × environment interaction. *Behavior Genetics, 29,* 433–444.

Kozlovsky, N., Matar, M. A., Kaplan, Z., Kotler, M., Zohar, J., & Cohen, H. (2007). The immediate early gene Arc is associated with behavioral resilience to stress exposure in an animal model of posttraumatic stress disorder. *European Neuropsychopharmacology, 18,* 107–116.

Kramer, D. A. (2004). Commentary: Gene–environment interplay in the context of genetics, epigenetics, and gene expression. *Journal of the American Academy of Child and Adolescent Psychiatry, 44,* 19–27.

Lang, U. E., Bajbouj, M., Sander, T., & Gallinat, J. (2007). Gender dependent association of the functional catechol-O-methyltransfera-seVal158Met genotype with sensation seeking personality trait. *Neuropsychopharmacology, 1350*, 1950–1955.

Lichtenstein, P., & Pedersen, N. L. (1997). Does genetic variance for cognitive abilities account for genetic variance in educational achievement and occupational status?: A study of twins reared apart and twins reared together. *Social Biology, 44*, 77–90.

Luecken, L., & Lemery, K. S. (2004). Early caregiving and physiological stress responses. *Clinical Psychology Review, 24*, 171–191.

Luthar, S. S., & Cicchetti, D. (2000). The construct of resilience: Implications for interventions and social policies. *Developmental Psychopathology, 12*, 857–885.

Luthar, S. S., Cicchetti, D., & Becker, B. (2000). The construct of resilience: A critical evaluation and guidelines for future work. *Child Development, 71*, 543–562.

Lykken, D. T., & Tellegen, A. (1996). Happiness is a stochastic phenomenon. *Psychological Science, 7*, 186–189.

Lyubomirsky, S., Sheldon, K. M., & Schkade, D. (2005). Pursuing happiness: The architecture of sustainable change. *Review of General Psychology, 9*, 111–131.

Maeng, S., Hunsberger, J. G., Pearson, B., Yuan, P., Wang, Y., Wei, Y., et al. (2008). BAG1 plays a critical role in regulating recovery from both manic-like and depression-like behavioral impairments. *Proceedings of the National Academy of Sciences USA, 105*, 8766–8771.

Maes, H. H., Neale, M. C., Martin, N. G., Heath, A. C., & Eaves, L. J. (1999). Religious attendance and frequency of alcohol use: Same genes or same environments: A bivariate extended twins kinship model. *Twin Research, 2*, 169–179.

Malhotra, A. K., Kestler, L. J., Mazzanti, C., Bates, J. A., Goldberg, T., & Goldman, D. (2002). A functional polymorphism in the COMT gene and performance on a test of prefrontal cognition. *American Journal of Psychiatry, 159*, 652–654.

Manke, B., McGuire, S., Reiss, D., Hetherington, E. M., & Plomin, R. (1995). Genetic contributions to adolescents' extrafamilial social interactions: Teachers, best friends, and peers. *Social Development, 4*, 238–256.

Martin, N. G., Eaves, L. J., Heath, A. C., Jardine, R., Feingold, L. M., & Eysenck, H. J.

(1986). Transmission of social attitudes. *Proceeding of the National Academy of Sciences USA, 83*, 4364–4368.

Masten, A., & Coatsworth, J. D. (1998). The development of competence in favorable and unfavorable environments: Lessons from research on successful children. *American Psychologist, 53*, 205–220.

Mayeux, R., Ottman, R., Maestre, G., Ngai, C., Tang, M. X., Ginsberg, H., et al. (1995). Synergistic effects of traumatic head injury and apolipoprotein-epsilon 4 in patients with Alzheimer's disease. *Neurology, 45*, 555–557.

McGrath, M., Kawachi, I., Ascherio, A., Colditz, G. A., Hunter, D. J., & De Vivo, I. (2004). Association between catechol-O-methyltransferase and phobic anxiety. *American Journal of Psychiatry, 161*, 1703–1705.

McGue, M., & Christensen, K. (2003). The heritability of depression symptoms in elderly Danish twins: Occasion-specific versus general effects. *Behavior Genetics, 33*, 83–93.

McGue, M., & Lykken, D. T. (1992). Genetic influence on risk of divorce. *Psychological Science, 6*, 368–373.

Moceri, V. M., Kukull, W. A., Emanuel, I., van Belle, G., & Larson, E. B. (2000). Early-life risk factors and the development of Alzheimer's disease. *Neurology, 54*, 415–420.

Moffitt, T. E. (1993). Adolescence-limited and life-course-persistent antisocial behavior: A developmental taxonomy. *Psychological Review, 100*, 674–701.

Montag, C., Buckholtz, J. W., Hartmann, P., Merz, M., Burk, C., & Reuter, M. (2008). COMT genetic variation affects fear processing: Psychophysiological evidence. *Behavioral Neuroscience, 122*, 901–909.

Nackley, A. G., Tan, K. S., Fecho, K., Flood, P., Diatchenko, L., & Maixner, W. (2007). Catechol-O-methyltransferase inhibition increases pain sensitivity through activation of both beta2- and beta3-adrenergic receptors. *Pain, 128*, 199–208.

Nes, R. B., Roysamb, E., Tambs, K., Harris, J. R., & Reichborn-Kjennerud, T. (2006). Subjective well-being: Genetic and environmental contributions to stability and change. *Psychological Medicine, 36*, 1033–1042.

Olsson, C. A., Anney, R. J., Lotfi-Miri, M., Byrnes, G. B., Williamson, R., & Patton, G. C. (2005). Association between the COMT Val158Met polymorphism and propensity to anxiety in an Australian population based longitudinal study of adolescent health. *Psychiatric Genetics, 15*, 109–115.

Olsson, C. A., Byrnes, G. B., Anney, R. J., Collins, V., Hemphill, S. A., Williamson, R., et al. (2007). COMT Val(158)Met and 5HTTLPR functional loci interact to predict persistence of anxiety across adolescence: Results from the Victorian Adolescent Health Cohort Study. *Genes, Brain and Behavior, 6*, 647–652.

Ostir, G. V., Markides, K. S., Black, S. A., & Goodwin, J. S. (2000). Emotional well-being predicts subsequent functional independence and survival. *Journal of the American Geriatric Society, 48*, 473–478.

Papaleo, F., Crawley, J. N., Song, J., Lipska, B. K., Pickel, J., Weinberger, D. R., et al. (2009). Genetic dissection of the role of catechol-O-methyltransferase in cognition and stress reactivity in mice. *Journal of Neuroscience, 28*, 8709–8723.

Pedersen, N. L., Plomin, R., Nesselroade, J. R., & McClearn, G. E. (1992). A quantitative genetic analysis of cognitive abilities during the second half of the life span. *Psychological Science, 3*, 346–353.

Pedersen, N. L., & Reynolds, C. A. (1998). Stability and change in adult personality: Genetic and environmental components. *European Journal of Personality, 12*, 365–386.

Perusse, D., Neale, M. C., Heath, A. C., & Eaves, L. J. (1994). Human parental behavior: Evidence for genetic influence and potential implication for gene–culture transmission. *Behavior Genetics, 24*, 327–335.

Pezawas, L., Meyer-Lindenberg, A., Drabant, E. M., Verchinski, B. A., Munoz, K. E., Kolachana, B. S., et al. (2005). 5-HTTLPR polymorphism impacts human cingulate–amygdala interactions: A genetic susceptibility mechanism for depression. *Nature Neuroscience, 8*, 828–834.

Pezawas, L., Verchinski, B. A., Mattay, V. S., Callicott, J. H., Kolachana, B. S., Straub, R. E., et al. (2004). The brain-derived neurotrophic factor val66met polymorphism and variation in human cortical morphology. *Journal of Neuroscience, 24*, 10099–10102.

Plomin, R., DeFries, J. C., & Loehlin, J. L. (1977). Genotype–environment interaction and correlation in the analysis of human variation. *Psychological Bulletin, 84*, 309–322.

Plomin, R., DeFries, J. C., McClearn, G. E., &

Rutter, M. (1997). *Behavioral genetics* (3rd ed.). New York: Freeman.

Plomin, R., Emde, R. N., Braungart, J. M., Campos, J., Corley, R., Fulker, D. W., et al. (1993). Genetic change and continuity from fourteen to twenty months: The MacArthur Longitudinal Twin Study. *Child Development, 64*, 1354–1376.

Plomin, R., Lichtenstein, P., Pedersen, N. L., & McClearn, G. E. (1990). Genetic influence on life events during the last half of the life span. *Psychology and Aging, 5*, 25–30.

Plomin, R., Pedersen, N. L., Lichtenstein, P., & McClearn, G. E. (1994). Variability and stability in cognitive abilities are largely genetic later in life. *Behavior Genetics, 24*, 207–215.

Pooley, E. C., Fineberg, N.. & Harrison, P. J. (2007). The met(158) allele of catechol-O-methyltransferase (COMT) is associated with obsessive compulsive disorder in men: Case-control study and meta-analysis. *Molecular Psychiatry, 12*, 556–561.

Reiss, D., Neiderhiser, J. M., Hetherington, E. M., & Plomin, R. (2000). *The relationship code: Deciphering genetic and social influence on adolescent development*. Cambridge, MA: Harvard University Press.

Reuter, M., Esslinger, C., Montag, C., Lis, S., Gallhofer, B., & Kirsch, P. (2008). A functional variant of the tryptophan hydroxylase 2 gene impacts working memory: A genetic imaging study. *Biological Psychology, 79*, 111–117.

Reuter, M., & Hennig, J. (2005). Association of the functional catechol-O-methyltransferase VAL158MET polymorphism with the personality trait of extraversion. *NeuroReport, 16*, 1135–1138.

Riese, M. L. (1990). Neonatal temperament in monozygotic and dizygotic twin pairs. *Child Development, 61*, 1230–1237.

Robinson, G. E., Fernald, R. D., & Clayton, D. F. (2008). Genes and behavior. *Science, 322*, 896–900.

Rutter, M. (2006). *Genes and behavior: Nature–nurture interplay explained*. Malden, MA: Blackwell.

Rutter, M., Moffitt, T. E., & Caspi, A. (2006). Gene–environment interplay and psychopathology: Multiple varieties but real effects. *Journal of Child Psychology and Psychiatry, 47*, 226–261.

Saudino, K. J., Pedersen, N. L., Lichtenstein, P.,

McClearn, G. E., & Plomin, R. (1997). Can personality explain genetic influences on life events? *Journal of Personality and Social Psychology, 72,* 196–206.

Seeman, T. E., Berkman, L. F., Charpentier, P. A., Blazer, D. G., Albert, M. S., & Tinetti, M. E. (1995). Behavioral and psychosocial predictors of physical performance: MacArthur studies of successful aging. *Journals of Gerontology: Biological Sciences and Medical Sciences, 50,* M177–M183.

Shanahan, M. J., & Hofer, S. M. (2005). Social context in gene–environment interactions: Retrospect and prospect. *Journals of Gerontology, 60,* 65–76.

Sheldrick, A. J., Krug, A., Markov, V., Leube, D., Michel, T. M., Zerres, K., et al. (2008). Effect of COMT val158met genotype on cognition and personality. *European Psychiatry, 23,* 385–389.

Shonkoff, J. P., & Phillips, D. A. (2000). *From neurons to neighborhoods: The science of early childhood development.* Washington, DC: National Academy Press.

Silberg, J. L., Pickles, A., Rutter, M., Hewitt, J., Simonoff, E., Maes, H., et al. (1999). The influence of genetic factors and life stress on depression among adolescent girls. *Archives of General Psychiatry, 56,* 225–232.

Silventoinen, K., Kaprio, J., Lahelma, E., & Koskenvuo, M. (2000). Relative effect of genetic and environmental factors on body height: Differences across birth cohorts among Finnish men and women. *American Journal of Public Health, 90,* 627–630.

Slaats-Willemse, D., Swaab-Barneveld, H., deSonneville, L., van der Meulen, E., & Buitelaar, J. (2003). Deficient response inhibition as a cognitive endophenotype of ADHD. *Journal of the American Academy of Child and Adolescent Psychiatry, 42,* 1242–1248.

Southwick, S. M., Vythilingam, M., & Charney, D. S. (2005). The psychobiology of depression and resilience to stress: Implications for prevention and treatment. *Annual Review of Clinical Psychology, 1,* 255–291.

Spotts, E. L., Neiderhiser, J. M., Towers, H., Hansson, K., Lichtenstein, P., Cederblad, M., et al. (2004). Genetic and environmental influences on marital relationships. *Journal of Family Psychology, 18,* 107–119.

Spotts, E. L., Pedersen, N. L., Neiderhiser, J. M., Reiss, D., Lichtenstein, P., Hansson, K., et al. (2005). Genetic effects on women's positive mental health: Do marital relationships and social support matter? *Journal of Family Psychology, 19,* 339–349.

Stein, M. B., Fallin, M. D., Schork, N. J., & Gelernter, J. (2005). COMT polymorphisms and anxiety-related personality traits. *Neuropsychopharmacology, 30,* 2092–2102.

Stone, A. A., Neale, J. M., Cox, D. S., Napoli, A., Vadlimarsdottir, V., & Kennedy-Moore, E. (1994). Daily events are associated with a secretory immune response to an oral antigen in men. *Health Psychology, 13,* 440–446.

Sublette, M. E., Baca-Garcia, E., Parsey, R. V., Oquendo, M. A., Rodrigues, S. M., Galfalvy, H., et al. (2008). Effect of BDNF val66met polymorphism on age-related amygdala volume changes in healthy subjects. *Progress in Neuro-Psychopharmacology and Biological Psychiatry, 32,* 1652–1655.

Suomi, S. J. (2000). A biobehavioral perspective on developmental psychopathology: Excessive aggression and serotonergic dysfunction in monkeys. In A. S. Sameroff, M. Lewis, & S. Miller (Eds., *Handbook of developmental psychopathology* (2nd ed., pp. 237–256). New York: Plenum Press.

Surtees, P. G., Wainwright, N. W. J., Willis-Owen, S. A. G., Sandhu, M. S., Luben, R., Day, N. E., et al. (2007). The brain-derived neurotrophic factor Val66Met polymorphism is associated with sense of coherence in a nonclinical community sample of 7335 adults. *Journal of Psychiatric Research, 41,* 707–710.

Taylor, W. D., Zuchner, S., McQuoid, D. R., Steffens, D. C., Blazer, D. G., & Krishnan, R. R. (2008). Social support in older individuals: The role of the BDNF val66met polymorphism. *American Journal of Medical Genetics B: Neuropsychiatric Genetics, 147,* 1205–1212.

Tellegen, A., Lykken, D. T., Bouchard, T. J., Wilcox, K. J., Segal, N. L., & Rich, S. (1988). Personality similarity in twins reared apart and together. *Journal of Personality and Social Psychology, 54,* 1031–1039.

Thapar, A., Harold, G., & McGuffin, P. (1998). Life events and depressive symptoms in childhood—shared genes or shared adversity?: A research note. *Journal of Child Psychology and Psychiatry, 39,* 1153–1158.

Truett, K. R., Eaves, L. J., Walters, E. E., Heath, A. C., Hewitt, J. K., Meyer, J. M., et al. (1994). A model system for analysis of family resemblance in extended kinships of twins. *Behavior Genetics, 24,* 35–49.

Vernon, P. A., Martin, R. A., Schermer, J. A., Cherkas, L. F., & Spector, T. D. (2008). Genetic and environmental contributions to humor styles: A replication study. *Twin Research and Human Genetics, 11,* 44–47.

Vernon, P. A., Martin, R. A., Schermer, J. A., & Mackie, A. (2008). A behavioral genetic investigation of humor styles and their correlations with the Big Five personality dimensions. *Personality and Individual Differences, 44,* 1116–1125.

Wade, T. D., & Kendler, K. S. (2000). The genetic epidemiology of parental discipline. *Psychological Medicine, 30,* 1303–1313.

Waldman, I. (2007). Gene–environment interactions reexamined: Does mother's marital stability interact with the dopamine receptor D2 gene in the etiology of childhood attention-deficit/hyperactivity disorder? *Development and Psychopathology, 19,* 1117–1128.

Walum, H., Westberg, L., Henningsson, S., Neiderhiser, J. M., Reiss, D., Igl, W., et al. (2008). Genetic variation in the vasopressin receptor 1a gene (AVPR1A) associates with pair-bonding behavior in humans. *Proceedings of the National Academy of Sciences USA, 105,* 14153–14156.

Weaver, I. C. G., Cervoni, N., Champagne, F. A., D'Alessio, A. C., Charma, S., Seckl, J., et al. (2004). Epigenetic programming by maternal behavior. *Nature Neuroscience, 7,* 847–854.

Werner, E., & Smith, R. (1992). *Overcoming the odds: High-risk children from birth to adulthood.* Ithaca, NY: Cornell University.

Wichers, M., Purcell, S., Danckaerts, M., Derom, C., Derom, R., Vlietinck, R., et al. (2002). Prenatal life and post-natal psychopathology: Evidence for negative gene–birth weight interaction. *Psychological Medicine, 32,* 1165–1174.

Winter, T., Kaprio, J., Viken, R. J., Karvonen, S., & Rose, R. J. (1999). Individual differences in adolescent religiosity in Finland: Familial effects are modified by sex and region of residence. *Twin Research, 2,* 108–114.

Winterer, G., Egan, M. F., Kolachana, B. S., Goldberg, T. E., Coppola, R., & Weinberger, D. R. (2006). Prefrontal electrophysiologic "noise" and catechol-O-methyltransferase genotype in schizophrenia. *Biological Psychiatry, 60,* 578–584.

Winterer, G., Musso, F., Vucurevic, G., Stoeter, P., Konrad, A., Seker, B., et al. (2006). COMT genotype predicts BOLD signal and noise characteristics in prefrontal circuits. *NeuroImage, 32,* 1722–1732.

Woo, J. M., Yoon, K. S., Choi, Y. H., Oh, K. S., Lee, Y. S., & Yu, B. H. (2004). The association between panic disorder and the L/L genotype of catechol-O-methyltransferase. *Journal of Psychiatric Research, 38,* 365–370.

Zautra, A. J., Hall, J. S., & Murray, K. E. (2008). Resilience: A new integrative approach to health and mental health research. *Health Psychology Review, 2,* 41–64.

Zhou, Z., Zhu, G., Hariri, A. R., Enoch, M. A., Scott, D., Sinha, R., et al. (2008). Genetic variation in human NPY expression affects stress response and emotion. *Nature, 452,* 997–1001.

Zubieta, J. K., Heitzeg, M. M., Smith, Y. R., Bueller, J. A., Xu, K., Xu, Y., et al. (2003). COMT val158met genotype affects mu-opioid neurotransmitter responses to a pain stressor. *Science, 299,* 1240–1124.

Zubieta, J. K., Ketter, T. A., Bueller, J. A., Xu, Y., Kilbourn, M. R., Young, E. A., et al. (2003). Regulation of human affective responses by anterior cingulate and limbic mu-opioid neurotransmission. *Archives of General Psychiatry, 60,* 1145–1153.

B

Cognitive, Affective, and Behavioral Models of Resilience

4

Positive Emotions as a Basic Building Block of Resilience in Adulthood

Anthony D. Ong
C. S. Bergeman
Sy-Miin Chow

More than two decades ago, Lazarus, Kanner, and Folkman (1980) suggested that under intensely stressful conditions, positive emotions may provide an important psychological time-out, sustain continued coping efforts, and restore vital resources that had been depleted by stress. Until recently, there has been little empirical support for these ideas. The empirical record for the adaptive function of positive emotions is beginning to accrue, however. Multiple studies have now shown that positive emotions have a wide range of beneficial downstream effects on individuals (for reviews, see Ashby, Isen, & Turken, 1999; Lyubomirsky, King, & Diener, 2005; Pressman & Cohen, 2005). Both theoretical and empirical work indicate that positive emotions promote flexibility in thinking and problem solving (Isen, Daubman, & Nowicki, 1987), counteract the physiological effects of negative emotions (Fredrickson & Levenson, 1998), facilitate adaptive coping (Folkman & Moskowitz, 2000), build psychological and social re-

sources (Keltner & Bonanno, 1997), and spark enduring well-being (Fredrickson & Joiner, 2002).

In this chapter, we outline the core assumptions and definitions that embody the concept of resilience. We then examine these assumptions by presenting a focused review designed specifically to highlight accumulating evidence that is consistent with the viewpoint that positive emotions represent a basic building block of resilience. We describe how this work has guided our own program of empirical research on positive emotions. Although this research involves multiple methods of data collection (i.e., longitudinal, diary, life history interviews), we outline findings derived from the daily diary process component of our work. In particular, we summarize findings from this research to illustrate the ways a daily process approach can unearth the dynamic character of resilience, as it unfolds both within individuals and across everyday life circumstances. We also present new data, building on the findings from our prior studies. Finally, drawing on these findings, as well as relevant work by others, we discuss priority recommendations for future research.

Historical Overview in Brief

Resilience has numerous meanings in prior research, but generally refers to a pattern of functioning indicative of "positive adaptation" in the context of "risk" or adversity. Underlying this broad definition are two specific conditions: (1) exposure to life risks and (2) evidence of positive adaptation despite threats to development. In early investigations of childhood resilience (e.g., Garmezy, Masten, & Tellegen, 1984; Rutter, 1987; Werner & Smith, 1982), *risk factors* were defined as discrete experiences (e.g., parental psychopathology, community violence) that carried high odds for maladjustment. Over the years (e.g., Luthar, 1999; Luthar & Cushing, 1999; Masten & O'Connor, 1989; Masten & Wright, 1998; Sameroff, Gutman, & Peck, 2003), the concept of risk has been broadened to include cumulative risk indices (e.g., tallies of adverse life events over time), acute trauma and chronic life difficulties (e.g., sexual abuse, neighborhood disorganization), and factors that forecast later maladjustment in the general population (e.g., low birthweight).

Positive adaptation, the second core component of resilience, represents adaptation that is substantially better than would be expected given exposure to significant risk. Although indicators of positive adaptation have varied across the context, population, and risk factor under study (for a review, see Luthar, 2006), extant conceptualizations have, in general, included three kinds of phenomena: good developmental outcomes despite high risk, sustained competence under stress, and recovery from trauma (Masten, Best, & Garmezy, 1990). Under each of these conditions, researchers have focused their attention on identifying *protective factors* that served to modify the adverse ef-

fects of risks in a positive direction. On the basis of early reviews of the childhood and adolescence literature, Garmezy (1985) described three major categories of protective factors: *individual attributes* (e.g., an engaging "easy" temperament and good self-regulation skills), *relationships* (e.g., parental warmth and trust, family cohesion, and close relationships with competent adults), and *external support systems* (e.g., quality neighborhoods and schools and connections to prosocial organizations). This set of protective factors has been remarkably reliable in predicting positive psychological functioning following adversity (Garmezy, 1987; Masten & Coatsworth, 1998; Rutter, 1987; Werner & Smith, 1992). The consistent support for these assets and resources led Masten (2001) to conclude that resilience emerges not from rare or extraordinary qualities and circumstances, but from "the everyday magic of ordinary, normative human resources in the minds, brains, and bodies of children, in their families and relationships, and in their communities" (p. 235).

At the other end of the life course is the growing literature on *optimal aging* (Baltes & Baltes, 1990; Rowe & Kahn, 1987; Schulz & Heckhausen, 1996) that has delineated distinct patterns of *developmental plasticity* (i.e., changes in adaptive capacity) across multiple life domains. This work underscores distinctions between resilience as *recovery* from adversity, and resilience as *maintenance* of development in the face of cumulative risks (for a review, see Staudinger, Marsiske, & Baltes, 1995). Other research has conceptualized resilience as distinct from the process of recovery (Bonanno, 2004). This perspective derives from studies demonstrating that resilience and recovery are distinct outcome trajectories that are empirically separable following highly aversive events, such as interpersonal loss (e.g., Bonanno et al., 2002) and psychological trauma (e.g., Bonanno, Galea, Bucciarelli, & Vlahov, 2006). Finally, several lines of adulthood research emphasize the need to assess positive outcomes (e.g., psychologi-

cal well-being, developmental growth) in response to challenge (Ryff & Singer, 2003a;
Ryff, Singer, Love, & Essex, 1998; Staudinger, Marsiske, & Baltes, 1993; Staudinger et
al., 1995). Studies within this tradition have
elaborated how age-graded influences (e.g.,
Baltes, 1987; Ryff & Heidrich, 1997), normative transitions (e.g., Smider, Essex, &
Ryff, 1996), non-normative events (e.g., Baltes, Reese, & Lipsitt, 1980; Tweed & Ryff,
1991), and chronic life difficulties (e.g., Baltes & Baltes, 1990; Singer & Ryff, 1999) are
linked to various aspects of adult mental and
physical health.

Recent reviews of the burgeoning research on child and adult resilience (Bonanno, 2005; Luthar & Brown, 2007; Ryff
& Singer, 2003a) have revealed important
parallels, as well as notable differences. Although a comprehensive review of the entire
evidentiary record across these two literatures is well beyond the scope of this chapter, we briefly highlight convergent themes
and guiding principles that shore up idiosyncratic viewpoints and approaches evident in
prior work.

From the perspective of human risk and
vulnerability, it is noteworthy that extant
studies of resilience have given limited empirical attention to the exact nature of the
stressors and challenges confronting resilient children and adults. As Ryff and her
colleagues note, in many instances, risk and
vulnerability are inferred from aversive or
otherwise unfavorable contexts (e.g., poverty, parental psychopathology, widowhood)
rather than empirically assessed (Ryff et al.,
1998). Additionally, within the developmental and adult literatures, most researchers
agree that it is important to consider adaptive functioning more broadly, beyond just
the avoidance of psychopathology or negative developmental outcomes (Masten et al.,
1990; Ryff & Singer, 2003a).

Both child and adult literatures (Bonanno, 2004; Luthar & Brown, 2007; Masten,
2001; Ryff & Singer, 2000) emphasize the
need to assess the relative contribution of
personality styles (e.g., ego resilience, posi-

tive self-concepts, hardiness) and environmental resources (e.g., access to supportive
relationships, close and nurturing family
bonds, quality relationships within the community) in response to challenge. Finally,
understanding of specific causal mechanisms
that underlie resilience is a central interest in
both the child and adult literatures (Luthar,
Cicchetti, & Becker, 2000; Rutter, 2000;
Ryff & Singer, 2003a; Ryff et al., 1998);
that is, rather than simply studying which
individual assets and social resources are
associated with positive adaptation, there is
growing awareness of the need to consider
how such factors contribute to resilience in
the face of challenge.

A Daily Process Approach to Studying Positive Emotions

A primary goal of our research has been to
investigate the daily context in which positive emotions arise in response to challenge.
Here we have adopted a daily process approach (i.e., diary methods) to examine how
the nature of stressors and the personality
of those involved can affect the experience
of positive emotion in later adulthood. This
approach involves intensive, day-to-day
monitoring of study variables, allowing us
to view change in fluctuating processes, such
as stress and mood, closer to real-time moments of change. In addition to providing
a framework in which to study inherently
intraindividual (within-person) questions
(Bolger, Davis, & Rafaeli, 2003), diary
methods confer specific methodological
advantages for the study of resilience and
positive emotions. As has been suggested
by others (e.g., Almeida, 2005), perhaps the
primary advantage of this methodology is its
ability to uncover dynamic processes (e.g.,
stress duration and recovery) that are of particular interest to resilience researchers. In
addition, diary methods allow individuals to
report their behavior and experiences over
the range of potentially stressful circumstances encountered in everyday life, thereby

facilitating ecologically valid research (Reis & Gable, 2000). Finally, diary designs have the potential for greater internal validity because the shorter lag between experience and reporting minimizes memory distortions (Stone, Shiffman, & DeVries, 1999).

In our research we have embarked on the study of positive emotions in everyday life by utilizing statistical methodologies that are responsive to dynamic changes over time. A major strength of the analytic approaches we utilize is the ability to model processes that may occur simultaneously within individuals and across contexts. This emphasis on multiple pathways and multiple levels of analysis is consistent with recent reviews of both child and adult resilience (Cicchetti & Dawson, 2002; Luthar & Brown, 2007; Masten, 2007; Ryff & Singer, 2003b). The contemporary statistical approaches we adopt (e.g., multilevel modeling, dynamic systems analysis) have enabled us to address a variety of questions, including some that are difficult, if not impossible, to address with cross-sectional methods. In particular, processes that involve patterns of change (e.g., cycles or rhythms), rates of change (e.g., duration or recovery), speed of change (e.g., nonlinear processes), and covariation in change (e.g., co-occurrence, lagged associations) are all ideally suited for study using multilevel modeling (MLM) and dynamic systems analysis.

Summary of Research Findings

Both the child and adult literatures on resilience have underscored the importance of personality characteristics that may protect individuals against stressful experiences. From the perspective of developmental processes, it is noteworthy that researchers have cautioned against viewing resilience as a stable personality trait. Commenting on the distinction between ego-resiliency and resilience, Luthar and colleagues (2000) noted, "The terms ego-resiliency and resilience differ on two major dimensions. Ego-resiliency

is a personality characteristic of the individual, whereas resilience is a dynamic developmental process. Second, ego-resiliency does not presuppose exposure to substantial adversity, whereas resilience, by definition, does" (p. 546). Recognizing that personality data may become especially powerful explanatory constructs when viewed in connection with dynamic processes that activate and make salient selective individual differences (Fleeson, 2004; Mischel, 2004), our program of research has emphasized the dynamic and coordinated interplay between both *trait* and *process* conceptualizations of resilience. In particular, our daily process research has explored the ways in which resilient personality styles can influence and support meaningful short-term adaptation to daily stress.

Positive Emotions and Personality Resilience

What personality styles are implicated in the generation and maintenance of positive emotions in the face of stress? As suggested earlier, one stable personality trait that has emerged as an important protective asset is *ego resiliency*, defined as the capacity to overcome, steer through, and bounce back from adversity (Block & Block, 1980; Block & Kremen, 1996). In longitudinal studies of personality, *ego-resilient* children were described as confident, perceptive, insightful, and able to have warm and open relations with others (Block, 1971, 1993). *Ego-brittle* children, by contrast, exhibited behavioral problems, depressive symptoms, and higher levels of drug use in adolescence (Block, Block, & Keyes, 1988; Block & Gjerde, 1990). Similar lines of research in adults have yielded evidence of the health benefits of personality resilience.

Personality Resilience and Stress Resistance

If certain personality styles are protective, then it should be possible to characterize such traits in terms of producing observable, coordinated changes in response to stress; that is, it should be possible to verify empirically the adaptive significance of personality in the context of stress (Bonanno, 2005; Curtis & Cicchetti, 2003; Ryff & Singer, 2003a). One way in which personality may play a crucial role in the stress process has been proposed by Zautra, Smith, Affleck, and Tennen (2001) in their dynamic model of affect (DMA). In contrast to other models of stress and coping, which view emotional adaptation entirely in terms of regulating psychological distress, the DMA takes into account the dynamic association between negative and positive emotions. The model predicts that under everyday circumstances, positive and negative emotions are relatively independent, whereas during stressful encounters, an inverse correlation between positive and negative emotions increases sharply, with negative emotions disproportionately outpacing positive ones (for a review, see Reich, Zautra, & Davis, 2003). One implication of the DMA is that the capacity for positive emotional engagement during times of stress may represent one potential pathway underlying stress resistance. According to this hypothesis, personality styles that embody the experience of positive emotions (i.e., personality resilience) should also seed flexible adaptation to stress.

In an initial investigation of the DMA, Ong, Bergeman, Bisconti, and Wallace (2006) examined the relationship between personality resilience and daily stress resistance in three independent samples of older adults. Personality resilience was predicted to carry with it important protective properties that would contribute to stress resistance, assisting high-resilient individuals in their ability to maintain positive emotional engagement effectively while under stress. To test the generalizability of findings, different measures of personality resilience (i.e., ego-resilience, hardiness) and daily distress (i.e., negative affect, anxiety and depressive symptoms) were used. Additionally, given that personality resilience may be negatively

correlated with neuroticism (Maddi et al., 2002), the extent to which the associations among trait resilience, daily stress, and emotion existed separately from their mutual associations with neuroticism was also examined.

Evidence supporting the stress resistance hypothesis was found across all three samples (Ong et al., 2006). Although relatively few key differences were observed between high-resilient individuals and their more vulnerable peers, those differences turned out to be revealing: During times of stress and uncertainty, high-resilient individuals' positive emotions (e.g., cheerful, peaceful, happy) appeared to sit side by side their negative emotions (e.g., anxious, worried, depressed) in relatively independent fashion. Put differently, the positive emotions of resilient individuals were not so easily erased by the negative emotions they experienced in the midst of stress. These findings provide support for the DMA (Zautra et al., 2001) by identifying an important personality style (i.e., personality resilience) underlying daily stress resistance. That is, the benefits conferred by positive emotions may be instantiated in personality styles characterized by positive emotions, bestowing on individuals the facility to experience the full richness and range of experience that makes up human emotional life. These findings also suggest that a more idiographic approach to understanding personality resilience may prove beneficial (Fleeson, 2001, 2004; Fleeson, Malanos, & Achille, 2002).

Personality Resilience and Stress Recovery

Given that resilient individuals are characterized by positive emotionality (Block & Kremen, 1996), it is possible that personality resilience may be associated with not only resistance to but also recovery from stressful life events. In a series of coordinated experimental and individual-difference studies, Fredrickson and colleagues (Fredrickson, Tugade, Waugh, & Larkin, 2003; Tugade,

Fredrickson, & Barrett, 2004) found that high-resilient individuals exhibited faster physiological and emotional recovery from stress. In one study (Tugade et al., 2004), higher personality resilience was linked to quicker cardiovascular recovery following a laboratory stressor. In another study (Fredrickson et al., 2003), higher personality resilience was associated with lower subsequent depressive symptoms.

In our work with older adults, we have hypothesized that *personality resilience*, the propensity to find meaning in difficult circumstances, would constitute an important route to understanding differential recovery from daily stress. To analyze recovery relationships, we examined lagged associations between daily stress and emotion. The results across several studies (Ong, Bergeman, & Bisconti, 2004; Ong et al., 2006) reveal that those high in personality resilience show weaker time-lagged effects of stress on psychological distress; that is, individuals high in personality resilience appear to recover more quickly and efficiently from daily stress than do their less resilient counterparts. In contrast, our analyses also reveal that, for less resilient individuals, the unpleasant experience of one daily stressful event tends to follow on the heels of another, thereby ratcheting up subsequent stress levels even higher.

Attention to Mechanisms

A major objective of our research has been to identify underlying causal mechanisms implicated in the effects of salient protective factors (Luthar et al., 2000; Rutter, 1987). Here our research has focused on the role of positive emotions as one important mechanism underlying resilient adaptation. Our efforts to date have largely explored the degree to which positive emotions account for the protective effects of personality resilience. Concretely, such efforts have involved mapping innovative methodological approaches onto increasingly complex, process-oriented models of resilience.

Protective Benefits of Positive Emotions

In terms of underlying mechanisms, our work has examined a conceptual model in which the effect of personality resilience is mediated through positive emotions (Ong & Bergeman, 2004). According to this model, the effect of personality resilience on adjustment to daily stress is hypothesized to be transmitted, at least partially, through the experience of daily positive emotions. Here we have turned to our research on widowhood for clues about the protective benefits of positive emotions.

Few life events affect adults more than the death of a spouse or life partner (Bonanno & Kaltman, 1999; Stroebe & Stroebe, 1983). Despite the distress and grief that the death of a loved one brings, however, there is considerable variability in individuals' responses to interpersonal loss; some individuals experience acute and enduring psychological distress, whereas others do not (Wortman & Silver, 1989; 1990). Accumulating evidence indicates that a substantial minority of bereaved individuals experience and express positive emotions far more frequently that might have been previously anticipated (Folkman, 1997; Ong et al., 2004). Ong and colleagues (2006) examined the hypothesis that among widows high in personality resilience, positive emotions would contribute to effective emotional recovery from stress. Results from MLM analyses confirmed this prediction. In support of the main hypothesis, our analyses revealed that personality resilience is associated with recovery from daily stress, and positive emotions may be the underlying mechanism by which high-resilient individuals achieve their adaptive outcomes.

Positive Emotions and the Resilience Cascade

Given that positive emotions appear to be an active ingredient in what it means to be "resilient" (Ong et al., 2006; Tugade & Fredrickson, 2004; Tugade et al., 2004), what are the salient mechanisms implicated in this association? Of particular relevance to researchers interested in compensatory models of resilience (e.g., Fergusson & Horwood, 2003; Sameroff et al., 2003) is the critical question of *how* personality resilience contributes to the experience of positive emotion. In our research with older adults, we have explored this question from a daily process perspective. Our work in this area builds on the seminal work of Suls and Martin (2005), who examined the mechanisms underlying vulnerability to neuroticism. From their analyses of the affective dynamics of neuroticism, Suls and Martin identified five fundamental ways in which individual differences in neuroticism could influence psychological distress: (1) hyperreactivity to minor hassles, (2) greater exposure to negative events, (3) appraisal of events as more harmful, (4) mood negative spillover, and (5) inability to adjust to recurring problems. Because these five elements appeared to represent integral components of a coordinated response to stress, Suls and Martin referred to them as the "neurotic cascade."

Our research (Ong, Bergeman, & Boker, in press) extends various aspects of Suls and Martin's framework by including positive dimensions of daily experience and their relationship to personality resilience. In doing so, we have borrowed terminology from previous research in an effort to capture the potential processes that may underlie daily positive experiences. Following recommendations by Zautra, Affleck, Tennen, Reich, and Davis (2005), we use the terms *differential engagement* and *responsiveness* to characterize daily positive events. Finally, in place of negative mood spillover, we examine the extent of positive mood *savoring* in response to daily positive events (Bryant, 2003; Bryant & Veroff, 2007).

Daily diary data on a sample of 300 older adults between the ages of 60 and 90 (*M* = 68.3 years, *SD* = 5.3 years) allowed us to explore potential mechanisms underlying the effects of personality resilience on daily positive emotions. Prior to the diary phase of the study, participants completed a battery of questionnaires that included measures of personality resilience using the Ego Resilience Scale (Block & Kremen, 1996) and neuroticism using the Neuroticism–Extraversion–Openness Personality Profile (NEO; Costa & McCrae, 1991). In addition, participants provided daily reports of their positive emotions using the daily form of the Positive and Negative Affect Schedule (PANAS; Watson, Clark, & Tellegen, 1988). The original PANAS comprises 10 items from the Positive Activation subscale (active, alert, attentive, determined, enthusiastic, excited, inspired, interested, proud, strong). In addition to these items, we included four additional low-arousal items (cheerful, satisfied, relaxed, self-assured) from selected octants of the mood circumplex (Feldman, 1995). Finally, daily positive events were measured using items from the Inventory of Small Life Events (ISLE; Zautra, Guarnaccia, & Dohrenwend, 1986). The ISLE assesses a wide range of everyday positive events in both interpersonal (spouse or significant others, family members, friends) and noninterpersonal life domains (health and finance). The scores were averaged across the five domains, yielding a daily index of positive events.

To suggest that personality can shape our responses to daily experience is to claim that personality styles, such as neuroticism, can set off a complex suite of coordinated responses, propelling a person to act in characteristic ways. There is diverse and abundant evidence that this is so (Bolger & Zuckerman, 1995; Suls & Martin, 2005). Our major aim was to test whether personality resilience would have similar predictive properties that are available within the individual that may be lawfully triggered by daily positive events. In particular, we investigated whether individuals with high personality resilience (compared to those low on the trait) would (1) engage more strongly with positive events, (2) show elevated responsiveness to positive events, and (3) exhibit greater positive mood savoring. Our findings supported each of our main predictions. Specifically, our first hypothesis was that high-resilient individuals would report greater engagement in positive events. Our analyses revealed that for each unit increase in personality resilience, the log-odds of occurrence of a positive event on an average day was .87, which corresponds to a probability of .71, a finding consistent with the *differential engagement hypothesis*.

Next we examined the current and lagged effects of positive events on positive mood (while adjusting for prior mood), whether differences in personality resilience moderated the event–mood relationship, and whether positive mood savoring (the influence of prior mood on present-day mood) mainly applied to high-resilient individuals. Consistent with expectation, higher levels of positive mood were positively associated with personality resilience and with positive event occurrence. More importantly, personality resilience moderated the positive event–mood association: Persons higher in personality resilience were more responsive to positive events when they occurred, a result that supports our *differential responsiveness hypothesis*. Finally, personality resilience moderated the strength of the time-lagged effect of positive emotions: High-resilient individuals were more likely to continue to be in a positive mood as long as 2 lags (days) later, a finding consistent with our *differential savoring hypothesis*. In short, positive emotions appear to stoke an upward spiral of positivity in resilient individuals (Ong et al., in press).

Summary and Conclusion

In this chapter, we have described a program of research on adulthood resilience from a daily process perspective. This research has yielded important clues about the nature of daily resilience as it unfolds in everyday life. We have argued that positive emotions constitute a "basic building block" of resilience. Overall, our research findings dovetail with

past research (e.g., Fredrickson & Levenson, 1998; Lazarus et al., 1980; Zautra, Johnson, & Davis, 2005) in demonstrating that positive emotions may function in the service of well-being by not only interrupting the ongoing experience of daily stress but also averting delays in adaptation to subsequent stressors. Additionally, our findings link up with prior research (e.g., Fredrickson et al., 2003; Tugade & Fredrickson, 2004) in demonstrating positive emotions' enduring connection to personality. Our data suggest that individual differences in personality resilience may constitute an important route to understanding differential resistance to and recovery from daily stress in later adulthood. In particular, personality resilience may contribute to positive adaptation by helping older adults sustain access to daily positive emotions, which in turn may lead to adaptive recovery from stress. Finally, our findings suggest that personality resilience is generative of other assets, catalyzing or setting into motion a *cascade* of positive experiences. Compared to those low in personality resilience, high-resilient individuals appear to exhibit greater engagement in, responsiveness to, and savoring of daily positive events. Taken together, these elements of daily experience may account for the robust effects of personality resilience on positive mood reported in prior research (Ong et al., 2006; Tugade & Fredrickson, 2004; Tugade et al., 2004).

In conclusion, although empirical research on positive emotions is steadily accumulating, a number of fundamental questions remain unanswered. For example, if positive emotions indeed constitute a basic building block of resilience, then should such emotions be viewed as having distinctive patterns of observable responses? That is, if positive emotions can be distinguished by their presumed specific causal mechanisms, then examining the observable outputs for specific positive emotions (e.g., joy, contentment, love) should give evidence of these distinctions. Why then is there little consistent evidence of strong correlations among self-report, behavioral, and physiological measures of discrete positive emotions? Do all positive emotions *broaden* the scope of momentary attention and *build* personal and social resources? If so, do they do so in varying degrees in the context of personal challenge and adversity? Is variation in positive emotional *states* isomorphic with variation in positive emotional *traits*? If so, is such variation evident across cultures? That is, do the effects of positive emotions (on the face, in the voice, in the body, or in experience) run similarly *between*, as well as *within*, individuals? It would be misleading to say that these questions have been overlooked by psychology, but perhaps they should be given much more scholarly attention in defining the paradigm that guides future research.

Finally, given that positive emotions are fleeting and the "broader mindsets" that they produce are fleeting (Fredrickson, 2001), one may reasonably ask what are the enduring, adaptive benefits of such emotions? We have suggested that positive emotions exist in significant measure to promote adaptive flexibility and to teach individuals to take advantage of opportunities that exist in the environment during times of relative calm. The resources that ensue from such opportunities (e.g., personality resilience, engagement in positive events), we argue, are beneficial to both the individual and to society during times of uncertainty. In particular, we contend that the importance of positive emotions lies, for the most part, in the future benefits that accrue from the process of experiencing positive emotion itself rather than achieving any short-term goal.

If our hypothesis is true, it makes us realize more deeply how much our future happiness is knit up by our momentary experience of positive emotions. More than simply reflecting our current success and satisfaction with life, positive emotions are vital to preparing us for an uncertain future by beckoning us to test the boundaries of what we know; to generate creative solutions to looming threats, both small and large; and to expect that behind every stressor we experience lurks unseen, myriad opportunities for transformative growth.

Acknowledgments

Preparation of this chapter was supported in part by grants from the National Institute on Aging (Nos. 1 R01 AG023571-A1-01 and 1 R01 AG-2357-A1-01).

References

Almeida, D. M. (2005). Resilience and vulnerability to daily stressors assessed via diary methods. *Current Directions in Psychological Science, 14*, 64–68.

Ashby, F., Isen, A. M., & Turken, A. U. (1999). A neuropsychological theory of positive affect and its influence on cognition. *Psychological Review, 106*, 529–550.

Baltes, P. B. (1987). Theoretical propositions of life-span developmental psychology: On the dynamics between growth and decline. *Developmental Psychology, 23*, 611–626.

Baltes, P. B., & Baltes, M. M. (Eds.). (1990). *Successful aging: Perspectives from the behavioral sciences.* New York: Cambridge University Press.

Baltes, P. B., Reese, H. W., & Lipsitt, L. P. (1980). Life-span developmental psychology. *Annual Review of Psychology, 31*, 65–110.

Block, J. (1971). *Lives through time.* Berkeley, CA: Bancroft Books.

Block, J. (1993). Studying personality the long way. In R. S. Parke & D. C. Funder (Eds.), *Studying lives through time: Personality and development* (pp. 9–41). Washington, DC: American Psychological Association.

Block, J., Block, J. H., & Keyes, S. (1988). Longitudinally foretelling drug usage in adolescence: Early childhood personality and environmental precursors. *Child Development, 59*, 336–355.

Block, J., & Gjerde, P. F. (1990). Depressive symptoms in late adolescence: A longitudinal perspective on personality antecedents. In A. S. Masten & J. E. Rolf (Eds.), *Risk and protective factors in the development of psychopa-*

thology (pp. 334–360). New York: Cambridge University Press.

Block, J., & Kremen, A.-M. (1996). IQ and ego-resiliency: Conceptual and empirical connections and separateness. *Journal of Personality and Social Psychology, 70,* 349–361.

Block, J. H., & Block, J. (1980). The role of ego-control and ego-resiliency in the organization of behavior. In W. A. Collins (Ed.), *The Minnesota Symposia on Child Psychology* (Vol. 13, pp. 39–101). Hillsdale, NJ: Erlbaum.

Bolger, N., Davis, A., & Rafaeli, E. (2003). Diary methods: Capturing life as it is lived. *Annual Review of Psychology, 54,* 579–616.

Bolger, N., & Zuckerman, A. (1995). A framework for studying personality in the stress process. *Journal of Personality and Social Psychology, 69,* 890–902.

Bonanno, G. A. (2004). Loss, trauma, and human resilience: Have we underestimated the human capacity to thrive after extremely aversive events? *American Psychologist, 59,* 20–28.

Bonanno, G. A. (2005). Resilience in the face of potential trauma. *Current Directions in Psychological Science, 14,* 135–138.

Bonanno, G. A., Galea, S., Bucciarelli, A., & Vlahov, D. (2006). Psychological resilience after disaster: New York City in the aftermath of the September 11th terrorist attack. *Psychological Science, 17,* 181–186.

Bonanno, G. A., & Kaltman, S. (1999). Toward an integrative perspective on bereavement. *Psychological Bulletin, 125,* 760–776.

Bonanno, G. A., Wortman, C. B., Lehman, D. R., Tweed, R. G., Haring, M., Sonnega, J., et al. (2002). Resilience to loss and chronic grief: A prospective study from preloss to 18-months postloss. *Journal of Personality and Social Psychology, 83,* 1150–1164.

Bryant, F. B. (2003). Savoring Beliefs Inventory (SBI): A scale for measuring beliefs about savouring. *Journal of Mental Health, 12,* 175–196.

Bryant, F. B., & Veroff, J. (2007). *Savoring: A new model of positive experience.* Hillsdale, NJ: Erlbaum.

Cicchetti, D., & Dawson, G. (2002). Editorial: Multiple levels of analysis. *Development and Psychopathology, 14,* 417–420.

Costa, P. T., & McCrae, R. R. (1991). *NEO PI-R professional manual.* Odessa, FL: Psychological Assessment Resources.

Curtis, W., & Cicchetti, D. (2003). Moving research on resilience into the 21st century: Theoretical and methodological considerations in examining the biological contributors to resilience. *Development and Psychopathology, 15,* 773–810.

Feldman, L. A. (1995). Variations in the circumplex structure of mood. *Personality and Social Psychology Bulletin, 21,* 806–817.

Fergusson, D. M., & Horwood, L. (2003). Resilience to childhood adversity: Results of a 12-year study. In S. S. Luthar (Ed.), *Resilience and vulnerability: Adaptation in the context of childhood adversities* (pp. 130–155). New York: Cambridge University Press.

Fleeson, W. (2001). Toward a structure- and process-integrated view of personality: Traits as density distributions of states. *Journal of Personality and Social Psychology, 80,* 1011–1027.

Fleeson, W. (2004). Moving personality beyond the person–situation debate: The challenge and the opportunity of within-person variability. *Current Directions in Psychological Science, 13,* 83–87.

Fleeson, W., Malanos, A. B., & Achille, N. M. (2002). An intraindividual process approach to the relationship between extraversion and positive affect: Is acting extraverted as "good" as being extraverted? *Journal of Personality and Social Psychology, 83,* 1409–1422.

Folkman, S. (1997). Positive psychological states and coping with severe stress. *Social Science and Medicine, 45,* 1207–1221.

Folkman, S., & Moskowitz, J. T. (2000). Positive affect and the other side of coping. *American Psychologist, 55,* 647–654.

Fredrickson, B. L. (2001). The role of positive emotions in positive psychology: The broaden-and-build theory of positive emotions. *American Psychologist, 56,* 218–226.

Fredrickson, B. L., & Joiner, T. (2002). Positive emotions trigger upward spirals toward emotional well-being. *Psychological Science, 13,* 172–175.

Fredrickson, B. L., & Levenson, R. W. (1998). Positive emotions speed recovery from the cardiovascular sequelae of negative emotions. *Cognition and Emotion, 12,* 191–220.

Fredrickson, B. L., Tugade, M. M., Waugh, C. E., & Larkin, G. R. (2003). What good are positive emotions in crisis?: A prospective study of resilience and emotions following the terrorist attacks on the United States on September 11,

2001. *Journal of Personality and Social Psychology, 84*, 365–376.

Garmezy, N. (1985). Stress-resistant children: The search for protective factors. In J. E. Stevenson (Ed.), *Recent research in developmental psychopathology: Journal of Child Psychology and Psychiatry book supplement* (pp. 213–233). Oxford, UK: Pergamon Press.

Garmezy, N. (1987). Stress, competence, and development: Continuities in the study of schizophrenic adults, children vulnerable to psychopathology, and the search for stress-resistant children. *American Journal of Orthopsychiatry, 57*, 159–174.

Garmezy, N., Masten, A. S., & Tellegen, A. (1984). The study of stress and competence in children: A building block for developmental psychopathology. *Child Development, 55*, 97–111.

Isen, A. M., Daubman, K. A., & Nowicki, G. P. (1987). Positive affect facilitates creative problem solving. *Journal of Personality and Social Psychology, 52*, 1122–1131.

Keltner, D., & Bonanno, G. A. (1997). A study of laughter and dissociation: Distinct correlates of laughter and smiling during bereavement. *Journal of Personality and Social Psychology, 73*, 687–702.

Lazarus, R. S., Kanner, A. D., & Folkman, S. (1980). Emotions: A cognitive–phenomenological analysis. In R. Plutchik & H. Kellerman (Eds.), *Theories of emotion* (pp. 189–217). New York: Academic Press.

Luthar, S. S. (1999). *Poverty and children's adjustment*: Thousand Oaks, CA: Sage.

Luthar, S. S. (2006). Resilience in development: A synthesis of research across five decades. In D. J. Cohen & D. Cicchetti (Eds.), *Developmental psychopathology: Risk, disorder, and adaptation* (pp. 739–795). Hoboken, NJ: Wiley.

Luthar, S. S., & Brown, P. J. (2007). Maximizing resilience through diverse levels of inquiry: Prevailing paradigms, possibilities, and priorities for the future. *Development and Psychopathology, 19*, 931–955.

Luthar, S. S., Cicchetti, D., & Becker, B. (2000). The construct of resilience: A critical evaluation and guidelines for future work. *Child Development, 71*, 543–562.

Luthar, S. S., & Cushing, G. (1999). Neighborhood influences and child development: A prospective study of substance abusers' offspring. *Development and Psychopathology, 11*, 763–784.

Lyubomirsky, S., King, L., & Diener, E. (2005). The benefits of frequent positive affect: Does happiness lead to success? *Psychological Bulletin, 131*, 803–855.

Maddi, S. R., Khoshaba, D. M., Persico, M., Lu, J., Harvey, R., & Bleecker, F. (2002). The personality construct of hardiness: II. Relationships with comprehensive test of personality and psychopathology. *Journal of Research in Personality, 36*, 72–85.

Masten, A. S. (2001). Ordinary magic: Resilience processes in development. *American Psychologist, 56*, 227–238.

Masten, A. S. (2007). Resilience in developing systems: Progress and promise as the fourth wave rises. *Development and Psychopathology, 19*, 921–930.

Masten, A. S., Best, K. M., & Garmezy, N. (1990). Resilience and development: Contributions from the study of children who overcome adversity. *Development and Psychopathology, 2*, 425–444.

Masten, A. S., & Coatsworth, J. (1998). The development of competence in favorable and unfavorable environments: Lessons from research on successful children. *American Psychologist, 53*, 205–220.

Masten, A. S., & O'Connor, M. J. (1989). Vulnerability, stress, and resilience in the early development of a high risk child. *Journal of the American Academy of Child and Adolescent Psychiatry, 28*, 274–278.

Masten, A. S., & Wright, M. O. D. (1998). Cumulative risk and protection models of child maltreatment. *Journal of Aggression, Maltreatment and Trauma, 2*, 7–30.

Mischel, W. (2004). Toward an integrative science of the person. *Annual Review of Psychology, 55*, 1–22.

Ong, A. D., & Bergeman, C. S. (2004). Resilience and adaptation to stress in later life: Empirical perspectives and conceptual implications. *Ageing International, 29*, 219–246.

Ong, A. D., Bergeman, C. S., & Bisconti, T. L. (2004). The role of daily positive emotions during conjugal bereavement. *Journals of Gerontology B: Psychological Sciences and Social Sciences, 59*, P168–P176.

Ong, A. D., Bergeman, C. S., Bisconti, T. L., & Wallace, K. (2006). Psychological resilience, positive emotions, and successful adaptation to stress in later life. *Journal of Personality and Social Psychology, 91,* 730–749.

Ong, A. D., Bergeman, C. S., & Boker, S. M. (in press). Resilience comes of age: Defining features in later adulthood. *Journal of Personality.*

Pressman, S. D., & Cohen, S. (2005). Does positive affect influence health? *Psychological Bulletin, 131,* 925–971.

Reich, J. W., Zautra, A. J., & Davis, M. C. (2003). Dimensions of affect relationships: Models and their integrative implications. *Review of General Psychology, 7,* 66–83.

Reis, H. T., & Gable, S. L. (2000). Event-sampling and other methods for studying everyday experience. In C. M. Judd & H. T. Reis (Eds.), *Handbook of research methods in social and personality psychology* (pp. 190–222). New York: Cambridge University Press.

Rowe, J. W., & Kahn, R. L. (1987). Human aging: Usual and successful. *Science, 237,* 143–149.

Rutter, M. (1987). Psychosocial resilience and protective mechanisms. *American Journal of Orthopsychiatry, 57,* 316–331.

Rutter, M. (2000). Resilience reconsidered: Conceptual considerations, empirical findings, and policy implications. In S. J. Meisels & J. P. Shonkoff (Eds.), *Handbook of early childhood intervention* (2nd ed., pp. 651–682). New York: Cambridge University Press.

Ryff, C. D., & Heidrich, S. M. (1997). Experience and well-being: Explorations on domains of life and how they matter. *International Journal of Behavioral Development, 20,* 193–206.

Ryff, C. D., & Singer, B. (2000). Interpersonal flourishing: A positive health agenda for the new millennium. *Personality and Social Psychology Review, 4,* 30–44.

Ryff, C. D., & Singer, B. (2003a). Flourishing under fire: Resilience as a prototype of challenged thriving. In J. Haidt & C. L. M. Keyes (Eds.), *Flourishing: Positive psychology and the life well lived* (pp. 15–36). Washington, DC: American Psychological Association.

Ryff, C. D., & Singer, B. (2003b). Thriving in the face of challenge: The integrative science of human resilience. In P. L. Rosenfield & F. Kessel (Eds.), *Expanding the boundaries of health and social science: Case studies in interdisciplinary innovation* (pp. 181–205). London: Oxford University Press.

Ryff, C. D., Singer, B., Love, G. D., & Essex, M. J. (1998). Resilience in adulthood and later life: Defining features and dynamic processes. In J. Lomranz (Ed.), *Handbook of aging and mental health: An integrative approach* (pp. 69–96). New York: Plenum Press.

Sameroff, A., Gutman, L. M., & Peck, S. C. (2003). Adaptation among youth facing multiple risks: Prospective research findings. In S. S. Luthar (Ed.), *Resilience and vulnerability: Adaptation in the context of childhood adversities* (pp. 364–391). New York: Cambridge University Press.

Schulz, R., & Heckhausen, J. (1996). A life span model of successful aging. *American Psychologist, 51,* 702–714.

Singer, B., & Ryff, C. D. (1999). Hierarchies of life histories and associated health risks. In M. Marmot & N. E. Adler (Eds.), *Socioeconomic status and health in industrial nations: Social, psychological, and biological pathways* (pp. 96–115). New York: New York Academy of Sciences.

Smider, N. A., Essex, M. J., & Ryff, C. D. (1996). Adaptation of community relocation: The interactive influence of psychological resources and contextual factors. *Psychology and Aging, 11,* 362–372.

Staudinger, U. M., Marsiske, M., & Baltes, P. B. (1993). Resilience and levels of reserve capacity in later adulthood: Perspectives from life-span theory. *Development and Psychopathology, 5,* 541–566.

Staudinger, U. M., Marsiske, M., & Baltes, P. B. (1995). Resilience and reserve capacity in later adulthood: Potentials and limits of development across the life span. In D. J. Cohen & D. Cicchetti (Eds.), *Developmental psychopathology: Risk, disorder, and adaptation* (Vol. 2, pp. 801–847). Oxford, UK: Wiley.

Stone, A. A., Shiffman, S. S., & DeVries, M. W. (1999). Ecological momentary assessment. In E. Diener & D. Kahneman (Eds.), *Well-being: The foundations of hedonic psychology* (pp. 26–39). New York: Russell Sage Foundation.

Stroebe, M. S., & Stroebe, W. (1983). Who suffers more?: Sex differences in health risks of the widowed. *Psychological Bulletin, 93,* 279–301.

Suls, J., & Martin, R. (2005). The daily life of the garden-variety neurotic: Reactivity, stressor exposure, mood spillover, and maladaptive coping. *Journal of Personality, 73,* 1–25.

Tugade, M. M., & Fredrickson, B. L. (2004). Resilient individuals use positive emotions to bounce back from negative emotional experiences. *Journal of Personality and Social Psychology, 86*, 320–333.

Tugade, M. M., Fredrickson, B. L., & Barrett, L. F. (2004). Psychological resilience and positive emotional granularity: Examining the benefits of positive emotions on coping and health. *Journal of Personality, 72*, 1161–1190.

Tweed, S. H., & Ryff, C. D. (1991). Adult children of alcoholics: Profiles of wellness amidst distress. *Journal of Studies on Alcohol, 52*, 133–141.

Watson, D., Clark, L. A., & Tellegen, A. (1988). Development and validation of brief measures of positive and negative affect: The PANAS scales. *Journal of Personality and Social Psychology, 54*, 1063–1070.

Werner, E. E., & Smith, R. (1982). *Vulnerable but invincible: A study of resilient children.* New York: McGraw-Hill.

Werner, E. E., & Smith, R. S. (1992). *Overcoming the odds: High risk children from birth to adulthood*: Ithaca, NY: Cornell University Press.

Wortman, C. B., & Silver, R. C. (1989). The myths of coping with loss. *Journal of Consulting and Clinical Psychology, 57*, 349–357.

Wortman, C. B., & Silver, R. C. (1990). Successful mastery of bereavement and widowhood: A life-course perspective. In M. M. Baltes & P. B. Baltes (Eds.), *Successful aging: Perspectives from the behavioral sciences* (pp. 225–264). New York: Cambridge University Press.

Zautra, A. J., Affleck, G. G., Tennen, H., Reich, J. W., & Davis, M. C. (2005). Dynamic approaches to emotions and stress in everyday life: Bolger and Zuckerman reloaded with positive as well as negative affects. *Journal of Personality, 76*, 1511–1538.

Zautra, A. J., Guarnaccia, C. A., & Dohrenwend, B. P. (1986). Measuring small life events. *American Journal of Community Psychology, 14*, 629–655.

Zautra, A. J., Johnson, L. M., & Davis, M. C. (2005). Positive affect as a source of resilience for women in chronic pain. *Journal of Consulting and Clinical Psychology, 73*, 212–220.

Zautra, A. J., Smith, B., Affleck, G., & Tennen, H. (2001). Examinations of chronic pain and affect relationships: Applications of a dynamic model of affect. *Journal of Consulting and Clinical Psychology, 69*, 786–795.

5

Personal Intelligence and Resilience

Recovery in the Shadow of Broken Connections

John D. Mayer
Michael A. Faber

Imagine awakening feeling rested and healthy, clear of mind, and looking forward to the day's events. Each of us depends on our body, our relationships, and our social situations for our day-to-day functioning. The connections between our selves—our personalities—and our surrounding systems are crucial to our well-being.

Personality is the individual's master psychological system. It oversees and organizes mental subsystems, such as motives, thoughts, and self-control. Moreover, personality governs the connections between the mind on the one hand, and the body and ongoing social situations on the other. For personality to function well, it must be in tune with all the environmental systems that surround it: the brain and the body that support personality, the stream of social situations that a person encounters, and the groups to which that person belongs. Solid connections in these areas make it easier for a person to make adjustments in overall functioning when such adaptations are needed.

Much of the time, personality juggles the psychological demands placed on it with fluency. Yet each of us also can face setbacks and struggles that require hardiness in the face of adversity. In two cases examined here, life circumstances jeopardized a person's connections to his surrounding systems:

- Hamilton Jordan, a presidential advisor, was diagnosed as a young man with the first of six cancers he would fight throughout his adult life. He describes being in tears after the first diagnosis and cradling his 2½-year-old son in his arms, grateful that his child could not fully appreciate what was happening to them (Jordan, 2001).
- Sammy, a second grader, was transferred

to an Oakland, California, school after his mother's divorce.[1] Sammy lost contact with his father; changed cultures, from the Southern town in which he grew up to a more urban Californian environment; and needed to make new friends and to catch up academically with his peers (Dyson, 1997).

Hamilton Jordan's diagnosis meant that his body might fail him; Sammy's transition to the new Oakland school meant that his social connections had been disconnected—at least temporarily. *Resilience* is a term psychologists use to refer to people's ability to cope with and find meaning in such stressful life events, in which individuals must respond with healthy intellectual functioning and supportive social relationships (Richardson, 2002). When our brains and bodies are healthy, when we interact well with others (and they with us), and when we—and society—maintain a reasonable psychosocial contract, we basically are functioning well. But things rarely go entirely well all the time. Most of us face disruptions in our connections over time. When these connections falter and the failure is substantial, resilience is needed to resolve the disruptions and reintegrate protective factors into our lives (Richardson, 2002; van Hoof & Raaijmakers, 2003).

This chapter focuses in particular on how personal intelligence—an ability to reason about one's own and others' personal information and personality—can promote resilience. Resilience itself is examined in two contexts: a biopsychological connection between personality and an individual's health, and a psychosocial contract between personality and an individual's social relationships. Both health and social connectedness are often stable for long periods of time. Cleavages in these connections, however, can occur unexpectedly at any time. The forms of resilience necessary for coping with disruptions to the two spheres are somewhat different. They share in common, however,

the idea that a certain degree of flexible thinking—a personal intelligence—can help in coming up with solutions.

Personality, Stressors, and Resilience: A Brief Background

Personality and Its Surroundings

Resilience is needed when a person's life connections are challenged. As an individual's most global and overarching psychological system, personality is responsible for the integrated functioning of an individual's mental processes—his or her motives, self-concept, hopes and dreams, and developmental progress. Personality is most likely to function well when it has strong, healthy connections to its surrounding systems, for example, healthy connections to the body and good social interactions.

Figure 5.1 identifies an individual's personality (middle left), including the operation of a person's larger psychological systems (e.g., motives, emotions, self-concept). Underlying overall personality are the brain and other biological systems that give rise to the individual's psychological processes and capabilities. Their position is depicted beneath personality and its subsidiary psychological systems to indicate that such biological systems are "lower level," or more molecular than personality itself; yet the healthy functioning of these smaller systems is essential to a well-connected personality. Similarly, we depend on our setting—our home, our street, our school or office—to be secure places for us. "All the world's a stage," Shakespeare noted, and to that end, each person possesses some props—clothes and jewelry, a briefcase or backpack—and other items with which to play a part on that stage.

Beyond our setting, each of us depends on our smooth interaction with a series of situations so as to maintain ourselves and our well-being. These situations include, for example, doing the laundry, making plans with a family member or friend, presenting a report to a supervisor, and the like (Figure 5.1, middle right). Personality must function fluidly in these situations; the particular situation can support and assist personality or challenge it.

Finally, we all are supported by—and work to maintain—memberships in the groups and societies of which we are a part. We are not just islands unto ourselves, but rather are members of larger communities (Figure 5.1, top). We are members of our families of origin and of new families of our own making through marriage and offspring. We form other groups as well: friends, enemies, links to our MySpace page.

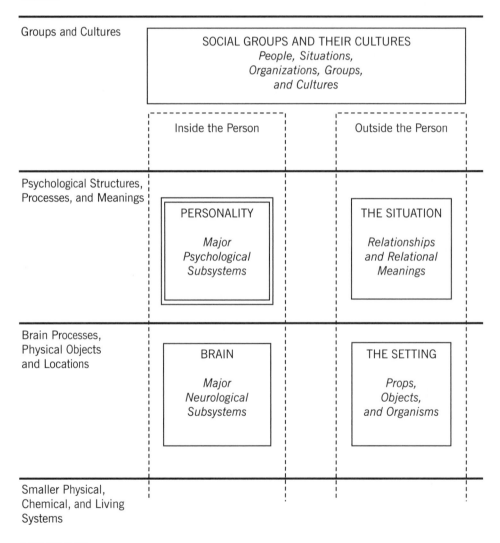

FIGURE 5.1. A structural model of personality amid its neighboring systems. From Mayer (2005, Figure 1). Copyright 2005 by the American Psychological Association. Reprinted by permission.

We are citizens of a town, a state, a nation. We have political, ethnic, and religious identifications that may place us in one group or another (Deaux, Reid, Mizrahi, & Ethier, 1995). We may identify with world civilization as a whole.

The position of personality amid its surroundings, however, speaks as well to personality's vulnerabilities. A weakening or severing of any connection between personality and its surrounding systems, such as the loss of a family member (group environment), or encountering an unsafe setting can place the person at risk. In general, then, personality's coherent functioning is threatened by a failure of any of its connecting systems: by genetic defects that influence the brain, by a chronic setting of poverty, by interactions with a pathogenic boss, or by prolonged or permanent disruptions of the family and broader community. When this happens, resilience is one way in which a robust personality can cope with the problem and restore the individual's psychological functioning to health.

Personality: Risk versus Resilience

Resilience research grew from studies of at-risk children: children who experienced risks, such as divorce and parental drug abuse, that were believed to predispose them to various forms of psychopathology (e.g., Benson, 1997; Richardson, 2002). Initially, researchers focused almost entirely on using risk factors to predict children's later life outcomes. In the course of such studies, however, researchers' attention was drawn to the substantial number of children with severe risk factors, including poverty, large family size, maladaptive temperament, community disruptions, schizophrenic relatives, and so forth, who nonetheless turned out to be healthy, functioning, happy adults (Garmezy, Masten, & Tellegen, 1984; Rutter, 1985; Werner & Smith, 1992).

One key study followed 200 severely at-risk children for nearly 30 years. The children had faced perinatal stress, poverty, daily disruptions to their routine, and severe mental health problems among their parents. Nonetheless, 72 of 200 children did very well as adults (Werner & Smith, 1992). These researchers wondered whether there existed resilience factors that counteracted the risk factors so as to promote positive outcomes, and, if so, what those resilience factors were. They began to turn their attention to the study of resilience, in addition to risk factors.

Summary: The Conditions that Elicit Resilience

Resilience, then, is revealed when an individual is stressed by having his or her unique personal connections severed or placed at risk. Such connections exist in relation to four key systems surrounding personality: the individual's (1) brain and body, (2) setting, (3) ongoing situations and interactions, and (4) social groups. This fourfold arrangement represents a model of the personality's surroundings (Mayer, 1995) and can be used to catalogue and classify various stressors.

Table 5.1 illustrates examples of stressors that can potentially disrupt connections, classified by the four systemic areas that interact with personality. For example, disruptions between personality and the brain and body accompany events such as contracting a mild virus (e.g., a cold) or, more seriously, a chronic illness (Table 5.1, column 2). Disruptions to a person's setting arise when an individual moves or suffers a small financial setback, or, more severely, experiences long-term conditions of poverty or of war (Table 5.1, column 3). Disruptions between personality and the situation involve examples such as chronic stress with one's spouse or family (Table 5.1, column 4). Finally, stressors involving group membership might include an individual's drop in status within, or expulsion from, a group (Table 5.1, column 5). In each instance, the person's level of connection is diminished as a consequence, and stress ensues. In these cases, resilience often is called for in order for the individual to recover and grow.

TABLE 5.1. Risk Factors Catalogued According to the Areas Surrounding Personality

	Areas surrounding personality			
	Brain and body	Setting	Situational interactions	Group memberships
	Examples of associated risk factors			
Mild stressor	Temporary physical Injury	Financial setback	Job interview	Mild group disapproval
Moderate stressor	Moderate injury or illness	Geographic stressor (mild flooding)	Mild public embarrassment	Loss of status within a group
Severe stressor	Severe chronic illness	War, extreme poverty	Ongoing marital distress	Expulsion from a group

Personality Factors Contributing to Resilience

Approaches to Studying Resilience

To date, research has roughly divided individual resilience factors into internal personality factors and factors related to the personality's surrounding systems. Among the personality factors have been social responsibility (conscientiousness), adaptability, tolerance, and achievement orientation; factors concerning the surrounding environment have included the presence of supportive caretakers and community resources, such as recreation centers (Werner & Smith, 1992). For example, Hjemdal, Friborg, Stiles, Rosenvinge, and Martinussen (2006) identified internal factors predictive of resilience, such as personal competence and social competence, and external factors, such as family cohesion and social resources. Moreover, at least some of the internal personality qualities studied today in the positive psychology movement can be regarded as a continuation and outgrowth of resilience research; such factors include gratitude, self-control, forgiveness, creativity, and faith (McCullough & Snyder, 2000; Seligman & Csikszentmihalyi, 2000).

Although one can consider each resilience factor individually, there are limits to such an approach. First, some specific resilience factors likely overlap with others in the same individual, as might be the case with forgiveness and gratitude (i.e., it seems likely that a person who forgives would be more likely to express gratitude). Similarly, optimism and faith would likely co-occur. Still other protective factors may conflict with one another—as might conscientiousness and creativity! The idea that combinations of resilience factors might be more important than specific ones themselves has prompted a second phase of theoretical work on resilience. The process of resilience is one that involves disruption and reintegration (e.g., Flach, 1997; Richardson, Neiger, Jensen, & Kumpfer, 1990). This second phase of theoretical work asks what personality (and community) processes foster and ultimately draws together a group of especially resilient factors.

It seems clear that certain worldviews, communicated successfully by a community, may provide such resilient qualities. For example, in poor black communities in the United States, the Black Church, which emphasizes factors such as forgiveness, gratitude, optimism, and achievement, may provide an external support that weaves together such a vision for an individual (Regnerus & Elder, 2003). Yet such religious factors come in many variations; certain variations may be less helpful, and some can discourage personal growth by, for example, emphasizing a "shoot low" perspective for the individual so as to stay out of trouble (e.g., Suskind, 1998, p. 68).

Are there factors within personality itself that help foster productive worldviews as well? A number of personality psychologists and resilience researchers have believed so, but the understanding of such personal development is incomplete. There has been a split in vision among theorists about how best to frame such a determinant of personal growth. Some psychologists suggest there is an innate growth mechanism that propels a person toward positive development. This approach, which is similar to self-actualization, as proposed by Carl Rogers and Abraham Maslow, describes resilience sometimes as a "spiritual source or innate resilience" and states that "there is a force within everyone that drives them to seek self-actualization, altruism, wisdom, harmony with a spiritual source of strength" (Richardson, 2002, p. 313). These views consider growth, in essence, to be a basic psychological drive. However, a second viewpoint, which might be referred to as the *planful* perspective on resilience, views such growth as the product of a thoughtful, reasoned approach to life. It is this latter viewpoint on which we focus in discussing the role of personal intelligence as it pertains to resilient functioning.

Personal Intelligence as a Factor in Resilience

The planful perspective on resilience emphasizes not so much an innate propensity to thrive and develop as it does the ability to problem-solve about life problems in an active way that promotes personal psychological growth and maturity. The concept of psychological mindedness, dating from the 1940s, represents such a resilience factor. Psychologically minded individuals were said to possess a constellation of abilities that made them better able than others to both learn about and change themselves. In particular, these individuals wanted to understand "relationships among thoughts, feelings, and actions, with the goal of learning the meanings and causes of his experiences and behavior" (Appelbaum, 1973, p. 36). People high in such abilities were said to exhibit an interest in others and what moti-

vates them, and an orientation that included a focus on future life planning (Appelbaum, 1973; McCallum & Piper, 1997).

Years later, Block and Block (1980, p. 48) described a related concept, ego resilience, as

> resourceful adaptation to changing circumstances and environmental contingencies, analysis of the "goodness of fit" between situational demands and behavioral possibility, and flexible invocation of the available repertoire of problem-solving strategies. ...

Howard Gardner (1983) also introduced at about this time the paired concepts of intrapersonal and interpersonal intelligences, which involved a complex of abilities, including the group capacities to reason about one's feelings, oneself, and society. Epstein (1998) added to these concepts the idea of *constructive thinking*: a constellation of thought processes that involved the capacity to carry out adaptive coping and to avoid superstitious, pessimistic, and self-defeating thought. There are, in other words, a number of theories related to problem solving about the self in its context.

A more recent concept—personal intelligence—draws together many ideas from some of those earlier theoretical formulations, and applies the intelligence concept to personality and personal information (Mayer, 2008). The personal intelligence concept depends, in part, on a growing convergence across theoretical perspectives as to what the personality system is like and how it functions (Buss, 2001; Funder, 2006; Mayer, 2005; McAdams & Pals, 2006; McCrae & Costa, 1999; Roberts, Kuncel, Shiner, Caspi, & Goldberg, 2007). Drawing together those consensual approaches, the theory states that

> personal intelligence involves the abilities: (a) to recognize personally-relevant information from introspection and from observing oneself and others, (b) to form that information into accurate models of personality, (c) to guide one's choices by using personality information

where relevant, and (d) to systematize one's goals, plans, and life stories for good outcomes. (Mayer, 2008, p. 215)

The presence of these abilities may be expressed in an individual's life in unique ways (Mayer, 2008, 2009), as we will see.

Personal Intelligence Compared to Emotional and Other Intelligences

Personal intelligence is part of a larger group of intelligences referred to as "hot" that include the social and emotional intelligences. For most of the 20th century, psychologists favored the study of "cool" (as opposed to hot) intelligences. The cool intelligences involve abstract reasoning about information that is typically general and impersonal. Verbal intelligence, for example, is concerned with word and propositional meanings; perceptual–organizational intelligence is concerned with identifying and reasoning about visual patterns. By contrast, hot intelligences concern the capacity to reason with information that is accompanied by psychic pleasure or pain (Mayer, Roberts, & Barsade, 2008). Examples of these intelligences include social intelligence, which involves reasoning about one's own and others' social situational behaviors; emotional intelligence, which involves reasoning about emotions, emotional information, and their meanings; and personal intelligence, as developed here, which concerns reasoning about personal information, one's self-concept, and life plans, among other areas.

Personal, social, and emotional intelligences are thus distinct members of the hot intelligence group; however, personal intelligence is broader than emotional intelligence. *Emotional intelligence* (EI) is defined as the capacity to reason about emotions and emotional knowledge, and to use emotions to enhance thought (Mayer et al., 2008). In contrast, *personal intelligence* (PI) addresses an individual's understanding of not only emotions, but also of his or her motives, self-concepts, dreams, imaginings, and other internal experiences and mental models of the self and others (Mayer, 2008). PI is also different than (but complementary to) social intelligence. PI focuses on inner personal experience and personal information in oneself and others. By contrast, social intelligence is relatively outer directed and involves reasoning about situations, interactions, social skills, and the interactions among groups (Weis & Süß, 2007).

Its initial theoretical development suggests that PI, in particular, describes specific inner qualities relevant to a person's resilience. The next section of this chapter examines two individuals who needed resilience in their lives, and how PI might have contributed to each person's response to challenging circumstances.

Life Falls Apart and Comes Together Again: PI in Two Brief Cases

PI concerns problem solving about personality and personal information. Resilience, in turn, concerns dealing with situations in which a person's life connections fall apart, and the individual must cope somehow. How might PI apply? Personal intelligence concerns four areas: identifying personal information, developing self- and other-models of personality, using such information to guide choices, and systematizing one's life. These areas of PI may be relevant to resilient responding when life's connections are strained or broken.

Identifying Personal Information

PI involves the capacity to identify accurate information about oneself based on one's own introspections and others' feedback. In regard to one's own personality this sometimes involves a certain amount of cleverness because the people surrounding us often may want to conceal or sugarcoat their complete and honest feedback to avoid hurt feelings, personal embarrassment, or unpleasant realities.

For Hamilton Jordan, a time arose during a visit to his doctor's office when, as he described it, he knew something was wrong. His doctor had sent him to the hospital for an X-ray rather than performing it himself in his office. A few hours after returning to the doctor's office from the hospital, his doctor spoke on the phone to the radiologist. Jordan (2001) recounts:

I strained to hear, but all I could make out was, "I understand, yes ... I understand."

He hung up the phone, turned away as if to avoid contact, slid the X-rays out of the large brown envelope, turned them upright one by one and lined them up on the illuminated viewer. ... "Hamilton, I hate to tell you this, but you have an abnormal chest film."

He paused to watch me as his words sank in. "This spot here is some kind of mass ... some kind of growth."

"Could it be cancerous growth?" I asked quietly.

"Yes," he said slowly, picking his words carefully. (p. 5)

Jordan's story includes an evocative personal account of his own altered feelings and awareness in response to the news. His ability to access his own internal mental states is a key part of personal intelligence. Jordan recounts:

I was stunned and just sat there, staring at the film. I felt like someone had suddenly pulled a plug and all the energy and feeling was flowing from my body. I had a surreal sense of standing apart from this bizarre scene and watching myself sitting in the examination room, talking with my doctor friend, asking predictable questions. (pp. 4–5)

Jordan's medical diagnosis represented an attenuation of his psychobiological connection—a breach between mind and body. However, perhaps due to his PI, his resilience response began with a detailed awareness of his situation.

Another part of PI involves seeking accurate information about oneself. Jordan sought accurate medical information and guidance from the start. When a physician told him there existed a reasonably effective treatment option for his condition, Jordan asked, "Reasonably [effective], doctor? What does that mean?" And after the doctor replied somewhat indirectly, Jordan persisted, exclaiming to the doctor, "Just quantify it for me!" Receiving yet another unsatisfactory response, Jordan insisted further that he wanted a precise, accurate answer. It was then the doctor told him his chance of surviving for 5 years was about 25% (Jordan, 2001, pp. 3–4). The pursuit of accurate feedback also is a key part of PI.

Although not everyone may be able to be this assertive (and not everyone may wish for this level of accurate information at the moment of hearing such news), accurate knowledge can be life-preserving. Although optimism generally predicts good health outcomes, the distortions of unrealistic optimism can be dangerous in medical and behavioral health contexts. Smokers, for example, who are unrealistically optimistic about their health status are less likely than other smokers to plan to stop smoking (Dillard, McCaul, & Klein, 2006). Similarly, students who are unrealistically optimistic about their health problems learn less about disease prevention and are less motivated to exercise (Davidson & Prkachin, 1997).

Jordan's monitoring of information also allowed for the correct evaluation of erroneous reports concerning his medical condition. A dramatic but amusing example of this occurred as he sat in his hospital room with his mother and sister, awaiting his diagnosis. A picture of him appeared on a local TV channel, and when he turned up the volume, he heard, "CBS has learned that former Carter aide Hamilton Jordan ... has been diagnosed with inoperable lung cancer" (Jordan, 2001, p. 2). After a moment of panic he realized that if his doctor (with whom he had just spoken) did not yet know what he had, CBS News probably did not know either. Such successful, quick, and accurate filtering of information reduced Jordan's stress and no doubt contributed to his resilience over time.

Developing Models of the Self and Others

A second area of PI involves developing accurate models of the self and others. The question "Who am I?" is one of the big questions of antiquity and of the modern day, of psychology and of personality as well (Mayer, 2007). To answer this question, each individual must develop an identity, or multiple identities (to fit specific contexts). This can be a lifelong project of discerning and filtering ideas of who one is, who one is not, and who one wants to be.

Identification occurs when an individual aspires to be the kind of person he or she perceives another as being, and alters his or her personality accordingly (Block & Turula, 1963). People often identify with admired others, and watching how such admired others behave may provide clues as to how to cope with new demands, reflecting an individual's capacity to adapt (Sanford, 1955). In healthy instances, individuals who are more identified are more resilient to environmental changes because they have internalized some of the strengths of admired others (Block & Turula, 1963).

Historically, many theorists believed that identity is crystallized in adolescence. Today, however, identity development is believed to begin before and to continue well beyond adolescence (Cramer, 2004; van Hoof & Raaijmakers, 2003). In this lifespan approach, the act of identification involves a person taking on as one's own another's values, attitudes, and behaviors, and integrating them to enhance his or her psychological security. To the extent that the target of identification has lived well, this integration can provide useful guidance during difficult times (van Hoof & Raaijmakers, 2003).

Personal identifications are a bit different from social identifications with peer groups, which are usually established along demographic or membership characteristics (e.g., socioeconomic status, activities/inter-ests, vocations, political affiliations, ethnic/religious groups, stigmatized groups, etc.; Deaux et al., 1995). Personal identifications more clearly involve an internal comparison and a judgment of the individual's possible selves (Block & Turula, 1963; Petrocelli & Smith, 2005). Group identifications, by contrast, involve assimilation and the perception of homogeneity—the subordination rather than the refining of the unique individual (De Cremer, 2004; Deaux et al., 1995). Although the process of developing a group identity is essential for establishing belongingness and social support, for some of the same reasons it cannot replace a strong and definitive personal identity. For example, in some instances, threats to one's personal identity are considered more dangerous to an individual than threats to his or her group identity (Gaertner, Sedikides, & Graetz, 1999). This seems to make sense both logically and evolutionarily; a focused attack on an individual has more immediate relevance to that person's survival than does a more diffuse attack on a larger group, to which any member(s) could conceivably respond on behalf of the group or the embattled individual. It must therefore be of surpassing importance to protect the people, values, and attitudes with which we identify individually because we alone are accountable when those values and attitudes are put to the test, as in the case of stressful life events that require resilient coping.

It is the richness of one's own self-depiction—through self-knowledge, creativity, and traits such as openness to experience—that predicts the fullness of one's identification with others (Clancy & Dollinger, 1993; Dollinger & Clancy, 1993). Even the person's use of consumer goods can play a role beyond the product's immediate usefulness in signifying the development of personal identification; particularly emblematic are things such as clothes, music choice, favorite TV shows, and slang (Rattansi & Phoenix, 1997).

The identification process begins as children start to understand some of the elements of personality, such as general typologies of individuals both real and fictional, then gradually shape them into more realistic images of themselves and understandings of others. These childhood images of personality can include imaginary beings, as well as real ones. Whether real or imagined, these characters help to teach us the existence of individual differences and the different forms personality can take. Understanding the possibilities of such individual differences can help a person develop a more accurate and useful identity. A good sense of identity, in turn, promotes successes in maintaining personal achievements, such as one's marriage and occupational satisfaction (Pals, 1999).

Resilience and Personal Identification with PI: The Case of Sammy

One young child's experience illustrates how resilience and learning about personality-relevant information can grow together. Sammy began the second grade in a new school. He knew no one and was enrolled well after the official beginning of classes. He needed an imaginative world at least for a while to provide some stability in a world full of real disruptions. Sammy's mother recently had brought him, along with two younger daughters, to his new neighborhood in Oakland, California, following her divorce. The transition severed Sammy's connections to his father, to his old school and his friends there, and to his earlier community in the Deep South. He was isolated now in the new school, and needed to establish some new kind of life.

Parents and/or caretakers are the first figures with whom a child tends to identify, followed by other close, admired persons. Cramer (2004) suggests that separation from or loss of a parent may be a catalyst for insecurity, confusion, and anxiety. Facing such isolation, Sammy had to find a source of identification that would allow him some security and the ability to forge new connections with his classmates. He accomplished

this through his fondness for the superhero characters the children all knew from the mass media. By identifying with these popular characters, Sammy not only found an effective coping mechanism for himself but was also able to make new friends by sharing experiences with them through imaginative play with popular fictional characters.

Psychologists often distinguish between *inner-focused coping* (changes in the self) and *surround-focused* or *behavioral coping*, which focuses on making changes in the environment (Folkman & Lazarus, 1980). Lacking the power to influence his environment, Sammy's initial identification with superheroes can be considered inner-focused coping—changes to his inner personality. One of Sammy's chief means of inner coping was to replace his real-but-lost connections to his friends and his father with connections to imaginary beings—specifically, to the superheroes of the X-Men and Ninja Turtles stories (Dyson, 1997). Although inner coping usually is hidden, in this case, a group of educators and psychologists observed Sammy and charted the progress in his school writing and conversations.

Commentary on PI and Sammy's Coping Strategies

Sammy's choice of thinking about and imagining superheroes was unlikely to have been accidental or haphazard. People distinguish between types of characters and tend to resonate quite differently to different sorts of actors. For example, one series of research studies indicates that people are drawn to one of five or so key types of archetypal characters in the popular media that permeate our lives. These archetypes include the Knower (which includes magician- and sage-like characters), the Carer (which includes lovers and caregivers), the Striver (which includes heroes), the Conflictor (which includes outlaws and shadow figures), and the Everyperson (persons like the rest of us) (Faber & Mayer, 2009).

The hero—the character with which Sammy resonated—belongs to the Striver group. These archetypes exist to triumph within their world—to carry out difficult and heroic tasks to overcome challenges and defeat threats, to achieve great things, and to become an inspiration to those that follow. Such Striver figures are very attractive to children who acutely perceive injustices and often suffer from their own powerlessness to repair them. Thus, playing superhero Strivers allows children an outlet for dealing with their powerlessness. A person's resonance with the Striver, in particular, can be distinguished from his or her responsiveness to other characters (e.g., Knowers or Carers), even across different representations of archetypal themes, such as those portrayed in film, art, and music (Faber & Mayer, 2009). Figure 5.2 shows examples of Knower, Carer, and Striver archetypes, each spanning two forms of media. Examples of the Knower embody a general archetypal character who values knowledge, wisdom, or aesthetic beauty. People who resonate favor-

ably toward such prototypical characters are likely to identify with them in their real lives, as well as with what they represent: Many of them may feel drawn to become artists, doctors, or teachers. Other archetype clusters, such as the Carer (lower left) and Striver (lower right), also have their own distinctive characteristics, and the people who gravitate toward them are likewise apt to adopt those characteristics (Faber & Mayer, 2009).

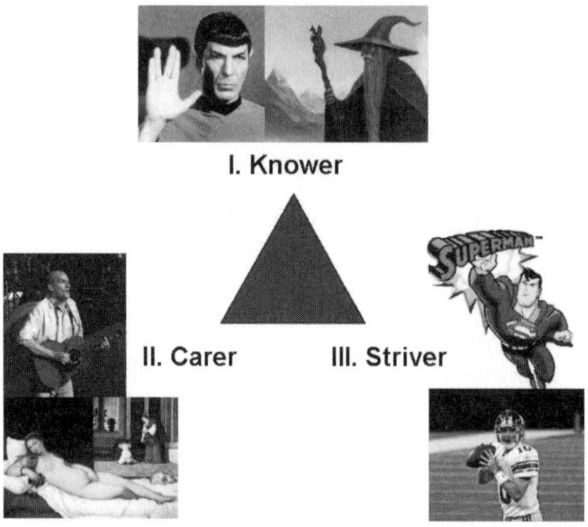

Although these identifications likely are more or less automatic in young children, identification can be viewed as an active process by which personality changes (Sanford, 1955). Those with demonstrable PI can effectively reason about such objects of identification and learn about personality from them. When children are under stress, they may rely on these imaginative identifications as a strategy to create attachments when others cannot be found. In her study of children who write about superheroes, Dyson (1997) remarked that many children use superheroes

FIGURE 5.2. Clockwise from top left: Knower images: Mr. Spock and Gandalf the Wizard (created by D. E. Phillips); Striver images: Superman and Eli Manning (photo by W. K. Hunter); Carer images: *Venus of Urbino* (painted by Titian) and James Taylor (photo by P. Keleher). All images used under license from creative commons; downloaded April 24, 2009, from *creativecommons.org/about/licenses*.

to achieve a sense of personhood and social belonging, of control and agency in a shared world. In making use of these symbols, children could assume identities within stories that revealed dominant ideological assumptions about relations between people—between boys and girls, adults and children, between people of varied heritages physical demeanors, and societal powers. These stories reflected the immediate values and interests of some children. (p. 2)

Use of Self-Models to Guide Choices

People with higher PI (relative to those lower in it) may be better able to use their knowledge of characters and characterization to fit within an environment. In Sammy's case, his interest and knowledge of superheroes began to interest other students in his class. Socioanalytic theorists talk about how social roles—including imaginary roles such as superheroes—help define relationship interactions among children (Hogan, 1982).

In Sammy's case, some of his peers became interested in playing superhero roles with him. Sammy used his ability to characterize superheroes to write increasingly sophisticated stories that he and his peers could enact. His new friends relied on Sammy's understanding of how such superheroes (and supervillains) interacted. On an occasion when Sammy failed to produce a story, his classmates were sorely disappointed. An observer recorded the child "Margaret" narrating one of Sammy's more disappointing stories ("Once upon a time there was X-Men, the bad guys, and they tried to destroy X-Men.") The observer recorded the following:

(The children [both boys and girls] begin to play out a mock battle, but, after a few minutes, they stop and stare at each other. ... Sammy's stories are always very long—but not this time, for some reason. The children sit down, grumbling about the short story.)
SAMMY: Ms. S. said we have 5 minutes and I couldn't finish it. I'll finish it tomorrow. Maybe we could play outside. ... Maybe at recess if I finish we could play X-Men. (Dyson, 1997, p. 63)

Sammy's uncharacteristic failure to produce a story in this instance reflected how important his storytelling had been in establishing connections among the children. Sammy effectively used his knowledge of personality-related information to entertain himself and his peers—to create friendship opportunities, to guide himself, and to fit into the world in a way tailored to meet his needs at that time in his development after the loss of earlier relationships. Moreover, he was able to change what had begun as inner coping through the use of personal fantasy to coping aimed at creating a new social group.

A similar (although more adult) form of coping occurred for Hamilton Jordan. Biopsychological challenges often first demand a considerable degree of inner coping. What makes such illnesses as Jordan's so insidious is that their course is only partially (if at all) under one's control. PI here focuses on acceptance and coping, as well as a special awareness of what is important. In respect to inner coping, Jordan employed a number of ways of framing and reframing the challenges he faced. As is the case for others who face such challenging stress, the consequences can be bracing:

A life threatening disease like cancer is a strange blessing that casts our life and purpose in sharp relief. ... I never want to forget the raw fear of cancer and the prospect of death. Because if I am ever able to simply block out those memories and set my emotions aside, I will lose the ironic blessing, the sense of purpose and focus that cancer has given my own life. (Jordan, 2001, p. 216)

This is, however, a resilient response; others understandably react to such news with a sense of isolation, discouragement, and despair. The personality attributes (and life context) that determine one's response go far beyond PI itself, and also include issues such as one's emotional disposition, prior experiences with illness, and the specific impact of the illness itself on one's health and well-being. Still, Jordan's resilient response was not isolated. When discussing such responses, Jordan's friend who was battling a brain tumor told him, "There is no such thing as a bad day!" (Jordan, 2001, p. 216).

With inner coping may come new ways to view oneself. Jordan developed an alternative identity as a successfully coping cancer patient—successful in the sense of having survived multiple cancers for a considerable time. He used that new sense of identity as a springboard for various life choices during his illnesses. Dorothy Jordan, Hamilton's wife and a pediatric oncology nurse, had begun a nonprofit camp called Camp Sunshine for children with cancer. Hamilton was drawn into the project because of his connection to his wife and his own bouts with cancer (Jordan, 2001). Again, in this instance, his own experiences with cancer and his acceptance of it indicated how using accurate self-knowledge—including one's evolving identity as a cancer patient and cancer survivor—can help to establish a new set of positive connections to the surrounding social world. It appears likely that others sense when an individual is using positive coping and are drawn to such successful individuals, both to learn how to do the same for themselves, and because such successes make the individual a better companion.

Systematizing Goals, Plans, and Life Stories

The fourth part of PI involves the ability to systematize one's goals, plans, and life stories in a meaningful fashion. When there are challenges in one's environment, as happens after a loss, people often have to rethink their life stories and what they mean. Reasoning about their autobiographies also helps individuals define themselves more generally (Bluck, Alea, Habermas, & Rubin, 2005; Pillemer, 2003). As people recall their life experiences, they have the more general opportunity to systematize their goals, plans, and autobiographical stories to create a personal sense of coherency and meaning from their lives (Erikson, 1963; Frankl, 1963; McAdams, 2006).

People recall events to see whether their "beliefs or values have changed" and to understand "who I am now" (Bluck et al., 2005, p. 104), as well as to find meaning in their pursuits and life stories. This meaning typically involves a sense of generating something to help the next generation, be it rearing a family or producing work to assist other people (Erikson, 1963). In a review of motivational research on writers (both professional and otherwise), Kellogg (1994, p. 103) emphasized the contributions of not only general intelligence but also of the meaning making that writing brings with it. According to Kellogg, making meaning defines our species, and writing provides a means for such meaning making. These observations suggest that a key contribution of the study of actors and writers (for this purpose) is to highlight their capacity to empathize with different characters, their tendency to observe carefully the mannerisms and

expressions of others, and their willingness to use writing, for example, as a method of meaning making in their lives.

Meaning making is an ongoing life process, and there is no reason to believe that it does not start early in life. Sammy's superhero stories were written at a second-grade level: His meaning making regarded the forces of good versus evil and the hero's capacity to triumph, and the relationships he built more generally plainly involved some elementary systematizing of his life needs at that time. Moreover, his interests and goals, which in part included superheroes, were organized to promote his social relationships. A similar process, but at a more sophisticated adult level, occurred for Hamilton Jordan. Jordan's authoring of his memoir is itself representative of his organizing and systematizing the information of his life.

Discussion

Connections and Resilience

To be resilient, a person must maintain productive interactions with his or her biological and social surroundings: his or her own body and its health, on the one hand, and the surrounding setting, situations, and societies, on the other. Making connections and maintaining good interactions may depend in part on PI, which comprises four abilities: (1) to recognize personality-relevant information accurately, (2) to form models of one's own and others' personalities, (3) to guide one's choices with such information, and (4) to systematize one's goals, plans, and life story for good outcomes (Mayer, 2008).

The need for resilience arises when there is a break in one or more key connections between an individual and his or her surrounding systems—a decline in health in the biological sphere, or a disconnection in interpersonal relations. In this chapter, we examined resilience in response to such disconnections in relation to both health and social interactions. Two cases illustrated such interrupted connections: The first involved Hamilton Jordan's struggles with cancer, and the second, the young boy Sammy, who had begun school in a new community after his mother's divorce. In each case, resilience involved moving from a state of lesser connection to one of greater connection.

These movements are illustrated in Figures 5.3 and 5.4. Figure 5.3 illustrates the potential movement from a broken connection—an extreme threat to health—back to full health. Figure 5.4 represents the potential movement from extreme social isolation back to social integration. Personality can survive and thrive without going all the way back to a fully connected relationship either to health or to social interactions; the successful movement and satisfaction with one's progress toward those goals, however, represents resilience. Each individual area of PI can contribute to such a journey toward reconnection.

The first area of PI—recognizing personality-relevant information—involves the capacity to accurately perceive and filter information about personality. It is important to identifying the relevant challenges and opportunities during times of personal adversity that may call for resilience. The more accessible and undistorted the information, the better off the individual may be.

Second, PI helps individuals form accurate mental models of themselves and others. Personal losses often involve separations from important others in one's life, due to events such as divorce, illness, war, or death. In this chapter we focused in particular on models of respected, admired, and even idealized others that may accompany such losses. Such role identifications represent models of others that can provide a compensatory relationship at a distance for personal losses, and in this way bring out one's strengths in adversity. This in turn is likely to lead to better developmental outcomes: For example, highly identified individuals experience higher levels of work success, community and political involvement, and family/marital success than others (Cramer, 2004). Even if someone experiences upheaval and

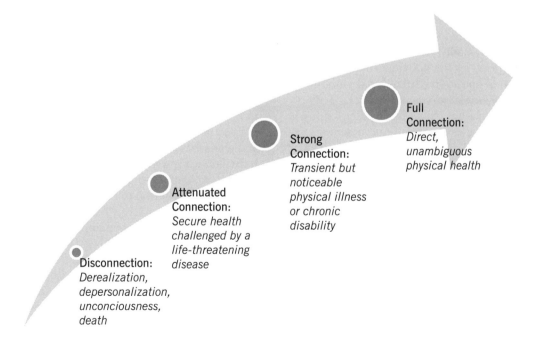

FIGURE 5.3. The range of connectedness between personality and underlying biological health.

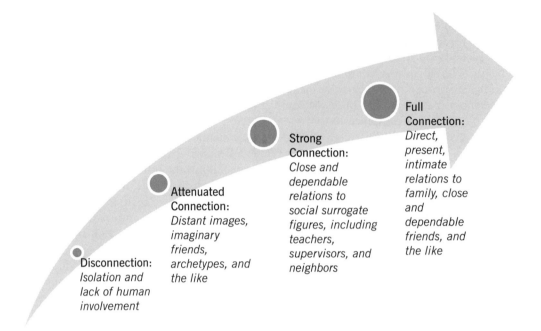

Full Connection: *Direct, present, intimate relations to family, close and dependable friends, and the like*

Strong Connection: *Close and dependable relations to social surrogate figures, including teachers, supervisors, and neighbors*

Attenuated Connection: *Distant images, imaginary friends, archetypes, and the like*

Disconnection: *Isolation and lack of human involvement*

FIGURE 5.4. The range of connectedness between personality and interactions with others.

separation from a significant caretaker—as Sammy did in leaving behind his father—an internalization of a role model's values keeps that person psychologically present in the observer's mind. Identifying with another person (whether real or imagined) in this way provides the individual with a veritable guiding spirit—the archetypal embodiment of one's own personal ideal self. This process is made possible by forming highly accurate models of the self and others.

Third, PI helps to guide an individual's choices when encountering difficult situations—a process that is key to resilient coping. Understanding the context of a problem—even implicitly—helps the person frame the situation appropriately and allows him or her to take on the needed role to resolve the problem successfully. The realization that his superhero stories meant as much to his peers as they did to him allowed Sammy to draw on the general appeal of the X-Men and the Ninja Turtles to forge new connections with the children at his new school. It was his awareness of the situation and his implicit self-knowledge that allowed Sammy to know what had to be done if he wanted to cope socially and emotionally with his initial isolation. Similarly, Hamilton Jordan's struggles with cancer allowed him a new willingness to help others with the same disease and to give them strength and support. In so giving, he was rewarded in return by the new connections he made in life.

Fourth, PI helps with systematizing goals and plans for future functioning; it allows the individual to construct a better life story. A mature person with high PI is likely not only to be able to recognize relevant problems and cope with them but also to construct meaning from the ordeal. For example, Hamilton Jordan was able to synthesize these aspects of his situation through his own PI, and in composing his memoirs (Jordan, 2001), he provided others in similar circumstances an inspirational blueprint: a blow-by-blow account of how they, too, might cope with such adversity. This systematizing goes beyond the perception of personality-relevant information, beyond forming models of oneself and others, and beyond making choices. The ability to form a coherent story involves capacities to discover a possible significance in events; to identify the productive aspects of one's own (and others') actions, and ultimately to be satisfied with some sort of personal growth.

Future Research in PI and Resilience

At present, research into PI is just beginning. The outline of an empirically informed theory of PI has been established (Mayer, 2008, 2009). Typically, the next stage in establishing the concept is the development of relevant measurement instruments. The "gold standard" for measurement in intelligence involves ability testing (Mayer et al., 2008), and this will likely be the case for PI as it has been for other intelligences, both cool and hot. People higher in PI, for example, ought to be better able than others to understand which traits are most likely to co-occur in a person. For instance, individuals high in PI should be able to recognize that a person's innovative qualities imply that he or she is more likely to be tolerant, relative to others, than to be loyal. Some preliminary data collected along these lines present an encouraging picture regarding the existence of PI.

If PI exists as hypothesized and is a factor that contributes to an individual's resilience, then it may provide a buffer against personal risks and impaired connections with one's surroundings. Like most personality variables that have not yet been extensively studied, the degree to which PI is heritable or influenced by environmental factors is unknown. Most people are likely to possess a sufficient amount of PI (or other compensatory intelligences) to be able to acquire new learning in the area of personality. It is likely, therefore, that teaching people about personal information, personality in general, its functions, and how to systematize plans and goals could provide a buffering effect against some forms of risk. It is likely that some educational programs in coping

with risk—for example, coping with medical disease or social loss—already do this. Developing curricula based more explicitly on a theory of PI may improve the coherence of such teachings and render the programs based on those teachings more effective. These are, however, speculations, until more is known.

Empirical research is still needed to determine whether, for example, people with highly accurate and informed self-knowledge make better use of such knowledge than others to repair and maintain their personal connections. For example, experimental groups might be administered mild stressors of varying personal relevance to see how people with relatively accurate or inaccurate self-models respond. Or, as another example, resilient and nonresilient choices might be assessed through behavioral studies. Even existing stories and personal narratives of difficult life situations could be coded for self-knowledge and compared to similar, nonstressful life stories. Such future research may make clearer the potential contributions of PI to an individual's response to and recovery from significant life stresses.

Note

1. Sammy's real name and other identifying details were changed from the original case in Dyson (1997).

References

Appelbaum, S. A. (1973). Psychological-mindedness: Word, concept and essence. *International Journal of Psycho-Analysis, 54*, 35–46.

Benson, P. I. (1997). *All kids are our kids.* Minneapolis, MN: Search Institute.

Block, J., & Turula, E. (1963). Identification, ego control, and adjustment. *Child Development, 34*, 945–953.

Block, J. H., & Block, J. (1980). The role of ego-control and ego-resiliency in the organization of behavior. In W. A. Collins (Ed.), *Development of cognition, affect, and social relations:*

The Minnesota Symposia on Child Psychology (Vol. 13, pp. 39–101). Hillsdale, NJ: Erlbaum.

Bluck, S., Alea, N., Habermas, T., & Rubin, D. C. (2005). A tale of three functions: The self-reported uses of autobiographical memory. *Social Cognition, 23*, 91–117.

Buss, D. M. (2001). Human nature and culture: An evolutionary psychological perspective. *Journal of Personality, 69*, 955–978.

Clancy, S. M., & Dollinger, S. J. (1993). Identity, self, and personality: I. Identity status and the five-factor model of personality. *Journal of Research on Adolescence, 3*, 227–245.

Cramer, P. (2004). Identity change in adulthood: The contribution of defense mechanisms and life experiences. *Journal of Research in Personality, 38*, 280–316.

Davidson, K., & Prkachin, K. (1997). Optimism and unrealistic optimism have an interacting impact on health-promoting behavior and knowledge changes. *Personality and Social Psychology Bulletin, 23*, 617–625.

Deaux, K., Reid, A., Mizrahi, K., & Ethier, K. A. (1995). Parameters of social identity. *Journal of Personality and Social Psychology, 68*, 280–291.

De Cremer, D. (2004). The closer we are, the more we are alike: The effect of self-other merging on depersonalized self-perception. *Current Psychology, 22*, 316–325.

Dillard, A. J., McCaul, K. D., & Klein, W. M. P. (2006). Unrealistic optimism in smokers: Implications for smoking myth endorsement and self-protective motivation. *Journal of Health Communication, 11*(Suppl. 1), 93–102.

Dollinger, S. J., & Clancy, S. M. (1993). Identity, self, and personality: II. Glimpses through the autophotographic eye. *Journal of Personality and Social Psychology, 64*, 1064–1071.

Dyson, A. H. (1997). *Writing superheroes.* New York: Teachers College Press.

Epstein, S. (1998). *Constructive thinking: The key to emotional intelligence.* New York: Praeger.

Erikson, E. H. (1963). *Childhood and society* (2nd ed.). New York: Norton.

Faber, M. A., & Mayer, J. D. (2009). Resonance to archetypes in media: There's some accounting for taste. *Journal of Research in Personality, 43*, 307–322.

Flach, F. F. (1997). *Resilience: How to bounce back when the going gets tough.* New York: Hatherleigh Press.

Folkman, S., & Lazarus, R. S. (1980). An analysis of coping in a middle-aged community sample. *Journal of Health and Social Behavior, 21*, 219–239.

Frankl, V. E. (1963). *Man's search for meaning: An introduction to logotherapy.* Oxford, UK: Washington Square Press.

Funder, D. C. (2006). Towards a resolution of the personality triad: Persons, situations, and behaviors. *Journal of Research in Personality, 40*, 21–34.

Gaertner, L., Sedikides, C., & Graetz, K. (1999). In search of self-definition: Motivational primacy of the individual self, motivational primacy of the collective self, or contextual primacy? *Journal of Personality and Social Psychology, 76*, 5–18.

Gardner, H. (1983). *Frames of mind: The theory of multiple intelligences.* New York: Basic Books.

Garmezy, N., Masten, A. S., & Tellegen, A. (1984). The study of stress and competence in children: A building block for developmental psychopathology. *Child Development, 55*, 97–111.

Hjemdal, O., Friborg, O., Stiles, T. C., Rosenvinge, J. H., & Martinussen, M. (2006). A new scale for adolescent resilience: Grasping the central protective resources behind healthy development. *Measurement and Evaluation in Counseling and Development, 39*, 84–96.

Hogan, R. (1982). A socioanalytic theory of personality. In M. M. Page (Ed.), *Nebraska Symposium on Motivation* (pp. 55–89). Lincoln: University of Nebraska Press.

Jordan, H. (2001). *No such thing as a bad day.* Atlanta, GA: Longstreet Press.

Kellogg, R. T. (1994). *The psychology of writing.* New York: Oxford University Press.

Mayer, J. D. (1995). The system–topics framework and the structural arrangement of systems within and around personality. *Journal of Personality, 63*, 459–493.

Mayer, J. D. (2005). A tale of two visions: Can a new view of personality help integrate psychology? *American Psychologist, 60*, 294–307.

Mayer, J. D. (2007). Big questions of personality psychology. *Imagination, Cognition and Personality, 27*, 3–26.

Mayer, J. D. (2008). Personal intelligence. *Imagination, Cognition and Personality, 27*, 209–232.

Mayer, J. D. (2009). Personal intelligence expressed: A theoretical analysis. *Review of General Psychology, 13,* 46–58.

Mayer, J. D., Roberts, R. D., & Barsade, S. G. (2008). Human abilities: Emotional intelligence. *Annual Review of Psychology, 59,* 507–536.

McAdams, D. P. (2006). *The redemptive self: Stories Americans live by.* New York: Oxford University Press.

McAdams, D. P., & Pals, J. L. (2006). A new Big Five: Fundamental principles for an integrative science of personality. *American Psychologist, 61,* 204–217.

McCallum, M., & Piper, W. E. (Eds.). (1997). *Psychological mindedness: A contemporary understanding.* Mahwah, NJ: Erlbaum.

McCrae, R. R., & Costa, P. T., Jr. (1999). A five-factor theory of personality. In L. A. Pervin & O. P. John (Eds.), *Handbook of personality: Theory and research* (2nd ed.). New York: Guilford Press.

McCullough, M. E., & Snyder, C. R. (2000). Classical sources of human strength: Revisiting an old home and building a new one. *Journal of Social and Clinical Psychology, 19,* 1–10.

Pals, J. L. (1999). Identity consolidation in early adulthood: Relations with ego-resiliency, the context of marriage, and personality change. *Journal of Personality, 67,* 295–329.

Petrocelli, J. V., & Smith, E. R. (2005). Who I am, who we are, and why: Links between emotions and causal attributions for self- and group discrepancies. *Personality and Social Psychology Bulletin, 31,* 1628–1642.

Pillemer, D. B. (2003). Directive functions of autobiographical memory: The guiding power of the specific episode. *Memory, 11,* 193–202.

Rattansi, A., & Phoenix, A. (1997). Rethinking youth identities: Modernist and postmodernist frameworks. *Identity, 5,* 97–123.

Regnerus, M. D., & Elder, G. H. (2003). Staying on track in school: Religious influences in high- and low-risk settings. *Journal for the Scientific Study of Religion, 42,* 633–649.

Richardson, G. E. (2002). The metatheory of resilience and resiliency. *Journal of Clinical Psychology, 58,* 307–321.

Richardson, G. E., Neiger, B., Jensen, S., & Kumpfer, K. (1990). The resiliency model. *Health Education, 21,* 33–39.

Roberts, B. W., Kuncel, N. R., Shiner, R., Caspi, A., & Goldberg, L. R. (2007). The power of personality: The comparative validity of personality traits, socioeconomic status, and cognitive ability for predicting important life outcomes. *Perspectives on Psychological Science, 2,* 313–345.

Rutter, M. (1985). Resilience in the face of adversity: Protective factors and resistance to psychiatric disorder. *British Journal of Psychiatry, 147,* 98–611.

Sanford, N. (1955). The dynamics of identification. *Psychological Review, 62,* 106–118.

Seligman, M. E. P., & Csikszentmihalyi, M. (2000). Positive psychology. *American Psychologist, 55,* 5–14.

Suskind, R. (1998). *A hope in the unseen: An American odyssey from the inner city to the Ivy League.* New York: Broadway Books.

van Hoof, A., & Raaijmakers, Q. A. (2003). The search for the structure of identity formation. *Identity, 3,* 271–289.

Weis, S., & Süß, H.-M. (2007). Reviving the search for social intelligence—a multitrait–multimethod study of its structure and construct validity. *Personality and Individual Differences, 42,* 3–14.

Werner, E., & Smith, R. (1992). *Overcoming the odds: High risk children from birth to adulthood.* Ithaca, NY: Cornell University Press.

6

The Resilient Personality

Andrew E. Skodol

The effects of life events and chronic stressors on people experiencing them are not uniform. Although psychosocial stressors may contribute to the occurrence of psychopathology, evidence also suggests that stress and adversity may lead to personal growth and improved functioning. These observations have prompted examination of individual differences among people experiencing stress in an attempt to understand why some develop distress and disability and others exhibit resilience in the face of adversity (Rutter, 1985). Understanding individual differences that protect some people from developing psychopathology in the face of adversity has profound implications for education, childrearing, treatment development, and the prevention of mental disorders.

Stress–Diathesis Model of Psychopathology

Theories of the causes of mental disorders are many. In most cases, etiology in psycho-

pathology can be assumed to be multifactorial. Most mental disorders are likely to be caused by a predisposition or vulnerability at the level of brain biochemistry and experience with acute life events or chronic stressful life circumstances. Such a model helps to explain why a person with a strong family history of depression, for example, may be asymptomatic for long periods but experience depression after a loss. In a population-based survey of female twin pairs, severely stressful events, such as the death of a close relative, assault, serious marital problems, or divorce, significantly predicted the onset of major depression in the month of occurrence. For individuals at highest genetic risk for depression, the probability of onset of major depression was significantly higher after stressful events than that for individuals at lowest genetic risk, suggesting "genetic control of sensitivity to the depression-inducing effects of stressful life events" (Kendler et al., 1995, p. 883). Overall sensitivity to stressful life events may be moderated by a functional variant in the serotonin transporter gene (Caspi et al., 2003), which may make individuals more sensitive even to mild stressors (Kendler, Kuhn, Vittum, Prescott, & Riley, 2005). High levels of cumulative lifetime exposure to adversity have also been causally implicated in the onset of depressive and anxiety disorders (Turner & Lloyd, 2004). Some disorders, however, may be caused exclusively by disease processes that directly alter brain structure and function, or by exogenous or environmental factors, such as drugs or toxins. A few disorders may be the result of solely psychosocial stressors.

Resilience

Psychobiological, personality, and social-behavioral factors have been identified that together may serve to protect a person from stress (Charney, 2004). *Resilience* refers to individual differences or life experiences that help people to cope positively with adversity, make them better able to deal with stress in the future, and confer protection from the development of mental disorders under stress (Richardson, 2002). Certain positive personality traits or character strengths that have been identified appear to be associated with adaptive outcomes in relation to the stresses of both common, normal developmental tasks and less common, abnormal adverse experiences. Maternal warmth, a stimulating environment, and an outgoing childhood temperament have been shown to be associated with resilience to socioeconomic deprivation, indicating that resilience itself is influenced by both genetic and environmental factors (Kim-Cohen, Moffitt, Caspi, & Taylor, 1994).

Many overlapping, but not identical, terms and concepts have been used to describe resilient personality traits and character strengths. This chapter attempts to synthesize these concepts and review research supporting the contention that they mitigate the effects of stress exposure on psychopa-

thology, highlighting limitations of existing research. Finally, some clinical implications of defining and identifying the resilient personality are discussed.

Two interrelated types of individual differences discussed in this chapter are personality and coping processes. *Personality* refers to constellations of traits or attributes that determine how people perceive, think about, and relate to themselves and the environment (American Psychiatric Association, 2000). Personality includes both fundamental behavioral predispositions, such as emotionality, activity, and sociability, commonly referred to as *temperament* (Buss & Plomin, 1986), and to more complex organizing and integrative systems that include cognitive and emotional components (Rutter, 1987). Personality traits are assumed to be relatively stable over time and relatively consistent across situations.

Coping refers to specific processes in which a person engages expressly for the purpose of dealing with stress (Folkman & Moskowitz, 2004; Lazarus & Folkman, 1984; Pearlin & Schooler, 1978). Coping involves cognitive, behavioral, and emotional responses. In contrast to personality, coping strategies may or may not be characteristic of a person, or consistent across stressful situations or functional roles. Personality and coping should be related, however, because certain personality traits predispose individuals to or are associated with the use of certain coping strategies and not others. Personality traits, coping processes, or a combination of both, are likely either to ameliorate or aggravate the impact of adverse experiences.

Resilient Personalities

Resilient personalities are characterized by traits that reflect a strong, well-differentiated, and integrated sense of self (*self-structure*) and traits that promote strong, reciprocal interpersonal relationships with others (Garmezy, 1991; Greef & Ritman, 2005; Rutter, 1987; Shiner, 2000). Together these traits contribute to high levels of adaptive functioning. As such, they may be thought of as reciprocals of *personality disorders*, which are inflexible and maladaptive patterns of perceiving, thinking, and relating, characterized by deficits in self-concept and in the capacity for interpersonal relationships (Bender & Skodol, 2007). It should be noted, however, that many of these concepts of personality strengths and deficits are most applicable to "Western" cultures and societies. Most research on adaptive capacities and resilience has been conducted in Western populations, in which individualism and self-reliance are highly valued. In other cultures, in which relationships to the family, the community, or the social group, and religion or spirituality are highly valued, the balance between individual and collective resources and efficacy may shift significantly in determining resilience to stress (Hollifield et al., 2008; Paton et al., 2008).

Sense of Self

A strong sense of self is evidenced by self-esteem, self-confidence or self-efficacy, self-understanding, a positive future orientation, and the ability to manage negative behaviors and emotions. Some of these traits have been subsumed under the concepts of "hardiness" and "ego-resilience." In psychodynamic terms, adaptive defense mechanisms are utilized.

Self-Esteem

Self-esteem is a sense of self-worth, self-respect, and self-acceptance that is usually linked to an expectation of success in life.

Self-Confidence/Self-Efficacy

A resilient personality is characterized by a belief in one's own abilities to manage life's challenges and situations effectively. Thus, self-confidence or self-efficacy is a prerequisite for resilience (Lin, Sandler, Ayers, Wolchik, & Luecken, 2004; Rutter, 1987). Resilient people have what has been termed an *internal locus of control*; that is, they believe that events that occur in their lives are most often influenced in large degree by their own behaviors and not a result of "fate," "bad luck," or another person's actions. An internal locus of control also contributes to the belief that problems can be solved as a result of one's own efforts, which generally leads to more effective coping strategies. A resilient person is optimistic and hopeful about the outcome of even difficult situations, such as a physical illness or the loss of a significant other (Peterson, 2000; Seligman, 2002). Self-confidence and self-efficacy are negatively correlated with personality traits of neuroticism (five-factor model; FFM) and negative emotionality (three-factor model; TFM), which represent tendencies to see and react to the world as threatening, problematic, and distressing, and to view oneself as vulnerable (Campbell-Sills, Cohan, & Stein, 2006). Self-confidence and self-efficacy are positively correlated with extraversion (FFM) and positive emotionality (TFM), tendencies to engage and confront the world with confidence in success (Nakaya, Oshio, & Kaneko, 2006). Although successful in their relationships with others, resilient people are also characterized by autonomy and self-reliance, in that they do not depend solely on others for meeting their needs or solving their problems. According to Cloninger's biosocial theory of personality, low self-directedness is related to personality disorders (Cloninger, Svrakic, & Przybeck, 1993); therefore, a highly self-directed person should be resilient.

Self-Understanding

Another characteristic of the resilient personality is an understanding of oneself as a person. Thus, resilient people have insight into their motivations, their emotions, and their strengths and weaknesses. Self-understanding gives resilient people a strong sense of personal identity; they see themselves as coherent personalities with meaning and purpose to their lives (Alim et al., 2008). Formation of a personal identity is a critical initial task of adult development (Cohen & Crawford, 2005). Accurate conscious perception and monitoring of one's own emotions is an important aspect of what has been called "socioemotional intelligence" (Goleman, 1995). There often is also a spiritual side to the resilient person, who sees him- or herself in the context of a broader world order. The resilient person is excited and motivated by the process of self-discovery.

Positive Future Orientation

Resilient people plan for the future. They are motivated to achieve and to be successful in diverse aspects of life (Masten et al., 1999; Werner & Smith, 1992). They are goal-directed, industrious, and productive (Clausen, 1991). They show determination and persistence in the pursuit of personal goals, while maintaining a sense of balance in their lives and the ability to sustain effort over time. Although generally optimistic about the outcomes of their efforts, they are also flexible in their ability to adapt to challenges, limitations, and changing life circumstances, and can accept setbacks with equanimity (Southwick, Vythilingam, & Charney, 2005).

Control of Negative Behavior and Emotion

Resilient people are responsible, conscientious, and generally exhibit a high degree of personal integrity (Benson, 1997). They tend to be honest and honorable, and they possess a strong set of values to which they strive to adhere. They have good control over impulses and do not tend toward spontaneous and unpremeditated acts, without regard to the potential consequences of their actions (Baumeister & Exline, 2000). The ability to delay gratification and adaptively displace and channel impulses is also characteristic of emotional intelligence. Resilient people are able to experience pleasure and other positive emotions, and often have a good sense of humor. A subjective sense of well-being is associated with low levels of neuroticism and high levels of extraversion, and with self-efficacy, agency, and autonomy.

Hardiness

Hardiness is a personality construct that comprises *control* (a tendency to feel and act as if one is influential rather than helpless in the face of external forces), *commitment* (a tendency to be involved, and to find purpose and meaning in life's activities and encounters rather than to feel alienation), and *challenge* (a belief that change is normal in life, and that the anticipation of change is an opportunity for growth rather than a threat to security) (Kobasa, Maddi, & Kahn, 1982).

Ego Resilience

The *ego resilience* concept was developed to describe personality traits that facilitate flexible and resourceful adaptation to life stressors, modulation of impulses, and adaptation to novel situations (Gjerde, Block, & Block, 1986). Some of the traits that fall within the rubric of ego resilience include social poise and presence, curiosity, competence, insight, and humor. Four prototypical groups of traits within the construct have been identified: confident optimism, productive activity, insight and warmth, and skilled expressiveness (Klohnen, 1996).

Defense Mechanisms

Defense mechanisms are automatic psychological processes that protect people against anxiety and awareness of internal or external stressors or dangers (Vaillant, 1992). The defense mechanisms of affiliation, altruism, anticipation, humor, self-assertion, self-observation, and sublimation are adaptive and likely to characterize the resilient personality. *Affiliation* involves dealing with emotional conflict or stressors by turning to others for help or support. *Altruism* is a dedication to meeting the needs of others. *Anticipation* is the experience of emotions in advance of future events and considering realistic alternative responses or solutions. *Humor* as a defense emphasizes the amusing or ironic aspects of a conflict or a stressor. *Self-assertion* is an expression of feelings and thoughts directly, in a way that is not coercive or manipulative. *Self-observation* is reflection on one's own thoughts, feelings, motivation, and behavior, and responding appropriately. *Sublimation* is the channeling of potentially maladaptive feelings or impulses into socially acceptable behavior (American Psychiatric Association, 2000).

Interpersonal Skills

Individuals with a strong sense of self are often appealing to others. Resilient personalities, however, also possess specific interpersonal skills that promote the development and maintenance of relationships that assist in coping with stressful life experiences. These "prosocial" personality traits may be grouped under the general concepts of sociability, emotional expressiveness, and interpersonal understanding. Combined with the traits of emotional awareness and control over impulses described earlier, these interpersonal skills complete the definition of emotional intelligence.

Sociability

Resilient people are naturally more sociable, gregarious, and extraverted than the norm. They tend to be gracious, cordial, affable, and genial. They are more likely to meet people, to form friendships easily, and to enjoy companionship, thus acquiring an extended social network. They are high on the FFM trait of agreeableness. Resilient people have good interpersonal communication skills. In times of stress, they have access to more social support, a fundamental component of resilience, even though they also are capable of being self-reliant.

Emotional Expressiveness

The ability to express one's emotions appropriately to others leads to stronger interpersonal relationships and to the effective use of these relationships at times of stress (Alim et al., 2008). Resilient people are able to convey warmth and other feelings openly and to trust other people with their most intimate feelings.

Interpersonal Understanding

Resilient people are empathic (Cowan, Wyman, & Work, 1996). They are able to perceive and experience the feelings of others, and to communicate this understanding to others. They tend to be unselfish and altruistic, having genuine interest in the welfare of others. These traits lead others to want to be in relationships with them, to trust them, and in turn to want to be of assistance to them.

Measurement

A number of scales have been developed to measure resilience or aspects of resilience, but none are comprehensive or have achieved widespread use. Some measure resilient personality traits in the context of other resilience factors, while others focus more exclusively on the resilient personality. An example of the former is the Resilience Scale for Adults (RSA), which covers five dimensions: personal competence, social competence, family coherence, social support, and personal structure (Friborg, Hjemdal, Rosenvinge, & Martinussen, 2003). Personal competence or strength was found to be related to the personality trait of emotional stability, social competence to extroversion and agreeableness, and personal structure to conscientiousness (Friborg, Barlaug, Martinussen, Rosenvinge, & Hjemdal, 2005). An example of the latter is the Connor–Davidson Resilience Scale (CD-RISC). A factor analysis in a general population sample yielded five factors: (1) personal competence, high standards, and tenacity; (2) trust in one's instincts, tolerance of negative affect, and strengthening effects of stress; (3) positive acceptance of change and secure relationships; (4) control; and (5) spiritual influences (Connor & Davidson, 2003). A Dispositional Resilience Scale (Bartone, Ursano, Wright, & Ingraham, 1989) was developed to measure the construct of hardiness. The Resilience Scale (RS; Wagnild & Young, 1993) measures perseverance, self-reliance, meaningfulness, existential aloneness, and equanimity.

Coping

Coping refers to specific thoughts and behaviors that a person uses to manage the internal and external demands of situations appraised as stressful, in order to be protected from psychological harm (Folkman & Moskowitz, 2004; Lazarus & Folkman, 1984; Pearlin & Schooler, 1978). Coping involves cognitive, behavioral, and emotional responses, and may or may not be consistent across stressful situations or functional roles. A distinction has been made between *coping style*, a general style of interacting related to personality (see below), and *coping response*, a stress-specific pattern in which an individual's perceptions, emotions, and behaviors prepare for adapting and changing (Beutler & Moos, 2003; Moos & Holahan, 2003). As conceptualized by Pearlin and Schooler (1978), coping can take three forms: modification or change of the stressful situation, control of the meaning of the experience to neutralize its stressful nature, or management of the emotional sequelae of the experience.

According to the model of Lazarus and Folkman (1984), a person initially makes a cognitive appraisal of harm, threat, or challenge embodied by a stressor. *Harm* refers to damage already done, a loss, for example; *threat* is the anticipation of harm; *challenge* represents demands that can be met. Next, there is a secondary appraisal of the extent to which the stressful situation might be changed or must be accepted. These appraisals are followed by either of two major broad styles of coping: problem-focused or emotion-focused. *Problem-focused coping* refers to efforts to resolve a threatening problem or diminish its impact by taking direct action. *Emotion-focused coping* refers to efforts to reduce the negative emotions aroused in response to a threat by changing the way the threat is attended to or interpreted. These types of coping can co-occur and interact: For example, emotion-focused coping may reduce distress to an extent that facilitates problem-focused coping, and problem-focused coping may reduce threat to an extent that also relieves emotional distress.

Measurement

Coping has traditionally been assessed by retrospective self-report measures, for example, the Coping Responses Inventory (Moos, 1993), the Ways of Coping Questionnaire (Folkman & Lazarus, 1988), and the COPE Inventory (Carver, Scheier, & Weintraub, 1989), and, more recently, by ecological momentary assessment (real-time) techniques (Stone et al., 1998).

Personality and Coping

Three important questions can be asked about personality and coping as factors promoting resilience:

1. What is the relationship of personality traits to coping styles or strategies?
2. What is the evidence for personality traits as protective factors in preventing negative outcomes in the face of adversity?
3. What is the evidence that personality factors have protective effects, independent of situational coping?

Research on the effects of personality and coping on the outcome of stressful experiences has suffered from a number of problems: using cross-sectional or retrospective designs, ignoring prior symptom (or disorder) status, combining heterogeneous stressors, using college student samples, and limited measurement of a range of resilient personality traits and other potentially mediating factors, such as coping strategies and the availability of social supports. Thus, the measurement of the outcome of the stressful experience and the personality or coping factor presumed to attenuate the effect of the stressor on the outcome have been confounded, with the result that the direction of causality between personality and psychopathology is ambiguous. Furthermore, because of the limitations imposed by sample selection and particular stressors, the results of any single study may not generalize widely.

Relationship of Personality Traits to Coping

As stated earlier, personality characteristics should affect the repertoire of coping strategies available to the individual. Personality traits might increase or decrease a person's appraisal of an experience as stressful or actually influence his or her coping response. A perception that a person has the necessary resources to handle a situation should reduce the perceived threat or increase the perceived efficacy of coping efforts. A negative perception would have the opposite effect. People high on the trait of extraversion or positive emotionality would likely engage with a problem and be action oriented in their approach to coping, while those who are high on the trait of neuroticism or negative emotionality would likely make negative appraisals and cope maladaptively, with distancing, distraction, or escape. People who are conscientious might be expected to carefully plan out their strategy rather than to act immediately in problem solving situations.

Persons high on self-esteem, optimism, or internal locus of control have been found to have more positive appraisals of stressful events (Holahan & Moos, 1991; Schiaffino & Revenson, 1992) and to be more likely to use problem-focused coping than emotion-focused coping because they believe that they can influence the outcome of a stressful situation for the better (Fleishman, 1984; Holahan & Moos, 1986; Smith, Pope, Rhodewalt, & Poulton, 1989; Taylor et al., 1992). Persons high on neuroticism relied more on emotion-focused coping (Bolger, 1990; Carver et al., 1989). Terry (1994) found that self-esteem was related to problem-focused coping for work-related problems appraised as controllable. Simeon and colleagues (2007) found that resilience was negatively correlated with harm avoidance and positively correlated with reward dependence from the Tridimensional Personality model in a sample of healthy volunteers. Lower optimism was associated with greater and lasting maternal fear appraisals in a study of children undergoing stem cell transplantation (DuHamel et al., 2007).

Resilient Personality as a Protective Factor

Some accumulated research supports the hypothesis that the resilient personality protects against the development of psychopathology in the face of adversity. The research that is most informative is longitudinal in design, and these studies are the focus of the illustrative review that follows.

In two cohorts of adolescent boys followed for 60 years or until death, use of mature, "healthy" defense mechanisms, such as humor, suppression, and anticipation, before 50 years of age predicted successful aging (Vaillant & Mukamal, 2001). Members of one of the groups had inner-city backgrounds characterized by considerable psychosocial adversity; the other group comprised Harvard graduates. In both groups, quality of aging, subjective life satisfaction, and objective mental health were associated with maturity of defenses. Included in life satisfaction was satisfaction with marriage, children, job or retirement, and friends. Objective mental health was measured by ratings of quality of marriage, job success, job satisfaction, no early retirement, vacations, social activities, no use of psychiatrists, and no use of tranquillizers.

Several adaptive capacities often associated with the resilient personality have been found to predict successful functioning in multiple domains for a school-based sample over a 20-year developmental period, from childhood (8–12 years) through emerging adulthood (17–23 years) years and into young adulthood (28–36 years) (Masten et al., 2004). Specifically, academic achievement, social competence, good conduct, intimate and reciprocal romantic relationships, and success and reliability in work were associated with traits of planfulness/future motivation and autonomy, and with good stress coping skills. Some specificity was found: Academic attainment was associated with planfulness, achievement motivation, and future orientation; success in romantic relationships was predicted by autonomy—an index of self-reliance, self-directedness, emotional independence, and independent decision making.

Resilient personality traits—specifically, confidence and optimism, insight and warmth, productive activity, and social interaction skills—at age 16 showed a dose–response relationship with a decreasing likelihood of developing psychiatric disorders, suicide attempts, violent or criminal behaviors, interpersonal difficulties, and educational or occupational problems by age 22 in the epidemiological Children in the Community Study (Bromley, Johnson, & Cohen, 2006). High levels of ego resilience in this study protected youth against the development of psychiatric disorders even if they experienced two or more negative life events.

Positive achievement experiences and positive interpersonal experiences during childhood and adolescence were significantly associated with remission from avoidant (AVPD) and schizotypal (STPD) personality disorders over a 4-year period in the Collaborative Longitudinal Personality Disorders Study (Skodol et al., 2007). Achievement motivation and social skills competency are often-mentioned aspects of resilience and positive youth development. The greater the number of positive experiences and the broader the developmental period (i.e., childhood and adolescence) they spanned, the better the prognosis of these personality disorders. Positive childhood experiences in the achievement and relationship domains predicted remission from AVPD and STPD (relationship experiences only) even in the presence of physical, sexual, and verbal abuse and neglect.

Optimism during pregnancy was associated with decreased depression severity 6 and 12 months postpartum in a sample of women having their first child (Grote & Bledsoe, 2007). Optimism was also protective of women who experienced significant financial, spousal, and physical stress during pregnancy.

Children from the Environmental Risk Longitudinal Study, a nationally representative sample of twin pairs and their families in England and Wales, were evaluated for individual, family, and neighborhood characteristics that would distinguish resilient and nonresilient children who were physically maltreated (Jaffee, Caspi, Moffitt, Polo-Thomas, & Taylor, 2007). Individual personality strengths included above average intelligence, sociability, and self-control. Consistent with a cumulative stressors model of adaptation, individual strengths did not distinguish between resilient and nonresilient children under conditions of high family and neighborhood stress. The authors concluded that, for children in multiproblem families, personal resources might not be sufficient for successful adaptation.

An epidemiological sample from the Isle of Wight Study was assessed in adolescence and followed up in midlife (Collishaw et al., 2007). Individuals who reported a history of child abuse who exhibited resilience against the development of later psychopathology scored significantly lower on the trait of neuroticism than nonresilient individuals and had better adolescent peer relationships and adult love relationships. Thus, personality strength and quality of interpersonal relationships were protective in the context of childhood abuse.

Personality traits from the Temperament and Character Inventory (TCI) were studied in relationship to symptoms of posttraumatic stress disorder following a firestorm in California (North, Hong, Suris, & Spitznagel, 2008). Intrusion and hyperarousal symptoms were prevalent and associated with the maladaptive personality traits of high harm avoidance and low self-directedness. The generally healthy personality profiles of survivors reflected their psychological resilience.

Optimism about the future course of their child's disease was correlated to lower psychological distress and passive reaction patterns correlated to higher distress in a sample of parents followed for 5 years after their child's treatment for cancer (Maurice-Stam, Oort, Last, & Grootenhuis, 2008).

Independence of Personality and Coping Effects

Do personality traits and coping styles have independent effects on the pathogenic aspects of stress? In a community sample, McCrae and Costa (1986) found that both neuroticism and coping were related to distress, but that coping showed no effect when neuroticism was statistically controlled. The study was retrospective, however, and asked how subjects coped with an event that occurred over a year earlier. Thus, subjects may have reported on typical coping styles, more consistent with their personalities, than on the specific strategy they employed at the time the stressful event occurred. Scheier, Carver, and Bridges (1994) demonstrated that optimism continued to be significantly correlated with aspects of coping, including planning, active coping, positive reinterpretation, and seeking support, and with symptoms of depression (negatively) when other personality traits were controlled. Campbell-Sills and colleagues (2006) found that resilience was

negatively associated with neuroticism and positively related to extraversion and conscientiousness. Coping styles also predicted variance in resilience, above and beyond personality traits. Task-oriented coping was positively related to resilience and mediated the relationship between conscientiousness and resilience. Emotion-oriented coping was associated with low resilience. Resilience itself was shown to moderate the relationship between the adversity of childhood emotional neglect and current psychiatric symptoms.

From retrospective or cross-sectional studies, whether personality traits mediate the effects of coping efforts or vice versa is not clear. How personality traits and coping independently impact positive health outcomes and adaptation to stressful events has also been the subject of longitudinal research.

In a longitudinal study of college students taking the Medical College Admissions Test, Bolger (1990) found that neuroticism was related to anxiety, but that ineffective coping mediated over half of the effect. This suggests that neuroticism leads people to cope ineffectively, and that ineffective coping in turn leads to increased distress.

Traits of optimism and locus of control, along with cognitive appraisals and coping, were evaluated as predictors of distress in a longitudinal study of women with breast cancer who were undergoing surgery (Stanton & Snider, 1993). After prebiopsy distress and age were controlled, only cognitive avoidance coping was a significant predictor. In another longitudinal study of breast cancer patients, Carver and associates (1993) found that optimism (vs. pessimism) was inversely related to anxiety, depression, and anger over a 1-year period following surgery. Coping strategies of acceptance, denial, and behavioral disengagement mediated the effects (of pessimism) on distress.

The relationships between hardiness, cognitive appraisals, and problem solving or emotion-focused coping and mental health after combat training were evaluated in Israeli military recruits (Florian, Mikulincer, & Taubman, 1995). The relationship between hardiness and mental health was mediated by appraisals and by coping strategies.

Personality resources, including self-esteem, dispositional optimism, and perceived control, were evaluated as predictors of distress, well-being, and decision satisfaction in a large group of women undergoing abortion (Major, Richards, Cooper, Cozzarelli, & Zubek, 1998). The mediating effects of both cognitive appraisals and postabortion coping on outcome were assessed. Women who had resilient personality traits appraised their abortions as less stressful and had higher perceptions of self-efficacy for coping with the abortion. More positive appraisals predicted greater acceptance/reframing coping and less avoidance/denial, venting, support seeking, and religious coping. Acceptance/reframing predicted better outcomes on all measures of postabortion adaptation; avoidance/denial and venting predicted poorer outcomes on all measures.

Although not entirely consistent, the results of these studies suggest independent roles for personality traits and coping behaviors on the outcome of stressful events.

Clinical Implications

Considerable attention in clinical evaluations of psychiatric patients is paid to eliciting histories of childhood abuse and neglect, especially for patients with evident personality psychopathology. For many, however, adverse childhood experiences have less of an impact on mental health outcomes than might be expected. Less attention is paid to exploring factors that might mitigate the deleterious effects of childhood maltreatment, or other adversities, and protect vulnerable children from developing personality disorders or promoting recovery.

Traditionally, personality assessment in clinical evaluations is focused on pathological personality traits that are components of

personality disorders (Skodol, 2005). Thus, the focus of an assessment might revolve around emotional expressivity, either constricted or excessive. Patients with schizoid personalities are cold and detached; those with obsessive–compulsive personalities express their feelings in controlled and stilted ways. In contrast, patients with borderline personalities are emotionally labile and react very strongly, particularly in interpersonal contexts, with a variety of intensely dysphoric emotions, such as depression, anxiety, irritability, and anger. Patients with histrionic personalities display rapidly shifting emotions that appear dramatic and exaggerated but are shallow in comparison to the intense emotional expressions of patients with borderline personalities.

As work has evolved on personality and personality disorder assessment and classification for DSM-V, serious consideration is being given to including a trait-based assessment as part of a revised dimensional approach to personality psychopathology (Skodol & Bender, 2009; Skodol, Bender, & Oldham, 2009). Core traits under consideration include emotional lability, submissivenes, social withdrawal, callousness, aggression, perfectionism, impulsivity, irresponsibility, and cognitive dysregulation, among others. These traits are viewed as the building blocks for major personality disorder prototypes and also as clinically relevant descriptors for personality problems of an infinite variety that could apply to any patient.

In light of the discussion of the potentially protective aspects of certain personality traits in this chapter, an argument can be made for the inclusion of a second set of traits in DSM-V that would direct clinical attention to the resilient personality. It would seem clinically useful to assess all patients on traits such as self-esteem, self-efficacy, optimism, achievement motivation, persistence, sociability, altruism, and emotional expressiveness. These assessments would be defined not as the absence of pathological personality traits but as the presence of healthy and adaptive ones. Of course, more study would be necessary to demonstrate which of these traits had the greatest utility in helping clinicians to determine treatment approaches and to predict prognoses. Then again, the same requirement applies to any selected set of pathological traits.

Resilient personality traits may have direct significance for treatment and prevention. Early intervention, with treatments designed to foster personal strengths and competencies and to develop interpersonal skills, could have a beneficial effect on young patients (Garber, 2006; Shiner, 2000). An increase in resilience in primary care outpatients, in general psychiatric outpatients, and in patients in clinical trials for generalized anxiety disorder and posttraumatic stress disorder was associated with greater improvement during treatment (Connor & Davidson, 2003). Stress management programs to enhance adaptation and promote resilience have been designed to improve the emotional well-being of patients with cancer by reducing depression and enabling them to remain engaged in their pursuits (Carver, 2005). And youth programs promoting social, emotional, cognitive, behavioral, and moral competencies may ultimately help prevent the development of psychopathology in vulnerable youth (Commission on Positive Youth Development, 2005).

References

Alim, T. N., Feder, A., Graves, R. E., Wang, Y., Weaver, J., Westphal, M., et al. (2008). Trauma, resilience, and recovery in a high-risk African-American population. *American Journal of Psychiatry, 165*, 1566–1575.

American Psychiatric Association. (2000). *Diagnostic and statistical manual of mental disorders* (4th ed., text rev.). Washington, DC: American Psychiatric Association.

Bartone, P. T., Ursano, R., Wright, K., & Ingraham, L. (1989). The impact of military air disaster on the health of assistance workers. *Journal of Nervous and Mental Disease, 177*, 317–328.

Baumeister, R. F., & Exline, J. J. (2000). Self-control, morality, and human strength. *Journal of Social and Clinical Psychology, 19*, 29–42.

Bender, D. S., & Skodol, A. E. (2007). Borderline personality as a self–other representational disturbance. *Journal of Personality Disorders, 21*, 500–517.

Benson, P. L. (1997). *All kids are our kids.* Minneapolis, MN: Search Institute.

Beutler, L. E., & Moos, R. H. (2003). Coping and coping styles in personality and treatment planning: Introduction to the special series. *Journal of Clinical Psychology, 59*, 1045–1047.

Bolger, N. (1990). Coping as a personality process: A prospective study. *Journal of Personality and Social Psychology, 59*, 525–537.

Bromley, E., Johnson, J. G., & Cohen, P. (2006). Personality strengths in adolescence and decreased risk of developing mental health problems in early adulthood. *Comprehensive Psychiatry, 47*, 315–324.

Buss, A. H., & Plomin, R. (1986). *Temperament: Early developing personality traits.* Hillsdale, NJ: Erlbaum.

Campbell-Sills, L., Cohan, S. L., & Stein, M. B. (2006). Relationship of resilience to personality, coping, and psychiatric symptoms in young adults. *Behaviour Research and Therapy, 44*, 585–599.

Carver, C. S. (2005). Enhancing adaptation during treatment and the role of individual differences. *Cancer, 104*(Suppl. 11), 2602–2607.

Carver, C. S., Pozo, C., Harris, S. D., Noriega, V., Scheier, M. F., Robinson, D. S., et al. (1993). How coping medicates the effect of optimism on distress: a study of women with early stage breast cancer. *Journal of Personality and Social Psychology, 65*, 375–390.

Carver, C. S., Scheier, M. F., & Weintraub, J. K. (1989). Assessing coping strategies: A theoretically based approach. *Journal of Personality and Social Psychology, 56*, 267–283.

Caspi, A., Sugden, K., Moffitt, T. E., Taylor, A., Craig, I. W., Harrington, H., et al. (2003). Influence of life stress on depression: Moderation by a polymorphism in the 5-HTT gene. *Science, 301*, 386–389.

Charney, D. S. (2004). Psychobiological mechanisms of resilience and vulnerability: Implications for successful adaptation to extreme stress. *American Journal of Psychiatry, 161*, 195–216.

Clausen, J. S. (1991). Adolescent competence and the shaping of the life course. *American Journal of Sociology, 96,* 805–842.

Cloninger, C. R., Svrakic, D. M., & Przybeck, T. R. (1993). A psychobiological model of temperament and character. *Archives of General Psychiatry, 50,* 975–990.

Cohen, P., & Crawford, T. (2005). Developmental issues. In J. M. Oldham, A. E. Skodol, & D. S. Bender (Eds.), *American Psychiatric Press textbook of personality disorders* (pp. 195–211). Washington, DC: American Psychiatric Publishing.

Collishaw, S., Pickles, A., Messer, J., Rutter, M., Shearer, C., & Maughan, B. (2007). Resilience to adult psychopathology following childhood maltreatment: Evidence from a community sample. *Child Abuse and Neglect, 31,* 211–229.

Commission on Positive Youth Development. (2005). The positive perspective on youth development. In D. L. Evans, E. B. Foa, R. E. Gur, H. Hendin, C. P. O'Brien, M. E. P. Seligman, et al. (Eds.), *Treating and preventing adolescent mental health disorders* (pp. 497–527). New York: Oxford University Press.

Connor, K. M., & Davidson, J. R. (2003). Development of a new resilience scale: The Connor–Davidson Resilience Scale (CD-RISC). *Depression and Anxiety, 18,* 76–82.

Cowan, E. L., Wyman, P. A., & Work, W. C. (1996). Resilience in highly stressed urban children: Concepts and findings. *Bulletin of the New York Academy of Medicine, 73,* 267–284.

DuHamel, K. N., Rini, C., Austin, J., Ostroff, J., Parsons, S., Martini, R., et al. (2007). Optimism and life events as predictors of fear appraisals in mother of children undergoing hematopoietic stem cell transplantation. *Psycho-Oncology, 16,* 821–833.

Fleishman, J. A. (1984). Personality characteristics and coping patterns. *Journal of Health and Social Behavior, 25,* 229–244.

Florian, V., Mikulincer, M., & Taubman, O. (1995). Does hardiness contribute to mental health during a stressful real-life situation?: The role of appraisal and coping. *Journal of Personality and Social Psychology, 68,* 687–695.

Folkman, S., & Lazarus, R. S. (1988). *The Ways of Coping Questionnaire.* Palo Alto, CA: Consulting Psychologists Press.

Folkman, S., & Moskowitz, J. T. (2004). Coping: Pitfalls and promise. *Annual Review of Psychology, 55,* 745–774.

Friborg, O., Barlaug, D., Martinussen, M., Rosenvinge, J. H., & Hjemdal, O. (2005). Resilience in relation to personality and intelligence. *International Journal of Methods in Psychiatric Research, 14,* 29–42.

Friborg, O., Hjemdal, O., Rosenvinge, J. H., & Martinussen, M. (2003). A new rating scale for adult resilience: What are the central protective resources behind health adjustment? *International Journal of Methods in Psychiatric Research, 12,* 65–76.

Garber, J. (2006). Depression in children and adolescents: Linking risk research and prevention. *American Journal of Preventive Medicine, 31*(6, Suppl. 1), S104–S125.

Garmezy, N. (1991). Resiliency and vulnerability to adverse developmental outcomes associated with poverty. *American Behavioral Scientist, 34,* 416–430.

Gjerde, P. F., Block, J., & Block, J. H. (1986). Egocentrism and ego resiliency: Personality characteristics associated with perspective-taking from early childhood to adolescence. *Journal of Personality and Social Psychology, 51,* 423–434.

Goleman, D. (1995). *Emotional intelligence.* New York: Bantam Books.

Greef, A. P., & Ritman, I. N. (2005). Individual characteristics associated with resilience in single-parent families. *Psychological Reports, 96,* 36–42.

Grote, N. K., & Bledsoe, S. E. (2007). Predicting postpartum depressive symptoms in new mothers: The role of optimism and stress frequency during pregnancy. *Health and Social Work, 32,* 107–118.

Holahan, C. J., & Moos, R. H. (1986). Personality, coping, and family resources in stress resistance: A longitudinal analysis. *Journal of Personality and Social Psychology, 51,* 389–395.

Holahan, C. J., & Moos, R. H. (1991). Life stressors, personal and social resources, and depression: A 4-year structural model. *Journal of Abnormal Psychology, 100,* 31–38.

Hollifield, M., Hewage, C., Gunawardena, C. N., Kodituwakku, P., Bopagoda, K., & Weerarathnege, K. (2008). Symptoms and coping in Sri Lanka 20–21 months after the 2004 tsunami. *British Journal of Psychiatry, 192,* 39–44.

Jaffee, S. R., Caspi, A., Moffitt, T. E., Polo-

Thomas, M., & Taylor, A. (2007). Individual, family, and neighborhood factors distinguish resilient from non-resilient maltreated children: A cumulative stressors model. *Child Abuse and Neglect, 31*, 231–253.

Kendler, K. S., Kessler, R. C., Walters, E. E., MacLean, C., Neale, M. C., Heath, A. C., et al. (1995). Stressful life events, genetic liability, and onset of an episode of major depression in women. *American Journal of Psychiatry, 152*, 833–842.

Kendler, K. S., Kuhn J. W., Vittum, J., Prescott, C. A., & Riley, B. (2005). The interaction of stressful life events and a serotonin transporter polymorphism in the prediction of episodes of major depression: A replication. *Archives of General Psychiatry, 62*, 529–535.

Kim-Cohen, J., Moffitt, T. E., Caspi, A., & Taylor, A. (1994). Genetic and environmental processes in young children's resilience and vulnerability to socioeconomic deprivation. *Child Development, 75*, 651–668.

Klohnen, E. C. (1996). Conceptual analysis and measurement of the construct of ego-resiliency. *Journal of Personality and Social Psychology, 70*, 1067–1079.

Kobasa, S. C., Maddi, S. R., & Kahn, S. (1982). Hardiness and health: A prospective study. *Journal of Personality and Social Psychology, 42*, 168–177.

Lazarus, R. S., & Folkman, S. (1984). *Stress, appraisal, and coping.* New York: Springer.

Lin, K. K., Sandler, I. N., Ayers, T. S., Wolchik, S. A., & Luecken, L. J. (2004). Resilience in parentally bereaved children and adolescents seeking preventive services. *Journal of Clinical Child and Adolescent Psychology, 33*, 673–683.

Major, B., Richards, C., Cooper, M. L., Cozzarelli, C., & Zubek, J. (1998). Personal resilience, cognitive appraisals, and coping: An integrative model of adjustment to abortion. *Journal of Personality and Social Psychology, 74*, 735–752.

Masten, A. S., Burt, K. B., Roisman, G. I., Obradovic, J., Long, J. D., & Tellegen, A. (2004). Resources and resilience in the transition to adulthood: Continuity and change. *Development and Psychopathology, 16*, 1071–1094.

Masten, A. S., Hubbard, J. J., Gest, S. D., Tellegen, A., Garmezy, N., & Ramirez, M. (1999). Competence in the context of adversity: Pathways to resilience and maladaptation from childhood to late adolescence. *Development and Psychopathology, 11*, 143–169.

Maurice-Stam, H., Oort, F. J., Last, B. F., & Grootenhuis, M. A. (2008). Emotional functioning of parents of children with cancer: The first five years of continuous remission after the end of treatment. *Psycho-Oncology, 17*, 448–459.

McCrae, R. R., & Costa, P. T. (1986). Personality, coping, and coping effectiveness in an adult sample. *Journal of Personality, 54*, 385–405.

Moos, R. H. (1993). *Coping Responses Inventory.* Odessa, FL: Psychological Assessment Resources.

Moos, R. H., & Holahan, C. J. (2003). Dispositional and contextual perspectives on coping: Toward an integrative framework. *Journal of Clinical Psychology, 59*, 1387–1403.

Nakaya, M., Oshio, A., & Kaneko, H. (2006). Correlations of Adolescent Resilience Scale with Big Five personality traits. *Psychological Reports, 98*, 927–930.

North, C. S., Hong, B. A., Suris, A., & Spitznagel, E. L. (2008). Distinguishing distress and psychopathology among survivors of the Oakland/Berkeley firestorm. *Psychiatry, 71*, 35–45.

Paton, D., Gregg, C. E., Houghton, B. F., Lachman, R., Lachman, J., Johnson, D. M., et al. (2008). The impact of the 2004 tsunami on coastal Thai communities: Assessing adaptive capacities. *Disasters, 32*, 106–119.

Pearlin, L. I., & Schooler, C. (1978). The structure of coping. *Journal of Health and Social Behavior, 19*, 2–21.

Peterson, C. (2000). The future of optimism. *American Psychologist, 55*, 44–55.

Richardson, G. E. (2002). The metatheory of resilience and resiliency. *Journal of Clinical Psychology, 58*, 307–321.

Rutter, M. (1985). Resilience in the face of adversity: Protective factors and resistance to psychiatric disorder. *British Journal of Psychiatry, 147*, 598–611.

Rutter, M. (1987). Psychosocial resiliency and protective mechanisms. *American Journal of Orthopsychiatry, 57*, 316–329.

Scheier, M. F., Carver, C. S., & Bridges, M. W. (1994). Distinguishing optimism from neuroticism (and trait anxiety, self-mastery, and self-esteem): A reevaluation of the Life Orientation Test. *Journal of Personality and Social Psychology, 67*, 1063–1078.

Schiaffino, K. M., & Revenson, T. A. (1992). The role of perceived self-efficacy, perceived control, and causal attributions in adaptation to rheumatoid arthritis: Distinguishing mediator from moderator effects. *Personality and Social Psychology Bulletin, 18*, 709–718.

Seligman, M. E. P. (2002). *Authentic happiness.* New York: Free Press.

Shiner, R. L. (2000). Linking childhood personality with adaptation: Evidence for continuity and change across time into late adolescence. *Journal of Personality and Social Psychology, 78*, 310–325.

Simeon, D., Yehuda, R., Cunill, R., Knutelska, M., Putnam, F. W., & Smith, L. M. (2007). Factors associated with resilience in healthy adults. *Psychoneuroendocrinology, 32*, 1149–1152.

Skodol, A. E. (2005). Manifestations, clinical diagnosis, and comorbidity. In J. M. Oldham, A. E. Skodol, & D. S. Bender (Eds.), *The American Psychiatric Publishing textbook of personality disorders* (pp. 57–87). Washington, DC: American Psychiatric Publishing.

Skodol, A. E., & Bender, D. S. (2009). The future of personality disorders in DSM-V? *American Journal of Psychiatry, 166*, 388–391.

Skodol, A. E., Bender, D. S., & Oldham, J. M. (2009). Future directions: Toward DSM-V. In J. M. Oldham, A. E. Skodol, & D. S. Bender (Eds.), *Essentials of personality disorders* (pp. 37–61). Washington, DC: American Psychiatric Publishing.

Skodol, A. E., Bender, D. S., Pagano, M. E., Shea, M. T., Yen, S., Sanislow, C. A., et al. (2007). Positive childhood experiences: Resilience and recovery from personality disorder in early adulthood. *Journal of Clinical Psychiatry, 68*, 1102–1108.

Smith, T. W., Pope, M. K., Rhodewalt, F., & Poulton, J. L. (1989). Optimism, neuroticism, coping, and symptom reports: An alternative interpretation of the Life Orientation Test.

Journal of Personality and Social Psychology, 56, 640–648.

Southwick, S. M., Vythilingam, M., & Charney, D. S. (2005). The psychobiology of depression and resilience to stress: Implications for prevention and treatment. *Annual Review of Clinical Psychology, 1*, 255–291.

Stanton, A. L., & Snider, P. R. (1993). Coping with a breast cancer diagnosis: A prospective study. *Health Psychology, 12*, 16–23.

Stone, A. A., Schwartz, J. E., Neale, J. M., Shiffman, S., Marco, C. A., Hickox, M., et al. (1998). A comparison of coping assessed by ecological momentary assessment and retrospective recall. *Journal of Personality and Social Psychology, 74*, 1670–1680.

Taylor, S. E., Kemeny, M. E., Aspinwall, L. G., Schneider, S. G., Rodriguez, R., & Herbert, M. (1992). Optimism, coping, psychological distress, and high-risk sexual behavior among men at risk for acquired immunodeficiency syndrome (AIDS). *Journal of Personality and Social Psychology, 63*, 460–473.

Terry, D. (1994). Determinants of coping: The role of stable and situational factors. *Journal of Personality and Social Psychology, 66*, 895–910.

Turner, R. J., & Lloyd, D. A. (2004). Stress burden and lifetime incidence of psychiatric disorders in young adults: Racial and ethnic contrasts. *Archives of General Psychiatry, 61*, 481–488.

Vaillant, G. E. (1992). *Ego mechanisms of defense: A guide for clinicians and researcher.* Washington, DC: American Psychiatric Press.

Vaillant, G. E., & Mukamal, K. (2001). Successful aging. *American Journal of Psychiatry, 158*, 839–847.

Wagnild, G. M., & Young, H. M. (1993). Development and psychometric validation of the Resilience Scale. *Journal of Nursing Measures, 1*, 165–178.

Werner, E., & Smith, R. (1992). *Overcoming the odds: High risk children from birth to adulthood.* Ithaca, NY: Cornell University Press.

7

Resilience in Response to Loss

Kathrin Boerner
Daniela Jopp

Loss represents an integral but also challenging part of human development. However, some people seem to respond to loss with striking resilience. In fact, research evidence, primarily from studies on bereavement, shows that resilience is a more common response to coping with loss than previously thought. This is striking given that a core element of traditional bereavement theories, which can be traced back to Freud's notion of the psychological function of grief (Freud, 1917/1957), is the assumption that healthy adjustment to the loss of a loved one requires a certain amount of struggle and emotional turmoil, also referred to as "working through one's grief." Nevertheless, empirical bereavement research points to substantial interindividual differences. There is strong and consistent evidence from multiple studies that this kind of processing is neither a prerequisite for positive adaptation nor necessarily the most common response to loss (e.g., Bonanno, 2004; see Wortman & Boerner, 2006, for a review).

A similar impression can be gleaned from research on losses other than bereavement, such as the loss of health or other resources in old age (e.g., Greve & Staudinger, 2006; Staudinger, Marsiske, & Baltes, 1995). To gain a more complete picture of resilience and related factors, this chapter seeks to go beyond a bereavement-based perspective on resilience in response to loss by also describing reactions to loss in the context of a catastrophic event and the decline in resources experienced in old age.

If resilience is indeed a common and ordinary phenomenon (Masten, 2001), why is it so vital to consider this phenomenon further when it comes to coping with loss? First, it is important to have a realistic assessment and understanding of common patterns in response to loss. Without this sort of evidence-based accuracy, the wrong expectations for people who experience loss easily arise, and being confronted with such expectations can be particularly unhelpful (Wortman & Boerner, 2006). Second, problematic adaptation cannot be fully understood without a deeper understanding of health and resilience (Bonanno, 2004), or of the individual's potential for resilience. Third, learning from those who are resilient after a loss can inform what others who have more difficulties may need to learn or may benefit from. Thus, insights about resilience are important for the development of prevention and intervention programs that help people maintain optimal functioning by stimulating and enhancing their capacity for resilience, if possible (Kelley, 2005; Pransky, 2003).

When it comes to the study of resilience, two general research approaches can be distinguished (Greve & Staudinger, 2006). The *process-oriented approach* investigates how aspects of the person (e.g., abilities) and environment (e.g., social support) are connected with consequences of certain adversities and risks. In this tradition, resilience is typically understood as the result of a process in which person and environment aspects have enabled a person to overcome difficulties, and he or she therefore fares better than nonresilient persons. In contrast, the *person-oriented approach* looks at resilient persons and attempts to determine what distinguishes them from those who are not resilient. In this context, resilience is mostly seen as quasi-invulnerability against adversity. In addition, most of this research has focused on resilience as an emotional response (e.g., Moskowitz, Folkman, & Acree, 2003; Staudinger & Fleeson, 1996); far less attention has been paid to the notion of functional resilience (e.g., Berkman et al., 1993). Moreover, there is a shared understanding that research on resilience needs to consider changes over time. Ideally, resilience is investigated with prospective studies that capture a person's experiences before and after the loss (Bonanno, 2004). Since an individual's life history and the point in time at which a loss is experienced play important roles, theoretical concepts and empirical studies on resilience also need to be embedded in a lifespan/course framework (Greve & Staudinger, 2006; Litz, 2005). In the follow-

ing sections, we describe what characterizes resilience in response to loss to assess how common it is, and to identify what contributes to resilience in the face of loss. We then discuss definitions and occurrence of resilience, as well as mechanisms and factors that might explain resilience. We conclude with consideration of issues related to resilience that require further attention and a discussion of practical implications of this work.

What Characterizes Resilience in Response to Loss?

The concept of resilience is generally understood to involve successful adaptation in the face of adversity, and for our purpose, adversity is characterized by the experience of loss. According to Hobfoll's (1989, 1998) conservation of resource theory, loss of any kind of resource that is valued by individuals triggers a stress reaction because people generally strive for maintenance or improvement of their resources. They also try to limit their losses by mobilizing their remaining resources, which is thought to mitigate the adverse effect of the loss. Based on this most general definition of loss, resilient individuals are less affected by resource loss, or are able to limit the impact of resource loss. However, beyond this core idea, the literature on resilience in response to loss provides a number of varying conceptualizations, with no clear consensus.

The main points of contention seem to be whether resilience includes recovery and growth processes. Whereas some authors, such as Garmezy (1991), define resilience as capacity for recovery and maintenance of functioning after incapacity, more recent publications separate the two aspects. Bonanno (2004), for example, defines resilience as "ability to maintain a stable equilibrium" (p. 20), reflecting an individual's capacity of stress resistance. He stresses that resilience and recovery are different concepts in the sense that they imply different trajectories of adaptation. Whereas resilience can involve some initial distress following a loss (e.g., Bonanno, Moskowitz, Papa, & Folkman, 2005), the dominant pattern is a relatively stable, positive emotional state before and after the loss, without any substantial downward peaks. In contrast, the pattern of recovery typically involves a clearly identifiable time of "not doing well" in response to loss, which is then followed by recovery or a "return to normal" (e.g., Bonanno, 2005). The key idea for this latter notion of resilience is the "ability to bounce back" from setbacks in life. In a more integrative manner, Roisman (2005) sees recovery as a special case of resilience, and suggests viewing resilience as a "family of loosely connected phenomena involving adequate (or better) adaptation in the context of adversity" (p. 264).

The next question, then, is whether the notion of growth through adversity is a part of resilience, as has been suggested by some authors. Based on his work with children, Masten (2001) proposed that the term resilience reflects the phenomenon of positive adaptation after balancing out negative circumstances. Ryff and colleagues also go beyond adapting to negative factors in her definition of resilience, which includes "maintenance, recovery, or improvement in mental or physical health following challenge" (Ryff, Singer, Love, & Essex, 1998, p. 74). However, Greve and Staudinger (2006) have argued that although growth phenomena may refer to resilience in terms of resistance capacity, they can also indicate completely different processes (e.g., growth can be stimulated by individuals setting developmental/learning goals); subsuming these phenomena under the concept of resilience may therefore be misleading. We agree with this position and further propose that the issue of whether recovery processes should be considered as instances of resilience is more a question of how narrowly the concept is defined. If resilience represents successful adaptation to major loss and life changes, then maintaining levels of well-being and functioning despite setbacks probably reflects resilience in the strictest sense. However, a life course of having experienced negative reactions to adversity but then being able to bounce back certainly reflects some degree of resilience in the grand scheme of things. Furthermore, we concur with Greve and Staudinger that loss management ought to be considered as another form of resilience. The authors suggest this for the case of old age, a time in life during which irreversible losses involving loved ones, as well as bodily, mental, and/or social functions, often accumulate. In this context, successful adaptation can mean adapting to a lower state of functioning, but the level of adaptation would have to be higher than one could have predicted given the adversity with which the individual has to cope. We contend that, depending on the nature of the loss, loss management can be an important pillar of resilience, even earlier in life.

Independent of the kind of trajectory that is thought to reflect resilience, there is no consensus about whether resilience should be viewed as an effect (outcome) or cause (antecedent) (Kaplan, 1999; Ryff et al., 1998). For resilience to be viewed an outcome, adjustment indicators in terms of well-being, distress, and functioning would have to be in place to judge a person as being resilient. To explain the cause of resilience, one would look for adaptive processes, resources, or other external conditions. In contrast, resilience can also be viewed as the cause of an outcome, such as emotional well-being. As Greve and Staudinger (2006) pointed out, the latter involves the risk of engaging in circular logic. For example, one could say that resilience in response to the death of a loved one might have been due to a person's coping capacity. One could also argue that this person adjusted so well because of his or her inner strength or resilience. However, the latter view would still leave us with the question of what constitutes this inner strength, and this may very well be the person's coping capacity. In other words, no matter what perspective one takes, the question of what explains resilience remains, and depending on the research question of interest, the concept of resilience may appear more on the "explanatory" or on the "to be explained" side of a conceptual model.

How Common Is Resilience in Response to Loss?

A question of central interest is whether individuals are likely to be resilient when faced with a loss. In the following sections, we address this question with respect to the three types of loss we are highlighting: bereavement, catastrophic event, and age-related decline.

Loss Due to Bereavement

The bulk of studies relevant to the investigation of resilience in response to loss can be found in the bereavement literature. Several longitudinal bereavement studies provide evidence regarding the occurrence of resilient responses to the death of a loved one. For instance, evidence for "minimal" grief, which involves scoring low in distress consistently over time, was found for 26% of parents in a study on loss of a child from SIDS (Wortman & Silver, 1987). In studies of conjugal loss, the following percentages of participants had minimal grief: 41% (Bonanno, Keltner, Holen, & Horowitz, 1995), 57% (Bournstein, Clayton, Halikas, Maurice, & Robins, 1973), 30% (Vachon et al., 1982), 78% (Lund et al., 1986), and 65% (Zisook & Shuchter, 1986).

In a prospective study on conjugal loss among older adults that included data from 3 years preloss to 18 months postloss (Bonanno et al., 2002; Bonanno, Wortman, & Nesse, 2004), nearly half of the participants (46%) experienced low levels of distress consistently over time (i.e., resilient group). Another trajectory in this study referred to as "depressed–improved" reflected elevated distress before the loss and improvement after the loss (10%). Several other recent studies provide convergent evidence for the resilience and depressed–improved patterns identified by Bonanno and colleagues. In a

study of older adult caregivers, for example, nearly half of the sample had low levels of depression both before and after the partner's death (Zhang, Mitchell, Bambauer, Jones, & Prigerson, 2008). Caregiver studies have further supported the existence of the depressed–improved pattern (e.g., Schulz et al., 2003). Both the resilient and depressed–improved patterns were also observed in a prospective study of gay men (Bonanno, Moskowitz, et al., 2005).

Taken together, the available data shows that "minimal" grief in response to the loss of a loved one is rather common. The number of respondents failing to show elevated distress or depression at the initial or final time point was sizable, ranging from one-fourth to over three-fourths of the sample. In fact, a recent comparison of nonbereaved and bereaved individuals who lost either a child or spouse (Bonanno, Moskowitz, et al., 2005) showed that slightly more than half of the bereaved did not significantly differ in terms of distress level from the matched sample of married individuals when assessed at 4 months and 18 months postloss. It should be noted that experiencing a resilient trajectory does not mean that there was no distress at any moment after the loss; rather, despite brief spikes in distress around the time of the death (Bonanno, Moskowitz, et al., 2005) or a short period of daily variability in levels of well-being (Bisconti et al., 2004), people who showed these patterns had generally low distress levels and managed to function at or near their normal levels (Bonanno, 2005). In this context, it is also important to note that resilience is more than the mere absence of symptoms (Bonanno, 2004). For example, in several studies, bereaved individuals who exhibited resilience in terms of low distress levels were also more likely than other bereaved people to experience and express positive emotion while talking about the loss (Bonanno & Keltner, 1997; Bonanno et al., 1995). Moreover, resilient individuals were also rated as better adjusted both pre- and postloss compared to more symptomatic bereaved individuals, when evaluated anonymously by their close friends (Bonanno, Moskowitz, et al., 2005).

One of the main concerns in the bereavement literature, when it comes to so-called "resilient responses" to loss, has been that those who do not become distressed or depressed following a major loss will experience a delayed grief reaction, or that physical health problems will emerge at some point in the future. Data from the longitudinal studies described earlier fail to support this view. In two studies, there were no respondents showing a delayed grief reaction (Bonanno et al., 1995; Bonanno & Field, 2001; Zisook & Shuchter, 1986). In the remaining studies, the percentage of respondents showing delayed grief ranged from 0.02% to 5.1% (Boerner, Wortman, & Bonanno, 2005; Bournstein et al., 1973; Lund, Caserta, & Dimond, 1986; Vachon et al., 1982; Wortman & Silver, 1987). Thus, these studies demonstrate that "delayed grief" does not occur in more than a small percentage of cases. Nor do physical symptoms appear to emerge among those who fail to experience distress soon after the loss. Both the Boerner and colleagues (2005) and Bonanno and Field (2001) studies are particularly convincing on this point because conjugally bereaved individuals were assessed over 4- and 5-year periods, respectively, with multiple outcome measures.

Loss Due to Catastrophic Events

Besides bereavement, research has also addressed adult resilience in the context of other critical life events (e.g., catastrophic event) as well as with respect to aging, both of which can be conceptualized as instances of resource loss. Although there are unique aspects to these types of losses (e.g., in that catastrophic events usually come without warning, whereas aging is a continuous, generally rather slow-advancing process that can be anticipated to some extent), both involve the loss of basic resources. For example, individuals who experience an earthquake or a terrorist attack are likely to suffer

not only from health consequences, if injured, but also from loss of other resources, such as friends, family, or financial means. They may have to give up their job, and they are at risk to lose psychological resources, such as feelings of security or the sense of a just world. In a large-scale study on terrorism in Israel, Hobfoll, Canetti-Nisim, and Johnson (2006) showed that exposure to terrorism was significantly related to loss in psychosocial resources (e.g., feeling less in control of one's life), as well as to symptoms of posttraumatic stress disorder (PTSD) and depression. Interestingly, this exposure was also linked to gain in psychosocial resources (e.g., hope and purpose in life), pointing to the possibility of positive outcomes that may be a part of resilience or at least enhance resilience.

Being the victim of a violent act, such as a terrorist attack, represents an extreme case of a critical life event. Nevertheless, studies show that a substantial number of people demonstrate rather high levels of resilience in response to such events. For instance, in their study on reactions of New Yorkers to the 9/11 terrorist attacks, Bonnano, Galea, Bucciarelli, and Vlahov (2006) found that even among strongly exposed individuals (i.e., compound exposure of having lost a friend or relative in the attack and seeing the attack in person), at least one-third showed resilience, as defined by none or one PTSD symptom. In other groups with less exposure, resilience was observed in up to 50% of participants. Parallel findings were reported with respect to depression; those individuals identified as resilient, based on minimal PTSD symptoms, had lower depression levels compared to not only the rest of the sample but also the average of U.S. nonclinical samples (Bonanno, Galea, Bucciarelli, & Vlahov, 2007).

Loss Due to Age-Related Decline

The process of aging can involve a multitude of losses, including the loss of social roles and social network members, decline in physical energy and health, and restrictions in cognitive capacity. However, empirical evidence suggests that a majority of old and very old individuals seem able to maintain a rather high level of well-being in spite of such losses (e.g., Jopp & Smith, 2006; Smith, Fleeson, Geiselmann, Settersten, & Kunzmann, 1999; Staudinger & Fleeson, 1996). Therefore, the concept of resilience in old age has recently received increasing attention (e.g., Greve & Staudinger, 2006; Ryff et al., 1998; Staudinger et al., 1995). In particular, there is a growing interest in clarifying the point at which the multitude of loss experiences at the very end of the lifespan may exceed the individual's capacity for adaptation (e.g., Baltes & Smith, 2003), which should result in fewer very old resilient individuals compared to preceding phases of old age. Although data on very old individuals are still limited, it seems to be the case that even centenarians affected by multiple severe restrictions maintain a surprisingly high level of well-being (Jopp & Rott, 2006). Findings further showed that centenarians felt at least as happy as middle-aged and older adults, which strongly speaks against a systematic breakdown of resilience mechanisms in very old age.

What Contributes to Resilience in the Face of Loss?

Research has addressed various factors that account for resilience in the face of loss. Empirical studies usually cover various different aspects and characteristics, rarely using the same set of predictors more than once, or applying systematic comparison across studies or loss types. Therefore, our focus herein is on those factors that have consistently been found to play a role in predicting resilience outcomes in at least one of the three loss contexts (i.e., bereavement, catastrophic event, and aging). We group predictors into the following categories: loss characteristics, intrapersonal factors, interpersonal factors, and coping and emotion regulation.

Loss Characteristics

Cause of death and circumstances around the death are generally considered as important predictors of bereavement outcomes. Specifically, resilience is unlikely if the death of a loved one was sudden and violent (Kaltman & Bonanno, 2003; Murphy, Johnson, Chung, & Beaton, 2003). Resilience as manifested in minimal distress trajectories is also less likely, if a lengthy illness was the cause of the death and the bereaved person was the caregiver. Findings consistently indicate that strain related to caregiving affects caregivers adversely before the death, and that the majority of caregivers experience relief and stress reduction after the death of the care recipient (Schulz et al., 2003). Consistent with this evidence, findings show that resilient bereaved spouses are more likely not to have provided direct care to an ill spouse (Bonanno et al., 2002). Rather, those who had an ill spouse or cared for him or her were more often found in the depressed–improved group.

The type of relationship a person had with the deceased, as well as the quality of the relationship, also represents important factors related to resilience. Resilience seems unlikely in response to the death of a child, particularly if the death occurred under sudden or violent circumstances. Rather, experiencing intense distress is considered as normative. For example, in her study on the violent death of a child, Murphy (1996) found that 4 months after the loss, over 80% of the mothers and 60% of the fathers rated themselves as highly distressed. The quality of relationship plays an essential role especially in the context to close relationships. In Bonanno's studies, resilient bereaved spouses tended to evaluate their marriage as positive and reported low degrees of dependency on the spouse, as well as lower general interpersonal dependency (e.g., Bonanno et al., 2002). Thus, resilience seems more likely among partners who are positively connected but not overly dependent on each other.

The nature and circumstances of a catastrophic event are also likely to play a role for resilience. As shown by Bonanno and colleagues (2006, 2007), types of exposure to the 9/11 terrorist attacks were related to the percentage of resilient individuals. For instance, 56% of the individuals who saw the attack were resilient, whereas resilience was only observed in 33% of those who were physically injured in the attacks. Compound exposure, combining loss of a friend or relative with having seen the attacks or having been involved in the rescue efforts, was also related to smaller likelihood of resilience. Furthermore, catastrophic events seem to be more likely to result in PTSD if the event is the result of purposeful human behavior (Charuvastra & Cloitre, 2008). For instance, the highest lifetime risk to develop PTSD was associated with sexual and physical assault and robbery (Frans, Rimmö, Aberg, & Frederikson, 2005). In a prospective study with residents from the same Israeli community, terror attack survivors develop PTSD twice as often as survivors of traffic accidents (Shalev & Freedman, 2005). There is further evidence that multiple exposure to events increases the risk of PTSD (e.g., Frans et al., 2005), and that negative events experienced after war trauma increases soldiers' risk for maladjustment (e.g., King, King, Fairbank, Keane, & Adams, 1998). Thus, experiencing more severe or multiple losses seems to decrease the chance of a resilient reaction in this context.

With respect to aging, one can assume that the nature and circumstances of the loss can also have an impact. For example, the nature of health-related loss and the controllability of the health problem are likely to affect a person's response to the loss. Furthermore, age-related losses in different domains of functioning and living (e.g., loss of cognitive capacity or of social network members) may all vary with respect to their importance for the individual, the extent to which they interfere with valued goals, and to which the individual can compensate for them. However, we are not aware of studies that have specifically assessed and systematically investigated different types of age-associated loss with respect to resilience. This may be due to the fact that a particular age-associated loss rarely happens in isolation but rather is accompanied by and intertwined with other losses. Therefore, one could assume that another decisive factor modulating resilience to age-related loss is the number and kind of events occurring simultaneously. If, for example, age-related loss is experienced in multiple domains of living (e.g., simultaneous retirement, heart condition, and loss of spouse), this may put additional strain on the individual and is likely to further reduce the chance of a resilient reaction pattern.

Intrapersonal Factors

Age and Gender

Chronological age and gender are often-examined factors in the context of resilience. However, it should be noted that they represent no causal mechanism per se but are carrier variables, most likely influential due to other characteristics closely related to them, such as health issues with respect to age or role aspects with respect to gender. It is also important to keep in mind that both are likely to interact with all or most of the factors reviewed in this section potentially contribute to resilience. For example, older adults who lose a spouse tend to report less distress than younger adults who lose a spouse (Miller & Wortman, 2002). That older bereaved partners in general fare better has been discussed in the context of the timing of the loss. Experiencing a loss at a point in the lifespan when loss is considered normative can help in dealing with the loss. It is, for instance, seen as normal if children survive their parents. If the sequence of dying is reversed, then the death is likely to create more distress. In old age, it also is common that one partner dies and the other survives. Nevertheless, even normative losses represent a situation that requires adaptation and can cause difficulties for the individual. Empirical findings also show that women are more likely to be resilient when their husbands die (Stroebe, Stroebe, & Schut, 2001). At the same time, resilience is less often observed in women who lose a child (Rubin & Malkinson, 2001). Both might be related to gender roles rather than to gender itself.

When it comes to catastrophic events, one might assume that being older involves additional risks because older individuals tend to have fewer resources at their disposal to manage a crisis, such as loss of the household due to a flood. Nevertheless, older adults might also have fewer expectations about how well they should deal with difficulties or what life should offer to them and they might not be in situations where they have to perform fully, such as the workplace. Therefore, being older might also be a facilitating factor in dealing with loss. As was found for other losses, older individuals were more likely to be resilient in Bonanno's 9/11 study. Being age 65 and older increased the chance for resilience threefold in comparison to young individuals ages 18–24 years (Bonanno et al., 2007). At the same time, women were less often found to be resilient compared to men. In fact, women's likelihood of belonging to the group of resilient individuals was less than half that of men.

In the context of aging, some evidence suggests that older individuals fare better with respect to coping with age-related changes. For example, several studies have found that individuals report stable levels of well-being despite the increase in resource loss with advanced age (e.g., Smith et al., 1999), and despite the fact that older adults seem rather realistic in terms of acknowledging and reporting losses (Connidis, 1989; Steverink, Westerhof, Bode, & Dittmann-Kohli, 2001). Older adults also seem to hold more elaborate concepts about development and aging (Heckhausen, Dixon, & Baltes, 1989; Jopp, Berendonk, et al., 2009), which might account for their ability to deal with losses better. Moreover, findings reveal that in very old age, some life aspects become less important for people's overall quality of life, and that

this is often the case for those aspects that have become worse (e.g., health; Jopp, Rott, & Oswald, 2008). Therefore, age-associated change in evaluation of age-related losses might represent one mechanism subsumed under the variable chronological age.

Gender has also been investigated in the context of adaptation to age-related loss but was mostly found to be unrelated to the experience of aging as loss (Steverink et al., 2001). There is some evidence that females are likely to report lower levels of subjective well-being in old and very old age (e.g., Pinquart & Sörensen, 2001), but this effect tends to be rather small. Regarding inconsistencies in findings for younger individuals, it has been argued that women might experience both more positive and more negative affect, and that the well-being measure used (e.g., life-satisfaction vs. depression) could therefore explain some of the variation (e.g., Diener, Suh, Lucas, & Smith, 1999). In old age, selection effects may also play a role, as suggested by stronger gender differences in very old compared to young-old individuals (Pinquart & Sörensen, 2001): Women are more likely to experience age-related chronic health conditions due to higher life expectancy; old men are more likely to be in a better physical condition because they represent a positive selection of their age group, which means that they have to deal with fewer restrictions. Thus, there seem to be confounds among age, gender, and selection effects.

Mental and Physical Health

In all three loss contexts addressed here, preloss mental and physical health seem to be important for resilience. There is consistent evidence across studies that resilient individuals are unlikely to have a history of prior mental health problems (e.g., Bonanno, Boerner, & Wortman, 2008; see Schulz, Boerner, & Hebert, 2008, for a review). Research evidence from studies on catastrophic events and on aging paints a similar picture. For instance, in a study on the survivors of the Enschede Fireworks disaster in the Netherlands, prior psychological problems, including depression, were significant predictors of postdisaster mental health problems (Dirkzwager, Grievink, van der Velden, & Yzermans, 2006). Similarly, when it comes to development of depressive symptomatology in advanced age, findings indicate that the risk for receiving a depression diagnosis is elevated for individuals with a prior depression episode (e.g., Cole & Dendukuri, 2003; Schoevers et al., 2003).

With respect to physical health, concurrent health and physical functioning (e.g., subjective health, instrumental activities of daily living; Hardy, Concato, & Gill, 2004) have been found to characterize resilient individuals who experienced a stressful life event (e.g., death or illness of a relative or friend). Similarly, prior physical health problems were associated with a reduced likelihood for resilience in studies of catastrophic events (e.g., 9/11 study: Bonanno et al., 2007; Enschede Fireworks study: Dirkzwager et al., 2006). Resilience in old and very old age was also found to be strongly determined by age-associated physical loss. For instance, about one-third of the age-related variance in aging satisfaction, a cognitive facet of well-being, was explained by physical constraints (Staudinger & Fleeson, 1996). Individuals who experienced their aging predominantly as loss were also more likely to report lower subjective health, whereas those who experienced aging as continuous growth were more likely to report better health (Steverink et al., 2001).

Personality

Considering their biological foundation, presence since birth, and considerable stability, personality traits are especially interesting in research on resilience, since they are likely to influence adaptation before and after the loss (e.g., Folkman & Lazarus, 1988). Personality factors have been addressed in various studies on bereavement, but overall they have been less useful in predicting grief trajectories compared to other variables (e.g., prior mental health, or loss characteristics discussed earlier). Nevertheless, there is evidence to suggest that resilient individuals tend to be characterized by higher extraversion and lower neuroticism levels (e.g., Bonanno et al., 2002). A similar impression can be gleaned from survivor studies of different catastrophic events (e.g., forest fire, civil war, and burn survivors); a more resilient reaction pattern typically is seen in persons with higher extraversion and lower levels of neuroticism (e.g., Aidman & Kollara-Mitsinikos, 2006; Fauerbach, Lawrence, Schmidt, Munster, & Costa, 2000; McFarlane, Clayer, & Bookless, 1997; Riolli, Savicki, & Capani, 2002). Extraversion and neuroticism also seem to be important for resilience in the aging context. For instance, in their work on the Berlin Aging Study, Staudinger, Freund, Linden, and Maas (1999) found that old and very old individuals with higher levels of extraversion reported higher satisfaction with their aging. Neuroticism, by contrast, was related to lower levels of aging satisfaction. Similarly, in a study with centenarians, Jopp and Rott (2006) were able to show that very old individuals with higher levels of extraversion were happier.

Resilient individuals are also likely to score high on measures of optimism. For instance, Moskowitz and colleagues (2003) found that optimism predicted fewer depressive symptoms and more positive states of mind in bereaved gay male caregivers following the death of a partner. Furthermore, bereaved spouses' worldviews prior to the loss may have allowed them to accept the death more readily (e.g., they scored higher on beliefs in a just world and acceptance of death; Bonanno et al., 2002). Again, similar findings emerge for the context of catastrophic events, including studies investigating adaptation among victims of the Kosovo crisis (Riolli et al., 2002), the 1999 earthquake in Turkey (Sumer, Karanci, Berument, & Gunes, 2005), as well as the Enschede Fireworks disaster (Van der Velden et al., 2007).

Thus, positive, optimistic attitudes towards life, as well as the willingness to accept certain negative facts of life, are likely to be found among the resilient. Complementing research on the positive effect of optimism for psychological adjustment to critical events, optimism also remains a crucial predictor of resilience in old age. Even centenarians, who, as a group, have experienced many more losses than younger adults, were found to profit from an optimistic outlook on life. German centenarians, who reported higher levels of optimistic outlook also indicated higher levels of happiness (Jopp & Rott, 2006).

One personality aspect that has received attention in the context of bereavement and catastrophic events is self-enhancement. Individuals characterized as self-enhancers seem to fare better in loss situations. Tending toward self-serving biases in perception and attribution, such as overstating one's positive qualities, self-enhancers also seem to have higher self-esteem and to deal better with traumatic situations. Self-enhancers confronted with the premature death of a spouse or civil war in Bosnia were given higher ratings on their functioning by mental health experts (e.g., Bonanno, Field, Kovacevic, & Kaltman, 2002). Comparable findings on the benefit of trait self-enhancement also emerged in a study on resilience in the aftermath of the 9/11 terrorist attacks (Bonanno, Rennicke, & Dekel, 2005). Again, resilient individuals were high on the trait of self-enhancement, which went along with ratings of better adjustment before the event and more positive affect, and less often felt restricted in talking about their emotions. However, the relation between self-enhancement and positive affect was qualified by the degree of exposure to physical danger: The relation of self-enhancement and positive affect was only observed in individuals who did not experience high levels of physical danger.

Another personality feature addressed in the context of resilience is attachment style. This research is based on the notion that securely attached people tend to have positive and realistic views of themselves, and to regard other people as dependable and reliable, whereas insecurely attached people see themselves in a less positive light and lack basic trust in others (Mikulincer & Shaver, 2003). Consequently, it is assumed that secure attachment comes with greater capacity to adapt to aversive events. In the bereavement context, Fraley and Bonanno (2004) found that securely attached persons were more likely to show a resilient trajectory. However, this was also the case for the dismissive–avoidant style, referring to a tendency to minimize importance of relationships. These latter individuals coped as well as the securely attached. Also in line with the prediction of greater adaptation capacity, in a study with high-exposure survivors of the 9/11 terrorist attacks, Fraley, Fazzari, Bonanno, and Dekel (2006) showed that securely attached persons exhibited fewer symptoms of PTSD and depression than insecurely attached persons. In addition, their friends considered them better adjusted than most people they knew, even prior to 9/11.

Interpersonal Factors

Social support seems generally to be a protective resource that does not necessarily distinguish between those who experience a loss (e.g., bereaved) and those who do not (e.g., nonbereaved control group). However, when different grief trajectory groups were compared (e.g., Bonnano et al., 2002), the resilient group clearly had more support from friends and relatives before the loss than most of the other trajectory groups, in particular those with long-term adjustment problems.

There is also considerable evidence for the important role of social support in the context of catastrophic events, mostly from studies on PTSD risk following such events, suggesting that individuals with more support are less likely to develop PTSD (Berwin, Andrews, & Valentine, 2000; Ozer, Best, Lipsey, & Weiss, 2003). Similarly, in

Bonanno and colleagues' (2007) 9/11 study, individuals reporting low levels of support were less likely to be resilient. Addressing further the mechanisms underlying this effect, Charuvastra and Cloitre (2008) concluded in their comprehensive review on the role of social relations in PTSD that the effects of social support seem to be more consistent for lack of support compared to its presence, perhaps due to the fact that benefits of support might depend on who provides support, whether the support matches the victim's needs, how support is perceived, and how network members view the event.

With respect to resilience in the face of aging, social factors were also found to play a role. For instance, individuals exhibited higher levels of well-being when they had persons available who would help in difficult situations (Perrig-Chiello, 1997). Social resources also become increasingly important with advancing age. Comparing old and very old individuals, the very old were more likely to be resilient (as indicated by higher levels of attachment to life) if they reported more frequent phone contacts (Jopp, Rott, & Oswald, 2008). The number of social network partners also had a significant effect on centenarians' well-being, both directly and mediated by an optimistic outlook on life (Jopp & Rott, 2006). Moreover, social support has been identified as an important predictor of well-being in older adults with chronic, progressive vision loss (Reinhardt, Boerner, & Horowitz, 2009). Thus, availability and adequacy of social support is a likely part of resilient responses to loss.

Coping and Emotion Regulation

When it comes to coping with bereavement, one important aspect to consider is what is often referred to as the processing of the loss or *grief processing*, which can include thinking and talking about the deceased, cherishing memories, or searching for meaning. Bonanno and colleagues (2002) found that resilient persons showed relatively low

levels of grief processing, but that they, at the same time, scored high on comfort from positive memories and low on avoidance. The latter finding indicates that low levels of grief processing are not indicative of denial or indifference toward the deceased. Consistent with these earlier findings, Bonanno, Moskowitz, and colleagues (2005) found more recently that both grief processing and deliberate avoidance predicted poorer long-term adjustment in response to parental and spousal loss, and that initial grief processing predicted later grief processing. This suggests that those who engage in much grief processing early on are also likely to do so later, and that they are less likely to show a resilient trajectory.

Another interesting aspect of coping with loss in the context of bereavement is emotion regulation. Bonanno, Papa, LaLande, Westphal, and Coifman (2004) found that resilient individuals show a higher capacity for flexible emotion regulation, as indicated by the ability to enhance or suppress emotional expression effectively in an experimental setting. Similarly, Coifman, Bonanno, Ray, and Gross (2007) found evidence that *repressive coping* (i.e., directing one's attention away from a negative affective experience) may promote resilience after spousal loss. In fact, both bereaved and nonbereaved individuals who exhibited signs of repressive coping (measured as discrepancy between the affective experience and sympathetic nervous system response) had fewer symptoms of psychopathology, fewer health problems/somatic complaints, and were rated as better adjusted by friends than those who did not show repressive coping.

An important part of emotion regulation is the ability not to let negative emotions "take over" entirely or "spread" to the extent that the experience of positive moments becomes impossible. Thus, it is not surprising that resilient individuals were found to have the ability to experience positive and negative affect at the same time, which means that they could maintain a relative independence of positive and negative affect (Coifman, Bonanno, & Rafaeli, 2007). Hence, resilient individuals may be able to experience the negative aspects of a loss, while also enjoying moments of emotional uplift, even during the phase of dealing with the loss. This may also enable them to be more positive in social situations, making them more enjoyable as social partners. Or, as stated by Bonanno and Keltner (1997), they might minimize the impact of the loss while "increasing continued contact with and support from important people in the social environment" (p. 134).

Coping concepts related to emotion regulation that have recently been proposed by Bonanno (2005) as contributors to resilience are pragmatic coping and adaptive flexibility, which in some instances are referred to as "ugly coping." The idea is that there may be successful ways of coping with isolated stressors or events that are not adaptive under normal circumstances. For example, although research has demonstrated the health benefits of expressing stress-related negative emotions, this benefit does not necessarily exist in the case of bereavement, and resilient bereaved individuals tend to express fewer negative feelings compared to other bereaved persons (Bonanno & Keltner, 1997). As further examples of pragmatic coping, Bonanno cites self-enhancement and dismissive–avoidant attachment. In our view, there is little adaptive flexibility in these examples because they seem to represent trait-like features. These features happened to be advantageous in certain situations, but they are not an expression of pragmatism or flexibility. However, one could argue that flexible emotion regulation represents Bonanno's idea of pragmatic coping.

Bonanno's concept of pragmatic or flexible coping involves the idea that the adaptiveness of the coping effort depends on the coping challenge, and that what may not be adaptive in one situation may be very adaptive in another. This is also one of the core assumptions of all major theories of lifespan development that have specified and empirically supported adaptive processes that serve to cope with major loss and life change. These lifespan theories propose both active, problem-solving efforts aimed at ending or improving an adverse situation, and inner adjustments to loss situations that allow the person to remain resilient even in the face of permanent loss. Such inner adjustments can include modifications of one's goals or preferences, lowering of personal standards, or positive reappraisals of stressful situations. As Greve and Staudinger (2006) pointed out, such "accommodative" processes (Brandtstädter & Renner, 1990; Brandtstädter & Rothermund, 2002; see also Baltes & Freund, 2003) lead to an altered view of a person's self, goals, and life situation, and are thus qualitatively different from defensive avoidance strategies: "This approach actually makes the problem go away permanently; denying the existence of a sickness does not cure it, but looking at it in relative terms makes it bearable. This is why we should not interpret denial and suppression as processes of resilience" (p. 826). Thus, accommodative coping is thought to be particularly beneficial when a person is faced with permanent loss. Since these types of loss are common in old age, it is not surprising that accommodative coping has been identified as important predictor of resilience in old age (e.g., Brandtstädter, 1999).

In terms of specific irreversible losses, accommodative coping has been found to be beneficial for middle-aged and older adults with chronic, progressive vision loss and related disability; those who engaged in accommodative coping were less likely to experience mental health problems as a result of the loss (Boerner, 2004). Similarly, coping activities, such as "giving up responsibility," have been found to be of adaptive value among older adults confronted with situations that do not allow for change but require acceptance of the loss (Staudinger et al., 1999). Supportive of this claim are findings on old and very old individuals with low resources and high somatic risks, for whom giving up goals or activities was protective in terms of maintaining positive levels of well-being (Jopp & Smith, 2006; Staudinger et al., 1999).

What Still Needs Further Attention?

Research on adult resilience to loss has generated a considerable number of studies whose findings contribute to an increasingly better understanding of how adults react to loss, as exemplified in work on resilience in the context of bereavement, catastrophic events, and age-associated loss. Nevertheless, this research has also resulted in new questions that need to be addressed in future research.

One intriguing question that has been raised more recently is whether there could be some downsides to a resilient response to loss. For instance, findings from two studies by Bonanno and colleagues suggest that self-enhancers might benefit from their trait in terms of resilience but not necessarily with respect to their social relationships. At the very least, self-enhancers were rated rather unfavorably by other individuals (e.g., as less honest and more self-centered; Bonanno et al., 2002). There are several possible explanations for this finding. It could be that resilient individuals are misunderstood by their social environment as a result of the same characteristics that enable them to be resilient, such as flexible emotion regulation or the ability to experience positive and negative affect at the same time. The failure to demonstrate obvious distress may violate other people's expectations for how a person should be responding to a loss. This may result in social partners' withdrawal from the resilient person and in subsequent loss of social support structures for this person. On the other hand, it could also be that some of the characteristics related to resilience indeed have negative consequences for social partners. For example, it is possible that the

same qualities that make resilient persons less vulnerable to outside stressors also make them less sensitive to other people's needs. This could have a negative impact on their close relationships.

Another intriguing question is what happens in families, or other social groups, when one person shows a low distress pattern after a loss, whereas other members in this social system experience intense distress. In such a case, would those who are more distressed be likely to benefit from the presence or availability of a resilient person? Or would the lack of congruence in the experience of individual members be more likely to lead to misunderstandings and individual coping efforts that interfere with one another? These questions have considerable importance in certain loss situations, for example, when couples are confronted with the death of a child. One spouse may feel uncomfortable expressing feelings of distress about the loss, if the partner appears not to be distressed (e.g., Wortman, Battle, & Lemkau, 1997). Future work addressing these questions would make an important contribution because people rarely face a loss in a social vacuum. The best way to test these ideas would be to draw on prospective data of couples or multiple family members, in which each person's perspective on the relationship could be assessed. Such data would provide the opportunity to learn what the deceased person thought about his or her relationship with the "resilient person."

Another interesting aspect that should be addressed in future research is whether resilience tends to be event-specific, or whether individuals are likely to be resilient across different loss situations. When comparing resilience to loss across bereavement, catastrophic events, and age-associated loss, the studies we reviewed indicated that some characteristics might be beneficial in all loss situations, such as flexible emotion regulation. However, other factors might be more beneficial in the context of certain losses, or might even represent a risk factor in another loss context. The classic example for the latter situation is gender, with women being generally more resilient in the case of losing a spouse but less resilient when losing a child. Exploring the differential effects of such factors might help us to gain more insight into the mechanisms underlying resilience. In addition, depending on the characteristics of a loss, the factors related to resilience might also differ. For instance, adaptation to retirement might benefit from proactive planning and development of alternative life goals, whereas consequences of a catastrophic event can only be anticipated to a certain extent and, due to their nature, are likely to exceed all expectations (e.g., tsunami in Asia, 2004). Depending on the nature of the loss, one might assume that specific constellations of factors related to resilience may be more beneficial than others.

One important contributor to resilience that, to date, seems to be conceptually and empirically underdeveloped in the literature on resilience in response to loss is coping. Although there have been recent suggestions to conceptualize coping processes that may be critical for resilience (e.g., adaptive flexibility; Bonanno, 2005), such efforts have remained fairly unconnected to well-advanced and empirically supported theories of lifespan development that have contributed greatly to explaining how people successfully cope with loss and major life change (Boerner & Jopp, 2007). We believe that research on resilience in response to loss would benefit immensely from conceptual guidance in terms of the constructs formulated in these theories, and the related predictions that address under which circumstances a particular coping direction may be more likely and adaptive. A stronger and more theoretically guided focus on coping should also include attention to how individuals develop their coping skills. This directly ties into the question of how resilience in response to loss comes about. Although the early resilience research examined chil-

dren, this work focused mostly on whether specific characteristics or trait profiles were related to resilience. Yet how, for example, children develop coping strategies that enable them to be resilient has rarely been examined. To what extent may individuals acquire characteristics, capacities, or skills to be resilient in the face of loss as a part of their learning history in the primary family context or, more broadly, through education and cultural contexts?

To address the latter part of this question, cross-cultural differences in resilience need to be addressed further. There are some hints that ethnicity and cultural background relate to the expression of resilience. In a cross-cultural study, Chinese participants seemed to recover more quickly from bereavement in terms of emotional adjustment compared to Americans, but they also reported more somatic complaints (Bonanno, Moskowitz, et al., 2005). Culturally shaped spiritual convictions may also have an impact on how individuals deal with loss. For example, for a person who believes that life is suffering and death is transcendence, as seen in Zen Buddhism, the experience of loss may be easier to bear. There may also be culturally shaped implications of particular losses. For example, in many cultures, the loss of one's husband involves loss of not only status and financial support but also of respect and basic human rights, which is likely to make coping more difficult. Cultures also differ substantially in prevalent attitudes toward aging, which can make dealing with age-related loss more or less difficult. Moreover, resilience may have different meanings in different cultures. To date, the bulk of research on resilience in response to loss has been conducted from a Western perspective, with corresponding study populations. It is likely that this has resulted in a portrayal of resilience that is biased by Western values, with a focus on the importance of maintaining high levels of functioning and well-being in the face of adversity. Thus, exploring in more detail whether and how resilience in response to loss and the meanings associated with resilience vary by culture might help us to gain a better understanding of the influence of culturally shaped factors, such as attitudes and expectations toward loss experiences.

Biological aspects of resilience may also be more important than expected so far. In their review, Curtis and Cicchetti (2003) have convincingly argued that research on resilience in the past decades has focused mainly on psychosocial correlates and conditions of resilience processes. They argue for expanding the scope of the concept of resilience to include the biological level, to focus on biological contributors to resilience, and to examine whether resilience is, at least to some extent, dependent on biophysiological factors. There is some evidence for persistent alteration of stress mechanisms and brain functioning from early trauma. Early life stress apparently produces a sensitization of the cortical corticotropin-releasing neuronal system and the hypothalamic–pituitary–adrenal axis stress response, as shown in preclinical studies (e.g., Coplan et al., 2001; Van Oers, de Kloet, & Levine, 1998). Victims of child abuse were also found to show changed corticotropin responses to a standard psychosocial stressor (Heim et al., 2000). Furthermore, recent studies have shown that traumatic stress can alter the brain structurally and functionally. These changes are assumed to be caused by an increasing neuronal fear network that results from exposure to different types of traumatic events (Kolassa & Elbert, 2007). Addressing resilience in response to loss by physiological methods and the means of brain research represents a fascinating avenue that can complement and potentially enrich the ongoing efforts in psychosocial research to improve our understanding of what resilient responses to loss can involve, and what after all makes them possible. The approach of combining physiological and psychosocial factors into more complex models to predict resilience will allow us better to define the mediating and moderating mechanisms that enhance resilience in the face of loss.

Taken together, the available literature shows that similar forms of resilience can be found in response to different types of loss situations, such as bereavement, catastrophic events, and age-related decline. It is also clear that there is some overlap in factors that may contribute to resilience (i.e., loss characteristics, intra- and interpersonal factors, and coping and emotion regulation). Future research should try to identify event-specific versus universal correlates of resilience across different types of loss, and these correlates ideally should include both psychosocial and biological aspects. Moreover, the gist of our current understanding of resilience in response to loss centers on the benefits of resilience in the context of Western values. To complement this picture, we need to know more about possible downsides of such resilience (e.g., negative social implications), and about different meanings and implications of resilience that may emerge when the phenomenon is considered outside the realm of Western values and perspectives. Furthermore, research evidence demonstrates that there are ways to cope that involve a certain degree of adaptive flexibility that makes resilient responses to loss more likely. However, we need to gain a better understanding of the nature of such coping mechanisms, and of how they are developed and shaped over the course of a person's life. Finally, we need more research that considers the dynamic interplay between the different factors that have been found to contribute to resilience. Besides considering which factors might be more important for resilience than others (e.g., when comparing personality to biological predictors), it is important to examine the ways in which the impact of some factors is enhanced or diminished due to their functional relations with other factors. Despite the considerable complexity that such integrative approaches involve when addressing the system of factors contributing to resilience rather than single predictors, they represent a promising avenue to further our understanding about resilience in response to loss.

References

Aidman, E. V., & Kollara-Mitsinikos, L. (2006). Personality disposition in the prediction of posttraumatic stress reactions. *Psychological Reports*, 99, 569–580.

Baltes, P. B., & Freund, A. M. (2003). Human strengths as the orchestration of wisdom and selective optimization with compensation. In L. G. Aspinwall & U. M. Staudinger (Eds.), *A psychology of human strengths: Fundamental questions and future directions for a positive psychology* (pp. 23–35). Washington, DC: American Psychological Association.

Baltes, P. B., & Smith, J. (2003). New frontiers in the future of aging: From successful aging of the young old to the dilemmas of the fourth age. *Gerontology*, 49, 123–135.

Berkman, L. F., Seeman, T. E., Albert, M., Blazer, D., Kahn, R., Mohs, R., et al. (1993). High, usual and impaired functioning in community-dwelling older men and women: Findings from the MacArthur Foundation Research Network on Successful Aging. *Journal of Clinical Epidemiology*, 46, 1129–1140.

Berwin, C. R., Andrews, B., & Valentine, J. D. (2000). Meta-analysis of risk factors for posttraumatic stress disorder in trauma-exposed adults. *Journal of Consulting and Clinical Psychology*, 68, 748–766.

Boerner, K. (2004). Adaptation to disability among middle-aged and older adults: The role of assimilative and accommodative coping. *Journals of Gerontology: Psychological Sciences and Social Sciences*, 59B, P35–P42.

Boerner, K., & Jopp, D. (2007). Improvement/maintenance and reorientation as central features of coping with major life change and loss: Contributions of three life-span theories. *Human Development*, 50, 171–195.

Boerner, K., Wortman, C. B., & Bonanno, G. (2005). Resilient or at risk?: A four-year study of older adults who initially showed high or low distress following conjugal loss. *Journals of Gerontology B: Psychological Sciences and Social Sciences*, 60B, P67–P73.

Bonanno, G. A. (2004). Loss, trauma, and human resilience: Have we underestimated the human capacity to thrive after extremely aversive events? *American Psychologist*, 59, 20–28.

Bonanno, G. A. (2005). Resilience in the face of potential trauma. *Current Directions in Psychological Science*, 14, 135–138.

Bonanno, G. A., Boerner, K., & Wortman, C. B. (2008). Trajectories of grieving. In M. Stroebe, R. Hansson, H. Schut, & W. Stroebe (Eds.), *Handbook of bereavement research and practice: 21st century perspectives* (pp. 287–307). Washington, DC: American Psychological Association Press.

Bonanno, G. A., Field, N., Kovacevic, A., & Kaltman, S. (2002). Self-enhancement as a buffer against extreme adversity: Civil war in Bosnia and traumatic loss in the United States. *Personality and Social Psychology Bulletin*, 28, 184–196.

Bonanno, G. A., & Field, N. P. (2001). Evaluating the delayed grief hypothesis across 5 years of bereavement. *American Behavioral Scientist*, 44, 798–816.

Bonanno, G. A., Galea, S., Bucciarelli, A., & Vlahov, D. (2006). Psychological resilience after disaster: New York City in the aftermath of the September 11th terrorist attack. *Psychological Science*, 17, 181–186.

Bonanno, G. A., Galea, S., Bucciarelli, A., & Vlahov, D. (2007). What predicts psychological resilience after disaster?: The role of demographics, resources, and life stress. *Journal of Consulting and Clinical Psychology*, 75, 671–682.

Bonanno, G. A., & Keltner, D. (1997). Facial expressions of emotion and the course of conjugal bereavement. *Journal of Abnormal Psychology*, 106, 126–137.

Bonanno, G. A., Keltner, D., Holen, A., & Horowitz, M. J. (1995). When avoiding unpleasant emotion might not be such a bad thing: Verbal–autonomic response dissociation and midlife conjugal bereavement. *Journal of Personality and Social Psychology*, 46, 975–985.

Bonanno, G. A., Moskowitz, J. T., Papa, A., & Folkman, S. (2005). Resilience to loss in bereaved spouses, bereaved parents, and bereaved gay men. *Journal of Personality and Social Psychology*, 88(5), 827–843.

Bonanno, G. A., Papa, A., Lalande, K., Westphal, M., & Coifman, K. (2004). The importance of being flexible: The ability to both enhance and suppress emotional expression predicts long-term adjustment. *Psychological Science*, 15, 482–487.

Bonanno, G. A., Rennicke, C., & Dekel, S. (2005). Self-enhancement among high-exposure survivors of the September 11th terrorist attack:

Resilience or social maladjustment? *Journal of Personality and Social Psychology, 88*(6), 984–998.

Bonanno, G. A., Wortman, C. B., Lehman, D., Tweed, R., Sonnega, J., Carr, D., et al. (2002). Resilience to loss, chronic grief, and their pre-bereavement predictors. *Journal of Personality and Social Psychology, 83*, 1150–1164.

Bonanno, G. A., Wortman, C. B., & Nesse, R. M. (2004). Prospective patterns of resilience and maladjustment during widowhood. *Psychology and Aging, 19*, 260–271.

Bournstein, P. E., Clayton, P. J., Halikas, J. A., Maurice, W. L., & Robins, E. (1973). The depression of widowhood after thirteen months. *British Journal of Psychiatry, 122*, 561–566.

Brandtstädter, J. (1999). Sources of resilience in the aging self. In F. Blanchard-Fields & T. Hess (Eds.), *Social cognition and aging* (pp. 123–141). New York: Academic Press.

Brandtstädter, J., & Renner, G. (1990). Tenacious goal pursuit and flexible goal adjustment: Explication and age-related analysis of assimilative and accommodative strategies of coping. *Psychology and Aging, 5*, 58–67.

Brandtstädter, J., & Rothermund, K. (2002). The life course dynamics of goal pursuit and goal adjustment: A two-process framework. *Developmental Review, 22*, 117–150.

Charuvastra, A., & Cloitre, M. (2008). Social bonds and posttraumatic stress disorder. *Annual Review of Psychology, 59*, 301–328.

Coifman, K. G., Bonanno, G. A., Ray, R. D., & Gross, J. J. (2007). Does repressive coping promote resilience?: Affective–autonomic response discrepancy during bereavement. *Journal of Personality and Social Psychology, 92*, 745–758.

Cole, M. G., & Dendukuri, N. (2003). Risk factors for depression among elderly community subjects: A systematic review and meta-analysis. *American Journal of Geriatric Psychiatry, 160*, 1147–1156.

Connidis, I. (1989). The subjective experience of aging: Correlates of divergent views. *Canadian Journal of Aging, 8*, 7–18.

Coplan, J., Smith, E., Altemus, M., Scharf, B., Owens, M., Nemeroff, C., et al. (2001). Variable foraging demand rearing: Sustained elevations in cisternal cerebrospinal fluid corticotropin-releasing factor concentrations in adult primates. *Biological Psychiatry, 50*, 200–204.

Curtis, W. J., & Cicchetti, D. (2003). Moving research on resilience into the 21st century: Theoretical and methodological considerations in examining the biological contributors to resilience. *Development and Psychopathology, 15*, 773–810.

Diener, E., Suh, E. M., Lucas, R. E., & Smith, H. L. (1999). Subjective well-being: Three decades of progress. *Psychological Bulletin, 125*, 276–302.

Dirkzwager, A. J. E., Grievink, L., van der Velden, P., & Yzermans, C. J. (2006). Risk factors for psychological and physical health problems after a man-made disaster. *British Journal of Psychiatry, 189*, 144–149.

Fauerbach, J. A., Lawrence, J. W., Schmidt, C., Munster, A. M., & Costa, P. T. (2000). Personality predictors of injury-related posttraumatic stress disorder. *Journal of Nervous and Mental Disease, 188*, 510–517.

Folkman, S., & Lazarus, R. S. (1988). Coping as a mediator of emotion. *Journal of Personality and Social Psychology, 54*, 466–475.

Fraley, R. C., & Bonanno, G. A. (2004). Attachment and loss: test of three competing models on the association between attachment-related avoidance and adaptation to bereavement. *Personality and Social Psychology Bulletin, 30*, 878–890.

Fraley, R. C., Fazzari, D. A., Bonanno, G. A., & Dekel, S. (2006). Attachment and psychological adaptation in high exposure survivors of the September 11th attack on the World Trade Center. *Personality and Social Psychology Bulletin, 32*, 538–551.

Frans, Ö., Rimmö, P.-A., Aberg, L., & Frederikson, M. (2005). Trauma exposure and posttraumatic stress disorder in the general population. *Acta Psychiatrica Scandinavica, 111*, 291–299.

Freud, S. (1957). Mourning and melancholia. In J. Strachey (Ed.), *The standard edition of the complete works of Sigmund Freud* (Vol. 14, pp. 152–170). London: Hogarth Press. (Original work published 1917)

Garmezy, N. (1991). Resilience in children's adaptation to negative life events and stressed environments. *Pediatric Annals, 20*, 459–466.

Greve, W., & Staudinger, U. M. (2006). Resilience in later adulthood and old age: Resources and potentials for successful aging. In D. Cicchetti & D. J. Cohen (Eds.), *Developmen-*

tal psychopathology (2nd ed., pp. 796–840). Hoboken, NJ: Wiley.

Hardy, S. E., Concato, J., & Gill, T. M. (2004). Resilience of community-dwelling older persons. *Journal of the American Geriatrics Society, 52*, 257–262.

Heckhausen, J., Dixon, R. A., & Baltes, P. B. (1989). Gains and losses in development throughout adulthood as perceived by different adult age groups. *Developmental Psychology, 25*, 109–121.

Heim, C., Newport, D. J., Heit, S., Graham, Y. P., Wilcox, M., Bonsall, R., et al. (2000). Increased pituitary–adrenal and autonomic responses to stress in adult women after sexual and physical abuse in childhood. *Journal of the American Medical Association, 284*, 592–597.

Hobfoll, S. E. (1989). Conservation of resources: A new attempt at conceptualizing stress. *American Psychologist, 44*, 513–524.

Hobfoll, S. E. (1998). *Stress, culture, and community. The psychology and philosophy of stress*. New York: Plenum Press.

Hobfoll, S. E., Canetti-Nisim, D., & Johnson, R. J. (2006). Exposure to terrorism, stress-related mental health symptoms, and defensive coping among Jews and Arabs in Israel. *Journal of Consulting and Clinical Psychology, 2*, 207–218.

Jopp, D., & Rott, C. (2006). Adaptation in very old age: Exploring the role of resources, beliefs, and attitudes in centenarians' happiness. *Psychology and Aging, 21*, 266–280.

Jopp, D., Rott, C., & Oswald, F. (2008). Valuation of life in old and very old age: The role of socio-demographic, social, and health resources for positive adaptation. *The Gerontologist, 48*, 646–658.

Jopp, D., & Smith, J. (2006). Resources and life-management strategies as determinants of successful aging: On the protective effect of selection, optimization, and compensation. *Psychology and Aging, 21*, 253–265.

Jopp, D., Wozniak, D., Damarin, A. K., Ehret, S., Stanek, S., Berendonk, C., et al. (2009). *Successful aging: Definitions and determinants reported by young, middle-aged, and older Germans*. Manuscript submitted for publication.

Kaltman, S., & Bonanno, G. A. (2003). Trauma and bereavement: Examining the impact of sudden and violent deaths. *Journal of Anxiety Disorders, 17*, 131–147.

Kaplan, H. B. (1999). Toward an understanding of resilience: A critical review of definitions and models. In M. D. Glantz & J. L. Johnson (Eds.), *Resilience and development: Positive life adaptations* (pp. 17–83). Dordrecht: Kluwer Academic.

Kelley, T. M. (2005). Natural resilience and innate mental health. *American Psychologist, 60*(3), 265.

King, L. A., King, D. W., Fairbank, J. A., Keane, T. M., & Adams, G. A. (1998). Resilience-recovery factors in post-traumatic stress disorder among female and male Vietnam veterans: Hardiness, post-war social support, and additional stressful life events. *Journal of Personality and Social Psychology, 74*, 420–434.

Kolassa, I.-T., & Elbert, T. (2007). Structural and functional neuroplasticity in relation to traumatic stress. *Current Directions in Psychological Science, 16*, 321–325.

Litz, B. T. (2005). Has resilience to severe trauma been underestimated? *American Psychologist, 60*(3), 262.

Lund, D. A., Caserta, M. S., & Dimond, M. F. (1986). Impact of bereavement on the self-conceptions of older surviving spouses. *Symbolic Interaction, 9*, 235–244.

Masten, A. (2001). Ordinary magic: Resilience processes in development. *American Psychologist, 56*, 227–238.

McFarlane, A. C., Clayer, J. R., & Bookless, C. L. (1997). Psychiatric morbidity following a natural disaster: An Australian bushfire. *Social Psychiatry and Psychiatric Epidemiology, 32*, 261–268.

Mikulincer, M., & Shaver, P. R. (2003). The attachment behavioral system in adulthood: Activation, psychodynamics, and interpersonal processes. In M. P. Zanna (Ed.), *Advances in experimental social psychology* (Vol. 35, pp. 53-152). New York: Academic Press.

Miller, E., & Wortman, C. B. (2002). Gender differences in mortality and morbidity following a major stressor: The case of conjugal bereavement. In G. Weidner, S. M. Kopp, & M. Kristenson (Eds.), *NATO Science Series: Series I. Life and Behavioural Sciences: Heart disease: Environment, stress and gender* (Vol. 327, pp. 251–266). Amsterdam: IOS Press.

Moskowitz, J. T., Folkman, S., & Acree, M. (2003). Do positive psychological states shed light on recovery from bereavement?: Findings from a 3-year longitudinal study. *Death Studies, 27,* 471–500.

Murphy, S. A. (1996). Parent bereavement stress and preventive intervention following the violent deaths of adolescent or young adult children. *Death Studies, 20,* 441–452.

Murphy, S. A., Johnson, L. C., Chung, I., & Beaton, R. D. (2003). The prevalence of PTSD following the violent death of a child and predictors of change 5 years later. *Journal of Traumatic Stress, 16,* 17–25.

Ozer, E. J., Best, S. R., Lipsey, T. L., & Weiss, D. S. (2003). Predictors of posttraumatic stress disorder and symptoms in adults: A meta-analysis. *Psychological Bulletin, 129,* 52–73.

Perrig-Chiello, P. (1997). *Wohlbefinden im Alter: Körperliche, psychische und soziale Determinanten und Ressourcen* [Well-being in old age: Physical, psychological and social determinants and resources]. München: Juventa.

Pinquart, M., & Sörensen, S. (2001). Gender differences in self-concept and psychological well-being in old age: A meta-analysis. *Journals of Gerontology: Psychological Sciences and Social Sciences, 56B,* P195–P213.

Pransky, J. (2003). *Prevention from the inside-out.* Cabot, VT: First Books.

Reinhardt, J. P., Boerner, K., & Horowitz, A. (2009). Personal and social resources and adaptation to chronic impairment over time. *Aging and Mental Health, 13,* 367–375.

Riolli, L., Savicki, V., & Capani, A. (2002). Resilience in the face of catastrophe: Optimism, personality, and coping in the Kosovo crisis. *Journal for Applied Social Psychology, 32,* 1604–1627.

Roisman, G. I. (2005). Conceptual clarifications in the study of resilience. *American Psychologist, 60*(3), 264.

Rubin, S. S., & Malkinson, R. (2001). Parental response to child loss across the life cycle: Clinical and research perspectives. In M. S. Stroebe, R. O. Hansson, W. Stroebe, & H. Schut (Eds.), *Handbook of bereavement research: Consequences, coping, and care* (pp. 219–240). Washington, DC: American Psychological Association.

Ryff, C. D., Singer, B., Love, G. D., & Essex, M. J. (1998). Resilience in adulthood and later life: Defining features and dynamic processes. In J. Lomranz (Ed.), *Handbook of aging and mental health: An integrative approach* (pp. 69–96). New York: Plenum Press.

Schoevers, R. A., Beekman, A. T. F., Deeg, D. J. H., Hooijer, C., Jonker, C., & van Tilburg, W. (2003). The natural history of late-life depression: Results from the Amsterdam Study of the Elderly (AMSTEL). *Journal of Affective Disorders, 76,* 5–14.

Schulz, R., Boerner, K., & Hebert, R. S. (2008). Caregiving and bereavement. In M. S. Stroebe, R. O. Hansson, H. Schut, & W. Stroebe (Eds.), *Handbook of bereavement research and practice: 21st century perspectives* (pp. 265–285). Washington, DC: American Psychological Association.

Schulz, R., Mendelsohn, A. B., Haley, W. E., Mahoney, D., Allen, R. S., Zhang, S., et al. (2003). End of life care and the effects of bereavement among family caregivers of persons with dementia. *New England Journal of Medicine, 349,* 1891–1892.

Shalev, A. Y., & Freedman, S. (2005). PTSD following terrorist attacks: A prospective evaluation. *American Journal of Psychiatry, 162,* 1188–1191.

Smith, J., Fleeson, W., Geiselmann, B., Settersten, R. A., Jr., & Kunzmann, U. (1999). Sources of well-being in very old age. In P. B. Baltes & K. U. Mayer (Eds.), *The Berlin Aging Study: Aging from 70 to 100* (pp. 450–471). New York: Cambridge University Press.

Staudinger, U. M., & Fleeson, W. (1996). Self and personality in old and very old age: A sample case of resilience? *Development and Psychopathology, 8,* 867–885.

Staudinger, U. M., Freund, A. M., Linden, M., & Maas, I. (1999). Self, personality, and life regulation: Facets of psychological resilience in old age. In P. B. Baltes & K. U. Mayer (Eds.), *The Berlin Aging Study: Aging from 70 to 100* (pp. 302–328). New York: Cambridge University Press.

Staudinger, U. M., Marsiske, M., & Baltes, P. B. (1995). Resilience and reserve capacity in later adulthood: Potentials and limits of development across the life span. In D. Cicchetti & D. J. Cohen (Eds.), *Developmental psychopathology: Vol. 2. Risk, disorder, and adaptation* (pp. 801–847). New York: Wiley.

Steverink, N., Westerhof, G., Bode, C., & Dittmann-Kohli, F. (2001). The personal experience of aging, individual resources, and subjective well-being. *Journals of Gerontology: Psychological Sciences and Social Sciences, 56B*, P364–P373.

Stroebe, M., Stroebe, W., & Schut, H. (2001). Gender differences in adjustment to bereavement: An empirical and theoretical review. *Review of General Psychology, 5*, 62–83.

Sumer, N., Karanci, A. N., Berument, S. K., & Gunes, H. (2005). Personal resources, coping self-efficacy, and quake exposure as predictors of psychological distress following the 1999 earthquake in Turkey. *Journal of Traumatic Stress, 18*, 331–342.

Vachon, M. L. S., Rogers, J., Lyall, W. A., Lancee, W. J., Sheldon, A. R., & Freeman, S. J. J. (1982). Predictors and correlates of adaptation to conjugal bereavement. *American Journal of Psychiatry, 139*, 998–1002.

Van der Velden, P. G., Kleber, R. J., Fournier, M., Grievink, L., Drogendjik, A., & Gersons, B. P. R. (2007). The association between dispositional optimism and mental health problems among disaster victims and a comparison group: A prospective study. *Journal of Affective Disorders, 102*, 35–45.

Van Oers, H., de Kloet, E., & Levine, S. (1998). Early vs. late maternal deprivation differentially alters the endocrine and hypothalamic responses to stress. *Developmental Brain Research, 111*, 245–252.

Wortman, C. B., Battle, E. S., & Lemkau, J. P. (1997). Coming to terms with sudden, traumatic death of a spouse or child. In R. C. Davis & A. J. Lurigio (Eds.), *Victims of crime* (pp. 108–133). Thousand Oaks, CA: Sage.

Wortman, C. B., & Boerner, K. (2007). Reactions to the death of a loved one: Myths of coping versus scientific evidence. In H. S. Friedman & R. C. Silver (Eds.), *Foundations of health psychology* (pp. 285–324). Oxford, UK: Oxford University Press.

Wortman, C. B., & Silver, R. C. (1987). Coping with irrevocable loss. In G. R. VandenBos & B. K. Bryant (Eds.), *Cataclysms, crises, and catastrophes: Psychology in action* (Master Lecture Series, Vol. 6, pp. 189–235). Washington, DC: American Psychological Association.

Zisook, S., & Shuchter, S. R. (1986). The first four years of widowhood. *Psychiatric Annals, 16*, 288–294.

8

Psychopathology as Dysfunctional Self-Regulation

When Resilience Resources Are Compromised

Paul Karoly

Current interest in the concepts of human resilience and positive adjustment has developed partly as a reaction to what many would view as a cross-disciplinary overemphasis on human adaptive failure—psychopathology. For example, as noted by Vaillant (2003), psychiatry, as well as clinical psychology, social work, nursing, and allied mental health disciplines, has traditionally been so descriptively focused on symptom expression that the characterization of mental health has typically been subtractive in nature (i.e., defined as the *absence* of symptoms). However, contemporary clinical science has been actively seeking to shed itself of its reliance on subjective, value-laden, and purely descriptive constructs, and to adopt a stronger empirical and theoretical stance anchored in biology (especially neurophysiology, biochemistry, genetics, and evolutionary theory; cf. Baron-Cohen, 1997; Caspi & Moffitt, 2006; Frith, 2008; Hyman, 2007; Meyer-Lindenberg & Weinberger, 2006; Peled, 2004) but cutting across multiple

analytic levels. Importantly, as the diverse mental health disciplines have become more multileveled and conceptual, the concepts of resilience and psychopathology have drawn closer together.

One manifestation of biological psychiatry's quest for a new identity is its movement toward a conceptual base in basic and applied neuroscience, built around the core assumptions that the human brain is a neural activity pattern processor, and that mental disorders develop chiefly from malfunctions of neural control (Hestenes, 1998; Kandel, 1998). The concept of *control*, as used by Hestenes (1998) and others, equates roughly to terms denoting the pursuit of "order," such as regulation, modulation, synchronization, and discrepancy management. Therefore, health, adjustment, adaptive success, normality, competence, and the like, can be understood as biopsychosocial conditions emanating from the mind/brain's capacity for the efficient and orderly processing of complex patterns of activity.

146

The premises of this chapter are consistent with the tenets of neuroscience across its cognitive, behavioral, affective, and social facets, and with those of control systems and social-cognitive theory, particularly in the sense that humans and their changing ecological niches are taken to represent complex transactional systems within which adaptive success and failure are probabilistic "outcomes," dependent upon the same set of component control structures and processes, but operating differently (Ford, 1987; Urban, 1987). Nonetheless, to psychiatry's somewhat monolithic neural control failure model must be added the following assumptions: (1) that the structures and processes upon which adaptive systems are built are jointly linked to the complex experiential transactions (the social dynamics of daily life), as well as to the processes taking place at the genetic/cellular level[1] and in complex nervous system tracts, and (2) that successful adaptation is dependent upon the transactional system's emergent capacity for self-regulation (i.e., the explicit and implicit pursuit of multiple goals over time and across changing contexts) (Bandura, 1986; Boekaerts, Pintrich, & Zeidner, 2000; Karoly, 1993a, 1993b, 1999, 2006; Murphy, 2001). This expanded conception should help to integrate better the mental health disciplines, particularly bridging clinical psychology, psychiatry, and neuroscience because, although it is certainly fair to assert that formative genetic and environmental influences meet at the level of the neuron (see Josiassen, 1993), the pragmatic import of these fateful meetings emerges only during "the actual life of the actor as culturally situated and as aimed at goals that may finally be dispositive" (Robinson, 2000, p. 42).

The approach to be illustrated in this chapter is what I call a situated neurocognitive motivational (SNM) model, and it is built on the foundational assumption that multilevel self-regulatory mechanisms, pivoting on goal processes that operate effectively within the social ecology of everyday life, define "normal functioning." Moreover, when com-paratively high levels of flexible and efficient self-regulation are in evidence, the foundations of *resilience* come into sharper focus. By logical extension, then, self-regulatory mechanisms can also provide the conceptual blueprints for apprehending failures of adjustment. Viewed within this light, resilience and adaptive failure should no longer be seen as polar opposites, but as the yin and the yang of human self-regulation.

In this chapter, I endeavor to illustrate how failures of situational, neural, and intrapersonal modulation of resilience resources—*dysfunctional self-regulation*—can serve as the etiological bedrock of most forms of psychopathology as articulated by the psychiatric community using the current *Diagnostic and Statistical Manual of Mental Disorders* (DSM-IV-TR; American Psychiatric Association, 2000). Less focal but nonetheless very important is the notion that the remediation or prevention of regulatory dysfunctions and a fuller appreciation of healthy living also depend on the insights gleaned from the self-regulation model herein presented.

Self-Regulation: Definition and Conceptual Introduction

I have succinctly defined *self-regulation* as the explicit and implicit pursuit of multiple goals over time and across changing contexts. Despite the apparent simplicity of this working definition, the concept of self-regulation remains controversial, partly as a result of long-standing philosophical debates and partly stemming from the inevitable divergence among contemporary theories. First, self-regulation has been erroneously set in opposition to "determinism" and conflated with the philosophy of "free will" by numerous scholars over the years. Second, self-regulation has been simplistically contrasted with "external regulation"—as though one could readily draw a sharp dividing line between intrapersonal and contextual sources of influence as opposed to recognizing the causal triadic reciprocity among intrapsychic, environmental, and behavioral forces (Bandura, 1984, 1986). Finally, a contrast of a more recent vintage is that which casts self-regulation as the opposite of "automaticity." I briefly address each of these somewhat misguided perspectives before moving forward.

To the degree that self-regulation is equated with "willpower" or volitional freedom, it runs afoul of a host of philosophical and practical objections that also line up squarely against folk psychology and commonsense ideas about free choice and moral responsibility. Willpower, for example, is a concept that is often used in a circular fashion, much like the psychoanalytic idea of "ego strength"; that is, a patient might be said to be a fire-setter because of poor ego strength, and the rationale for believing that ego-strength is deficient is the fact that the patient sets fires. The same sort of reasoning applies to the willpower concept whenever it is used to "explain" why people do or do not stay on their diets or abolish bad habits. Nonetheless, the concepts of willpower (free will) and volition can be interpreted as acceptable synonyms for self-regulation, provided that (1) a model of the concept's "working parts" is logically and empirically established before the fact, and (2) neither is viewed as the "opposite" of determinism. In fact, occupying the pole diametrically opposed to deterministic thinking is the epistemic position of nondeterminism, or *acausality*. Likewise, the true opposite of *free will* (volition, self-regulation) is the doctrine of *nonagentic mechanism*, the belief that all causes are entirely mechanical and non-person-centered (Howard, 2008). Consequently, one can logically espouse both self-regulation and deterministic thinking.

The notion that "external control" is a developmentally early mode of life management that must eventually be replaced by self-determination has a long historical provenance. Nonetheless, although adults in our society must take responsibility for their actions and decisions, such "ownership" does

not (indeed cannot) completely liberate them from environmental influences or free them from the causal press of genetics, temperament, or nonconscious forces. Thus, *self-regulation* is a relative term, and the *self* prefix should never be read as implying personal hegemony or total independence from external forces. As Bandura (1984) has noted, the self-regulating system is both a "product and producer of influences" (p. 508). One important implication of a reciprocal deterministic stance is that self-regulation as a process can appropriately be studied in a controlled laboratory environment, such that when it is played out under an experimenter's instructions or surveillance, it does not somehow become a false or watered down version of "real" self-regulation.

In the first two examples of mistaken ideas about the topic of self-regulation, an implicit enemy of understanding was either–or thinking. In recent years, another dichotomy has arisen, built around cognitive psychology's distinction between controlled versus automatic processing (Schneider & Chein, 2003). Advocates of the power of automatic processes have asserted that involuntary or effortless habits hold sway over our actions, emotions, and choices (see Bargh, 2007; Winkielman & Berridge, 2004). Such a stance implies that the self-reflective, conscious, or "controlled" processes inherent in the notion of self-regulation represent at best a marginal set of psychological constructs whose importance has been overblown, or at worst an epiphenomenon. Whereas one can dispute the technical, logical, and the polemical aspects of the contemporary work on automaticity (see De Houwer, 2006; Katzko, 2006; Kihlstrom, 2008), acknowledgment of the *dual process* nature of control seems reasonable. Thus, rather than construing automatic processes as the obverse of self-regulatory processes, consider that self-regulation occurs in two forms: the deliberative or conscious form (the main focus of this chapter) and the automatic form (Karoly, in press).

A Descriptive Model of Self-Regulatory Components and Targets, and Some of Its Underlying Assumptions

Self-regulation can be articulated at multiple analytic levels. Moreover, it is time-dependent, activated and bounded by external circumstance and by the functioning of biogenetic and somatic systems, and has developed to influence a host of meaningful adaptive targets. In light of its inherent complexity, the topic of self-regulation has usually been approached in a piecemeal fashion, with investigators seeking to carve out of a systematic process manageable pieces that remain to be neatly and consensually tied together. To aid in my exposition, I offer a rendering (see Figure 8.1) of the essential elements of the regulatory process. Each shaded box represents what I call episodically *modifiable factors*—online constituents of self-regulation that, although routinely functioning in a relatively stable manner, are nonetheless capable of being influenced by each other, as well as by transitional events,

deliberate interventions, and/or the passage of time. The targets of self-regulatory processes are also listed within a shaded box. The goal systems component is centrally featured because of its presumed connectivity to all of the surrounding functional elements.

Regulatory Components: A Selective Overview

In Figure 8.1, nine functions (in shaded boxes) are depicted as leading to various to-be-regulated targets. Each of the functions plays a causal role, in conjunction with the others, in choreographing the system's operation. I consider several of these functional components in this section. Later, when discussing particular patterns of regulatory disturbance that manifest as DSM-defined disorders, I reintroduce many of these components.

Within classical cybernetic and control models (Ford, 1987; Powers, 1973), the place to begin is with the *feedback loop*, the key analytic unit upon which system dynam-

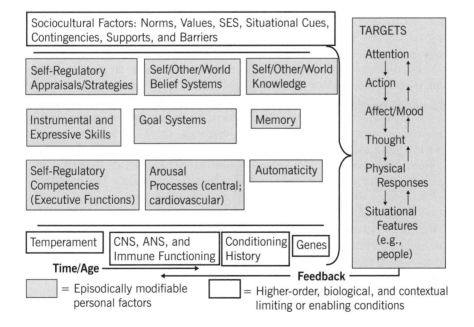

FIGURE 8.1. Descriptive model of self-regulatory components and targets.

ics are built. In Figure 8.1, feedback is indicated by the arrow moving backward from the bottom of the Targets box. This arrow represents the environmental information, also known as *knowledge of results*, that is made available to the self-regulating system for course corrections or for validating that the system is on the right path. Of course, we need to specify what is being fed back to the system because this process is the presumed *activator* of the diverse functions depicted in Figure 8.1. Indeed, it might appear that I have presented a model of a system that just seems to "sit there," with no reason to turn on.

The impetus for movement (not specifically shown) is what control theorists call *error* (or, more correctly, an *error signal*), a mismatch or discrepancy between what an individual expects (to see, to hear, to feel, to happen, etc.) and what is presently occurring at the person–environment interface. Traditional social learning accounts (see Karoly & Kanfer, 1982) posit that self-regulation happens when external supports or cues become unavailable, or when habitual modes of responding fail to bring about the desired consequences. Yet these are but two aspects of discrepancy or error. Traditional models of psychopathology posit major and minor life disruptions, called *stressful life events*, as the precipitants of compensatory reactivity. Yet these events are likewise aspects of experiential discrepancy that may be sufficient but not always necessary for regulatory system activation. In fact, within an SNM perspective, *stress* can be broadly defined as any environmental or intrapsychic event or process that disturbs or threatens to undermine an actor's directional path or goal trajectory, and that comes to operate as an error signal within a self-regulatory system whose prime function it is to reduce, eliminate, or compensate for the perceived mismatch, and sometimes to quell occurrent physiological hyperarousal. Thus, role confusion, repeated task failure, social rejection, imagined offenses by significant others, goal conflict, and the like, can serve as stressors, in ad-

dition to the high-intensity, life-threatening, physically taxing, or excessively demanding sorts of situations frequently discussed in the clinical literature. I return to this point later in this chapter when I discuss the concept of resilience.

Goal Systems

Although not indicated by a specific arrow in Figure 8.1, the information (sensory, motor, perceptual, cognitive, etc.) about directional movement that is fed back to the self-regulating human is processed at the functional juncture marked Goal Systems. This function is subserved, in the literal sense, by neural and biochemical activity in the frontal and prefrontal cortex, and the hypothalamus, as well as in supportive allocortical brain structures, such as the hippocampus, the amygdala, and the anterior cingulate cortex, and in the brainstem (cf. Lewis & Todd, 2007; Luu & Tucker, 2003; Miller & Cohen, 2001; Owen, 2006; Posner, Rothbart, Sheese, & Tang, 2007). In a representational sense, what I am calling *goal systems* can be understood as a set of hypothetical mechanisms designed to perform several key roles in the regulatory process.

Because the idea of *regulation* for free-ranging humans typically means self-adjustments that permit individuals to achieve repeatable consequences through variable means in the service of short- and long-term goals, at least three prerequisite operations must be enacted: action, perception, and comparison (see Powers, 2004). A specific goal (e.g., "To lose 15 pounds") serves as a reference, command, or set-point signal that specifies (or feeds forward) the system's objective(s). Whether acted upon by internal states (e.g., hunger) or external events (a waiter holding out the dessert tray), the goal ("To lose 15 pounds") has the potential to direct a person's attention to relevant stimuli, to invoke instrumental and expressive actions that are consistent with it (smilingly waving off the waiter's offer of dessert), and to inspire a congratulatory comparative judgment ("Although it was difficult, I'm proud that I did the right thing!"). Unfortunately, the fact that a person has a specific goal in mind does not invariably lead to action or cognition in accordance with that goal. Therefore, within the current framework, additional activational states, meditational processes, and enabling and disabling boundary conditions must be stipulated in order to construct a systematic account of regulatory success and/or failure in the real world.

In recent years, a great deal of conceptual and research effort has been expended on opening up the territory that both encompasses and borders the *goal* construct (Austin & Vancouver, 1996; Bogdan, 1994; Emmons, 1999; Karoly, 1999; Little, 1983). This is as it should be, in light of the centrality to human adjustment of the so-called *governing functions*, defined as a set of selective, organizational, and evaluative capabilities that focus on three key regulatory concerns: (1) *direction*—what state or outcome is desired; (2) *regulation*—how goals are selected, prioritized, and monitored; and (3) *control*—how skills and knowledge come to implement action plans in an efficient and flexible manner (see Ford, 1987). As should be apparent, goals fall under the aegis of the *directive function*. However, goal-relevant thinking ranges over a wider array of motivational operations, including (but not limited to) selection, prioritization, monitoring, and control. Because pursuing goals across changing settings and over long stretches of time is what living creatures do, it is not surprising that the cognitive architecture of goal-relevant thinking is as intricate as its lifespan navigational mission.

At present, goals are typically assessed along three fundamental dimensions: content, evaluative characteristics, and structure (see Austin & Vancouver, 1996, for a review). Construing self-regulated movement toward goals as a *journey*, the *content* of a goal simply reflects the nature of the intended destination. Thus, the "I want to lose 15 pounds" goal would be considered a "health goal" or a "self-improvement" goal. Wanting to make more friends or to be a better friend would be classified as "social" or "interpersonal" goals. Other categories include vocational, school-related (academic), familial, recreational, spiritual, and environmental goals, and the like (see Emmons, 1999).

Although I would contend that an excellent way truly to understand another person is by determining what specific goals he or she is pursuing, it is also the case that, at least in Western cultures, the categories of goals that people typically seek are relatively small in number. Each person works toward his or her "personalized" set of goals focused on specific outcomes and in a distinct priority ordering, but the between-person commonalities remain clearly discernible. Thus, if challenged to guess the goals of the crowd at Yankee Stadium, one would more often be right than wrong by predicting that any random adult fan was currently trying to lose weight, reduce financial debt, exercise more, earn a better wage, or spend more time with family. Consequently, another vehicle for appraising goals is to determine not just *what* people want, but *how* they want.

The "how" of goal cognition involves both the explicit and implicit evaluative appraisals that people make of their journeys (also called *goal topography*) and the patterned relations among goal appraisals—*goal structures* (Austin & Vancouver, 1996; Emmons, 1999; Karoly, 1999, in press; Little, 1983). Evaluative appraisals or rating dimensions used to describe goals can be quite varied, but they tend to be stable indicators of the rater's higher-order, schematic understanding of the intended journeys, and they often act as moderators of the links between life events and various adjustment-related outcomes. For example, whether individuals evaluate their goal(s) as involving either the possibility of approaching positive outcomes or avoiding negative ones appears to have a discernible impact on the experience and outcome of the goal pursuit process (see Higgins & Spiegel, 2004; Karoly & Newton, 2006). And, finally, structural aspects of goal cognition pertain to derived indices of goal-related thinking—such as when a person's goals are listed along the rows and columns of a matrix, and the degree to which each goal either helps or interferes with each of the others is then rated (thus yielding indices of goal facilitation and goal conflict) (see Emmons, 1999). In general, goal content, various rating dimensions, and structural measures, such as conflict and goal differentiation, operate as goal system mechanisms when they possess the ability differentially to impact future goal attainment. Whether these goal-centered elements play a determinative role in the individual's navigation of the motivational landscape greatly depends on their internal organization, their connections to allied self-regulatory functions, and the availability of situational cues, supports, or affordances. Thus, it should be kept in mind that goals and goal systems are, by themselves, insufficient as explanations or predictors of action.

Self-Regulatory Competencies

Life would be much simpler if people pursued only one goal at a time, and if the world consistently provided its denizens the assistance to attain this one goal precisely when and where they needed it. But such ideal circumstances are rarely found in the natural world. Moving toward multiple, distant, and sometimes conflicting aspirations usually requires sensitivity to the changing world around us and a capacity to make adjustments or "trade-offs" between seemingly incompatible foci of awareness. For example, we not only need to be able to "shield" our focal goal(s) from environmental distractions but also to stay alert for any new growth and development opportunities that this same environment may bring. We need to focus our attention on our current activities but not forget about the goals we have put "on hold." We must mobilize our cognitive and emotional commitments toward those ends we are striving to attain but

not become so strongly or rigidly invested that we cannot disengage when the situation so warrants. Because we humans are awash in a sea of options, our brains must balance flexibility with control. To manage the higher-order fine-tuning of our motivational lives requires a set of evolved, hardwired capacities that are often labeled *executive functions* (EFs). These functions, labeled *self-regulatory competencies*, are depicted in Figure 8.1.

Discussed most regularly in the neuropsychology literature, EFs are often simply presented as lists of component skills for which there are no prototypical or process pure measures (Burgess, 1997). For present purposes, I follow Barkley (2001) by conceptualizing *executive functioning* as a class of evolved mental faculties that manifest as behavioral responses directed toward the self for the purpose of changing or modifying future outcomes. Included in this class are *inhibitory control* (the ability to override dominant response tendencies), working memory, task–set switching, discrepancy/error monitoring, attention control, and planning. Whereas Barkley also lists self-directed affect, and receptive and expressive language on his list of EFs, I have placed "instrumental and expressive skills" and "arousal processes" in separate boxes, and consider affect control as a "target" of the system rather than as a distinct skill. Temporary or permanent deficits in executive functioning brought about through biogenetic or experiential means, or both, are hypothesized to be among the critical determinants of psychological disorders (see below).

An important point to bear in mind is that the measurement of EFs requires the use of performance tests that are usually timed, often computer generated, and for which norms or comparative data are or can be made available. One can more readily ascertain a person's attributions about his or her ability to inhibit impulsive actions, plan for the future, keep track of errors, and so forth, but such experience-based, personal reckonings fall into yet a third category of self-regulatory component—*self-regulatory appraisals/strategies.*

Self-Regulatory Appraisals/Strategies

From the perspective of measurement convenience, it is not surprising that the literature on self-regulation has focused the bulk of its attention on self-rated regulatory abilities as opposed to performance-based skills. However, in addition to ease of measurement, self-appraisals of personal skills and action strategies have a long and distinguished tenure in cognitive and social-cognitive psychology. Probably the most studied of such appraisals are *self-efficacy* expectations (see Bandura, 1997). Whereas it might require a bit of imagination to conjecture about the links between goal constructs, EF deficits, and psychopathology, the idea that misguided or inaccurate self-appraisals can precede psychological disorder is somewhat more transparent. In general, beliefs about one's ability to exert control or display personal agency, or to engage in specific strategies to enhance one's advantage in situations where control is "up for grabs," are important elements of this particular functional component.

Another key element pertains to what control theorists describe as the process of comparing system input to a preset standard or reference—the so-called *comparator function* (Carver & Scheier, 1998; Ford, 1987; Karoly, 1995; Powers, 1973). The comparison process rarely operates in a precise, machine-like fashion. Thinking about one's actions in comparison to a standard can be activated by focusing attention on oneself or on the task at hand, but the comparator might not always be so engaged. Moreover, the standards used to make one's comparison may be too high (strict) or too low (lenient) for the well-being of the system.

Not all appraisals relevant to self-regulation pertain directly to the regulatory process per se. The box in Figure 8.1 labeled Self/Other/World Belief Systems encompasses other cognitive activities that have been found to play important moderating roles in overall system performance. For example, people are socialized to believe many things about themselves, the workings of the world, and the inclinations of the people in it (whether the world is a safe place; whether certain people can be trusted; how to deal with failures, mistakes, and disappointments; etc.) The process of self-regulated goal pursuit cannot help but be affected by people's causal attributions, hedonic preferences, prejudices, accurate and flawed self-assessments, and personal philosophies. However, in the interest of space, this function is not further elaborated here.

Automaticity

Sometimes overlooked in models of self-regulation that pivot upon conscious awareness and decision making, the role of nonconscious factors must be acknowledged if we are to achieve a complete understanding of how self-regulation works and how it can go awry. As noted previously, automaticity is often presented as an adversary of conscious or deliberate self-regulation. However, when viewed as a type of self-regulation, automaticity proves to be not only a means of conserving cognitive resources but, as with the tendency to form goals in the first place, also a mechanism for simplifying a world that routinely presents us with a superabundance of choices. Both the failure to automate and the rigid adherence to automatic patterns can present serious adaptive problems.

Some Foundational Assumptions

If our purpose is to comprehend the workings of self-regulation, aptly describable as "a system of multiple layers of interacting control" (Toates, 2006, p. 76), then we must begin with the broad assumption that system control is both feedback– and feed forward–based, and is hierarchically organized, reflecting both higher-order, mainly conscious components and stimulus-bound, automatic components (Ford, 1987; Powers, 1973; Toates, 2006).

Moreover, to address not only the determinants of goal-directed movement but also the *potential for* goal-directed movement, particularly when people are "stuck" in patterns of maladaptive action or maladaptive inaction, we must also seek to understand the sources of *system flexibility*. In the present analysis, *flexibility* refers to the capacity to overcome systemic inertia, to multitask when necessary, to reconfigure one's goals and means, and/or to override automaticity in the service of counteracting self-defeating habits. Here I assume that the construct of motivational or regulatory *flexibility* can be usefully interpreted both as a stable individual-difference factor and an emerging, systems-centered characteristic. Among the threats to regulatory flexibility and, hence, potential risk factors for psychopathology are poorly developed or overtaxed executive skills (working memory, inhibitory capacity, error monitoring, etc.) and varied structural aspects of goal organization, such as between-goal interference/conflict and an extreme overinvestment in certain goals (what I have termed *meaning saturation*).

Third, a viable self-regulatory system is also an efficient system. By *efficient* I mean something akin to the contemporary environmentalist idea of *sustainability* (i.e., the capacity of a system to conserve resources [not waste] and to generate some resource reserves for future use) (see Barnett, Salmond, Jones, & Sahakian, 2006). More than half a century ago, in fact, Wishner (1955) proposed that efficiency could be used to characterize degrees of psychological disturbance. Wishner focused on efficiency in meeting the requirements of everyday tasks as a measure of psychological health. Substituting "goals" for "tasks," his analysis is certainly compatible with the current motivational framework. Moreover, not meeting the requirements necessary to attain one's valued goals readily becomes an index of psychopathology. To operationalize his index of efficiency–inefficiency, Wish-

ner chose to highlight the relation between diffuse and focused behavior. This energy-centered analysis yielded the following equation:

$$E = (F/D, P)$$

with *efficiency* defined as a function of focal to diffuse activity combined with productivity (*P*), or environmental impact. To transport this conception usefully outside the confines of the laboratory and into the clinical world, Wishner further suggested that one would need to examine the "motives" of the individual, and the degree of concordance between these motives and the demands of the tasks/goals at hand. It is worth noting that Wishner's ideas are highly consistent with contemporary notions of "person–environment fit" and "self-concordance" (Sheldon, 2007).[2]

Intriguing though it may be, Wishner's (1955) efficiency construct captures only a part of what I have in mind. Consistent with the clinical data (some of which I review later in this chapter), the brand of inefficiency that pervades a majority of DSM disorders has less to do with general "wheel spinning" and more to do with the active and vigorous pursuit of what I call *compensatory goals*, and in a manner that overshadows the person's interest in and capacity for the pursuit of prior normative strivings. The systematic waste of personal resources (time, energy, money, and personal passion) on pursuing and justifying goals that were established in response to complex, ambiguous, forcefully imposed, or inadequately mastered role or task requirements, along with a strong resistance to giving up or modifying these pursuits, defines what I mean by motivational *inefficiency*. The reader need only picture the sorts of activities associated with persons diagnosed as *obsessive–compulsive* to appreciate the appropriateness of the inefficiency notion as it is here defined (see also my discussion of clinical disorders below).

Not pictured in Figure 8.1 are the factors that give rise to the pursuit of specific goals.

What factors undergird the maintenance or revision of self-regulated goal trajectories?

Taking a very long view, it is reasonable to propose a simple answer: Humans are evolutionarily designed to pursue goals and to react strongly to serious threats to goal attainment; therefore, as Locke and Latham (1990) have said, "The ultimate biological basis of goal-directed action is the organism's need to sustain its life by taking the actions its nature requires" (p. 3).

At a more immediate or proximal cause level, the antecedents of self-regulation have been articulated by different theorists in varied ways. Some have suggested that self-regulation unfolds in the service of basic needs or under the guidance of traits or self-conceptions (e.g., Deci & Ryan, 2000), and that it varies in strength in proportion to how closely the individual's goals cleave to dictates of these plenary forces. By contrast, the SNM framework takes a more down-to-earth, ecologically grounded view of directional movement. Under the aegis of control systems and dynamical models (Carver & Scheier, 1998; Ford, 1987; Powers, 1973; Toates, 1998), often assailed by humanists as too "mechanical" or "robotic" to capture human nature, the current approach assumes that historical and current events, cultural teachings and norms, genetics and biology, personal knowledge and memory, and many other background forces combine with the functions listed in Figure 8.1 to shape personal trajectories over time and across settings.

Note that Figure 8.1 lists one of the targets of regulation as Situational Features (e.g., people). This aspect of the model merits our careful attention. Despite the person-centeredness that adheres to the term *self*-regulation, the fact remains that individuals often regulate themselves in order to influence others, and often seek to influence others so as to better manage themselves (Vohs & Ciarocco, 2004). Moreover, many of our most cherished goals are social in nature. Although the term may seem odd, *social self-regulation* is an important construct within the SNM because, like the passage of time, the social (group, family) matrix is an integral element of the functional system but is often overlooked.

Goal Episodes, Goal Episode Schemas, and Goal Episode Dynamics

The complexity of the self-regulatory system as articulated here is balanced somewhat by the relative simplicity of its foundational analytic units. The feedback loop, of which I have already spoken, is the best example. In addition, as has been described in basic research with animals, motivated behavior tends to "occur in bouts" (McSweeney & Swindell, 1999). In humans, bouts are better conceived as *episodes* (Karoly, 2008). Thus, goal or, more often, subgoal pursuit can be parsed into contextually bounded sequences of fairly discrete events with discernible start and end points during which the individual's attention, thoughts, feelings, and actions are momentarily integrated by virtue of their systematic relationship to the goal in question (see Derryberry & Rothbart [1997], Ford [1987], and Lewis & Todd [2005] for more thorough discussions of the self-organizing nature of human motivational systems).

The sequential enactment of goal episodes is the stuff of life and of autobiographical memory, with special salience afforded to episodes relating to goal frustration or failure and to goal success (Conway & Pleydell-Pearce, 2000). Social, identity-related, and other types of personally meaningful goal episodes that occur during times of stress or developmental transition (times when failure or threat of failure loom large), are likely to be reviewed, evaluated, and reframed in the service of retrospective and anticipatory coping. Such pre- and postepisode processing yields what I term *goal episode schemas* (GES). GES are roughly equivalent to what Ford (1987) has called *behavior episode schemas* (BES), with the slight difference being my recognition of goals as the key integrative elements rather than behaviors per se. Goal episodes, like Ford's behavior episodes, are hierarchically organized, with smaller scale events arrayed under larger scale events; divisible into instrumental, observational, or thought-based types; and typically encompass variable means enacted in a definable set of circumstances toward the attainment of a desired outcome(s). GES are the mental constructions (scripts, prototypes) of goal episodes, and thus are selective rather than accurate accounts of events. The function of GES, like BES, is to help organize perception, thought, and emotion, and to provide procedural knowledge for the execution of relevant context-bound action in the service of goal pursuit.

I presume that psychopathology of varied types develops in part from the content and structure of GES and from the dynamic relationships between GES and other self-regulatory functions (relations that I call *goal episode dynamics*, or GED). More specifically, the capacity of a self-regulatory system for effective life space navigation (i.e., goal pursuit in naturalistic settings), as well as for active resistance to destabilization (i.e., resilience), hinges on its context sensitivity, that is, its ability to monitor the external terrain for opportunities to engage in goal pursuit, to frame the goal pursuit problem to be solved, to model the course of its actions over time, to plausibly revise its models and plans in response to actual or anticipated error (discrepancy, interruption, delay, etc.), and to shield its focal pursuit(s) from distraction. The adequacy of the individual's GES to track the changing demands of the social and physical world efficiently and flexibly as they relate to desired personal trajectories (to map or coordinate inputs, internal signals, and outputs) figures prominently in self-regulatory success. Thus, in the current framework, context sensitivity, error monitoring, anticipatory acumen (also known as *mental time travel*), suppression of irrelevant information, and knowledge updating are among the critical intersystem dynamic mechanisms capable of orchestrating psychosocial risk, symptom creation, symptom maintenance, and posttreatment relapse.

Implications of a Goal-Centered Self-Regulatory Failure Model for Understanding Psychopathology

Flowing from the premise that self-regulatory dynamics can serve as a combined descriptive and explanatory platform for appraising both human adjustment and its failures is a set of interleaved implications that hold considerable promise for unifying clinical science. Several of these implications merit our attention.

First, the SNM perspective emphasizes that experiential transactions and biogenetic underpinnings are coequals in accounting for the multidimensional and fluid nature of human adaptive failures. Such a view contrasts sharply with *essentialism*, the philosophical doctrine that complex entities (including people) are what they are because of their *essences* or defining features. Clinical psychiatry and clinical psychology have been involved for many decades in the search for the varied *essences* of mental illness (see Ghaemi, 2003). Essentialist thinking has likewise given rise to reductionism and materialistic thinking to the degree that the major analytic or explanatory focus of modern clinical science tends to center almost exclusively on somatic mechanisms (Brendel, 2003) and on categorical nosologies that seek to "carve nature at its joints" (Ghaemi, 2003; Zachar, 2000). By contrast, the self-regulatory SNM model, being philosophically pluralistic and pragmatic, stresses the importance of specifying multiple causal pathways to both psychological disorder and health, including, but not limited to, genetic and experiential risk or resilience factors, temporally extended (developmental) influences, and situational and intrapsychic factors contributing to symptom specificity, symptom maintenance, relapse, or resistance.

However, central to the arguments of this chapter is yet another pathway that hinges upon what I call *functional–ecological unfolding* (i.e., the day-to-day shaping of symptoms and syndromes by self-regulatory mechanisms driving the ongoing person ×

situation exchange. This form of the person × situation exchange is partly accessible via experience sampling (diary-based) methodologies (see Bolger, Davis, & Rafaeli, 2003). And the transactional mechanisms of particular importance are those defined as GES and GED, as briefly articulated earlier.

Stated pointedly, the majority of the patterns described in current diagnostic manuals, the DSM-IV-TR and the *Psychodynamic Diagnostic Manual* (American Psychiatric Association, 2000; PDM Task Force, 2006), represent people's excessive, deficient, and/or disorganized efforts at *regulating* (maintaining and changing) their thoughts, decisions, feelings, perceptions, or actions. The term *disorder* implies nothing less than a person (or persons) experiencing one or more discrepancy-based regulatory disruptions that have eventuated in patterns of misdirected automaticity, goal-centered motivational compensation and justification, and/or the establishment of conflicted intention systems. Thus, within the SNM framework, *directional misguidance* and *degrees of context-specific task failure* replace personal "defect" or "disease" as central organizing features of psychopathology.

Should clinical scientists desire a simplifying organization that places diverse patterns of regulatory dysfunction into categories, I can tentatively suggest four classifications: (1) disorders deriving from disconnections among the major operative functions; (2) disorders stemming from adequately connected system components operating at low levels of flexibility and efficiency; (3) intact systems pursuing ill-fitting, deviant, or compensatory goals; and (4) focal dysfunctions in one or more of the individual components. Note that this listing is focused on putative causes rather than on "symptom" patterns per se. For comparative purposes, readers should consult the Ford and Urban (1998) four-category diagnostic system based on a control theoretical framework that roughly parallels the SNM model, but with a focus on behavioral manifestations. Finally, there is no reason to assume that these categories are non-overlapping or that the patterns of maladaptation they engender will be expressed in a unitary fashion. Any of the four can undergird what has previously been broadly designated as "underregulation" and "misregulation" (Baumeister & Heatherton, 1996) or under- and overregulation (Derryberry & Rothbart, 1997). The adequacy of this rudimentary typology is illustrated later.

Within the SNM framework, commonly observed symptoms might seem to lose some of their luster to the extent that they are derivative or consequential phenomena, secondary to self-regulatory system disruption. Of course, such a derived view of symptoms is hardly original, having been promulgated in the late 19th century by Breuer and Freud (1895). Nonetheless, symptoms remain at the phenomenal center of most forms of psychological suffering, and are nowhere demeaned in the present conceptual space.

Also emanating from the SNM perspective is an image of the person with (and without) psychological problems that emphasizes how goal-guided action, emotion, and cognition unite to create the possibilities for growth. This sensibility is, however, not unique to the current framework. Within clinical psychology (Shahar, 2006) and counseling psychology (Young, Valach, & Domene, 2005), efforts to mount a volition-centered assault on conceptualization, assessment, and intervention are now clearly in evidence.

Finally, the present articulation of the topic of self-regulated motivation stands in opposition to the widespread assumption, fueled in part by classical psychoanalytic writings and the legal system, that motivation is usually the *victim* of psychopathological states; that is, individuals are often presumed to be unable to modulate or master their feelings, thoughts, or actions, or muster the "will" to change because of their "mental illness." The present perspective, by contrast, conceives of self-regulatory dysfunctions as the unintentional *architects* of pathological adjustment (and thus perhaps is better aligned with ego or self psychology).

Illustrations from the DSM

As space limitations preclude any sweeping retooling of all the DSM categories, I illustrate the utility of the SNM model for several relatively prevalent forms of DSM-defined psychopathology, highlighting the etiological, triggering, or disorder-maintaining role of one or more of the previously discussed goal-based self-regulatory components.

Unipolar Depression

Although heterogeneity of symptom expression is the rule in clinical work, individuals who display excessive sadness, lethargy, feelings of worthlessness, loss of pleasure, and the like for several months at a time, and who therefore are typically diagnosed as having a *major depressive disorder*, constitute an especially diverse group whose members fall along a continuum of affective disability. In fact, the heterogeneity within the mood and personality disorders has recently prompted an attempt to organize them into a multidimensional spectrum model (e.g., Lara, Pinto, Akiskal, & Akiskal, 2006). For present purposes, the preferred simplifying strategy derives from the premises of the SNM model.

As a disorder of self-regulation, depression prominently features disruptions to emotion regulation and emotion processing, often occurring in the form of blocked appetitive motivation or dysfunctions of the positive arousal (behavioral activation) system (Fowles, 1994; Gray, 1987). As per the SNM model, emotion-based problems in depression necessarily co-occur with cognitive and behavioral ones, and involve neurologically, personally, and ecologically mediated goal dynamics at their core.

To serve as a conceptual launching pad for a consideration of reactive, unipolar depression, I start with an approach that shares many characteristics with social-cognitive and control systems theory, and with the present SNM model. In his neurocognitive theory of goal-based action control, Schneider (2006) elaborates upon many of the themes previously introduced here to describe precisely how the central nervous system and the goal system interact to yield clinical depression.

Schneider (2006) views depression, in the spirit of similar control system formulations (e.g., Carver & Scheier, 1998; Karoly, 1999; Klinger, 1977; Pyszczynski & Greenberg, 1987; Strauman, 1989), as a disorder wherein the selection and execution of actions are disturbed as the result of an individual's chronic nonattainment of important goals.[3] With goal failure (discrepancy, frustration) as the primary sensitizing experience, the depressed person typically embarks upon a stable pattern of dysfunctional goal cognition and pursuit (see also Kuhl & Helle, 1986) characterized by inactivity and avoidance, loss of attentional control, the development of negative expectations about the future, and the stress-induced prolonged emission of cortisol. This latter reaction pattern is particularly important because the continuous emission of cortisol is hypothesized eventually to produce central nervous system (e.g., executive function) damage.

Notably, Schneider's conception pivots on what he calls *goal–action episodes*, a construct akin to *goal episodes*, as discussed earlier in this chapter. Motor action representations are said to be intrinsically linked to "goal states" (i.e., intended states or events stored in memory; what I am simply calling goals) in the form of a goal–action episode. Similarly, the outcomes of goal–action episodes, whether actual or mentally simulated, give rise to emotions—positive emotions in response to success, and negative emotions in response to failure. In addition, goal–action episodes are presumed to compete with one another for the control of current action; that is, only one goal–action episode at a time can direct behavior; and the competition is, at least in part, regulated by stored probability (action–outcome) estimates that, in my model, are a key aspect of a person's anticipatory GES. Individuals keep track of or self-monitor single action–outcome sequences, as well as their repeated patterns over time (so-called *metamonitoring*). Metamonitoring is hypothesized to modify beliefs (GES) and to generate moods (cf. Carver & Scheier, 1998).

Although there is much to Schneider's (2006) formulation that I cannot here address, some of its major assertions (already tested or testable) about the causal and maintenance mechanisms in depression include the following: (1) Extended episodes of depressive mood and a focus on negative action–outcome expectancies/beliefs are precipitated by the metamonitoring of repeated goal pursuit failure; (2) the repeated activation of low probability estimates for future success constitutes stressful events that give rise to prolonged cortisol secretion, and eventually to damage of executive control systems in the brain, including the anterior cingulate, the amygdala, the hippocampus, and parts of the prefrontal cortex; and (3) state-dependent depressive mood leads to a reduction in approach-related actions and an increase in avoidance behavior.

With reference to my categorical account, Schneider's model would seem to highlight several paths. First, the precipitating pattern of repeated goal failure can be linked to any of the listed factors, with a disconnection between the components or a specific component weakness serving as the likely contributors. Second, a low level of system flexibility appears to be in evidence as regards the depressive's inability to override self-defeating metamonitoring. Third, cortisol-induced neural damage can be considered a focal dysfunction generated by the aforementioned processes. And, finally, the high avoidance and low approach behaviors would seem to be the joint consequence of compromised executive functions, high levels of arousal, negative GES, and automaticity converging to alter goal system content choices in favor of compensatory aspirations.

Obsessive–Compulsive Disorder

That cognition, emotion, action, and perception are blended in the unfolding of goal episodes is nowhere better illustrated than in the arcane, self-defeating patterns that characterize obsessive–compulsive disorder (OCD). The common concerns or content foci associated with OCD typically involve safety versus harm, personal responsibility, rules and rule violation, and a general insecurity about one's place in the world. Such concerns give rise to rigid patterns of behavior built around compensatory, order-themed goals designed to bring about the belief (however temporary) that some degree of control or mastery has been achieved. Although anxiety is usually considered the underlying precipitant of obsessive thinking and compulsive rituals (OCD is, after all, classified as an "anxiety disorder"), within the current framework, OCD is yet another form of self-regulatory abridgment. Without denying the anxiety-reducing effects of certain obsessive rituals and obsessive thoughts, without minimizing the role of fear and autonomic arousal, and acknowledging its link to negative affect and avoidance behaviors, the central building blocks of OCD are best articulated with reference to the multiple components displayed in Figure 8.1.

It is not by accident that *attention* is listed first under the self-regulatory targets (Figure 8.1). The failure to control attention or the tendency to focus attention for extended periods on a single information channel (typically the self) can be a source of adaptive difficulty (Ingram, 1990; Lyubomirsky, Tucker, Caldwell, & Berg, 1999). The voluntary modulation of attention, on the other hand, is a key source of adaptive flexibility (Derryberry, 2002). People with the symptoms of OCD clearly demonstrate diverse forms of context specific task failure. That is, they fail to do what others expect while rigidly pursuing a set of sometimes personally abhorrent goals (doing what they themselves would prefer not to do) partly as a result of the systematic breakdown of higher-order supervisory or executive control over attention, the automation of ritualistic habits, and pathogenic goal episode schemata and dynamics.

Note was earlier made of the person's need to coordinate inputs, internal states, and outputs for the sake of goal guidance; and it is generally believed that the prefrontal cortex (PFC) and its support structures provides the top-down control necessary to accomplish such coordination (Miller & Cohen, 2001). Disturbances to what I have termed *self-regulatory competencies* have been linked to an array of psychological disorders, with a growing body of neuropsychological evidence (e.g., Greisberg & McKay, 2003; Moritz et al., 2002; Purcell, Maruff, Kyrios, & Pantelis, 1998; Ursu, Stenger, Shear, Jones, & Carter, 2003; van Veen & Carter, 2006) suggesting that deficits in executive regulatory mechanisms are implicated in OCD.

For example, studies using functional magnetic resonance imaging (fMRI) or positron emission tomographic (PET) technology in people with OCD have reported correlations between OCD symptoms and abnormal activity in a number of brain areas, including orbitofrontal cortex, thalamus, and anterior cingulate cortex (ACC). The ACC is of particular interest because this structure has been hypothesized to serve either as an error detector or as a conflict (discrepancy) detector—functions attributed to the comparator process in feedback-based control theory formulations of self-regulation (Ford, 1987; Powers, 1973). Notably, Ursu and colleagues (2003) found that both conflict and error-related ACC activation tended to covary with OCD symptoms during a continuous performance task. When conflict, error, or discrepancies are detected, the efficient regulatory system should recruit attentional resources to manage the conflict, often by a focus on one set of action paths and suppression of the processing of irrelevant information. vanVeen and Carter (2006) have shown experimentally that during interference tasks, the ACC alerts the PFC to

exert its executive control. In persons with OCD, then, this error-monitoring → inhibition of irrelevancies process may be dysregulated, possibly instigating the inappropriate concern over error commission, the repetitive checking, and the tendency to focus on small, often irrelevant details that are so often a part of the clinical picture.

Of course, the whole clinical picture for OCD is invariably more complex. By referring to Figure 8.1 and presuming the functional interconnectedness of the pictured components, one can further hypothesize that disturbed action monitoring (contained within the Self-Regulatory Competencies box) leads to the formation of failure avoidant goals (the Goal Systems box), the pursuit of which becomes relatively mindless (or automatic) over time. Having formed goals that are predicated on the fear of making mistakes or breaking the rules (or, in control theory terms, experiencing intention–action discrepancies), it is probably the case that obsessive individuals eventually situate such goals at the top of their priority list, where they displace other normative pursuits, thus forming the basis of so-called "overvalued ideas" (Veale, 2002). The tendency of persons with OCD to persist in their error- or conflict-centered concerns, even in the face of counterevidence, might be attributed to a dysfunction in yet another executive function: selective attention (see Clayton, Richards, & Edwards, 1999).

Furthermore, if the commission of errors is somehow transformed or rescripted via thought-based (i.e., simulated) GES into the possibility of causing harm to oneself or others, then the goal system, in combination with the arousal system, may set about to monitor and then avoid perceived *danger* signals. Unfortunately, the same action monitoring dysfunction, as already described, will doom this enterprise as well. A neural circuitry model of the failed danger detection process in OCD, implicating a number of prefrontal and limbic structures, has recently been formulated by Szechtman and Woody (2004).

Some investigations of executive dysfunction in OCD rely not on direct neural assessments but on the use of performance tests.[4] Usually a subset of EF tests is administered to a sample of OCD patients or to persons with obsessive or compulsive habits determined to exist at subclinical levels, and their performance is compared against that of a matched control sample or other psychopathological groups. The kinds of self-regulatory deficits that can be identified depend, of course, on the executive skills included in the test battery. In one such study, Bannon, Gonsalvez, Croft, and Boyce (2006) set out to determine how active and remitted patients with OCD compared to those with panic disorder on a set of EF tests, and whether the executive deficiencies detected are stable dimensions of OCD or simply state-dependent side effects of symptom experience. Employing tests of inhibitory skill (the go/no-go task), task set switching (the Wisconsin Card Sorting Test), planning (the Tower of Hanoi), working memory (a dual-tracking task) and several others, these investigators confirmed that persons with OCD not only display deficits in task set shifting and inhibition but that these executive deficits are stable over time.

Addictive Disorders

Persons labeled as *addicts* are often described as impulsive, apparently animated by "urges" or "cravings" that either are not felt by other people or are not felt with the same urgency. Current research on the addictions has tended to emphasize the role of biogenetic and temperamental influences but has also begun to examine how these factors interact with online self-regulatory elements such as executive functioning and self-regulatory appraisals, as well as with critical environmental stressors or transitions to shape the symptomatic expressions of substance users and abusers. From an SNM perspective, the addiction problem is viewed as an emergent rather than a static phenomenon, deriving interactively from genetic and early environmental factors, and from activity in the neu-

ral and behavioral self-regulatory systems, physiology, and cultural and interpersonal influences. Thus, the so-called "addict" is neither the passive bearer of a "disease" nor the agile captain of his or her ship. Importantly, we hope that from the perspective of an integrative model, the commonalities across various addictive disorders (e.g., their power to co-opt energy previously devoted to normative pursuits, their influence on daily moods, decision-making capacities, and engagement in reckless/risky activities, as well as their relapse proneness) can be better understood (see Donovan, 1988).

Conceptions of addiction built upon self-regulatory processes are not uncommon because regulatory deficits, in the form of impaired control over emotions, decisions, and actions, have been linked, with varying degrees of consistency, to alcohol and drug abuse, tobacco smoking, and eating disorders (Curtin & Fairchild, 2003; Fillmore, 2003; Finn, 2002; Verdejo-Garcia, Rivas-Perez, Vilar-Lopez, & Perez-Garcia, 2007). But we should not overlook the importance of what I have called "deviant goals" in the creation of *maladaptive wanting* and its substance-seeking behavioral aftermath (see Robinson & Berridge, 1993). Whereas evolution sought to equip humankind with the hardwired means to survive hardship and navigate the ups and downs of life, the structure of modern industrialized societies seems to have made it possible for us to misappropriate our highly developed self-regulating brains and their supportive neurotransmitter systems for the pursuit of short-term hedonistic experiences (substance use) that may or may not be rewarding, and that may or may not ultimately kill us and those around us. We appear to accomplish this feat of self- and other-destructiveness by, among other things, distracting ourselves from the often painful antecedents of our self-indulgent habits and systematically discounting their future costs (Ainslie, 2006; Steele & Josephs, 1990).

Self-regulatory competencies or EFs are key players in both the etiology and maintenance of various addictive disorders because they undergird the intricate planning and self-deceptive mental machinations that often accompany the acquisition of addictive habits, and they bear the neurophysiological damage attendant to prolonged substance use. Fortunately, they may also ride to the rescue as "resilience resources," if developed to sufficient strength.

The work of Giancola and his associates (e.g., Giancola, 2000, 2004; Giancola, Parrott, & Roth, 2006) aptly illustrates the multiple roles performed by self-regulatory competencies in addictive pathology. Giancola has argued that the disruptive effects of alcohol on self-awareness, problem solving, attention allocation, and other aspects of information processing can be integrated around EF impairment. Focusing specifically on the link between alcohol intoxication and interpersonal aggression, Giancola has hypothesized that EF serves as a mediator; that is, alcohol consumption presumably disrupts higher-order self-regulatory skills, such as inhibition, attention, working memory, and the like, and this disruption leads to aggressiveness in a provocative environment. In addition, Giancola suggests that EF capacity can serve as a moderator of the aforementioned meditational link; that is, persons with low to moderate executive skills will be more likely to show aggression when under the influence of alcohol relative to persons with better developed skills. Employing a large battery of EF tests and a laboratory aggression paradigm involving the administration of electrical shocks to a fictitious opponent, Giancola has found support for his moderation hypothesis, but only for males, perhaps because of the laboratory aggression task that is used.

Implications for Primary Prevention and Resilience

Prevention science, charged with identifying the risks to adaptive functioning and strengthening people's resistance to these risks, has sometimes come under fire for its lack of a coherent model of psychopathology. Underlying this critique is the presumption that prevention advocates would have to know precisely how human adjustment "goes wrong" before they could design ways to forestall untoward outcomes (Heller, Wyman, & Allen, 2000). However, knowing *precisely* how human adaptive systems fail is a tall order for psychology,[5] particularly when we contemplate what modern medicine has accomplished without having a truly comprehensive model of illness or health. In this chapter I have argued for a perspective that, although incomplete, is sufficiently broad and possesses adequate precision about the process of life space navigation (i.e., self-regulation) to serve as a useful guide in our developing clinical efforts.

The SNM framework presumes that people act individually and collectively to regulate their lives by means of feedback and feed-forward mechanisms, and that they are capable of creating not only great distress and upheaval but also palpable social and personal advantage, order, and growth. Consequently, social and behavioral scientists and philosophers need not invent two widely disjunctive accounts of *good* and *evil*, *health* and *illness*, *competence* and *incompetence* to address the dualities inherent in the enterprise of living. This sentiment is mirrored in the work of Masten and Curtis (2000), who have argued that the concepts of competence and psychopathology can be integrated, not only because they share common intellectual roots and common interpretive problems, but also because the manifestations of adaptive and maladaptive behavior are strongly associated and mutually influential over time. That they share common mechanisms or a *final common pathway* is the theme that I wish to convey. I believe that the processes herein considered under the banner of self-regulation contain all the elements needed to erect a heuristically powerful account of resilience, wellness, flourishing, positive health, or human potential (see also Ryff & Singer, 1998).

Simply stated, if psychopathology is dysfunctional self-regulation, then *health* is functional self-regulation (i.e., the effective time- and context-bound operation of all the components shown in Figure 8.1 as they are applied to the normative tasks of everyday life). The capacity to bounce back after adversity or to be minimally affected by adversity—the condition typically labeled *resilience*—can be viewed as either the result of the *effective operation* of self-regulatory processes under conditions of stress or transition or, alternatively, as the result of *especially well-developed self-regulatory functions* under stressful or transitional conditions. Because there are currently no data to aid in choosing between these two closely connected self-regulatory formulations, I simply propose that the patterns of stress reactivity protection, arrayed under the descriptive banner of *resilience*, are facilitated by an intact self-regulatory system operating at high levels of flexibility and efficiency, and in relation to specific goals and to specific situational challenges/constraints and affordances. Systems-based resilience resources can act either to reduce the individual's sensitivity to threat or to enhance threat regulation, or both.

Understanding what differentiates persons who succumb to adversity from those who prevail, or perhaps even flourish, necessitates the identification of key psychosocial mediators, as well as the active and attended-to features of the environment. Such an understanding of resilience is consistent with Mischel and Shoda's (1995) influential cognitive–affective personality systems (CAPS) model (see also Freitas & Downey, 1998), as well as with the present multicomponent self-regulatory formulation. An important proviso of any transactional model of resilience is the presumption that demonstrating resilience in one context does not ensure its manifestation in another. As Freitas and Downey (1998) have pointed out, in accordance with the present perspective, as well as with the CAPS model, resilient outcomes are the joint result of inter-

nal mediators and situational affordances. Viewing resilience in such a dynamic manner may help to obviate the shortcomings of exclusively person-centered or trait-based (one size fits all) preventive interventions.

How then does self-regulation, operating under conditions of stress or transition, yield resilient rather than pathogenic outcomes? First, readers are reminded that resilience is often more likely than psychological deterioration under many sorts of adverse conditions (Bonanno, 2004). *Hedonic adaptation* (i.e., the reduction of affective intensity in response to extremely negative [or positive] events) (see Frederick & Loewenstein, 1999), psychological compensation (Backman & Dixon, 1992), the mobilization of well-learned coping skills, counterfactual ("Things could have been worse") thinking, the availability of social support, and the like, all contribute to understanding why exposure even to the most devastating traumas of warfare (e.g., service in Vietnam) yields current posttraumatic stress disorder (PTSD) prevalence rates of only about 15% for men and 8.5% for women (Ozer, Best, Lipsey, & Weiss, 2003). Yet, notably, it is also the case that offline enabling conditions, such as temperament and genetics (as listed in Figure 8.1), along with *noncompromised* or well-functioning regulatory components, such as executive skills, goal process cognition, well-honed instrumental and expressive abilities, and self-regulatory appraisals, can serve to augment and enable our acquired coping skills and our evolved physiological defenses. In the space remaining, I provide empirical illustrations of how some of these self-regulatory components help to buffer stress or upgrade resilience in the face of adversity or transition, in contrast to how their compromised versions have been shown to undergird the genesis of clinical disorders.

Focusing on children ages 8 to 17, classified as resilient and nonresilient based on a set of clinical indices, and currently living under impoverished conditions, Buckner, Mezzacappa, and Beardslee (2003) hypothesized that self-regulatory skills, reflecting what in my model are termed *self-regulatory competencies* or EFs, would predict resilience over and above the influence of relevant developmental factors such as age, intelligence, self-esteem, parental monitoring, and adversity. Using a Q-sort methodology, the authors fashioned a set of self-descriptive sorts tapping executive attention, inhibition, planfulness, emotional control, and related self-regulatory competencies. The findings supported the authors' contentions, with executive regulatory skills emerging as "the most potent independent predictor of resilience" (p. 154). That is, whereas all the variables in the regression analysis accounted for fully 69% of the variance in children's resilient adaptation, the zero-order correlation of self-regulation and resilience was itself .675, accounting for over 45% of the variance in this key dependent measure.

In light of the widely acknowledged risks to adjustment posed by normative life transitions (Arnett, 2001; Rutter, 1996; Stewart, 1982), Cantor and her colleagues have been investigating the transition to college and the psychological underpinnings of good versus poor social management of age-graded life tasks, under the broad assumption that personal vulnerability and resilience hinge on the individual's ability to engage actively in salient life task pursuits, with and without others. In one study, Zirkel and Cantor (1990) examined the effects on the college experience of different types of personal goals, including the goal concerned with achieving independence (being on one's own away from family) and with finding a personally meaningful identity. However, as noted earlier, the contents of people's goals are often less telling than their manner of construing or characterizing them; therefore, Zirkel and Cantor asked their subjects to self-generate goals, then rate each goal along various evaluative (topographic) dimensions, including perceived control over the goal, its difficulty, its stressfulness, its importance, its enjoyment, time invested in it, and the degree to which the respondent becomes absorbed in its pursuit (see Little, 1983). The investigators clustered the patterns of response to the independence and identity goals into those reflecting absorption in these life tasks (tasks rated as high in absorption, challenge, difficulty, time investment, etc.) versus non-absorption (tasks rated as relatively low in stressfulness, difficulty, and challenge, but high in control). When the absorbed and unabsorbed freshmen were followed via telephone interview into their junior year, their earlier patterns of goal construal were found to predict academic and social performance and perceived stress. Although both groups were very bright, high-achieving honor's students at the University of Michigan, those described as absorbed reported higher levels of stress and psychological symptoms, and lower levels of satisfaction with their academic and social performance relative to their unabsorbed peers. Thus, the goal-centered motivational frame of reference that characterized the unabsorbed students could be interpreted as providing a degree of protection from the adverse effects of overinvestment in the key life tasks of independence and identity seeking.

Finally, in a study by Windsor, Anstey, Butterworth, and Rodgers (2008), midlife adults were found to benefit from the stress-buffering potential of temperament-based self-regulatory tendencies. Specifically, Windsor and colleagues sought to show that neurologically grounded tendencies to approach desirable/rewarding stimuli, organized under the umbrella of the *behavioral approach system* (BAS), would buffer the effects of negative life events on perceptions of control. In addition, a second, independently operating *behavioral inhibition system* (BIS) is believed to give rise to avoidance of aversive events and the inhibition of goal-directed action. The authors further hypothesized that any protective effects of BAS sensitivities would vary as a function of BIS sensitivity. The data were collected as part of a large, community-based longitudinal survey of over 2,000 adults between 20 and 64 years old in two Australian cities. Results showed that, among other things, individuals high in BAS and low in BIS sensitivity maintained relatively high control perceptions irrespective of changes in negative life events, supporting the protective role of temperamental self-regulation.

Summary

A number of years have passed since Fowles (1994) summarized the advantages of a motivational approach to psychopathology. These included its relevance to emotional problems and its ready connection to neurochemical processes; to animal models; to pharmacological and genetic models; and to learning, ecological, and cognitive approaches. We can today add its relation to social, cognitive, and affective neuroscience, with special reference to EFs and its methodological ties to functional neuroimaging and naturalistic time sampling via momentary ecological assessment. Also of great importance is the emergence of a cohesive literature on goal cognition and goal pursuit, often organized under the aegis of the self-regulation of emotion, thought, or action, and applied creatively to the analysis of human psychopathology (e.g., Baumeister, 1997; Hamilton, Greenberg, Pysczcynski, & Cather, 1993; Kring & Werner, 2004; Mansell, 2005; Newman & Wallace, 1993).

This chapter, yet another brick in the edifice of experimental psychopathology, sought to establish a goal-centered self-regulatory model as a potentially unifying framework around which contemporary clinical science and practice could align. Built on basic conceptions articulated by Ford (1987), Powers (1973), Gray (1987), and others, the SNM perspective casts most or all of the varieties of psychopathology described in the psychiatric lexicon as different kinds of functional disorganization emerging out of the dynamic matrix statically depicted in Figure 8.1. Similarly, this perspective suggests that resilience, as a construct applied to understanding the emerging nature of health and successful adjustment to adversity, can likewise be written in the language of goal-guided self-regulation. Because most of the assertions put forward here have either been tested or are amenable to empirical verification, confidence in the integrative and practical utility of the SNM perspective on mental health, resilience, and psychopathology simply awaits the magisterial verdict of time.

Notes

1. The emerging field of *epigenetics*, in fact, assumes that life experiences are capable of altering gene expression, thereby influencing psychiatric disorders (see Higgins, 2008).
2. Using a diary-based data collection method with a focus on goals, one could compute an index of *Goal Pursuit Efficiency* by calculating the ratio of mean goal progress (across daily episodes or per week) over mean goal-related activity or effort (per day or per week). Such a metric would certainly honor the spirit of Wishner's original conception.
3. Within a distinct but compatible behaviorist framework, this goal-based failure formulation can be read as a loss of positive emotional stimulation (see Staats & Eifert, 1990).
4. It is important to keep in mind that performance tests (and clinical observations) provide the vital behavioral data from which neuropsychologists and other neuroscientists can determine the adaptive function of central nervous system structures and processes.
5. It may be seen as an even taller order for psychiatry, which for too long has held an "anti-etiological" mindset (Schaffner, 2002).

References

Ainslie, G. (2006). A selectionist model of the ego: Implications for self-control. In N. Sebanz & W. Prinz (Eds.), *Disorders of volition* (pp. 119–149). Cambridge, MA: MIT Press.

American Psychiatric Association (2000). *Diagnostic and statistical manual of mental disorders* (4th ed., text rev.). Washington, DC: Author.

Arnett, J. J. (2001). Conceptions of the transition to adulthood: Perspectives from adolescence through midlife. *Journal of Adult Development, 8,* 133–143.

Austin, J. T., & Vancouver, J. B. (1996). Goal constructs in psychology: Structure, process, and content. *Psychological Bulletin, 120,* 338–375.

Backman, L., & Dixon, R. A. (1992). Psychological compensation: A theoretical framework. *Psychological Bulletin, 112,* 259–283.

Bandura, A. (1984). Representing personal determinants in causal structure. *Psychological Review, 91,* 508–511.

Bandura, A. (1986). *Social foundations of thought and action: A social cognitive theory.* Englewood Cliffs, NJ: Prentice-Hall.

Bandura, A. (1997). *Self-efficacy: The exercise of control.* New York: Freeman.

Bannon, S., Gonsalvez, C. J., Croft, R. J., & Boyce, P.M. (2006). Executive functions in obsessive–compulsive disorder: State or trait deficits? *Australian and New Zealand Journal of Psychiatry, 40,* 1031–1038.

Bargh, J. A. (Ed.). (2007). *Social psychology and the unconscious: The automaticity of higher mental processes.* New York: Psychology Press.

Barkley, R. A. (2001). The executive functions and self-regulation: An evolutionary neuropsychological perspective. *Neuropsychological Review, 11,* 1–29.

Barnett, J. H., Salmond, C. H., Jones, P. B., & Sahakian, B. J. (2006). Cognitive reserve in neuropsychiatry. *Psychological Medicine, 36,* 1053–1064.

Baron-Cohen, S. (Ed.). (1997). *The maladapted mind: Classic readings in evolutionary psychopathology.* Hove, UK: Psychology Press.

Baumeister, R. F. (1997). Esteem threat, self-regulatory breakdown, and emotional distress as factors in self-defeating behavior. *Review of General Psychology, 1,* 145–174.

Baumeister, R. F., & Heatherton, T. F. (1996). Self-regulation failure: An overview. *Psychological Inquiry, 7,* 1–15.

Boekaerts, M., Pintrich, P., & Zeidner, M. (Eds.). (2000). *Handbook of self-regulation.* San Diego, CA: Academic Press.

Bogdan, R. J. (1994). *Grounds for cognition: How goal-guided behavior shapes the mind.* Hillsdale, NJ: Erlbaum.

Bolger, N., Davis, A., & Rafaeli, E. (2003). Diary methods: Capturing life as it is lived. *Annual Review of Psychology, 54,* 579–616.

Bonanno, G. A. (2004). Loss, trauma, and human resilience: Have we underestimated the human capacity to thrive after extremely aversive events? *American Psychologist, 59,* 20–28.

Brendel, D. H. (2003). Reductionism, eclecticism, and pragmatism in psychiatry: The dialectic of clinical explanation. *Journal of Medicine and Philosophy, 28,* 563–580.

Breuer, J., & Freud, S. (1895). Studies on hysteria. In J. Strachey (Ed.), *The standard edition of the complete psychological works of Sigmund Freud* (Vol. 2). London: Hogarth Press.

Buckner, J. C., Mezzacappa, E., & Beardslee, W. R. (2003). Characteristics of resilient youths living in poverty: The role of self-regulatory processes. *Development and Psychopathology, 15,* 139–162.

Burgess, P. W. (1997). Theory and methodology in executive function research. In P. Rabbitt (Ed.), *Methodology of frontal and executive function* (pp. 79–113). Hove, UK:Psychology Press.

Carver, C. S., & Scheier, M. F. (1998). *On the self-regulation of behavior.* New York: Cambridge University Press.

Caspi, A., & Moffitt, T. E. (2006). Gene–environment interactions in psychiatry: Joining forces with neuroscience. *Nature Reviews Neuroscience, 7,* 583–590.

Clayton, I. C., Richards, J. C., & Edwards, C. J. (1999). Selective attention in obsessive-compulsive disorder. *Journal of Abnormal Psychology, 108,* 171–175.

Conway, M. A., & Pleydell-Pearce, C. W. (2000). The construction of autobiographical memories in the self-memory system. *Psychological Review, 107,* 261–288.

Curtin, J. J., & Fairchild, B. A. (2003). Alcohol and cognitive control: Implications for regulation of behavior during response conflict. *Journal of Abnormal Psychology, 112,* 424–436.

Deci, E. L., & Ryan, R. M. (2000). The "what" and "why" of goal pursuits: Human needs and the self-determination of behavior. *Psychological Inquiry, 11,* 227–268.

De Houwer, J. (2006). Using the Implicit Association Test does not rule out an impact of conscious propositional knowledge on evaluative conditioning. *Learning and Motivation, 37,* 176–187.

Derryberry, D. (2002). Attention and voluntary self-control. *Self and Identity, 1,* 105–111.

Derryberry, D., & Rothbart, M. K. (1997). Reactive and effortful processes in the organization of temperament. *Development and Psychopathology, 9*, 633–652.

Donovan, D. M. (1988). Assessment of addictive behaviors: Implications of an emerging biopsychosocial model. In D. M. Donovan & G. A. Marlatt (Eds.), *Assessment of addictive behaviors* (pp. 3–48). New York: Guilford Press.

Emmons, R. A. (1999). *The psychology of ultimate concerns: Motivation and spirituality in personality.* New York: Guilford Press.

Fillmore, M. T. (2003). Drug abuse as a problem of impaired control: Current approaches and findings. *Behavioral and Cognitive Neuroscience Reviews, 2*, 179–197.

Finn, P. R. (2002). Motivation, working memory, and decision making: A cognitive–motivational theory of personality vulnerability to alcoholism. *Behavioral and Cognitive Neuroscience Reviews, 1*, 183–205.

Ford, D. H. (1987). *Humans as self-constructing living systems: A developmental perspective on behavior and personality.* Hillsdale, NJ: Erlbaum.

Ford, D. H., & Urban, H. B. (1998). *Contemporary models of psychotherapy: A comparative analysis.* New York: Wiley.

Fowles, D. C. (1994). A motivational theory of psychopathology. In W. D. Spaulding (Ed.), *Integrative views of motivation, cognition, and emotion: Nebraska Symposium on Motivation* (Vol. 41, pp. 181–238). Lincoln: University of Nebraska Press.

Freitas, A. L., & Downey, G. (1998). Resilience: A dynamic perspective. *International Journal of Behavioral Development, 22*, 263–285.

Frith, C. (2008). In praise of cognitive neuropsychiatry. *Cognitive Neuropsychiatry, 13*, 1–7.

Ghaemi, S. N. (2003). *The concepts of psychiatry: A pluralistic approach to the mind and mental illness.* Baltimore: Johns Hopkins University Press.

Giancola, P. R. (2000). Executive functioning: A conceptual framework for alcohol-related aggression. *Experimental and Clinical Psychopharmacology, 8*, 567–597.

Giancola, P. R. (2004). Executive functioning and alcohol-related aggression. *Journal of Abnormal Psychology, 113*, 541–555.

Giancola, P. R., Parrott, D. J., & Roth, R. M. (2006). The influence of difficult temperament on alcohol-related aggression: Better accounted for by executive functioning. *Addictive Behaviors, 31*, 2169–2187.

Gray, J. A. (1987). *The psychology of fear and stress.* New York: Cambridge University Press.

Greisberg, S., & McKay, D. (2003). Neuropsychology of obsessive–compulsive disorder: A review and treatment implications. *Clinical Psychology Review, 23*, 95–117.

Hamilton, J. C., Greenberg, J., Pyszczynski, T., & Cather, C. (1993). A self-regulatory perspective on psychopathology and psychotherapy. *Journal of Psychotherapy Integration, 3*, 205–248.

Heller, K., Wyman, M. F., & Allen, S. M. (2000). Future directions for preventive science: From research to adoption. In C. R. Snyder & R. E. Ingram (Eds.), *Handbook of psychological change: Psychotherapy processes and practices for the 21st century* (pp. 660–680). New York: Wiley.

Hestenes, D. (1998). Modulatory mechanisms in mental disorders. In D. J. Stein & J. Ludik (Eds.), *Neural networks and psychopathology* (pp. 132–164). New York: Cambridge University Press.

Higgins, E. S. (2008). The new genetics of mental illness. *Scientific American Mind, 19*, 40–47.

Higgins, E. T., & Spiegel, S. (2004). Promotion and prevention strategies for self-regulation: A motivated cognition perspective. In R. F. Baumeister & K. D. Vohs (Eds.), *Handbook of self-regulation: Research, theory, and applications* (pp. 171–187). New York: Guilford Press.

Howard, G. S. (2008). Whose will? How free? In J. Baer, J. C. Kaufman, & R. F. Baumeister (Eds.), *Are we free?: Psychology and free will* (pp. 260–274). New York: Oxford University Press.

Hyman, S. E. (2007). Can neuroscience be integrated into the DSM-V? *Nature Reviews Neuroscience, 8*, 725–732.

Ingram, R. E. (1990). Self-focused attention in clinical disorders: Review and a conceptual model. *Psychological Bulletin, 107*, 156–176.

Josiassen, R. C. (1993). Psychobiological reflections of adult psychopathology. In S. Bellack & M. Hersen (Eds.), *Psychopathology in adulthood* (pp. 57–88). Boston: Allyn & Bacon.

Kandel, E. R. (1998). A new intellectual framework for psychiatry. *American Journal of Psychiatry, 155*, 457–469.

Karoly, P. (1993a). Goal systems: An organizing framework for clinical assessment and treatment planning. *Psychological Assessment, 5,* 273–280.

Karoly, P. (1993b). Mechanisms of self-regulation: A system's view. *Annual Review of Psychology, 44,* 23–52.

Karoly, P. (1995). Self-control theory. In W. O'Donohue & L. Krasner (Eds.), *Theories of behavior therapy: Exploring behavior change* (pp. 259–285). Washington, DC: American Psychological Association.

Karoly, P. (1999). A goal systems-self-regulatory perspective on personality, psychopathology, and change. *Review of General Psychology, 3,* 264–291.

Karoly, P. (2006). Tracking the leading edge of self-regulatory failure: Commentary on "Where do we go from here?: The goal perspective in psychotherapy." *Clinical Psychology: Science and Practice, 13,* 366–370.

Karoly, P. (2008). Systematizing personal goals: The three R's. *European Health Psychologist, 10,* 29–31.

Karoly, P. (in press). Goal systems and self-regulation: An individual differences perspective. In R. Hoyle (Ed.), *The handbook of personality and self-regulation.* Malden, MA: Blackwell.

Karoly, P., & Kanfer, F. H. (Eds.). (1982). *Self-management and behavior change: From theory to practice.* New York: Pergamon Press.

Karoly, P., & Newton, C. (2006). Effects of approach and avoid mindsets on performance, self-regulatory cognition, and affect in a multi-task environment. *Cognitive Therapy and Research, 30,* 355–376.

Katzko, M. W. (2006). A study of the logic of empirical arguments in psychological research: "The automaticity of social behavior" as a case study. *Review of General Psychology, 10,* 210–228.

Kihlstrom, J. F. (2008). The automaticity juggernaut—or, are we automatons after all? In J. Baer, J. C. Kaufman, & R. F. Baumeister (Eds.), *Are we free?: Psychology and free will* (pp. 155–180). New York: Oxford University Press.

Klinger, E. (1977). *Meaning and void: Inner experience and the incentives in people's lives.* Minneapolis: University of Minnesota Press.

Kring, A. M., & Werner, K. H. (2004). Emotion regulation and psychopathology. In P. Philippot & R. S. Feldman (Eds.), *The regulation of emotion* (pp. 359–385). Mahwah, NJ: Erlbaum.

Kuhl, J., & Helle, P. (1986). Motivational and volitional determinants of depression: The degenerated intention hypothesis. *Journal of Abnormal Psychology, 95,* 247–251.

Lara, D. R., Pinto, O., Akiskal, K., & Akiskal, H. S. (2006). Toward an integrative model of the spectrum of mood, behavioral, and personality disorders based on fear and anger traits: I. Clinical implications. *Journal of Affective Disorders, 94,* 67–87.

Lewis, M. D., & Todd, R. M. (2005). Getting emotional: A neural perspective on emotion, intention, and consciousness. *Journal of Consciousness Studies, 12,* 210–235.

Lewis, M. D., & Todd, R. M. (2007). The self-regulating brain: Cortical–subcortical feedback and the development of intelligent action. *Cognitive Development, 22,* 406–430.

Little, B. R. (1983). Personal projects: A rationale and method for investigation. *Environment and Behavior, 15,* 273–309.

Locke, E. A., & Latham, G. P. (1990). *A theory of goal setting and task performance.* Englewood Cliffs, NJ: Prentice-Hall.

Luu, P., & Tucker, D. M. (2003). Self-regulation by the medial frontal cortex: Limbic representation of motive set-points. In M. Beauregard (Ed.), *Consciousness, emotional self-regulation and the brain* (pp. 123–161). Philadelphia: Benjamins.

Lyubomirsky, S., Tucker, K. L., Caldwell, N. D., & Berg, K. (1999). Why ruminators are poor problem solvers: Clues from the phenomenology of dysphoric rumination. *Journal of Personality and Social Psychology, 77,* 1041–1060.

Mansell, W. (2005). Control theory and psychopathology: An integrative approach. *Psychology and Psychotherapy: Theory, Research and Practice, 78,* 141–178.

Masten, A. S., & Curtis, W. J. (2000). Integrating competence and psychopathology: Pathways toward a comprehensive science of adaptation in development. *Development and Psychopathology, 12,* 529–550.

McSweeney, F. K., & Swindell, S. (1999). General-process theories of motivation revisited: The role of habituation. *Psychological Bulletin, 125,* 437–457.

Meyer-Lindenberg, A., & Weinberger, D. R. (2006). Intermediate phenotypes and genetic mechanisms of psychiatric disorders. *Nature Reviews Neuroscience*, 7, 818–827.

Miller, E. K., & Cohen, J. D. (2001). An integrative theory of prefrontal cortex function. *Annual Review of Neuroscience*, 24, 167–202.

Mischel, W., & Shoda, Y. (1995). A cognitive-affective system theory of personality: Reconceptualizing situations, dispositions, dynamics and invariance in personality structure. *Psychological Review*, 102, 246–268.

Moritz, S., Birkner, C., Kloss, M., Jahn, H., Hand, I., Haasen, C., et al. (2002). Executive functioning in obsessive–compulsive disorder, unipolar depression, and schizophrenia. *Archives of Clinical Neuropsychology*, 17, 477–483.

Murphy, D. (2001). Hacking's reconciliation: Putting the biological and sociological together in the explanation of mental illness. *Philosophy of the Social Sciences*, 31, 139–162.

Newman, J. P., & Wallace, J. F. (1993). Diverse pathways to deficient self-regulation: Implications for disinhibitory psychopathology in children. *Clinical Psychology Review*, 13, 699–720.

Owen, A. M. (2006). The human ventrolateral frontal cortex and intended action. In N. Sebanz & W. Prinz (Eds.), *Disorders of volition* (pp. 329–346). Cambridge, MA: MIT Press.

Ozer, E. J., Best, S. R., Lipsey, T. L., & Weiss, D. S. (2003). Predictors of posttraumatic stress disorder and symptoms in adults: A meta-analysis. *Psychological Bulletin*, 129, 52–73.

PDM Task Force. (2006). *Psychodynamic diagnostic manual*. Silver Spring, MD: Alliance of Psychoanalytic Organizations.

Peled, A. (2004). From plasticity to complexity: A new diagnostic method for psychiatry. *Medical Hypotheses*, 63, 110–114.

Posner, M. I., Rothbart, M. K., Sheese, B. E., & Tang, Y. (2007). The anterior cingulate gyrus and the mechanism of self-regulation. *Cognitive, Affective, and Behavioral Neuroscience*, 7, 391–395.

Powers, W. T. (1973). *Behavior: The control of perception*. Chicago: Aldine.

Powers, W. T. (2004). *Making sense of behavior: The meaning of control*. New Canaan, CT: Benchmark.

Purcell, R., Maruff, P., Kyrios, M., & Pantelis, C. (1998). Cognitive deficits in obsessive–compulsive disorder on tests of frontal–striatal function. *Biological Psychiatry*, 43, 348–357.

Pyszczynski, T., & Greenberg, J. (1987). Self-regulatory perseveration and the depressive self-focusing style: A self-awareness theory of reactive depression. *Psychological Bulletin*, 102, 122–138.

Robinson, D. N. (2000). Paradigms and the "myth of framework": How science works. *Theory and Psychology*, 10, 39–47.

Robinson, T. E., & Berridge, K. C. (1993). The neural basis of drug craving: An incentive sensitization theory of addiction. *Brain Research Reviews*, 18, 247–291.

Rutter, M. (1996). Transitions and turning points in developmental psychopathology: As applied to the age spans between childhood and mid-adulthood. *International Journal of Behavioral Development*, 19, 603–626.

Ryff, C. D., & Singer, B. (1998). The contours of positive human health. *Psychological Inquiry*, 9, 1–28.

Schaffner, K. F. (2002). Clinical and etiological psychiatric diagnoses: Do causes count? In J. Z. Sadler (Ed.), *Descriptions and prescriptions: Values, mental disorders and the DSMs* (pp. 271–290). Baltimore: Johns Hopkins University Press.

Schneider, W., & Chein, J. M. (2003). Controlled and automatic processing: Behavior theory and biological mechanisms. *Cognitive Science*, 27, 525–559.

Schneider, W. X. (2006). Action control and its failure in clinical depression: A neuro-cognitive theory. In N. Sebanz & W. Prinz (Eds.), *Disorders of volition* (pp. 275–306). Cambridge, MA: MIT Press.

Shahar, G. (2006). Clinical action: Introduction to the special section on the action perspective in clinical psychology. *Journal of Clinical Psychology*, 62, 1053–1064.

Sheldon, K. M. (2007). Considering "the optimality of personality": Goals, self-concordance, and multilevel personality integration. In B. R. Little, K. Salmela-Aro, & S. D. Phillips (Eds.), *Personal project pursuit: Goals, action, and human flourishing* (pp. 355–373). Mahwah, NJ: Erlbaum.

Staats, A. W., & Eifert, G. H. (1990). The paradigmatic behaviorism theory of emotions: Basis for unification. *Clinical Psychology Review*, 10, 539–566.

Steele, C. M., & Josephs, R. A. (1990). Alcohol myopia: Its prized and dangerous effects. *American Psychologist, 45,* 921–933.

Stewart, A. J. (1982). The course of individual adaptation to life changes. *Journal of Personality and Social Psychology, 42,* 1100–1113.

Strauman, T. J. (1989). Self-discrepancies in clinical depression and social phobia: Cognitive structures that underlie emotional disorders? *Journal of Abnormal Psychology, 98,* 14–22.

Szechtman, H., & Woody, E. (2004). Obsessive–compulsive disorder as a disturbance of security motivation. *Psychological Review, 111,* 111–127.

Toates, F. (1998). The interaction of cognitive and stimulus–response processes in the control of behaviour. *Neuroscience and Biobehavioral Reviews, 22,* 59–83.

Toates, F. (2006). A model of the hierarchy of behaviour, cognition, and consciousness. *Consciousness and Cognition, 15,* 75–118.

Urban, H. B. (1987). Dysfunctional systems: Understanding pathology. In M. E. Ford & D. H. Ford (Eds.), *Humans as self-constructing living systems: Putting the framework to work* (pp. 313–346). Hillsdale, NJ: Erlbaum.

Ursu, S., Stenger, V. A., Shear, M. K., Jones, M. R., & Carter, C. S. (2003). Overactive action monitoring in obsessive compulsive disorder: Evidence from functional magnetic resonance imaging. *Psychological Science, 14,* 347–353.

Vaillant, G. E. (2003). Mental health. *American Journal of Psychiatry, 160,* 1373–1384.

van Veen, V., & Carter, C. S. (2006). Conflict and cognitive control in the brain. *Current Directions in Psychological Science, 15,* 237–240.

Veale, D. (2002). Over-valued ideas: A conceptual analysis. *Behaviour Research and Therapy, 40,* 383–400.

Verdejo-Garcia, A., Rivas-Perez, C., Vilar-Lopez, R., & Perez-Garcia, M. (2007). Strategic self-regulation, decision-making and emotion processing in poly-substance abusers in their first year of abstinence. *Drug and Alcohol Dependence, 86,* 139–146.

Vohs, K. D., & Ciarocco, N. J. (2004). Interpersonal functioning requires self-regulation. In R. F. Baumeister & K. D. Vohs (Eds.), *Handbook of self-regulation: Research, theory, and application* (pp. 392–407). New York: Guilford Press.

Windsor, T. D., Anstey, K. J., Butterworth, P., & Rodgers, B. (2008). Behavioral approach and behavioral inhibition as moderators of the association between negative life events and perceived control in midlife. *Personality and Individual Differences, 44,* 1080–1092.

Winkielman, P., & Berridge, K. C. (2004). Unconscious emotions. *Current Directions in Psychological Science, 13,* 120–123.

Wishner, J. (1955). The concept of efficiency in psychological health and in psychopathology. *Psychological Review, 62,* 69–80.

Young, R. A., Valach, L., & Domene, J. F. (2005). The action–project method in counseling psychology. *Journal of Counseling Psychology, 52,* 215–223.

Zachar, P. (2000). *Psychological concepts and biological psychiatry: A philosophical analysis.* Philadelphia: Benjamins.

Zirkel, S., & Cantor, N. (1990). Personal construal of life tasks: Those who struggle for independence. *Journal of Personality and Social Psychology, 58,* 172–185.

9

Self-Complexity
A Source of Resilience?

Eshkol Rafaeli
Atara Hiller

In this chapter, we take a social-cognitive view to answering the question "What is it about me that makes me resilient?" By doing that, we equate "me" with the cognitive self, an entity hard to define and difficult to measure or study that has nevertheless been of great interest to psychologists, who, for over a century, have suggested that it plays a central role in thought, affect, behavior, as well as resilience. The self first appeared prominently in the writings of William James (1890), who distinguished between "the self as known" (the "me") and the "self as knower" (the "I"). This distinction between the experienced self and the experiential self exists today as well. Using the more recent terminology of social cognition, Linville and Carlston (1994) equated the "me" with the declarative knowledge we have about ourselves, and the "I" with the procedural knowledge that directs our actions, thoughts, and feelings. In this chapter, we focus on the former and, specifically, on

structural features of the self-concept that play some role in resilience and well-being.

From a social-cognitive view, a resilient self has the cognitive contents, structures, or mechanisms that help one withstand external stressors without serious debilitation. This view focuses less on teleological growth or poststressor advancement, and more on here-and-now coping. Thus, the majority of the work we review here treats resilience (or well-being) as involving temperate emotions, most commonly in reaction to external stressful life events. It then sets out to determine what structural qualities of the self promote this form of resilience.

The empirical study of the self originally focused on the belief that it is a unitary construct (Allport, 1955; Rogers, 1977; Wylie, 1974, 1979). The vast literature on self-esteem is in fact predicated on the notion that people have a unitary self, and that a single dimension of esteem can measure the valence of individuals' feelings about their (seemingly unified) self. Whereas some psychologists (James, 1890; Kelly, 1955) and sociologists (Mead, 1934) always held a multifaceted view of the self, an empirical treatment of this multifacetedness began only in the last four decades, with multidimensional models from social cognition (Higgins, 1987; Markus, 1977), narrative psychology (Gergen & Gergen, 1983), and psychodynamic theories (Westen, 1992). Social-cognitive models in particular view the self as comprising various aspects, roles, and perspectives. Each of these multiple "selves" reflects the information we have about ourselves as we are in that particular aspect of ourselves. Consequently, individual differences may exist both in the content (and overall valence associated with the self; i.e., self-esteem: Wylie, 1974), and in the organizational features or structure of this self-knowledge. Both content and structure may play important roles in well-being and resilience.

In a review of the self-concept literature, McConnell and Strain (2007) note that most attention to date has focused on self-content rather than structure. For instance, abundant work examines *self-enhancement*, or individuals' tendency to view themselves positively. For example, Brown (1998) found that people with high self-esteem tend to endorse more positive than negative traits for the self, and argued that this tendency is important for developing and maintaining greater subjective well-being in the face of stressors and negative feedback (Taylor & Brown, 1988, 1994). Supporting this idea, Taylor, Lerner, Sherman, Sage, and McDowell (2003) found that self-enhancers not only report better mental health but indeed have a better autonomic nervous system response to stress (as reflected by healthier hypothalamic–pituitary–adrenal [HPA] axis profiles), a finding that was mediated by their enhanced psychosocial resources (e.g., optimism, mastery, and extraversion). In contrast, others (e.g., Colvin & Block, 1994; Paulhus, 1998; Shedler, Mayman, & Manis, 1993) have found that self-enhancement is

related to poor mental health. For instance, Colvin, Block, and Funder (1995) found greater self-enhancement to predict psychological impairment and poorer social skills.

Research on self-enhancement (as well as other self-content-related phenomena; e.g., self-verification or self-assessment) has tended to treat the self as unitary, even as the position that the self is complex and multifaceted was gaining prominence, and a separate research tradition focused on self-structure emerged.

Cognitive Structure and Self-Structure

The study of the structure of self-knowledge has its roots in cognitive (especially cognitive structure) models of personality that emerged in the first half of the 20th century. These included Lewin's field theory (1935), the models of the Gestalt school, and the neurocognitive work of Hebb (1949). These earlier models were a strong influence on George Kelly's (1955) pioneering work on the psychology of *personal constructs*, a comprehensive theory of individual differences in the structure of social or self-knowledge, and of the psychological implications of such individual differences. In his theory, Kelly suggested that the distinctive constructs with which a person organizes the world are significant sources of individual differences in personality, emotion, and behavior. The set of constructs—or the construct system—used by any individual is that person's idiosyncratic theory of how the social world (or the intrapersonal world— i.e., the self) is organized. Construct systems can vary in their consistency, rigidity, and complexity—and these variations will determine how "useful" the construct system is in anticipating and responding to the world, and indeed, how resilient one is. To assess construct systems, Kelly developed the *repertory grid* technique, an interview method that elicits a person's idiographic constructs by identifying similarities and differences among triads of targets (which could be other people or aspects of the self). The theoretical notion of complexity within the personal constructs system was further elaborated by Bieri (1955; Tripodi & Bieri, 1966), who used the repertory grid technique to obtain cognitive complexity scores, and suggested that a construct system characterized by greater complexity would allow one to make better predictions of behavior (i.e., to respond more adaptively to one's environment).

Kelly's and Bieri's work was rich theoretically but depended on assessment techniques that were quite cumbersome to administer and score. A novel alternative approach to the study of cognitive complexity was presented by Scott (1962, 1969), who was interested in individuals' ability to change selectively their cognitive structure in response to environmental stimuli. Scott employed a trait-sorting task that could be scored using a variety of statistics, mostly measures of dispersion borrowed from information theory (Attneave, 1959). Scott's approach became the dominant one used in self-complexity research, and we return to it in greater detail later.

By the 1970s, several alternative conceptualizations of cognitive complexity were available; these included, in addition to the ones reviewed earlier, others by Crocket (1965), Wyer (1964), and Zajonc (1960). A review of this literature (Streufert & Streufert, 1978) found it to be so plagued with confusing, inconsistent terminology that it was impossible to generalize one theorist's conceptualization to another's theory. The term *complexity* was being used to describe the "beholder's" perceptual system (e.g., Kelly, 1955; Scott, 1962, 1969), as well as the "beheld" stimulus domain (e.g., Wyer, 1964; Zajonc, 1960). Moreover, the notion of complexity was used inconsistently, sometimes referring to one elemental feature of cognitive structure, *differentiation* (the degree to which a cognitive domain contains multiple distinct elements; e.g., Crocket, 1965), at other times to another elemental feature, *integration* (the degree of coherence, interrelatedness,

or unity of the cognitive domain), and at yet other times to some mixture of the two (e.g., Zajonc, 1960). This led to different indices of "complexity" that rarely were empirically related.

Researchers interested in *self*-complexity inherited the complex (or maybe simply disorganized?) legacy of cognitive complexity research; in keeping with this legacy, they proceeded to generate multiple, mostly unrelated models that did not speak clearly to one another. For example, Anderson (1992) studied *complexity variables*, indices of differentiation and centrality based on Zajonc's (1960) cognitive complexity work. Using Zajonc's task, elementary school children generated self-descriptive traits, sorted them into hierarchical groups, and determined which traits were related. The differentiation index refers to the total number of categories composing the schema (e.g., scholastic competence, athletic competence, social acceptance). Higher differentiation scores (i.e., more numerous categories) were expected to lead to less reactivity to positive or negative events because other self-aspects could be activated to maintain self-regard. The centrality index reflects the organization of the schema around one central issue. In Anderson's study, this issue was scholastic pursuits: Centrality scores are high when scholastic traits are strongly interrelated with other traits. Anderson found that both differentiation and centrality indexes were unrelated to participants' responses to self-relevant feedback.

Stein (1994) also adopted Zajonc's (1960) methods but formed an amalgam of two indices: differentiation (the number of attributes in the self-schema) and unity (the degree of dependence among the attributes included in the self-schema). If participants' self-schemas were both differentiated and not unified, and therefore less integrated, their complexity was higher. Participants had higher differentiation scores if they generated more characteristics about themselves, and lower unity scores if they indicated that changes in one characteristic did not change other characteristics. High complexity subjects responded more thoughtfully to feedback (as reflected by slower response times) and did not have much change in their self-esteem levels. Low complexity subjects had more of a change—interestingly, in the direction of more self-esteem following failure feedback. In other words, their responses appeared to be more defensive.

Rosenberg (1977), as well as Woolfolk and his colleagues (1999; Woolfolk, Novalany, Gara, & Allen, 1995), used the hierarchical classes clustering algorithm (HICLAS) method (described in Deboeck & Rosenberg, 1988) that derives from network theory. HICLAS represents the structure of cognitions by categorizing participants' responses into classes or clusters based on patterns of the co-occurrence of attributes within descriptions of others and of the self. Individuals are asked to describe their mothers, fathers, significant others, three other people important to them, and three acquaintances who are less important. They are also asked to describe 11 various aspects of themselves (e.g., "me as I actually am," "how I am with my mother," "me as I ideally would like to be," "me when I am depressed"). A minimum number of characteristics must be used in describing each target person or self-aspect. All of the descriptions are then combined into one randomized list, and respondents rate each of the other people and each of the self-aspects on each characteristic that they themselves provided; a 0- to 2-point scale is used, with 0 indicating that the item does not apply at all, and 2 indicating that the item applies to a great degree to the given person or self. This procedure yields a two-way matrix of targets (20 self-aspects and significant others) by attributes (a varying number of free-response characteristics generated by the subject), which is analyzed using HICLAS (Woolfolk et al., 1999). HICLAS studies repeatedly indicate the need to partition self-complexity into positive and negative constructs. They report an absence of any association between positive self-complexity and depression or self-

esteem, but a positive association between negative self-complexity and depression or low self-esteem (Gara et al., 1993; Woolfolk et al., 1995, 1999).

Self-complexity models based on the Zajonc (1960) or Rosenberg (1977) approaches represent an implicit way of studying complexity. In contrast, Evans (1994) used the self-report Self-Complexity Inventory (SCI) to measure self-complexity explicitly. In the SCI, eight stressful scenarios in particular domains (e.g., failing a test) are presented, and respondents are asked to rate the degree to which they would be affected both globally and in particular domains other than that portrayed in the scenario (e.g., parental relationships, peer acceptance, physical appearance).

The SCI was initially created to study self-complexity in adolescence, and was guided by Werner's *orthogenetic principle* (1948, 1957), which posits that development proceeds from a state of global undifferentiation through increasing differentiation and specificity, and ultimately to integration and consolidation. In terms of the self-concept, young children are thought to have simple, global, and undifferentiated self-concepts. As they mature, they develop and identify numerous distinct self-aspects reflecting various abilities, activities, and relationships; with time, these become integrated into a coherent identity. Marsh (1989) and his colleagues (Marsh, Barnes, Cairns, & Tidman, 1984; Marsh & Shavelson, 1985) provided evidence for this developmental view by showing that multiple self-aspects were more intercorrelated among young children than for older children and adolescents, indicating that adolescents are better able to distinguish among these aspects.

Evans (1994) argued that those adolescents who have not developed the abilities to distinguish their cognitive domains have greater psychological problems. According to developmental psychologists, the ability to differentiate among various domains of the self emerges around age 7 or 8 years (Harter, 1982). Cramer (1987) suggested that older children begin developing differentiated and more numerous self-aspects as a defense against the anxiety that results from growing older. Abela and Véronneau-McArdle (2002) explained that self-complexity develops together with the capacity for abstract reasoning and formal operational thought. At a certain age, the simplified and globally positive self-view characteristic of earlier childhood ceases to provide a good fit with the negative, as well as positive, self-relevant information they are receiving. To reconcile their shifting view of themselves, they begin to differentiate self-aspects from the global self. With different self-relevant experiences, individual differences in both the content and structure of these self-aspects emerge. Evans and Seaman's (2000) work supports the idea that one such individual difference, in the complexity of the self, is indeed associated with more mature defense strategies and higher global self-worth; specifically, those with less complex organization had immature defenses, as well as more externalizing and internalizing behaviors.

The SCI is more a measure of integration, assessing the degree to which particular domains of the self-concept are interrelated. Psychoanalytic theorists (e.g., Blatt & Lerner, 1983; Leigh, Westen, Barends, Mendel, & Byers, 1992) have also proposed models of self-complexity that emphasize integration over differentiation. To do so, they use open-ended interviews or projective measures (e.g., the Thematic Apperception Test; Murray, 1943) to code complexity as a function of a number of factors, including perspective taking, ambivalence, and elaboration present in the free responses. These models too suggest that self-complexity (i.e., complex *perceptual* tendencies) is related to psychological and chronological maturation.

More than 20 years after Streufert and Streufert's (1978) frustrated critique of the disorganized field of cognitive complexity, Rafaeli-Mor and Steinberg (2002) reviewed the extant literature on *self*-complexity, including the models summarized earlier, and came to the same conclusion with regards to this field. As had been the case with cognitive complexity, a consensual definition of self-complexity seemed impossible to obtain: Various models of self-complexity operationalized it very differently, some emphasizing the differentiation of the self-concept, others its integration, and still others a combination of both differentiation and integration. Nonetheless, among the various models of self-complexity, one operationalization stood out as both widely studied and visible: the social-cognitive model of self-complexity developed by Linville (1985, 1987). Linville's theory is notable for several reasons. First, it has piqued the most interest among clinical and social psychologists, and has generated the most extensive body of research. Her model is the only one that has achieved broad recognition within psychology—to the point of inclusion in undergraduate and graduate texts. Second, Linville's model has been used to address a wide range of resilience or well-being outcomes, including depression (Brown & Rafaeli, 2007; Linville, 1987), mood following trauma (Morgan & Janoff-Bulman, 1994), escape from self (Dixon & Baumeister, 1991), narcissism (Rhodewalt & Morf, 1995), response to domestic violence (Steinberg, Pineles, Gardner, & Mineka, 2003), self-esteem (Campbell, Chew, & Scratchley, 1991), and coping with the ups and downs of everyday life (Campbell et al., 1991; Cohen, Pane, & Smith, 1997; Constantino, Wilson, & Horowitz, 2006; Miller, Omens, & Delvadia, 1991). Finally, whereas most self-complexity models suggest that complex individuals process information differently and (in particular) respond in more moderate ways to life events, Linville's model has been unique in detailing the processes that bring about this relationship by bringing together the cognitive structure tradition of Scott (1969), Bieri (1955), and others, with the language of more modern social-cognitive approaches. For these reasons, we devote the majority of this review to this model, its predictions, and literature examining these predictions.

Linville's Self-Complexity Model

Linville's (1985) definition of *self-complexity* begins with the recognition that the self is not unitary, but instead comprises multiple "self-aspects," which may include social roles, relationships, physical features, types of activities, and goals. Each of these self-aspects includes (or is associated with) one or several attributes—typically, traits. For example, Mary might see herself as a mother, a union organizer, and a wife; as a mother, she might see herself as fierce, loving, and anxious; as a union organizer, as fierce and energetic; and as a wife, as content and playful. Linville defined *self-complexity* conceptually as having more numerous self-aspects (e.g., Mary has three; others may have as few as one, or as many as 20 or more), and having less redundancy or overlap among these self-aspects (in Mary's case, the only redundancy is due to the linkage of the trait "fierce" to two of her aspects—being a mother, and being a union organizer).

Self-complexity is thought to develop through processes of generalization and discrimination. The more one experiences varied roles, relationships, and situations, the more differentiated those self-aspects become. Increased differentiation is thought to allow more efficient processing of self-relevant information, more effective discrimination among the various demands of one's roles and situations, and quicker and more appropriate responses to those demands.

To measure self-complexity, Linville (1985, 1987) used a trait-sorting task similar to the one developed by Scott (1969) in his studies of cognitive complexity. Subjects are given a list of trait words and are asked to use those words to describe different aspects or roles in their lives. The subject is free to identify as many or as few piles of traits (i.e., self-aspects), and to use any trait once, multiple times, or never. The resultant distribution of traits into self-aspects is then summarized using the dimensionality statistic (H) (Attneave, 1959; Scott, 1969), an index borrowed from information theory. It measures the degree to which a given observation falls into numerous categories rather than only one. H is interpreted as the minimal number of independent binary attributes needed to reproduce a trait sort. In other words, it describes the number of dimensions that underlie the sort.

Earlier research by Linville (e.g., 1982) addressed *social* (rather than *self-*) categorization and judgments, and offered a social-cognitive take on a widely prevalent ingroup–outgroup phenomenon. This early work demonstrated that affective extremity toward outgroup members can occur as a consequence of the fact that people hold less complex knowledge structures for outgroups than for ingroups (with the groups based on factors such as age, race, or sex).

Linville (1985) imported this model from the realm of intergroup processes (and evaluations) to the realm of intrapersonal cognition (and affect). Following the same logic that applied to in- versus outgroups, she suggested that individuals who hold a more complex *self*-representation were likely to experience more subdued emotional reactions to self-relevant situations; those with more simple representations were expected to show higher affective extremity. Thus, the model suggests a trade-off between self-complexity and affective extremity. According to this trade-off, greater self-complexity is expected to moderate the impact of positive and negative events for two main reasons, having to do with (1) the relative proportion of the entire self-concept implicated and (2) the degree of spillover among overlapping self-aspects. The model makes the following assumptions: First, when a particular event occurs, it is expected to exert its effect on the self-aspect most relevant to it. For example, a fight with her husband will be most relevant to Mary's *wife* self-aspect. Second, the proportion of the entire self-concept that is "taken up" by the implicated self-aspect will be directly related to the strength of the event's effect. In Mary's case, her *wife* self-aspect takes up one-third of her self-concept; for someone with twice as many self-aspects, that proportion will only be one-sixth. Third, the activation of an implicated self-aspect may spread to other self-aspects, to the extent that these other aspects overlap or are associated with the implicated self-aspect. In Mary's case, no such spillover would occur from *wife* to the other two self-aspects; however, events affecting her in one of those two self-aspects (as a union organizer or a mother) would lead to some spillover of activation because these two self-aspects are linked by a common trait.

As thoughts and emotions from one aspect are activated, related self-aspects will also be activated depending on context, associated thoughts, recency and frequency of activation, and relation to already activated aspects, so that more of the self is affected (Linville, 1987). A self-concept characterized by greater complexity—that is, by more numerous and more independent self-aspects—will stem the flow of affective spillover and make the owner of that self-concept be less susceptible to extreme reactions to life events. In other words, those with greater self-complexity are more resilient in response to stressful events.

Early evidence for the affective spillover effect came from a study (Linville, 1985, Study 1) in which participants completed the trait-sorting task along with affect and self-evaluation questionnaires, and were then provided (false) feedback of success or failure following an analytical task putatively related to intelligence. After receiving this feedback, participants were asked to report their mood and self-evaluation again (because a purported computer glitch had resulted in lost data earlier on). Those higher in self-complexity responded less negatively to failure feedback, and less positively to success feedback, than those low in self-complexity. In another study, Linville (1985, Study 2) demonstrated that those high in self-complexity reported more stable daily moods (i.e., less mood variability) over a 2-week period. Finally, Linville (1987) expanded the hypothesized role of self-complexity and suggested that it would serve as a buffer against the negative effects of naturally occurring stressful life events. In a short-term (2 week) prospective study, she demonstrated that Time 1 self-complexity did in fact buffer the effects of Time 1 stressful events on both depressive and somatic symptoms, as well as on the incidence of various stress-related illnesses (e.g., flu, aches, or cramps) at Time 2.

The Status of Self-Complexity Literature

Linville's self-complexity (SC) model, and particularly the prediction that SC plays a moderating and stress-buffering role, has been met with great enthusiasm in clinical, developmental, and social-psychological circles, and has generated scores of studies attempting to replicate or expand it. Though the results of some replications (e.g., Kalthoff & Neimeyer, 1993, Study 1) supported the model, those of many others did not, and the overall picture has been quite mixed. Two reviews (Koch & Shepperd, 2004; Rafaeli-Mor & Steinberg, 2002) help to clarify the methodological and theoretical factors responsible for the mixed findings regarding SC and well-being, coping, and resilience.

To examine the SC–well-being association, Rafaeli-Mor and Steinberg (2002) carried out a two-pronged research synthesis on the broadest set of available studies that used Linville's operationalization and reported any positively or negatively valenced well-being outcome (including mood, self-esteem, or depression). Included in the synthesis were all published studies (and all obtainable unpublished work as well), beginning with Linville's (1985) earliest study, and ending in March 1998. The largest group of studies found (70 of them) reported simple associations (typically, correlations) between Linville's dimensionality index (the *H* statistic) and a well-being measure. These were included in a standard meta-analysis and subdivided into three groups: (1) those in which the entire sample had experienced some uniform stressor (e.g., childbirth: Gallant, 1991; failure feedback: Linville, 1985, Study 1, failure condition); (2) those in which the entire sample had experienced a uniform positive event (or "uplift"; e.g., success feedback: Linville, 1985, Study 1, success condition); and (3) those in which no uniform event was specified, so that only a zero-order correlations were available for meta-analytic aggregation.

The standard meta-analysis found results that failed to support Linville's (1985) stress-buffering model. When aggregated, the largest group of studies (Group 3—those with no uniform event) had a weak (but negative; mean weighted $r = -.04$) association between SC and well-being; those with greater complexity had more negative mood, less self-esteem, or more depressive symptoms. Though complexity was positively related to well-being in the uniform stressor group (Group 1), the aggregate effect size was very small (mean weighted $r = .03$), indicating very weak stress buffering. In contrast, complexity was moderately and negatively related to well-being in the uniform uplift group (Group 2; mean weighted $r = -.27$), suggesting that it serves more as a moderator of positive events than of negative events.

A more appropriate test of a stress-buffering effect is a prospective *diathesis–stress* design, which includes an interaction between the putative buffer (Linville's dimensionality index, in this case) and an index of stressors; Time 2 outcomes (e.g., depressive symptoms) can then be predicted based on the buffer, the stressor, and their interaction, while adjusting for the Time 1 level of the outcome. Unfortunately, this design does not lend itself easily to meta-analytic aggregation because it is usually impossible to obtain a standard effect size from different multiple regression interaction terms. Nonetheless, Rafaeli-Mor and Steinberg (2002) supplemented the meta-analysis of the larger group of studies with a second analytic prong: a simpler, more rudimentary vote-counting procedure on 24 studies that directly tested the hypothesized stress-buffering effect of SC, and that had reported interaction effects within regressions models. Vote counting in this case simply involved reporting whether a particular study's regression model supported or did not support the buffering hypothesis.

As with the standard meta-analysis, the results of the vote-counting procedure did not support the stress-buffering hypothesis. Though seven of the 24 studies found a significant buffering effect, four other studies found the reverse (a significant exacerbation effect), and the majority of studies failed to find any significant effect.

Following Rafaeli-Mor and Steinberg's (2002) research synthesis, Koch and Shepperd (2004) conducted a qualitative review of a smaller set of studies that examined the association between SC and coping with stress. This review was more sympathetic to Linville's (1985) hypothesis, and concluded that SC is indeed a buffer of stress. One major point of departure in the Koch and Shepperd review was their decision to focus only on studies using prospective diathesis–stress designs. In their view, the cross-sectional studies (which were found by Rafaeli-Mor & Steinberg [2002] to report mostly negative, though weak, associations between SC and well-being) were irrelevant for testing Linville's stress-buffering prediction. This exclusion seems inappropriate to us: After all, the cross-sectional associations suggest that for the average person, SC is mildly deleterious (cf. McConnell & Strain, 2007).

Even if we disregard Rafaeli-Mor and Steinberg's (2002) cross-sectional results, or the finding that SC had a stronger buffering effect on positive (uplift) than on negative (stressor) events, Koch and Shepperd (2004) do not provide any counterevidence to the results of the vote-counting procedure—the analysis aggregating only prospective studies of the sort found acceptable. That analysis did not find support for the stress-buffering model; moreover, additional prospective studies (e.g., Constantino et al., 2006; Rothermund & Meiniger, 2004; Schleicher &

McConnell, 2005) have also failed to find such support.

Despite this divergence in both methods and conclusions, the main thrust of both review articles was a search for potential factors in the designs or operationalizations used in the reviewed studies that could have affected the SC–resilience association. One such factor noted in both reviews is the valence of the traits used in the self-descriptive task which yields the SC scores. Rather than being a simple methodological issue, this factor brings up a fundamental question about the role of valence in the organization of self-knowledge. As we noted earlier (and as noted by others; e.g., McConnell & Strain, 2007), the interest in self-structure was originally a departure from the focus on the content of the self-concept. If valence (i.e., a feature of content) affects SC, we can no longer treat complexity as a purely structural variable. As it turns out, that is indeed the case.

Morgan and Janoff-Bulman (1994) were first to discuss the segregation of SC by valence. They examined the complexity of positive self-representations separately from that of negative self-representations in an investigation of SC's role in the lives of students who had (or had not) experienced trauma. Three separate dimensionality indices (H statistics) were computed: one for positive SC (P-SC), one for negative SC (N-SC), and one for overall SC (O-SC). Individuals who had been exposed to trauma did not differ from those who had not in their P-SC, N-SC, or O-SC. However, individuals who had experience with trauma and had high P-SC exhibited better adjustment; the same was not true for those with higher N-SC. In fact, N-SC was associated with poorer adjustment among those participants without a traumatic life event.

Another study (Woolfolk et al., 1995) similarly partitioned SC into partially independent positive and negative dimensions. They too found that N-SC was inversely related to self-esteem, and that depression is related to high N-SC and low P-SC. Thus, according

to both Morgan and Janoff-Bulman (1994) and Woolfolk and colleagues (1995), the more people perceive themselves with multiple negative self-aspects, the greater their levels of depression, and the lower the levels of self-esteem and adjustment to trauma.

Consistent with these findings, Rafaeli-Mor and Steinberg (2002) found a continuous effect for the valence content of the trait list used in SC tasks: Cross-sectional studies with a higher proportion of negative traits reported more negative associations between SC and well-being. However, prospective studies (i.e., those in Groups 1 and 2 detailed earlier) that included a greater proportion of negative traits had *stronger* buffering effects. In other words, if anything, it appears that it is the N-SC that buffers the impact of positive and negative events. We return to this issue of valence within the self-concept again at two later points (in discussing the problems with SC measurement, and in reviewing additional indices of self-structure). For now, we just wish to point out that these findings call into question an implicit part of the SC model—that complexity would buffer affective extremity regardless of the valence of the traits used in the SC task.

Several related factors that help to explain some of the heterogeneity of study results have to do with the internal validity versus external generalizability of the studies. Rafaeli-Mor and Steinberg (2002) found that more constrained and internally consistent studies obtained stronger associations between SC and well-being in the direction predicted. For example, when both SC and well-being were measured in the same session, they tended to be more strongly associated than if there was a time lag between them. Similarly, studies in which stressors were lab-induced (e.g., false feedback studies vs. ones using naturalistic stressors) also yielded stronger results in line with Linville's model. Finally, studies in which the well-being measure was of mood or emotion (i.e., relatively transitory and narrow constructs) resulted in findings similar to Linville, whereas those measuring self-esteem or depression (i.e., broader and more stable aspects of well-being) were less similar.

Identifying—and Solving—the SC Measurement Problem

Fortunately, the reviews of the SC literature, with their findings of partial or mixed support for the SC stress-buffering model have not had a chilling effect on this topic of research. Instead, they have stimulated multiple attempts at refining this compelling model. Several of these attempts have focused on the operationalization and measurement of SC, and particularly, on the problematic index (the H statistic) used in it. Why is this statistic so problematic? As Rafaeli-Mor and Steinberg (2002) noted, the short answer is that H was developed as a measure of dispersion or variability, and therefore may not truly capture complexity, at least not in the sense of either differentiation or integration. This statistic originated in information theory (Attneave, 1959), and was first used in psychology as a way of describing dimensionality within multidimensional models of knowledge structures (Scott, 1969). It is best suited for such multidimensional models; in contrast, Linville's (1985) model of multiple selves applies a categorical approach to self-knowledge. The two underlying mechanisms driving the SC stress-buffering process (i.e., the existence of alternative self-aspects and the degree of spreading activation among them) assume a hierarchical, categorical view of the self-schema.

In Scott's (1962, 1969) original research, the trait sort and H, the dimensionality statistic, were used to operationalize cognitive complexity as "the number of groups-worth of information ... represented as the dispersion of objects over a set of distinctions yielded by the category system" (Scott, 1962, p. 408). Importantly, Scott himself presented three caveats to the use of the dispersion measure in studying cognitive complexity. First, this statistic is limited in use to dichot-

omous attributes (whether a trait is included in the group or not). Second, H probably reflects a lower bound score of true cognitive dimensionality, since it is impossible to assess completely any particular category. Third, any tendency toward randomness in assignment of attributes (traits) to groups (in this case, self-aspects) will falsely inflate H: If the subject completing the sort task is not paying attention, then he or she may fail to match two groups that should be identical in his or her mind.

Despite these limitations, Scott (1962, 1969) indicated that H is a reliable and sound, albeit approximate, measure of the structure of cognition, and not dependent on the content of the attributes. While that may be true for H when it is used to index dimensionality in cognitive structure, it has been shown to be untrue when used to index SC, as the meta-analytic results reviewed earlier—particularly the results pertaining to valence within the trait sort—indicate.

To examine this question directly, Rafaeli-Mor, Gotlib, and Revelle (1999) examined the meaning and measurement of SC, and revealed two major problems with the H statistic. First, H proved to be very sensitive to the valenced content of the self-concept. To demonstrate this, the study used a "worst split-half" approach for establishing internal consistency (Revelle, 1979). In this approach, an index (in this case, H) is computed not only for randomly selected halves of a scale (or, in this case, the trait list) but also for halves created in a nonrandom way to maximize their difference; this nonrandom splitting was based on valence. In the random splitting, H demonstrated decent split-half reliability ($r = .85–.88$); however, in the valenced split, its reliability was not significantly different from zero ($r = .17$).

Another problem stems from the fact that the H statistic is a single value that is supposed to reflect two mechanisms that underlie the buffering effects of SC: the number of self-aspects and their distinctiveness. A similar idea was suggested by Linville (1987):

Self-representations may differ in terms of both the number of self-aspects and the degree to which distinctions are made among self-aspects. Two self-aspects are distinct to the extent to which they are represented by different cognitive elements. ... Greater self-complexity involves having more self-aspects and maintaining greater distinctions among self-aspects. (p. 664)

If these two components of complexity were strongly associated, the choice of a single index (e.g., H) might have been justified. As it turns out, the components are usually unrelated to each other, and H is a particularly bad measure of one of them.

To demonstrate this, Rafaeli-Mor and colleagues (1999) examined two straightforward component indices—one indexing the number of self-aspects (NSA), the other, indexing overlap among them (OL, defined as the average overlap between any two self-aspects over all possible pairs of self-aspects). Linville's H had the expected strong positive association with NSA ($r = .71$, $p < .001$—almost identical to Linville's [1987] own finding). In contrast, it had a moderate and countertheoretical positive association with the OL index as well ($r = .24$, $p < .01$): in other words, when self-aspects were *less* distinct, H levels were greater. Importantly, the two proposed component indices had higher split-half reliabilities both in the random and in the ("worst split-half") valenced splits (for NSA, $r = .97$–$.98$ and $.65$, respectively; for OL, $r = 90$–$.92$ and $.66$, respectively). In other words, unlike H, the separate component measures were not strongly affected by the valence of the traits used.

For these theoretical and empirical reasons, it appears that the H statistic might have been an inappropriate choice for the study of SC. The component indices proposed by Rafaeli-Mor and colleagues (1999) directly tap the two separate mechanisms proposed by Linville (1985); they do not have the same internal consistency problems, and,

unlike the H statistic, they assume the same categorical cognitive representation that is central to Linville's model.

To date, four groups have utilized Rafaeli-Mor and colleagues' (1999) component indices, all replicating the finding that the H statistic fails to capture the overlap or distinctiveness of self-aspects. One study (Luo & Watkins, 2008) focused mostly on measurement issues, but the others went on to investigate the roles of the component indices in resilience in the face of stress; we briefly review their results below.

Rothermund and Meiniger (2004) used the indices in two studies, pitting the predictions of the affective spillover model against those of an alternative model of stress buffering. Rather than the passive cognitive–affective process of spreaded activation, which may occur following any kind of event (as predicted by Linville), Rothermund and Meiniger suggested that individuals self-regulate using an active process of reorientation and positive reappraisal—but that they do so only when such regulation is needed, which is following negative events. According to this self-regulatory model, a large number of self-aspects (high NSA) promote efficient self-regulation by offering a greater choice of domains on which to focus one's attention and activities (i.e., a better framework for reorientation and positive reappraisal after the experience of negative events). In contrast, the model expects the second component of SC—low overlap or high distinctness among self-aspects—to have little effect on well-being (because both high and low OL may be beneficial for various reasons). Using a large undergraduate sample, Rothermund and Meiniger indeed found that the NSA index buffered the effects of negative life events on participants' depression, and that distinctness (low OL) had no such effect; furthermore, neither component buffered the effects of positive events. They also reported that those participants who had high NSA and a high level of negative life events increased their frequency of positive events, as would be expected according to the self-regulatory model (though not according to the spreaded activation model).

Constantino and colleagues (2006, Study 2) also used the component indices in a prospective design replicating that of Linville (1987). Neither component (nor their interaction) interacted with stress to predict depressive symptoms at Time 2 (though their model may not have included the necessary component, two-way interaction of NSA and OL). However, a follow-up analysis using only those participants who had not been depressed at Time 1 (i.e., for whom there could be an emergence of depression) proved more promising. Both the OL index itself, and the interaction of OL and stress predicted Time 2 depression levels. Also, though the NSA index did not buffer stress, it had a negative association with perceived stress—a finding that is consistent with that of Rothermund and Meiniger (2004).

One of Rothermund and Meiniger's (2004) key points is the need to examine SC (and its components) vis-à-vis various *types* of events (in their case, positive vs. negative). Brown and Rafaeli (2007) followed a similar strategy by investigating the impact of SC on stressors of various kinds: objective versus subjective, diffuse and minor versus acute and severe. In two prospective studies, these authors found a complex pattern of results indicating that the same structural properties may buffer us under one type of stress but exacerbate the effect of other types of stress. Specifically, NSA alone served as a buffer of low-level subjective stress (a finding similar to that of Rothermund and Meiniger); *high* OL among self-aspects alone served as a buffer of accumulated mundane stress; but *low* OL and the interaction of low OL and high NSA served as buffers of very severe stressors, such as loss or victimization (similar to Constantino et al., 2006).

Following Rafaeli-Mor and colleagues (1999), another thorough psychometric critique (Locke, 2003) further explained why H is not an appropriate measure for the social-cognitive model of SC (Linville, 1985)—or

for any other model attempting to measure the complexity of cognitive representations. By placing experimental constraints on the trait-sorting task, Locke (2003) demonstrated several fundamental problems with the index. First, H levels are affected by the number of traits endorsed. Though this relationship is curvilinear, it rises until the probability of endorsement reaches 50%, which occurs quite rarely (especially with negative traits). This likely explains why researchers (Morgan & Janoff-Bulman, 1994; Woolfolk et al., 1995, 1999) found P-SC and N-SC to differ in their ability to buffer stressors. Rather than well-being or depression being related substantively to variations in the organization of positive or negative traits, they may simply be related to the number of negative and positive traits endorsed, which themselves affect the H statistics used to index P-SC and N-SC.

Three additional problems noted by Locke (2003) also detract from the utility of the H statistic: (1) It confounds uncertainty between and within self-aspects, (2) confounds role numerosity and role independence, and (3) does not measure spillover or overlap accurately. The last two problems were similar to the ones identified by Rafaeli-Mor and colleagues (1999), and like those authors, Locke suggested that alternative indices of role numerosity and role OL be used if the SC model is ever to be accurately tested.

Locke (2003) explicitly approaches complexity from an information theory perspective, which leads to slightly different assumptions than those of both Linville (1985) and Rafaeli-Mor and colleagues (1999). For example, he assumes that nonendorsement of a trait (i.e., Mary failing to say that she is "ebullient" in a particular role) conveys the same amount of information as the endorsement of the trait. In pure information terms, this assumption is absolutely correct. However, in psychological terms, most cognitive and social-cognitive models examining objects and their features (e.g., Fazio, Sherman, & Herr, 1982; Tversky, 1977) do not support this assumption, and instead focus only on the *presence* of traits. Nonetheless, based on information theory assumptions, Locke suggests a modification of the OL index proposed by Rafaeli-Mor and his colleagues; to date, no study has tested this modified index, but such a test would be useful.

Other Approaches to the Study of Self-Structure

Although SC has garnered much research attention, it is only one of several models that tie the structure of the self to well-being. To conclude our review, we briefly discuss these other models, placing SC in relation to them within the broader framework of *self-concept differentiation and integration*—the degree to which the self contains a pluralism of multiple distinct elements, and the degree of unity, coherence, or interrelatedness among these elements (cf. Campbell, Assanand, & Di Paula, 2003; Rafaeli-Mor & Steinberg, 2002).

Differentiation (Pluralism) Approaches

The first component of SC—the number of distinct self-aspects—clearly speaks to differentiation. As such, it fits within a long tradition of research on the effects of having few versus abundant social roles, a tradition that predates the cognitive study of the self (e.g., Stryker, 1987; Thoits, 1983). Thoits noted that having few social roles is tied to social isolation, and therefore to poorer well-being. Similar conclusions emerge from George Brown and colleagues' work on social isolation and depression (e.g., Brown & Harris, 1978), which suggests that more varied social involvements are beneficial because they engender more opportunities for social contact and integration (Oatley & Bolton, 1985).

Using the number of self-aspects (obtained from the trait-sorting procedure) as a differentiation index addresses a shortcoming of the sociological tradition. In this tradition, identity accumulation and role involvement

are typically operationalized using a fixed set of roles. The method developed by Linville (1985) provides a straightforward index of differentiation, yet one emphasizing its idiographic psychological meaning. In addition, this method allows computation of another index of self-knowledge organization: an evaluative integration versus compartmentalization index.

Showers (1992) proposed the construct of *compartmentalization* to refer to the way in which positive information and negative information are either segregated (compartmentalized) or integrated across various self-aspects. In a *compartmentalized* organization, the traits associated with any self-aspect tend to be predominantly positive *or* negative. In contrast, an *evaluatively integrated* organization involves self-aspects that contain both positive *and* negative traits. Compartmentalization is indexed with the statistic *phi* (Φ) (or Cramer's V; Cramer, 1974), which calculates the extent to which the distribution of negative and positive traits across self-aspects deviates from what would be expected by chance. In early studies (Showers, 1992), compartmentalization was shown to interact with the differential importance of self-aspects: Individuals who emphasize self-aspects that are purely or predominantly positive in valence are more likely to activate positive information about themselves. As a consequence, they are less likely to be affected by negative events, and more likely to have high levels of self-esteem and low levels of depression. Those who emphasize self-aspects that are purely or predominantly negative in valence appear to be more strongly affected by stress, and more likely to feel depressed; however, if they maintain an evaluatively integrative self-concept, these strong reactions are moderated.

Subsequent studies (reviewed in Showers & Zeigler-Hill, 2007) have elaborated on this basic model to make the following dynamic predictions: Positively compartmentalized individuals (i.e., those with predominantly positive self-aspects) do have the highest levels of self-esteem but are also more vulnerable than integrated individuals to various daily events or to lab-induced social rejection (Zeigler-Hill & Showers, 2007). In other words, maintaining *evaluative integration* (i.e., a balanced view of positives and negatives in most of one's self-aspects) appears to be a source of resilience.

Self-concept compartmentalization may seem conceptually similar to SC, especially when the latter is partitioned into positive versus negative complexity (e.g., Morgan & Janoff-Bulman, 1994). In fact, the two are distinct, both theoretically and empirically. Showers, Abramson, and Hogan (1998) suggest that SC and compartmentalization are two different methods of coping with stress: Complex individuals may not need to compartmentalize, and compartmentalized ones may not need to have as much complexity. Indeed, several studies (e.g., Campbell et al., 2003; Luo & Watkins, 2008) found SC and compartmentalization to be unrelated, and though Campbell and her colleagues began their study with the assumption that compartmentalization is a pluralism/differentiation index, they conclude it by saying that it really does not map on either pluralism or unity, and instead, explores an issue that goes beyond these purely structural aspects of cognition.

Integration Approaches

OL among self-aspects, the second component of SC, is more an index of unity than of differentiation. As such, it is conceptually related to other indices of self-concept *integration*—indices that tap the degree to which the self is clear and coherent, and the extent to which self-aspects show internal consistency. *Self-concept integration* was described by Block (1961) as the outcome of successful psychological development and as an indication of psychological well-being. Drawing on Block's ideas, Donahue, Robins, Roberts, and John (1993; Roberts & Donahue, 1994) proposed the opposing concept of *self-concept differentiation* (SCD; the term

unfortunately creates confusion when considered as an integration and not a differentiation measure; *self-concept fragmentation* might have been a better term; cf. Campbell et al., 2003). SCD reflects lack of integration and is operationalized as the degree of unshared variance across social roles. To assess SCD, participants usually rate a set of attributes separately for a number of social roles or self-aspects; the degree of nonoverlap among role- or context-specific ratings is used as an index of SCD.

SCD has been shown to be related to depression, anxiety, and low self-esteem (Constantino et al., 2006; Donahue et al., 1993). It is also consistently related to other measures of self-concept unity (Campbell et al., 2003), particularly to the construct of self-concept clarity (Campbell, 1990) and to low self-discrepancies (Higgins, 1987).

Self-concept clarity is the degree to which the self is clearly and confidently defined, internally consistent, and temporally stable (Campbell, 1990). Though Campbell initially measured clarity using unobtrusive measures (e.g., reaction times, responses to pairs of antonyms), she and her colleagues (Campbell et al., 1996) later developed a 12-item self-report scale to measure it. Individuals low in clarity were found to have lower levels of self-esteem (Campbell, 1990; Campbell et al., 1996), were less positive about and more reactive to daily life events (Campbell et al., 1991), and were characterized by "chronic self-analysis," low internal state awareness, and a ruminative form of self-focused attention (Campbell et al., 1996).

Self-discrepancies were introduced by Higgins (1987) and his colleagues (Higgins, Bond, Klein, & Strauman, 1986; Strauman & Higgins, 1987), who defined them as the degree to which the real self differs from the ideal self or the ought self (i.e., one's *self-guides*, which may reflect one's own view and/or the internalized views of significant others). Higgins, Klein, and Strauman (1985) developed the Selves Questionnaire, in which participants list up to 10 traits for each of the self-states, according to their perspective and to the perspective of their mother, father, and a close friend. For a given pair of lists, self-discrepancy scores are computed by subtracting the number of characteristics that "match" from the number of characteristics that "mismatch." Higher scores indicate larger self-discrepancies. Higgins proposed that different types of self-discrepancies induce specific negative emotions. Higgins and colleagues (1985) and Strauman and Higgins (1987) found that an Actual–Ideal discrepancy results in feelings of dejection, whereas an Actual–Ought discrepancy results in feelings of agitation. The greater the accessibility and magnitude of a particular type of self-discrepancy, the more the individual will suffer the negative emotions associated with it. Those whose self-states are more concordant are expected to experience greater well-being.

To summarize, the work of Donahue, Campbell, Higgins, and their colleagues on a variety of self-concept unity variables indicates that a cohesive self is tied to less distress and better psychological well-being. Unlike the SC stress-buffering model (Linville, 1987), as well the evaluative compartmentalization model (Showers, 2000), these models' predictions are not specifically about resilience factors in response to stressors. Instead, they suggest a cross-sectional association between unity or integration and well-being.

It is important to keep in mind that *differentiation* (pluralism) and *integration* (unity) are not necessarily related to each other. In the extreme case—a complete absence of pluralism (i.e., the monolithic unitary self that was assumed to be the rule in early research)—integration is obviously constrained (or simply undefined). But within the normal range of differentiation (i.e., for individuals with fewer or more self-aspects), integration (i.e., the degree of overlap among self-aspects) may be high or low. Both our own research on the components of SC, and that of others (e.g., Campbell et al.'s review of various unity and pluralism measures) find this to be the case empirically as well.

However, most of the extant literature on SC has not distinguished between the pluralism component (number of self-aspects) and the unity component (overlap among them), and instead has relied on the unitary H statistic. As we have shown, this statistic provides an imperfect reflection of the first component, and an abysmal one of the second.

Conclusions and Future Directions for Self-Complexity Research

Close to half a century of cognitive complexity research and almost 25 years of social-cognitive attention to *self*-complexity have generated much interest but no firm conclusions regarding the role of integration, differentiation, or complexity in resilience. Conceptual confusion characterized these fields (cf. Rafaeli-Mor & Steinberg, 2002; Streufert & Streufert, 1978); when that seemed under control, measurement problems hit hard (cf. Locke, 2003; Rafaeli-Mor et al., 1999). As a consequence, despite an impressive amount of both theorizing and attempted empirical work, it remains unclear whether SC, differentiation of self-aspects, or unity among them are markers of emotional health, vulnerability factors, or buffers of stress-related responses. We conclude this chapter with some suggestions for a more informative future of SC research.

The first recommendation, one that we made a decade ago (Rafaeli-Mor et al., 1999) and still firmly stand by, is that researchers interested in this model must pay closer attention to the underlying cognitive model. If they share our understanding of this model, they need to choose measures that reflect it well; if they differ from us (as Locke [2003] does), they may wish to use modified indices. Instead, the majority of studies replicating and extending Linville's (1985) work simply adopted the faulty H statistic, and are therefore less informative than they should be. Given the high correlation between H and the number of self-aspects, they might tell us something about self-differentiation; they certainly tell us nothing about self-unity or the overlap between aspects. The solution, of course, is to calculate, test, and report the two component indices of complexity (NSA and OL). As we argued earlier, they are particularly good indices of differentiation and integration, respectively—better in some ways than other established measures of these concepts. This is because they are (1) less affected by valence, and (2) obtained from Linville's trait-sorting task, a task free of the value judgments inherent in measures such as Campbell's (1990) Self-Concept Clarity Scale.

Few published studies to date have used the component measures; many continue to use the faulty H statistic. Before any additional participants sit down to sort traits into self-aspects in new studies, we hope that the dozens of researchers who have published or unpublished trait-sort data will revisit their existing datasets and remedy the measurement problem by simply running the appropriate analyses on them. Once that happens, an accurate picture regarding SC as a resilience factor will be within reach.

Several of the researchers attempting to clarify the role of SC tried to do so by partitioning self-knowledge into positive and negative attributes, then computing H for each valenced set. Our review (and that of Locke, 2003) suggests that the conclusions drawn from these studies are probably artifactual. Nonetheless, as part of painting an accurate picture regarding SC, we hope to learn whether the two psychometrically valid components of complexity (NSA and OL) also differ in their effects when computed on valenced information.

Relatedly, the issue of valence within the self-system should certainly remain at the center of attention. As Rafaeli-Mor and Steinberg (2002) found, the valence make-up of the traits used in different SC studies was directly related to their results. To make sure valence is examined thoroughly, we (and others; e.g., Constantino et al., 2006; Zeigler-Hill & Showers, 2007) strongly suggest that researchers use balanced trait lists

with equal numbers of positive and negative traits.

If SC is a resilience factor, studies of various designs should show that. The most ubiquitous SC study is one reporting the cross-sectional association between SC and some well-being measure (cf. Rafaeli-Mor & Steinberg, 2002). Unlike other reviewers (e.g., Koch & Shepperd, 2004) we believe such studies could be very informative. For example, future research may show that having high differentiation (i.e., high NSA) is associated with better well-being (as was found by Constantino et al. [2006] with regard to perceived stress). If that is the case, we may conclude that apart from whatever stress-buffering role it plays (or does not play), NSA is a source of resilience.

Nonetheless, cross-sectional research should be supplemented by studies using other designs. One clearly informative design is the prospective diathesis–stress study. With such studies, we hope to see the suggestions of Brown and Rafaeli (2007) put into effect. In particular, we hope that future studies pay close attention to (1) the timing and nature of stressors (i.e., acute vs. chronic, severe vs. diffuse); (2) the careful probing of interaction effects (e.g., Aiken & West, 1991; Solomon & Haaga, 2003); and (3) the predictions of each SC component as a separate buffer of stress, as well as the joint buffering offered by the interaction of the two components.

But formidable progress in SC research will require it to go beyond blanket statements about the adaptive or maladaptive nature of complexity, whether obtained cross-sectionally or prospectively. What is needed are process studies, in which the underlying mechanisms of spillover (Linville, 1985) or of reorientation (Rothermund & Meiniger, 2004) are directly observed. In some ways, it is quite puzzling that no study to date has really examined the processing mechanisms behind SC. For example, to study the processes inherent in Linville's spillover prediction would require testing each of the following steps:

1. If a life event (e.g., lab-induced feedback) relevant to a particular self-aspect occurs, then that self-aspect and the attributes tied to it should become activated.
2. Once the self-aspect is activated, the individual's mood should be imbued by affect tied to the nature of the event (good vs. bad) the nature of the attributes, or some combination of the two.
3. The activation of the specific self-aspect spills over because of trait overlap, into related self-aspects; the more the overlap, the greater the spillover.
4. The overall mood should be a function of the total proportion of the self that is affected (i.e., depending on both NSA and OL).

Some researchers (e.g., Cohen et al., 1997; McConnell, Rydell, & Brown, 2007; Smith & Cohen, 1993) have begun moving in this direction; we hope others will as well.

Once the processing mechanisms underlying SC as a resilience factor are established, future research may profitably examine how different self-aspects, or different attributes within these aspects, may affect these processes and promote (or hinder) resilience. As McConnell and Strain (2007) note, all selves are not created equal; those self-aspects that are more important (Pelham, 1991), more central (Anderson, 1992), or more clearly defined (Campbell, 1990) may matter more; spillover may not be a symmetrical process.

Recent work on another prominent model of self-knowledge organization, namely, evaluative compartmentalization versus integration (Showers, 2000), raises the interesting possibility that structural properties are not trait-like, and should instead be considered as part of a dynamic model. According to such a model, individuals may *reorganize* their self-concept adaptively in response to life events or moods. Some evidence that this may occur with SC has been reported (Showers et al., 1998), but more evidence is needed. The implications of such findings are crucial to determining whether any stress-buffering benefits of SC predate the stressful

life events, or possibly are part of a resilient form of poststressor development.

Selves differ in males and females, are defined differently in various cultures (Gabriel & Gardner, 1999), and may change with age (Diehl, Hastings, & Stanton, 2001). To be able to speak to the generality of SC processes, a wider variety of samples reflecting diverse populations needs to be examined. Maybe most vital are samples of individuals with various forms of stress-related psychopathology or ones contending with ecologically significant, nontrivial stressors. For example, if SC is a resilience factor against stress-related depression (as predicted by Linville, 1987), we should ideally measure it before the onset of mental illness or the occurrence of traumatic events in individuals who are vulnerable to major disorders. Very few studies have examined SC in psychopathology at all, though some notable exceptions do exist: Showers and colleagues' (1998) sample was followed prior to first-onset depression; Taylor, Morley, and Barton (2007) assessed individuals with remitted bipolar disorder or major depression; and Gara and colleagues (1993) have done extensive research on SC in depression. Clearly, more clinical studies (applying what we now know about SC mechanisms and measurement) are needed.

We began by noting that a social-cognitive structural variable such as SC will confer resilience mostly in the stress-buffering sense, and not in the posttraumatic growth sense. Indeed, most of the research reviewed here, including Linville's (1985) original formulation of the SC model, as well as more recent responses to it, focuses on this aspect of resilience. Yet there are ways in which SC could speak to the issue of growth. For example, the developmental work (e.g., Abela & Veronneau-McArdle, 2002; Evans & Seaman, 2000) we reviewed suggests that greater SC is a marker for effective and appropriate development. The degree to which this development follows, or maybe even requires, adaptation to stressful life events is unknown, but it is a topic of great interest to students of both normative and disordered maturation of the self-system (cf. Harter, 1998). We hope future developmental research of this sort will help to clarify what happens to the self-concept (and to its complexity) in individuals whose response to stressors is a resilient one of growth and advancement.

Closing Words

SC has broad theoretical appeal. It may yet prove to be an important cognitive resilience factor as a buffer of stress, or possibly as a marker of poststress growth and adaptation. For that to happen, the conceptual and methodological problems we reviewed need to be addressed; happily, several research groups are doing just that. In the future, if SC is indeed found to be a source of resilience, we hope to see it incorporated into models applying social-cognitive research to foster well-being, for example, in cognitive therapy prevention and intervention approaches.

References

Abela, J. R. Z., & Veronneau-McArdle, M.-H. (2002). The relationship between self-complexity and depressive symptoms in third and seventh grade children: A short-term longitudinal study. *Journal of Abnormal Child Psychology, 30*(2), 155–166.

Aiken, L. S., & West, S. G. (1991). *Multiple regression: Testing and interpreting interactions.* Thousand Oaks, CA: Sage.

Allport, G. W. (1955). *Becoming.* New Haven, CT: Yale University Press.

Anderson, K. M. (1992). Self-complexity and self-esteem in middle childhood. In R. P. Lipka & T. M. Brinthaupt (Eds.), *Self-perspectives across the lifespan* (pp. 11–52). Albany: State University of New York Press.

Attneave, F. (1959). *Applications of information theory to psychology.* New York: Holt-Dryden.

Bieri, J. (1955). Cognitive complexity-simplicity and predictive behavior. *Journal of Abnormal and Social Psychology, 51*, 263–268.

Blatt, S. J., & Lerner, H. (1983). Investigations

in the psychoanalytic theory of object relations and object representations. In J. Masling (Ed.), *Empirical studies of psychoanalytic theory* (Vol. 1, pp. 189–249). Hillsdale, NJ: Erlbaum.

Block, J. (1961). Ego identity, role variability, and adjustment. *Journal of Consulting Psychology, 25*, 392–397.

Brown, G., & Harris, T. O. (1978). *Social origins of depression: A study of psychiatric disorder in women.* London: Tavistock.

Brown, G., & Rafaeli, E. (2007). Components of self-complexity as buffers for depressed mood. *Journal of Cognitive Psychotherapy: An International Quarterly, 21*, 308–331.

Brown, J. D. (1998). *The self.* New York: McGraw-Hill.

Campbell, J. D. (1990). Self-esteem and clarity of the self-concept. *Journal of Personality and Social Psychology, 59*, 538–549.

Campbell, J. D., Assanand, S., & Di Paula, A. (2003). The structure of the self-concept and its relation to psychological adjustment. *Journal of Personality, 71*, 115–140.

Campbell, J. D., Chew, B., & Scratchley, L. S. (1991). Cognitive and emotional reactions to daily events: The effects of self-esteem and self-complexity. *Journal of Personality, 59*, 473–505.

Campbell, J. D., Trapnell, P. D., Heine, S. J., Katz, I. M., Lavallee, L. F., & Lehman, D. R. (1996). Self-concept clarity: Measurement, personality correlates, and cultural boundaries. *Journal of Personality and Social Psychology, 70*, 141–156.

Cohen, L. H., Pane, N., & Smith, H. S. (1997). Complexity of the interpersonal self and affective reactions to interpersonal stressors in life and in the laboratory. *Cognitive Therapy and Research, 21*, 387–407.

Colvin, C. R., & Block, J. (1994). Do positive illusions foster mental health?: An examination of the Taylor and Brown formulation. *Psychological Bulletin, 116*, 3–20.

Colvin, C. R., Block, J., & Funder, D. C. (1995). Overly positive self-evaluations and personality: Negative implications for mental health. *Journal of Personality and Social Psychology, 68*, 1152–1162.

Constantino, M. J., Wilson, K. R., & Horowitz, L. M. (2006). The direct and stress-buffering effects of self-organization on psychological adjustment. *Journal of Social and Clinical Psychology*, 25, 333–360.

Cramer, H. (1974). *Mathematical methods of statistics*. Princeton, NJ: Princeton University Press.

Cramer, P. (1987). The development of defense mechanisms. *Journal of Personality*, 55, 597–614.

Crocket, W. H. (1965). Cognitive complexity and impression formation. In B. H. Maher (Ed.), *Progress in experimental personality research* (Vol. 2, pp. 47–90). New York: Academic Press.

Deboeck, P., & Rosenberg, S. (1988). Hierarchical classes: Model and data analysis. *Psychometrika*, 53, 361–381.

Diehl, M., Hastings, C. T., & Stanton, J. M. (2001). Self-concept differentiation across the life span. *Psychology and Aging*, 16, 643–654.

Dixon, T. M., & Baumeister, R. F. (1991). Escaping the self: The moderating effect of self-complexity. *Personality and Social Psychology Bulletin*, 17, 363–368.

Donahue, E. M., Robins, R. W., Roberts, B. W., & John, O. P. (1993). The divided self: Concurrent and longitudinal effects of psychological adjustment and social roles on self-concept differentiation. *Journal of Personality and Social Psychology*, 64, 834–846.

Evans, D. W. (1994). Self-complexity and its relation to development, symptomatology and self-perception during adolescence. *Child Psychiatry and Human Development*, 24, 173–182.

Evans, D. W., & Seaman, J. L. (2000). Developmental aspects of psychological defenses: Their relation to self-complexity, self-perception, and symptomatology in adolescents. *Child Psychiatry and Human Development*, 30, 237–254.

Fazio, R. H., Sherman, S. J., & Herr, P. M. (1982). The feature-positive effect in the self-perception process: Does not doing matter as much as doing? *Journal of Personality and Social Psychology*, 42, 404–411.

Gabriel, S., & Gardner, W. L. (1999). Are there "his" and "hers" types of independence?: The implications of gender differences in collective vs. relational interdependence for affect, behavior, and cognition. *Journal of Personality and Social Psychology*, 77, 642–655.

Gallant, M. M. (1991). *Transition to parenthood: The role of self-complexity*. Unpublished master's thesis, Wilfred Laurier University.

Gara, M. A., Woolfolk, R. L., Cohen, B. D., Goldston, R. B., Allen, L. A., & Novalany, J. (1993). Perception of self and other in major depression. *Journal of Abnormal Psychology*, 102, 93–100.

Gergen, K. J., & Gergen, M. (1983). Narrative of the self. In T. Sarbin & K. Scheibe (Eds.), *Studies in social identity* (pp. 254–273). New York: Praeger.

Harter, S. (1982). The perceived competence scale for children. *Child Development*, 53, 87–97.

Harter, S. (1998). The development of self-representations. In W. Damon (Series Ed.) & N. Eisenberg (Vol. Ed.), *Handbook of child psychology: Vol. 3. Social, emotional, and personality development* (5th ed., pp. 553–617). New York: Wiley.

Hebb, D. O. (1949). *The organization of behavior*. New York: Wiley.

Higgins, E. T. (1987). Self-discrepancy: A theory relating self and affect. *Psychological Review*, 94, 319–40.

Higgins, E. T., Bond, R. N., Klein, R., & Strauman, T. (1986). Self-discrepancies and emotional vulnerability: How magnitude, accessibility, and type of discrepancy influence affect. *Journal of Personality and Social Psychology*, 51(1), 5–15.

Higgins, E. T., Klein, R., & Strauman, T. (1985). Self-concept discrepancy theory: A psychological model for distinguishing among different aspects of depression and anxiety. *Social Cognition*, 3, 51–76.

James, W. (1890). *The principles of psychology* (Vol. 1). New York: Holt.

Kalthoff, R. A., & Neimeyer, R. A. (1993). Self-complexity and psychological distress: A test of the buffering model. *International Journal of Personal Construct Psychology*, 6, 327–349.

Kelly, G. A. (1955). *The psychology of personal constructs* (Vols. 1–2). New York: Norton.

Koch, E. J., & Shepperd, J. A. (2004). Is self-complexity linked to better coping?: A review of the literature. *Journal of Personality*, 72, 727–760.

Leigh, J., Westen, D., Barends, A., Mendel, M. J., & Byers, S. (1992). The assessment of complexity of representations of people using TAT and interview data. *Journal of Personality*, 60, 809–837.

Lewin, K. (1935). *A dynamic theory of personality: Selected paper.* New York: McGraw-Hill.

Linville, P. W. (1982). The complexity–extremity effect and age-based stereotyping. *Journal of Personality and Social Psychology, 42,* 193–211.

Linville, P. W. (1985). Self-complexity and affective extremity: Don't put all of your eggs in one cognitive basket. *Social Cognition, 3,* 94–120.

Linville, P. W. (1987). Self-complexity as a cognitive buffer against stress-related illness and depression. *Journal of Personality and Social Psychology, 52,* 663–676.

Linville, P. W., & Carlston, D. E. (1994). Social cognition and the self. In P. G. Devine, D. L. Hamilton, & T. M. Olstrom (Eds.), *Social cognition: Impact on social psychology* (pp. 143–193). San Diego, CA: Academic Press.

Locke, K. D. (2003). *H* as a measure of complexity of social information processing. *Personality and Social Psychology Review, 7,* 268–280.

Luo, W., & Watkins, D. (2008). Clarifying the measurement of a self-structural process variable: The case of self-complexity. *International Journal of Testing, 8,* 143–165.

Markus, H. (1977). Self-schemata and processing information about the self. *Journal of Personality and Social Psychology, 35,* 63–78.

Marsh, H. W. (1989). Age and sex effects in multiple dimensions of self-concept: Preadolescence to early adulthood. *Journal of Educational Psychology, 81,* 417–430.

Marsh, H. W., Barnes, J., Cairns, L., & Tidman, M. (1984). Self-Description Questionnaire: Age and sex effects in the structure and level of self-concept for preadolescent children. *Journal of Educational Psychology, 76,* 940–956.

Marsh, H. W., & Shavelson, R. J. (1985). Self-concept: Its multifaceted, hierarchical structure. *Educational Psychologist, 20,* 107–123.

McConnell, A. R., Rydell, R. J., & Brown, C. M. (2007). *On the presentation of self-concept: Multiple selves, their organization, and implications for affect.* Manuscript submitted for publication.

McConnell, A. R., & Strain, L. M. (2007). Content and structure of the self. In C. Sedikides & S. Spencer (Eds.), *The self in social psychology* (pp. 51–73). New York: Psychology Press.

Mead, G. H. (1934). *Mind, self, and society.* Chicago: University of Chicago.

Miller, M. L., Omens, R. S., & Delvadia, R. (1991). Dimensions of social competence: Personality and coping styles. *Personality and Individual Differences, 12,* 955–964.

Morgan, H. J., & Janoff-Bulman, R. (1994). Positive and negative self-complexity: Patterns of adjustment following traumatic versus non-traumatic life experiences. *Journal of Social and Clinical Psychology, 13,* 63–85.

Murray, H. A. (1943). *Thematic Apperception Test manual.* Cambridge, MA: Harvard University Press.

Oatley, K., & Bolton, W. (1985). A social-cognitive theory of depression in reaction to life events. *Psychological Review, 92,* 372–388.

Paulhus, D. L. (1998). Interpersonal and intrapsychic adaptiveness of trait self-enhancement: A mixed blessing? *Journal of Personality and Social Psychology, 74,* 1197–1208.

Pelham, B. W. (1991). On confidence and consequences: The certainty and importance of self-knowledge. *Journal of Personality and Social Psychology, 60,* 518–530.

Rafaeli-Mor, E., Gotlib, I. H., & Revelle, W. (1999). The meaning and measurement of self-complexity. *Personality and Individual Differences, 27,* 341–356.

Rafaeli-Mor, E., & Steinberg, J. (2002). Self-complexity and well-being: A review and research synthesis. *Personality and Social Psychology Review, 6,* 31–58.

Revelle, W. (1979). Hierarchical cluster analysis and the internal structure of tests. *Multivariate Behavioral Research, 14,* 57–74.

Rhodewalt, F., & Morf, C. C. (1995). Self and interpersonal correlates of the narcissistic personality inventory: A review and new findings. *Journal of Research in Personality, 29,* 1–23.

Roberts, B. W., & Donahue, E. M. (1994). One personality, multiple selves: Integrating personality and social roles. *Journal of Personality, 62,* 199–218.

Rogers, T. B. (1977). Self-reference in memory: Recognition of personality items. *Journal of Research in Personality, 1,* 295–305.

Rosenberg, S. (1977). New approaches to the analysis of personal constructs in person perception. In *Nebraska Symposium on Motiva-*

tion (Vol. 24, pp. 174–242). Lincoln: University of Nebraska Press.

Rothermund, K., & Meiniger, C. (2004). Stress-buffering effects of self-complexity: Reduced affective spillover or self-regulatory processes? *Self and Identity, 3,* 263–281.

Schleicher, D. J., & McConnell, A. R. (2005). The complexity of self-complexity: An associated systems theory approach. *Social Cognition, 23,* 387–416.

Scott, W. A. (1962). Cognitive complexity and cognitive flexibility. *Sociometry, 25,* 405–414.

Scott, W. A. (1969). Structure of natural cognitions. *Journal of Personality and Social Psychology, 12,* 261–278.

Shedler, J. A., Mayman, M., & Manis, M. (1993). The illusion of mental health. *American Psychologist, 48,* 1117–1131.

Showers, C. J. (1992). Compartmentalization of positive and negative self-knowledge: Keeping bad apples out of the bunch. *Journal of Personality and Social Psychology, 62,* 1036–1049.

Showers, C. J. (2000). Self-organization in emotional contexts. In J. P. Forgas (Ed.), *Feeling and thinking: The role of affect in social cognition* (pp. 283–307). New York: Cambridge University Press.

Showers, C. J., Abramson, L. Y., & Hogan, M. E. (1998). The dynamic self: How the content and structure of the self-concept change with mood. *Journal of Personality and Social Psychology, 75,* 478–493.

Showers, C. J., & Zeigler-Hill, V. (2007). Compartmentalization and integration: The evaluative organization of contextualized selves. *Journal of Personality, 75,* 1181–1204.

Smith, H. S., & Cohen, L. H. (1993). Self-complexity and reactions to a relationship breakup. *Journal of Social and Clinical Psychology, 12,* 367–384.

Solomon, A., & Haaga, D. A. F. (2003). Reconsideration of self-complexity as a buffer against depression. *Cognitive Therapy and Research, 27,* 579–591.

Stein, K. F. (1994). Complexity of the self-schema and responses to disconfirming feedback. *Cognitive Therapy and Research, 18,* 161–178.

Steinberg, J. A., Pineles, S. L., Gardner, W. L., & Mineka, S. (2003). Self-complexity as a potential cognitive buffer among abused women. *Journal of Social and Clinical Psychology, 22,* 560–579.

Strauman, T. J., & Higgins, E. T. (1987). Automatic activation of self-discrepancies and emotional syndromes: When cognitive structures influence affect. *Journal of Personality and Social Psychology, 53,* 1004–1014.

Streufert, S., & Streufert, S. C. (1978). *Behavior in the complex environment.* Washington, DC: Winston.

Stryker, S. (1987). Stability and change in self: A structural symbolic interactionist explanation. *Social Psychology Quarterly, 50,* 44–55.

Taylor, J. L., Morley, S., & Barton, S. B. (2007). Self-organization in bipolar disorder: Compartmentalization and self-complexity. *Cognitive Therapy and Research, 31,* 83–96.

Taylor, S. E., & Brown, J. D. (1988). Illusion and well-being: A social psychological perspective on mental health. *Psychological Bulletin, 103,* 193–210.

Taylor, S. E., & Brown, J. D. (1994). Positive illusions and well-being revisited: Separating fact from fiction. *Psychological Bulletin, 116,* 21–27.

Taylor, S. E., Lerner, J. S., Sherman, D. K., Sage, R. M., & McDowell, N. K. (2003). Portrait of the self-enhancer: Well adjusted and well liked or maladjusted and friendless? *Journal of Personality and Social Psychology, 84,* 165–176.

Thoits, P. A. (1983). Multiple identities and psychological well-being: A reformulation and test of the social isolation hypothesis. *American Sociological Review, 48,* 174–187.

Tripodi, T., & Bieri, J. (1966). Cognitive complexity, perceived conflict, and certainty. *Journal of Personality, 34,* 144–153.

Tversky, A. (1977). Features of similarity. *Psychological Review, 84,* 327–352.

Werner, H. (1948). *Comparative psychology of mental development.* New York: Follett.

Werner, H. (1957). The concept of development from a comparative and organismic point of view. In D. Harris (Ed.), *The concept of development* (pp. 125–248). Minneapolis: University of Minnesota Press.

Westen, D. (1992). The cognitive and the psychoanalytic self: Can we put our selves together? *Psychological Inquiry, 3,* 1–13.

Woolfolk, R. L., Gara, M. A., Ambrose, T. K., Williams, J. E., Allen, L. A., Irvin, S. L., et al. (1999). Self-complexity and the persistence of depression. *Journal of Nervous and Mental Disease, 187*(7), 393–399.

Woolfolk, R. L., Novalany, J., Gara, M. A., & Allen, L. A. (1995). Self-complexity, self-evaluation, and depression: An examination of form and content within the self-schema. *Journal of Personality and Social Psychology, 68,* 1108–1120.

Wyer, R. S., Jr. (1964). Assessment and correlates of cognitive differentiation and integration. *Journal of Personality, 32,* 495–509.

Wylie, R. (1974). *The self-concept* (Vol. 1). Lincoln: University of Nebraska Press.

Wylie, R. (1979). *The self-concept* (Vol. 2). Lincoln: University of Nebraska Press.

Zajonc, R. B. (1960). The process of cognitive tuning in communication. *Journal of Abnormal and Social Psychology, 61,* 159–167.

Zeigler-Hill, V., & Showers, C. J. (2007). Self-structure and self-esteem stability: The hidden vulnerability of compartmentalization. *Personality and Social Psychology Bulletin, 33,* 143–159.

10

Anchored by Faith
Religion as a Resilience Factor

Kenneth I. Pargament
Jeremy Cummings

In spite of the fact that the founding figures in psychology viewed religion as central to an understanding of human behavior, the field of psychology largely neglected religious issues for much of the 20th century. When religion was considered, it was often (1) viewed as a source of pathology, (2) measured by a few global religious items, and (3) explained in terms of purportedly more basic phenomena. The past 20 years have witnessed an important shift in this trend. The number of studies on religion has grown, and it has become clear through this research that religiousness can play a significant role in response to major life stressors.

This chapter begins with a conceptual background on religion and coping. We examine recent theoretical, empirical, and practical advances in studies of religion and adjustment to major life stressors. In so doing, we challenge stereotypes of religiousness as a defense or source of pathology. We assert instead that religiousness is a significant resilience factor for many peo-ple. We identify what it is about religiousness that helps many people withstand the effects of life crises. Rather than taking a reductionistic approach to religion, we suggest that religion has unique effects on resilience. In addition, we point to evidence that indicates religiousness itself is resilient to major life stressors; that is, in difficult times, religion is effective in helping people sustain their relationship with the sacred. It is also necessary to make a few cautionary comments about the complex nature of the links between religion and resilience. First, there is evidence that religiousness can help people move beyond prior levels of adjustment to achieve fundamental positive transformation. Second, some forms of religiousness may exacerbate rather than mitigate the effects of major life stressors. Finally, we conclude with an illustration of some promising approaches that integrate religious resources into interventions designed to enhance individual resilience to life stressors.

Conceptual Background

Defining religion has proven problematic for the social sciences. Definitions abound, but consensus is lacking. However, Pargament (1997) has developed a framework for understanding religion that is broad enough to account for a variety of phenomena, while retaining that which is distinctive about religion. According to this approach, *religion* is a "search for significance in ways related to the sacred" (Pargament, 1997, p. 32). This definition rests on the assumption that individuals are goal-directed beings, actively pursuing objects of importance to them (see Emmons, 1999). Although there are many types of significant objects, objects of religious significance are distinct from secular objects in that the former are sacred. *The sacred* is a term that encompasses concepts of God or some other higher power, as well as aspects of life that take on elevated attributes (e.g., transcendence, ultimacy, boundlessness) by virtue of their association with the divine. It is important to stress that this definition broadens the boundaries of religious study beyond traditional views of God to incorporate other, seemingly secular parts of life that are imbued with sacred meaning, from science and the self to marriage and parenting (Pargament & Mahoney, 2005). For instance, when parenthood is viewed as a commission received from God, this role takes on a sacred quality. What makes someone religious from the perspective of this definition is the individual's involvement in the search for either a sacred end or sacred pathways to attain another significant object.

With this definition in hand, Pargament (1997) goes on to explicate the connections between religion and the process of coping. He notes that although people tend to turn to their faith for help in times of greatest stress, the old adage that "there are no atheists in foxholes" is not accurate. In fact, some people are nonbelievers before they encounter crisis and remain nonbelievers during and after the crisis. The critical question, then, is what determines whether someone will involve religion in the process of coping. Pargament posits two key factors here: the degree to which religion is available to the individual, and the degree to which it is perceived as offering compelling solutions to the problems raised by the critical life event. Citing abundant empirical evidence that more religious people are more likely to make use of religious coping methods, he suggests that individuals with a deeper, more developed set of religious beliefs, practices, and relationships find their "religious orienting system" more available to them as a coping resource in difficult times. Not only that, individuals with a stronger religious orienting system are likely to find religious solutions to problems more compelling than alternative solutions. This is also the case for individuals who have more limited social and personal resources, such as older adults and disenfranchised groups in our society. Finally, religious solutions are particularly compelling when people face life's most serious problems, problems that point to the limits of human agency and control. Empirical evidence supports each of these assertions (Pargament, 1997).

There is a rich variety of religious resources, ranging from involvement in church institutional life (e.g., church attendance) and religious practices (e.g., prayer, meditation) to religious beliefs (e.g., life after death, God) and religious experiences (e.g., mysticism). Moreover, religion provides its adherents with a number of coping methods designed to deal with major life stressors, including religious support, support from God, benevolent religious reappraisals, purification rituals, rites of passage, and religious forgiveness. According to Pargament (1997), the choice of religious coping methods is shaped by multiple influences—the demands raised by a particular situation, the individual's religious orienting system, and the individual's goals or objects of significance in life.

With respect to this latter point, Pargament (1997) maintains that part of religion's power lies in its ability to serve several functions; that is, it can help people attain a variety of significant objects. In this chapter, we address four of these major religious functions. First, religion is commonly linked functionally to the search for meaning, the sense that there is an underlying reason for the universe in general or one's experiences in particular. Geertz (1966) described religion as a source of beliefs about the "general order of existence" that produce deep emotions and motivations within the individual. When successful, the pursuit of ultimate meaning can protect against the despair that may result from living in what is perceived to be an otherwise cold, arbitrary expanse of space. Not only that, a sense of religious meaning can provide the hope that unpleasant circumstances serve a greater purpose. Second, religion has been tied to the quest for emotional comfort or anxiety reduction. According to Freud (1927/1961), humans turn to religion because they are aware of their frailty and are easily overcome by worry in the face of uncontrollable forces in the universe. The perceived presence of a benevolent deity can allay the fears of the troubled and dry the tears of those who mourn. A third often-described function of religion is to promote a sense of social interconnectedness. For Durkheim (1912), religion's ability to unify a group of individuals into an organized social institution, with a common set of beliefs, values, and practices, was one of its key distinguishing characteristics. Involvement in a religious community can afford the member of the congregation and denomination interpersonal intimacy and social identity. Finally, and perhaps most importantly, people turn to religion for reasons that are spiritual in character; they seek a relationship with the sacred itself. Indeed, many religions teach that the greatest possible good is to commune with and know the true nature of the divine. Johnson (1959) expressed this sentiment eloquently: "It is the ultimate Thou whom the religious person seeks most of all" (p. 70).

It should be stressed that these functions of religion are not mutually exclusive. An individual can seek any or all of these ends. Furthermore, individuals can seek each of these destinations through a variety of spiritual pathways that involve diverse beliefs, practices, relationships, and emotions.

Before turning to religion's role in promoting resilience with respect to each of these four major religious functions, it is important to address a general stereotype about religion and coping that has run through much of the literature in psychology.

Religion as a Source of Strength Rather Than Weakness

Traditionally, psychologists have viewed religion in stereotypical terms. Freud (1927/1961) saw religion as a childish response to the need for safety and protection from the overpowering forces of nature. Through religion, he said, "we can breathe freely, can feel at home in the uncanny and can deal by psychical means with our senseless anxiety" (p. 20). Make no mistake about it, though, Freud argued the comfort achieved through religion was purchased at the price of competence and maturity. "Surely infantilism is destined to be surmounted," he wrote (p. 63). Similarly, B. F. Skinner (1971) maintained that "God is the archetype pattern of an explanatory fiction," one that, he believed, "becomes irrelevant when the fears which nourish it are allayed and the hopes fulfilled—here on earth" (pp. 165, 201).

In 1995, Pargament and Park confronted the view that religion is "merely a defense," an essentially immature, maladaptive attempt to reduce personal turmoil. In their review of the empirical and clinical literature, they acknowledged cases of religiously based denial of problems and religiously based passivity in the face of serious problems. However, they asserted that these examples may be the exception rather than the rule. Pargament and Park identified other, more constructive and more prevalent forms of religiousness. For example, they cited empirical studies indicating that rather than denying their difficulties, religious people often reappraise these situations in more benign spiritual terms, so that they are less threatening. Furthermore, they noted research that suggests religiousness is often tied to greater self-efficacy and active problem-solving approaches, instead of helpless dependence and passivity.

More recent studies confirm the role of religion in facing rather than denying painful life situations. For example, research suggests that religiousness is not a barrier to acknowledging troubling information. In a study of women seeking medical consultation for symptoms of breast cancer, self-rated religiousness/spirituality was negatively associated with the length of time the participants waited to visit the doctor after noticing breast symptoms (Friedman et al., 2006). Those women who perceived themselves as religious or spiritual did not deny threatening signs, but confronted their suspicions directly. Similarly, Prado and colleagues (2004) found that HIV-seropositive African American women who engaged in religious behaviors (e.g., attending religious services, praying, reading religious materials) were less likely to rely on avoidant coping methods, such as denial and suppression of thoughts.

Furthermore, claims that religiousness universally undermines one's sense of competence are unfounded. Yangarber-Hicks's (2004) study of individuals diagnosed with serious mental illness revealed those who lent more importance to religion also reported greater feelings of empowerment. As for specific religious approaches to problem solving, different approaches had different outcomes. Not surprisingly, waiting for God to solve problems and asking God for a miracle were generally accompanied by a lower sense of self-efficacy in the recovery process. However, working together *with* God toward recovery was associated with greater empowerment.

Research also suggests that religiousness may be especially conducive to personal agency in more stressful life situations.

Shortly after terrorist attacks in Istanbul, Fischer, Greitemeyer, Kastenmüller, Jonas, and Frey (2006) assessed levels of intrinsic religiousness (i.e., religious commitment) and self-efficacy among customers in a German café who had been informed of the attacks. Fischer and colleagues repeated the process in the same café 2 months later with different participants. In the first condition, those who reported higher levels of intrinsic religiousness also reported greater self-efficacy. In contrast, no such relationship was found in the second condition (2 months later). The researchers concluded that when issues of mortality were most salient, religion was most promotive of self-efficacy.

Apparently, then, religious people are no less, and perhaps even more, inclined to face their troubles and feel capable of dealing with them. Not only that, they appear to take more direct measures to solve problems. For instance, Canada and colleagues (2006) found a positive relationship between the endorsement of religious/spiritual beliefs and practices, and actively attempting to resolve problems among women with ovarian cancer. Similarly, a study of caregivers of family members with mental illness demonstrated that those who were highly personally religious tended to take better care of themselves (Murray-Swank et al., 2006). Finally, Yoshimoto and colleagues (2006) studied problem-solving skills in female partners of men with prostate cancer over a period of 10 weeks. Compared to women in couples in which only the female partner used religious coping, women in couples in which both partners used religious coping grew less impulsive and careless over time with respect to problem solving.

Taken as a whole, these studies make clear that religious people do not generally bury their heads in the sand or wait helplessly for someone else to solve their problems. In contrast to these stereotypes, the empirical evidence suggests that religious people are generally actively engaged in dealing with their personal tribulations. Moreover, their religiousness may enhance such efforts.

Beyond demonstrating that general religiousness is not characterized by defensiveness, passivity, or denial, research has shown that religiousness can be a source of strength, helping people adjust in the midst of crisis (e.g., Contrada et al., 2004; Cotton et al., 2006; Koenig, 2007). Heart surgery patients with strong religious beliefs tend to have less hostility prior to surgery and to experience fewer complications after the operation (Contrada et al., 2004). Koenig (2007) studied a sample of depressed cardiac patients and compared the most religious participants (in terms of religious attendance, prayer, Bible reading, and intrinsic religiousness) to the rest of the sample. After statistically accounting for numerous covariates, the most religious patients remitted from depression 53% faster than the other patients. Along similar lines, a meta-analysis of studies on religiousness and depressive symptoms indicated that religiousness is associated with less symptomatology; this relationship was stronger in samples experiencing greater stress (Smith, McCullough, & Poll, 2003). Thus, religiousness appeared to buffer the effects of stressors on symptomatology.

Higher levels of religiousness have also been linked directly to positive outcomes among samples dealing with life traumas. In the previously described study of heart surgery patients by Contrada and colleagues (2004), religious belief was associated with greater optimism. Similarly, Cotton and colleagues (2006) discovered that organizational religiousness, nonorganizational religiousness, and intrinsic religiousness were positively correlated with optimism in a sample of patients with HIV/AIDS. For victims of domestic violence, attendance at religious services was related to better quality of life (Gillum, Sullivan, & Bybee, 2006).

In light of these studies, it is clear that there is a connection between religion and resilience. However, these studies have made use of measures of global religiousness, which do not point clearly to the actual mechanisms by which religion produces its effects. More specific theoretical frameworks and measures are needed to shed light on religion's relationship to resilience. Below, we consider some of the progress in this direction with respect to four religious functions.

Religion and Meaning-Related Resilience

Park and Folkman (1997) proposed a model delineating how issues of meaning come into play in times of distress. Their model has particular implications for religion. They note that people are motivated to seek out meaning in life generally, and in stressful life situations in particular. In their model, Park and Folkman make a key distinction between global and situational meaning. *Global meaning* involves people's general beliefs, assumptions, and expectancies about the world and themselves. It also provides a set of goals that direct behavior. *Situational meaning* grows out of the experience of a life event and subsequent determination of the significance of the event—whether it is threatening or not—and the individual's ability to deal with it. According to Park and Folkman, incongruity between situational meaning and global meaning creates a pressure to reconcile the two by altering either the former or the latter; this process is known as *reappraisal*.

One facet of global meaning that is particularly relevant to religion is the belief that one's life has an ultimate purpose (Park & Folkman, 1997). Such a belief has important implications for how well one functions in life. Indeed, Krupski and his colleagues (2006) found that among low-income men with prostate cancer, those who indicated higher levels of belief in their life's meaning also tended to have a better quality of life in terms of both physical and mental outcomes. Religion is one possible source of global meaning, Park and Folkman noted. Many religions posit that a deity or other supernatural force guides the course of history and individual lives according to a greater plan. If secular meaning is associated with positive outcomes, as Krupski and colleagues found, one might expect religious meaning to be related to similar outcomes. Some research supports this hypothesis.

For example, researchers have looked into the ways people cope with the stresses of growing old. Krause (2003) set out to discover factors that might be tied to subjective well-being in what may be an otherwise daunting phase of life. To this end, Krause asked a nationwide sample of older adult Americans about how strongly they felt that God had a plan for their lives, and that their faith gave them a sense of direction. Endorsing a religiously based global meaning system was positively correlated with life satisfaction, self-esteem, and optimism. In other words, simply perceiving a spiritual significance to life may be a resource in the midst of trying times.

Park and Folkman (1997) do not limit religion's impact on meaning strictly to global systems; rather, they acknowledge that people can draw on religion as they interpret the meaning of specific situations in life. This process is particularly salient when stressors challenge the individual's sense of meaning. Nonreligious people might question their belief in a just world when it appears that innocent people suffer. The same problem is pertinent for individuals who believe in a loving, all-powerful God. Park and Folkman suggest that one solution to this dilemma is to reappraise the negative event positively, so that it fits with global meaning structures. In the religious context, this might be achieved by concluding that God has a purpose for allowing the suffering to occur.

There is evidence that religiousness may help individuals find meaning in tragedy. Murphy, Johnson, and Lohan (2003) followed a group of parents who each had lost a child to a violent death. Shortly after each child's death, Murphy and colleagues assessed these parents' reported levels of seeking God's help, putting trust in God, praying more than usual, and trying to find comfort in religion. They found that these means of religious coping predicted a greater ability to find meaning in the child's passing 5 years

after the death. Additional support for the relationship between religious meaning and well-being was found in a sample of Indian patients who had been in serious accidents (Dalal & Pande, 1988). Among those who were permanently disabled, attributing the accident to karma or to God's will was positively correlated with a scale assessing positive attitude, the expectation that they would recover, the belief that they must make efforts to recover, and plans for resuming their lives after the recovery process. This correlation held true both at the initial assessment and at a subsequent assessment 2 weeks later. One possible explanation for these results is that having a religiously based reason for one's suffering makes it easier to respond adaptively to that suffering.

A study of HIV-positive individuals is suggestive of the power of spirituality to facilitate the reconciliation of situational and global meaning through benefit finding, a concept closely related to reappraisal (Carrico et al., 2006). *Benefit finding* can be defined as identifying positive outcomes of an otherwise negative experience. Scores on a measure tapping faith in God, a sense of peace, religious behavior, and a compassionate view of others were associated with both positive reappraisal and agreement that having HIV brought benefits, such as discovering a sense of purpose, feeling closer to others, and learning to accept life's imperfections. Benefit finding and positive reappraisal in turn correlated negatively with depressive affective symptoms. Moreover, the negative relationship between spirituality and depressed mood was mediated by benefit finding and positive reappraisal. Hence, religiousness/spirituality is linked to global meaning and meaning making in specific life situations, which are in turn tied to lower levels of negative affect.

Whereas Carrico and colleagues (2006) demonstrated that religiousness/spirituality is consistent with secular forms of benefit finding and positive reappraisal, religion also provides a basis for the explicitly religious reframing of negative life events. In a study of hospice care providers, Mickley, Pargament, Brant, and Hipp (1998) identified several beneficial forms of positive religious reframing, including reappraising the stressor as an opportunity for spiritual growth or as the will of God. Of course, it is also possible to use one's religion to appraise a stressor negatively as evidence of an apathetic or unfair God; however, such undesirable appraisals are far less common (Mickley et al.). Some participants in Krause and colleagues' (2002) study of Japanese elders appear to have utilized benevolent religious reframing. Those who lost a loved one and believed in an afterlife were less likely to have hypertension 3 years after their loss than others who were bereaved and had no such belief. Afterlife belief may have protected its adherents from the injurious effects of their loss. As Krause and colleagues noted, the death of a loved one may be less damaging to those who expect to see their loved ones again on the other side of the grave.

Thus, it appears that religion plays a role in multiple levels of the meaning system. It may establish a foundational meaning system that orders the individual's understanding of the universe and particular events. When a situation does not fit the global meaning system, religion can also help put a positive spin on the stressor. Park and Folkman's (1997) framework provides a fruitful way to grasp the cognitive aspect of religion's contribution to resilience.

Religion and Emotional Resilience

Religious injunctions to cultivate positive emotions and overcome negative emotions are plentiful. For instance, the apostle Paul counseled early Christians, "Do not be anxious about anything" (Philippians 4:6, *New International Version* Bible [NIV]) and to "rejoice in the Lord always" (Philippians 4:4, NIV). Psychological theories have long echoed the belief that religion serves to stabilize individuals' emotional lives (e.g., Freud, 1927/1961). Indeed, many studies support

the notion that religion is linked to desirable emotional outcomes and suggest that religion may play a key role in promoting emotional resilience (e.g., Acklin, Brown, & Mauger, 1983; Koenig, 2007; Pargament et al., 1994).

One particularly productive line of research has focused on religion's relationship with depression and related negative affect. Hebert, Dang, and Schulz (2007) conducted a longitudinal study of depression and complicated grief in family caregivers of patients with dementia. Higher levels of attendance at religious services, prayer frequency, and importance of spirituality/religious faith when the caregivers were first assessed predicted lower levels of depression at follow-up; among bereaved participants, religious service attendance predicted less depression and complicated grief. In Koenig's (2007) longitudinal study of patients with congestive heart failure or chronic obstructive pulmonary disorder, both public and private forms of religiousness were associated with decreased time to remission of depression. Koenig noted that this effect was strongest for the most highly religious patients. Similarly, another study indicated that bereaved individuals with low levels of spiritual belief tended to resolve their grief more slowly than those with higher spiritual belief (Walsh, King, Jones, Tookman, & Blizard, 2002). In addition to global religiousness, positive religious coping appears to have salutary effects on depression. Positive religious coping was associated with less depression, both cross-sectionally and longitudinally, in a geriatric sample (Bosworth, Park, McQuoid, Hays, & Steffens, 2003).

Religiousness appears to be negatively related to other forms of negative affect as well. Kendler and colleagues (2003) found that social religiousness (e.g., church attendance and interaction with religious individuals) was associated with a reduced likelihood of receiving a diagnosis of generalized anxiety disorder. Attendance at religious services has also been tied to lower levels of anger and hostility in both cancer patients and patients receiving treatment for a nonthreatening condition (Acklin et al., 1983). Pargament and colleagues (1994) conducted a longitudinal study of the effects of various religious coping methods on emotions concerning the Gulf War in a college student sample. Spiritually based coping predicted lower scores on a scale assessing a range of negative emotions approximately 3 weeks after the initial questionnaire administration.

Of course, reduction in negative affect is not the only form of emotional resilience. Researchers are interested in factors that lead to increased positive affect, and religion is one such factor. One study of elderly widows revealed that more frequent attendance at religious services contributed significantly to a mixture of positive emotions, including excitement, pride, and pleasure, even after researchers controlled for sociodemographic variables and emotional support provided by family members (McGloshen & O'Bryant, 1988). Along with organizational religiousness, the way in which religious individuals hold their beliefs may have implications for emotional well-being. McIntosh, Inglehart, and Pacini (1990) assessed the degree to which Christian college students adjusting to the transition to college viewed their religious beliefs as central and open to questioning. Centrality and flexibility of beliefs were linked to greater esteem and happiness in college. Religious coping is yet another source of emotional uplift in trying times. In the previously described study of college students' emotional reactions to the Gulf War, religious support was related to higher positive affect cross-sectionally, and pleading for divine intervention was predictive of positive affect longitudinally (Pargament et al., 1994).

It should be noted that cross-sectional research occasionally finds positive correlations between religion and undesirable emotional outcomes. The *stress mobilization theory* (Pargament, 1997) is a potential explanation for such puzzling inconsistency. According to the theory, cross-sectional studies catch participants in the midst of

their distress when the more distressed participants are more likely to turn to religion as a coping resource, creating a temporary positive correlation between religiousness and distress. However, the theory predicts that if these participants were studied longitudinally, greater religiousness would be followed by reduced distress. As a matter of fact, longitudinal studies, such as those conducted by Hebert and colleagues (2007), Koenig (2007), and Pargament and colleagues (1994), confirm that religion is, in the long run, often beneficial emotionally.

Religion and Relational Resilience

It is often said that humans are social creatures. Implicit in this statement is the notion that people need relationships. The social psychology literature is replete with studies affirming that perceived social isolation is frequently accompanied by mental and physical illness, and shorter life length (see Hawthorne, 2008). Hence, it appears that involvement with other people is integral to quality of life. One place to which people often turn for social interaction is the religious community. In the best cases, a church can represent a strong network of caring persons who respond swiftly and appropriately to the needs of others throughout the lifespan.

Quite a few investigators have put this ideal to the test, empirically assessing the link between religiousness and relational resilience. For instance, Wink, Dillon, and Larsen (2005) looked at well-being in a sample of adults in their late 60s to mid-70s. They found that religiousness (as assessed by belief in God and an afterlife, prayer, and frequent attendance at a traditional place of worship) was positively correlated with social support (as indicated by number of people in one's social network, frequency of social contact, presence of a confidant, and whether one lives alone or with someone else). A study of battered women revealed that nonwhite women who attended church frequently and reported that their place of worship was a source of strength and comfort to them also reported higher levels of social support; no such relationship was found for white women (Gillum et al., 2006). Likewise, Watlington and Murphy (2006) found that being involved in public and private religious activities, as well as having spiritual experiences, was associated with greater social support. A longitudinal study following participants for 30 years appears to confirm the role of religious service attendance on relationships (Strawbridge, Shema, Cohen, & Kaplan, 2001). Participants who attended weekly and saw fewer than three family members or friends per month in 1965 were 62% more likely to have increased their number of social relationships in 1995; weekly attenders with three or more social relationships in 1965 were 37% less likely to have dropped below three relationships by 1995.

Research on attendance suggests at least one fairly obvious explanation for the link between religiousness and social support. It is only intuitive to presume that meeting regularly with fellow congregants will facilitate relationships, especially in a context where leaders and doctrines officially promote interpersonal connectedness and "bearing one another's burdens." This effect would not be unique to religion; any social club or activity could create similar bonds. But does this theory fully account for the religion–social support relationship? Prado and colleagues (2004) reported that although religiously involved individuals appear to use more social support in the coping process because they have more people available to support them, this indirect relationship does not exhaust the association between religious involvement and support in coping. Perhaps some aspect of religiousness, in addition to regular proximity to fellow congregants, contributes to relational resilience.

As a matter of fact, there are intrapsychic religious variables that also predict relational resilience. In a study of dialysis patients, O'Brien (1982) found that those who rated their faith as more important to them re-

ported higher levels of social interaction and lower levels of alienation. Not only was there more social contact for patients who valued their faith, but also the quality of their interactions was higher. General religious coping is another intrapsychic religious variable that predicts social support longitudinally in distressed populations (Koenig et al., 1992). In a cross-sectional study of patients with advanced cancer, higher levels of positive religious coping were associated with greater perceived support (Tarakeshwar et al., 2006). These findings suggest that there is more to religion's link to social support than meets the eye.

The relationships among religion, social support, and outcomes are somewhat complicated. The amount of support from clergy and church members has been tied to lower levels of depression and greater reports of secular and religious benefit finding among family members during the cardiac surgery of a loved one (VandeCreek, Pargament, Belavich, Cowell, & Friedel, 1999). However, whereas church-based emotional support has been found to buffer the effects of financial strain on self-rated health for black older adult participants, this relationship did not hold for white older adult participants (Krause, 2006a, 2006b). In the same study, those who reported attending church infrequently also reported receiving less emotional support, and support was a weaker buffer for infrequent (as opposed to frequent) attenders. These findings indicate that the social benefits of church attendance do not extend to all elderly attenders (i.e., those who are white or attend infrequently).

Interestingly, it appears that relational resilience may influence religious coping. Schottenbauer and colleagues (2006) found that secure attachment is associated with positive religious coping. Because the attachment relationship is presumed to precede coping with a life crisis, Schottenbauer and colleagues' findings suggest that establishing an adaptive attachment may set the foundation for beneficial religious coping methods. Apparently, those who enjoy a good relationship with human attachment figures often expect the same benevolence and protection from their divine attachment figure.

Religion and Religious Resilience

Society commonly values having a sense of meaning in life, positive affect, and social connectedness, and various facets of religiousness appear related to each of these types of resilience. Even so, it would be inappropriate to reduce religion solely to the pursuit of these goals. Pargament, Magyar-Russell, and Murray-Swank (2005) have argued that many religious individuals seek religious ends in themselves. These ends include, but are not limited to, closeness to God, closeness to a religious community, and fidelity to a religious way of life. Stressors often present a very real threat to religiousness, drawing the affected individual into a battle for what may be the most precious parts of life. The threatened or actual loss of such sacred objects may be highly distressing for the religious person.

There is, however, abundant evidence that religion itself tends to be resilient to stress. For instance, the death of a loved one can be particularly difficult for those who survive him or her. A prospective study by Hebert and colleagues (2007) addressed religious outcomes in caregivers of dementia patients who passed away during the course of the study. Caregivers reported that frequency of prayer and self-rated importance of spirituality/religious faith remained the same after their loss; in fact, caregivers attended religious services more frequently following the loss. Still, the ability to weather one storm with one's faith intact is not particularly surprising.

It could be argued that exposure to multiple stressors may lead to more of a drain on a person's religious reservoir. Falsetti, Resick, and Davis's (2003) findings contradict this notion: For individuals who had encountered traumatic events, experiencing more than one trauma was related to higher,

not lower, levels of intrinsic religiousness. In this sample, 70% of the participants reported no change in religious beliefs following their first (or only) trauma; 16% reported becoming less religious, whereas 13% reported becoming more religious. Of those who experienced multiple traumas, 73% reported no change in religiousness after the second event.

But perhaps prolonged suffering poses the greatest challenge to the resilience of religion. In contrast to this argument, Cotton and colleagues' (2006) longitudinal study of patients with HIV/AIDS revealed no significant changes in organized religious activities, nonorganized religious activities, overall spirituality, positive religious coping, or negative religious coping over a period of 12–18 months. Only intrinsic religiousness decreased, whereas feelings of meaning and peace increased. In short, there is evidence that acute, multiple, and persistent stressors do not necessarily lead to declines in religiousness.

It is also important to note that people who are more religious prior to stressful events appear to demonstrate greater religious resilience. Several studies by Ai and her colleagues illustrate this point (Ai, Park, Huang, Rodgers, & Tice, 2007; Ai, Peterson, Tice, & Koenig, 2004; Ai, Tice, Peterson, & Huang, 2005). Participants waiting to undergo cardiac surgery reported greater use of prayer as a coping method (i.e., indicated that prayer was important and helpful to them, and that they intended to use prayer to cope with the surgery) if they also reported having a strong religious faith (i.e., said that religion was important to them and described themselves as highly religious) (Ai et al., 2004). After the 9/11 terrorist attacks, graduate and undergraduate students in mental health classes were asked about the effects the attacks had on them and how they were coping (Ai et al., 2005). Stronger religious faith and greater use of prayer in coping were associated with *spiritual support*, which refers to feeling close to a higher power and experiencing love, peace, guidance, and strength through this relationship. Last, in another sample of preoperative cardiac surgery patients, general religiousness correlated moderately to very positively with positive religious coping (Ai et al., 2007).

It is perhaps intuitive that religious individuals use religious coping and experience positive religious outcomes. They have more invested in religion, so they should hold more tightly to it. Furthermore, their investment in religion pays dividends in the form of familiarity with adaptive religious coping methods. Thus, they are able to maintain that which is of utmost importance to them through the most trying times of life. Religion, then, appears to be able to help people in crisis conserve not only a sense of meaning, emotional comfort, and relationships but also religion itself.

Spiritual Transformation

Resilience is complex, and the term itself can be applied to different types of phenomena. Masten, Best, and Garmezy (1990) have described three classes of resilience: desirable outcomes in individuals who are at elevated risk for certain undesirable outcomes; continued positive functioning in spite of stressors; and a return to normal following a decline in functioning due to a traumatic event. Thus far, this chapter has presented religion as a resilience factor, stabilizing the afflicted and restoring homeostasis. Nevertheless, religion is a force for not only conservation but also transformation in stressful times (Pargament, 1997). To put it another way, religion can contribute to fundamental change in what the individual holds to be significant and the pathways the individual takes to significance.

Religiousness may contribute to perceptions of positive and profound change following major life stressors. In a study of people with HIV/AIDS, nonorganizational religious activities, intrinsic religiousness, and positive and negative religious coping were predictive of beliefs that one's life had improved

(Szaflarski et al., 2006). This relationship was stronger for participants with lower functioning in terms of health status and health concerns, suggesting that the stress associated with illness actually increased religion's positive effects on perceived improvement in quality of life. Among female sexual assault victims, religious coping has been associated with reports of positive life changes with respect to self, relationships, life philosophy or spirituality, and empathy (Frazier, Tashiro, Berman, Steger, & Long, 2004). Additionally, increases in religious coping over time have been accompanied by reports of more positive life changes (Frazier et al., 2004). Phillips and Stein (2007) investigated predictors of *stress-related growth*, which refers to perceived personal improvements resulting from a stressful experience. In their sample of people with schizophrenia or bipolar disorder, benevolent religious reappraisal (e.g., viewing one's mental illness as a part of God's plan) was positively correlated with stress-related growth.

In the previous section we described how individuals generally preserve their religiousness in the face of crisis. However, traumatic events can stimulate increases in religiousness as well. Forty-five percent of the participants in a study of people with HIV stated that their religiousness and spirituality increased after their diagnosis (Ironson, Stuetzle, & Fletcher, 2006). As noted earlier, Falsetti and colleagues (2003) discovered that people who experienced multiple traumas indicated higher levels of greater intrinsic religiousness. Nineteen percent of respondents who had multiple traumas reported growing more religious after the second event, whereas only 8% reported declines in religiousness. Thus, it seems that personal trials can serve as opportunities for religious growth. This may be especially true if the individual draws on religion as a source of strength. In studies of people facing a variety of major life stressors, a number of predictors, including traditional measures of religiousness, collaborative coping, and positive religious coping, have shown positive relationships with desirable religious outcomes (i.e., self-reported spiritual growth, increased closeness to God, and increased closeness to one's faith community) (Pargament et al., 1999; Smith, Pargament, Brant, & Oliver, 2000). One longitudinal study of people dealing with the trauma of a flood in the Midwest found that positive religious coping at the time of the initial survey was predictive of positive religious outcomes 4 months later (Smith et al., 2000). Perhaps those who find that their religious resources sustain them in dark times grow in the conviction that their faith is valuable and learn to integrate it better into their lives.

Spiritual Struggles

Although religion is largely a source of strength and resilience, there are occasions in which distress overwhelms the individual's religious orienting system, jeopardizing one's grasp on the sacred. Of course, those with a weaker religious orientation may be particularly vulnerable to the effects of major life stressors, but the most traumatic of life's events may cause religious turmoil and struggle for many people. During these times of spiritual struggle, the individual may take drastic, even harmful measures to prevent the sacred from slipping away or to restructure his or her relationship with the sacred. *Spiritual struggles* have been defined as "efforts to transform or conserve a spirituality that has been threatened or harmed (Pargament, Murray-Swank, Magyar, & Ano, 2005, p. 247). According to Pargament, Murray-Swank, and colleagues (2005), there are three main types of spiritual struggle: interpersonal, intrapsychic, and divine. *Interpersonal* spiritual struggles may take the form of doctrinal disputes between church members or of a person feeling rejected by a religious community, to name two examples. In *intrapsychic* struggle, the individual may wrestle with religious doubts, questioning the truth of core beliefs. This type of struggle may also manifest as opposition between religiously sanctioned and religiously proscribed desires (Exline & Rose, 2005). The last type of struggle is characterized by a troubled relationship with the *divine*. People may become angry with God due to perceived injustice, or they may feel as though God has abandoned them or is punishing them (Pargament, Murray-Swank, et al., 2005). In each case, apart from the stressors that elicit it, spiritual struggle can be a source of trouble in and of itself. Struggles of these kinds may be particularly contentious when people perceive that others fail to respect, honor, or protect a spiritual bond.

The Negative Religious Coping Scale, developed by Pargament, has been used to assess spiritual struggles in numerous studies and focuses primarily on divine struggles (McConnell, Pargament, Ellison, & Flannelly, 2006). High scores on this measure are often accompanied by negative psychosocial outcomes. Advanced cancer patients who make greater use of negative religious coping have reported lower overall, existential, and psychological quality of life (Tarakeshwar et al., 2006). For caregivers of terminally ill cancer patients, negative religious coping is predictive of greater caregiver burden, less satisfaction with the caregiver role, lower quality of life, and higher risk for major depressive disorder or an anxiety disorder; these relationships remained significant after researchers controlled for demographic variables (Pearce, Singer, & Prigerson, 2006). Negative religious coping has also been associated with more severe depression in a sample of depressed geriatric patients (Bosworth et al., 2003).

Just as religious resources may be especially helpful to people going through major life stressors, spiritual struggles may be especially problematic to people dealing with critical situations, in essence, making bad matters worse. For example, McConnell and colleagues (2006) examined the correlates of negative religious coping in a national sample that included both participants who had experienced an injury or serious illness in the preceding year and those who had not experienced such an event. For the entire sample, negative religious coping was associated with anxiety, phobic anxiety, depression, paranoid ideation, obsessive–compulsiveness, and somatization. However, the relationship between negative religious coping and anxiety, as well as phobic anxiety, was especially marked for those who had had an injury or illness. In a similar vein, Lonczak, Clifasefi, Marlatt, Blume, and Donovan (2006) studied correlates of religious coping in a correctional population. They found an interaction between experiencing stressful life events and pleading for divine intervention (a negative religious coping method), such that pleading exacerbated the ties between stressful life events and depression; the same interaction effect was found when predicting hostility from pleading and stress. The results of these two studies are consistent with the notion that spiritual struggles "make bad matters worse," increasing the negative outcomes of negative life stressors. It is therefore important to recognize that although religion is generally a resilience factor for people dealing with difficulties, it can also be a hindrance to recovery from stressful events.

Psychospiritual Interventions to Enhance Religious Contributions to Resilience

In recent years, a number of people have begun to move from research to practice in this domain of study (for a review, see Pargament, 2007). Considering the potential contributions of religion to resilience, incorporating religious resources into psychotherapy is an obvious next step. Several authors have demonstrated how these resources may be integrated into the process of change to enhance personal resilience. The findings are promising.

One approach to helping individuals struggling with a variety of life problems has attempted to integrate religion and spirituality into rational-emotive therapy (RET; Warnock, 1989; Johnson & Ridley, 1992).

Traditional RET presents the following model of distress. An activating event, such as a stressor, arises in a person's life. The individual responds with certain cognitive interpretations or beliefs, which in turn produce emotional and behavioral consequences in the individual. Irrational beliefs (i.e., those that are false) tend to produce negative consequences, such as anxiety, depression, and isolation. RET provides a framework for challenging irrational beliefs to replace maladaptive emotions and behaviors with adaptive ones.

Warnock (1989) has noted that religious beliefs, which are often very central to clients, can be both helpful and harmful. When a client highly values irrational religious beliefs, it may be necessary to confront those beliefs. Furthermore, religious traditions themselves often present logical and rational teachings that can be used to counteract irrational beliefs. Warnock demonstrates how Christian beliefs may be applied to RET for work with Christian clients.

One basic irrational belief, which has been named *demandingness*, entails the expectation that the individual must succeed at everything he or she does, that everyone must approve of the individual, and that life must always go the way one wants it to go. For Christian clients, a therapist might point out that Jesus was willing to provoke the wrath of contemporary religious authorities and proceeded to do so by contradicting them and breaking their traditions (Warnock, 1989). In addition, Jesus accepted the fact that suffering was a part of life, refusing to resist those who planned to take his life and telling his disciples that they would also be persecuted (Warnock, 1989). Such examples can normalize the struggles of a therapy client. In theory, if the client accepts suffering, he or she will find it less upsetting.

Another form of irrational belief occurs when clients exaggerate how bad their circumstances are. The more they tell themselves that the situation is awful or could not be worse, the worse they feel. Christian clients may benefit from being reminded that crucifixion is a particularly terrible fate (Warnock, 1989). Nevertheless, Jesus reacted relatively calmly in the face of death, submitting to the authorities. If Jesus had believed that crucifixion was the worst situation possible, he probably would have attempted to escape it. This account may encourage clients to view their problems as bearable by putting them into perspective.

Low frustration tolerance is also a common irrational response. People tell themselves that they cannot stand to have their desires thwarted. Perseverance becomes increasingly difficult when one's efforts seem to be of no avail. In this case, the therapist can direct the client's attention to Jesus's response to the apparent failure of his mission (Warnock, 1989). Most of those who heard Jesus's teachings did not understand or accept his true message, and many ridiculed him. In spite of this opposition, Jesus remained true to his convictions. Likewise, clients can learn to persevere despite frustration.

The fourth basic irrational response is *condemnation*, the tendency to blame oneself or others. Clients caught in the trap of condemnation make little progress; if they consider themselves irredeemably wicked, they have no hope of changing, and if they blame others, they may perceive themselves as having no responsibility for change. However, clients can be reminded that Jesus did not preach condemnation (Warnock, 1989). Although he acknowledged the sins of the adulteress and the woman at the well, he offered them the hope that they could indeed be free from their past failures. Therapists can use this principle to help clients release feelings of guilt and blame to move toward desired ends.

Johnson and Ridley (1992) conducted an exploratory study comparing RET with an explicitly Christian version of RET in a sample of participants who responded to an add for short-term counseling for depression. The Christian version utilized Biblical examples to challenge clients' irrational beliefs and also integrated other Christian con-

tent and prayer into the treatment. After six weekly, 50-minute sessions, both treatment groups exhibited significant declines in depressive symptoms, automatic negative self-statements, and irrational values. Although these results must be interpreted cautiously due to the exploratory nature of the study, they do suggest that conducting RET from a Christian perspective may not reduce the efficacy of the treatment. Because the effects were equivalent for the treatment groups, it may be preferable to work with clients within a framework that fits their religious beliefs.

Another example of an intervention that incorporates religious resources was developed by Siwy and Smith (1988). This group therapy targets individuals with interpersonal issues and is advertised as a Christian therapy, although non-Christians are also welcome. Prospective group members are typically referred by other therapists. Pretreatment screening comprises a review of the client with the referring therapist, psychological testing of the client, and an interview with the client conducted by the group cotherapists. The intervention is not designed for clients with severe psychotic or mood disorders that have not been stabilized. Group sizes range from five to eight clients, and each group meets weekly for 1.5-hour sessions.

The inner faith of the therapists and clients forms the basis for psychospiritual interventions (Siwy & Smith, 1988). Therapists mobilize religious resources, such as prayer and scripture reading, during sessions. In addition, clients may choose to discuss their thoughts about and relationship with God. Each individual is valued as a unique image of God and members are expected to treat each other with respect. Scapegoating is not permitted, whereas accurate empathy is cultivated for the sake of creating a sense of safety in the clients. Siwy and Smith explain that this therapeutic environment is necessary if clients are to relax their defenses and reveal their personal problems. The group members confront and challenge each other, but they also explore and affirm each individual's gifts. The goal of this process is to restore each client's ability to relate to others in a healthy manner.

The reviewed psychospiritual interventions are just two examples of a growing approach to the application of religion to individual suffering. Yet they suggest that religion can be effectively woven into psychotherapy. In fact, one recent meta-analysis indicated that participants in spiritually integrated treatments showed somewhat greater benefits than those in comparative interventions (Smith, Bartz, & Richards, 2007). More research certainly remains to be done on the outcomes of this integrative movement.

Summary

Religion represents a potent resilience factor. Far from encouraging defensiveness, denial, passivity, and pathology, religion is often associated with self-efficacy and the active confrontation of problems, along with a host of positive outcomes. However, the links between religion and resilience are neither simple nor straightforward.

Our review of the literature demonstrates that these two constructs have a complex, multifaceted relationship. Religion may provide people with a belief in the meaningfulness of life and life's stressors, which may, in turn, preserve psychological well-being. People experiencing stressful events also appear to benefit emotionally from religion; those who are more religious tend to have lower levels of negative affect and higher levels of positive affect. Furthermore, various forms of religiousness are associated with receiving more social support, and support of this kind can buffer the effects of stressors. Finally, in the face of adversity, people of faith show a remarkable ability to preserve their sense of connection with the sacred and their religious way of life.

However, religion is not simply a typical resilience factor. Whereas resilience is often conceived of as the maintenance of or return to normal functioning following a trauma, religiousness can be a catalyst for positive life changes and stress-related growth. Many religious individuals feel that their faith helps them use crisis as an opportunity to achieve highly valued outcomes, both secular and spiritual. However, religion's power for positive transformation is balanced by its potential for serious harm. Spiritual struggle can worsen the negative effects of stressful life events, decreasing quality of life and increasing negative affect.

It is surprising that researchers and practitioners have neglected or diminished the role of religion in stressful times for so many years. As the findings in this chapter indicate, religion can be a powerful force for resilience among people grappling with the most traumatic experiences in life. Yet there is a great deal more to be learned about the connections between religion and resilience. This knowledge will be essential in our efforts both to understand more fully the nature of resilience and to facilitate greater resilience among people in critical life situations.

References

Acklin, M. W., Brown, E. C., & Mauger, P. A. (1983). The role of religious values in coping with cancer. *Journal of Religion and Health*, 22, 322–333.

Ai, A. L., Park, C. L., Huang, B., Rodgers, W., & Tice, T. N. (2007, June). Psychosocial mediation of religious coping styles: A study of short-term psychological distress following cardiac surgery. *Personality and Social Psychology Bulletin*, 33(6), 867–882.

Ai, A. L., Peterson, C., Tice, T. N., & Koenig, H. G. (2004). Faith-based and secular pathways to hope and optimism subconstructs in middle-aged and older cardiac patients. *Journal of Health Psychology*, 9(3), 435–450.

Ai, A. L., Tice, T. N., Peterson, C., & Huang, B. (2005, June). Prayers, spiritual support, and positive attitudes in coping with the September 11 national crisis. *Journal of Personality*, 73(3), 763–791.

Bosworth, H. B., Park, K.-S., McQuoid, D. R., Hays, J. C., & Steffens, D. C. (2003). The impact of religious practice and religious coping on geriatric depression. *International Journal of Geriatric Psychiatry, 18*, 905–914.

Canada, A. L., Parker, P. A., de Moor, J. S., Basen-Engquist, K., Ramondetta, L. M., & Cohen, L. (2006). Active coping mediates the association between religion/spirituality and quality of life in ovarian cancer. *Gynecologic Oncology, 101*, 102–107.

Carrico, A. W., Ironson, G., Antoni, M. H., Lechner, S. C., Durán, R. E., Kumar, M., et al. (2006). A path model of the effects of spirituality on depressive symptoms and 24-h urinary-free cortisol in HIV-positive persons. *Journal of Psychosomatic Research, 61*, 51–58.

Contrada, R. J., Goyal, T. M., Cather, C., Rafalson, L., Idler, E. L., & Krause, T. J. (2004). Psychosocial factors in outcomes of heart surgery: The impact of religious involvement and depressive symptoms. *Health Psychology, 23*(3), 227–238.

Cotton, S., Puchalski, C. M., Sherman, S. N., Mrus, J. M., Peterman, A. H., Feinberg, J., et al. (2006). Spirituality and religion in patients with HIV/AIDS. *Journal of General Internal Medicine, 21*, S5–S13.

Dalal, A. K., & Pande, N. (1988). Psychological recovery of accident victims with temporary and permanent disability. *International Journal of Psychology, 23*, 25–40.

Durkheim, E. (1912). *The elementary forms of religious life.* New York: Free Press.

Emmons, R. A. (1999). *The psychology of ultimate concerns: Motivation and spirituality in personality.* New York: Guilford Press.

Exline, J. J., & Rose, E. (2005). Religious and spiritual struggles. In R. F. Paloutzian & C. L. Park (Eds.), *Handbook of the psychology of religion and spirituality* (pp. 315–330). New York: Guilford Press.

Falsetti, S. A., Resick, P. A., & Davis, J. L. (2003, August). Changes in religious beliefs following trauma. *Journal of Traumatic Stress, 16*(4), 391–398.

Fischer, P., Greitemeyer, T., Kastenmüller, A., Jonas, E., & Frey, D. (2006). Coping with terrorism: The impact of increased salience of terrorism on mood and self-efficacy of intrinsically religious and nonreligious people. *Personality and Social Psychology Bulletin, 32*(3), 365–377.

Frazier, P., Tashiro, T., Berman, M., Steger, M., & Long, J. (2004). Correlates of levels and patterns of positive life changes following sexual assault. *Journal of Consulting and Clinical Psychology, 72*(1), 19–30.

Freud, S. (1961). *The future of an illusion.* New York: Norton. (Original work published 1927)

Friedman, L. C., Kalidas, M., Elledge, R., Dulay, M. F., Romero, C., Chang, J., et al. (2006). Medical and psychosocial predictors of delay in seeking medical consultation for breast symptoms in women in a public sector setting. *Journal of Behavioral Medicine, 29*(4), 327–334.

Geertz, C. (1966). Religion as a cultural system. In M. Banton (Ed.), *Anthropological approaches to the study of religion* (pp. 1–46). London: Tavistock.

Gillum, T. L., Sullivan, C. M., & Bybee, D. I. (2006). The importance of spirituality in the lives of domestic violence survivors. *Violence Against Women, 12*(3), 240–250.

Hawthorne, G. (2008). Perceived social isolation in a community sample: Its prevalence and correlates with aspects of peoples' lives. *Social Psychiatry and Psychiatric Epidemiology, 43*(2), 140–150.

Hebert, R. S., Dang, Q., & Schulz, R. (2007). Religious beliefs and practices are associated with better mental health in family caregivers of patients with dementia: Findings from the REACH study. *American Journal of Geriatric Psychiatry, 15*(4), 292–300.

Ironson, G., Stuetzle, R., & Fletcher, M. A. (2006). An increase in religiousness/spirituality occurs after HIV diagnosis and predicts slower disease progression over 4 years in people with HIV. *Journal of General Internal Medicine, 21*, S62–S68.

Johnson, P. E. (1959). *Psychology of religion.* Nashville: Abingdon Press.

Johnson, W. B., & Ridley, C. R. (1992). Brief Christian and non-Christian rational-emotive therapy with depressed Christian clients: An exploratory study. *Counseling and Values, 36*(3), 220–229.

Kendler, K. S., Liu, X.-Q., Gardner, C. O., McCullough, M. E., Larson, D., & Prescott, C. A. (2003). Dimensions of religiosity and their relationship to lifetime psychiatric and substance use disorders. *American Journal of Psychiatry, 160*, 496–503.

Koenig, H. G. (2007). Religion and remission of depression in medical inpatients with heart failure/pulmonary disease. *Journal of Nervous and Mental Disease, 195*, 389–395.

Koenig, H. G., Cohen, J. J., Blazer, F. H., Pieper, C., Meador, K. G., Shelp, F., et al. (1992). Religious coping and depression among elderly, hospitalized medically ill men. *American Journal of Psychiatry, 149*, 1693–1700.

Krause, N. (2003). Religious meaning and subjective well-being in late life. *Journal of Gerontology B: Psychological Sciences and Social Sciences, 58*(3), S160–S170.

Krause, N. (2006a). Church-based social support and mortality. *Journals of Gerontology B: Psychological Sciences and Social Sciences, 61*(3), S140–S146.

Krause, N. (2006b). Exploring the stress-buffering effects of church-based and secular social support on self-rated health in late life. *Journals of Gerontology B: Psychological Sciences and Social Sciences, 61*(1), S35–S43.

Krause, N., Liang, J., Shaw, B. A., Sugisawa, H., Kim, H.-K., & Sugihara, Y. (2002). Religion, death of a loved one, and hypertension among older adults in Japan. *Journal of Gerontology B: Psychological Sciences and Social Sciences, 57*(2), S96–S107.

Krupski, T. L., Kwan, L., Fink, A., Sonn, G. A., Maliski, S., & Litwin, M. S. (2006). Spirituality influences health related quality of life in men with prostate cancer. *Psycho-Oncology, 15*, 121–131.

Lonczak, H. S., Clifasefi, S. L., Marlatt, G. A., Blume, A. W., & Donovan, D. M. (2006). Religious coping and psychological functioning in a correctional population. *Mental Health, Religion and Culture, 9*(2), 171–192.

Masten, A. S., Best, K. M., & Garmezy, N. (1990). Resilience and development: Contributions from the study of children who overcome adversity. *Development and Psychopathology, 2*(4), 425–444.

McConnell, K. M., Pargament, K. I., Ellison, C. G., & Flannelly, K. J. (2006). Examining the links between spiritual struggles and symptoms of psychopathology in a national sample. *Journal of Clinical Psychology, 62*(12), 1469–1484.

McGloshen, T. H., & O'Bryant, S. L. (1988). The psychological well-being of older, recent widows. *Psychology of Women Quarterly, 12*, 99–116.

McIntosh, D. N., Inglehart, M. R., & Pacini, R. (1990, April). *Flexible and central religious belief systems and adjustment to college.* Paper presented at the meeting of the Midwestern Psychological Association, Chicago.

Mickley, J. R., Pargament, K. I., Brant, C. R., & Hipp, K. M. (1998). God and the search for meaning among hospice caregivers. *Hospice Journal, 13*(4), 1–17.

Murphy, S. A., Johnson, L. C., & Lohan, J. (2003). Finding meaning in a child's violent death: A five-year prospective analysis of parents' personal narratives and empirical data. *Death Studies, 27*, 381–404.

Murray-Swank, A. B., Lucksted, A., Medoff, D. R., Yang, T., Wohlheiter, K., & Dixon, L. B. (2006). Religiosity, psychosocial adjustment, and subjective burden of persons who care for those with mental illness. *Psychiatric Services, 57*(3), 361–365.

O'Brien, M. E. (1982). Religious faith and adjustment to long-term hemodialysis. *Journal of Religion and Health, 21*, 68–80.

Pargament, K. I. (1997). *The psychology of religion and coping.* New York: Guilford Press.

Pargament, K. I. (2007). *Spiritually integrated psychotherapy: Understanding and addressing the sacred.* New York: Guilford Press.

Pargament, K. I., Cole, B., VandeCreek, L., Belavich, T., Brant, C., & Perez, L. (1999). The vigil: Religion and the search for control in the hospital waiting room. *Journal of Health Psychology, 4*(3), 327–341.

Pargament, K. I., Ishler, K., Dubow, E., Stanik, P., Rouiller, R., Crowe, P., et al. (1994). Methods of religious coping with the Gulf War: Cross-sectional and longitudinal analyses. *Journal for the Scientific Study, 33*, 347–361.

Pargament, K. I., Magyar-Russell, G. M., & Murray-Swank, N. A. (2005). The sacred and the search for significance: Religion as a unique process. *Journal of Social Issues, 61*(4), 665–687.

Pargament, K. I., & Mahoney, A. (2005). Sacred matters: Sanctification as a vital topic for the psychology of religion. *International Journal for the Psychology of Religion, 15*(3), 179–198.

Pargament, K. I., Murray-Swank, N. A., Magyar, G. M., & Ano, G. G. (2005). Spiritual struggle: A phenomenon of interest to psychology and religion. In W. R. Miller & H. D. Delaney (Eds.), *Judeo-Christian perspectives* on psychology: Human nature, motivation, and change (pp. 245–268). Washington, DC: American Psychological Association.

Pargament, K. I., & Park, C. (1995). Merely a defense?: The variety of religious means and ends. Journal of Social Issues, 51, 13–32.

Park, C. L., & Folkman, S. (1997). Meaning in the context of stress and coping. Review of General Psychology, 1(2), 115–144.

Pearce, M. J., Singer, J. L., & Prigerson, H. G. (2006). Religious coping among caregivers of terminally ill cancer patients: Main effects and psychosocial mediators. Journal of Health Psychology, 11(5), 743–759.

Phillips, R. E., & Stein, C. H. (2007). God's will, God's punishment, or God's limitations?: Religious coping strategies reported by young adults living with serious mental illness. Journal of Clinical Psychology, 63(6), 528–540.

Prado, G., Feaster, D. J., Schwartz, S. J., Pratt, I. A., Smith, L., & Szapocznik, J. (2004). Religious involvement, coping, social support, and psychological distress in HIV-seropositive African American mothers. AIDS and Behavior, 8(3), 221–235.

Schottenbauer, M. A., Klimes-Dougan, B., Rodriguez, B. F., Arnkoff, D. B., Glass, C. R., & Lasalle, V. H. (2006). Attachment and affective resolution following a stressful event: General and religious coping as possible mediators. Mental Health, Religion and Culture, 9(5), 448–471.

Siwy, J. M., & Smith, C. E. (1988). Christian group therapy: Sitting with Job. Journal of Psychology and Theology, 16(4), 318–323.

Skinner, B. F. (1971). Beyond freedom and dignity. New York: Knopf/Random House.

Smith, B. W., Pargament, K. I., Brant, C., & Oliver, J. M. (2000). Noah revisited: Religious coping by church members and the impact of the 1993 Midwest flood. Journal of Community Psychology, 28(2), 169–186.

Smith, T. B., Bartz, J. D., & Richards, P. S. (2007). Outcomes of religious and spiritual adaptations to psychotherapy: A meta-analytic review. Psychotherapy Research, 17, 643–655.

Smith, T. B., McCullough, M. E., & Poll, J. (2003). Religiousness and depression: Evidence for a main effect and the moderating influence

of stressful life events. Psychological Bulletin, 129(4), 614–636.

Strawbridge, W. J., Shema, S. J., Cohen, R. D., & Kaplan, G. A. (2001). Religious attendance increases survival by improving and maintaining good health behaviors, mental health, and social relationships. Annals of Behavioral Medicine, 23(1), 68–74.

Szaflarski, M., Ritchey, P. N., Leonard, A. C., Mrus, J. M., Peterman, A. H., Ellison, C. G., et al. (2006). Modeling the effects of spirituality/religion on patients' perceptions of living with HIV/AIDS. Journal of General Internal Medicine, 21, S28–S38.

Tarakeshwar, N., Vanderwerker, L. C., Paulk, E., Pearce, M. J., Kasl, S. V., & Prigerson, H. G. (2006). Religious coping is associated with the quality of life of patients with advanced cancer. Journal of Palliative Medicine, 9(3), 646–657.

VandeCreek, L., Pargament, K., Belavich, T., Cowell, B., & Friedel, L. (1999). The unique benefits of religious support during cardiac bypass surgery. Journal of Pastoral Care, 53(1), 19–29.

Walsh, K., King, M., Jones, L., Tookman, A., & Blizard, R. (2002). Spiritual beliefs may affect outcome of bereavement: Prospective study. British Medical Journal, 324, 1551–1555.

Warnock, S. D. M. (1989). Rational-emotive therapy and the Christian client. Journal of Rational-Emotive Therapy and Cognitive-Behavior Therapy, 7(4), 263–274.

Watlington, C. G., & Murphy, C. M. (2006). The roles of religion and spirituality among African American survivors of domestic violence. Journal of Clinical Psychology, 62(7), 837–857.

Wink, P., Dillon, M., & Larsen, B. (2005). Religion as moderator of the depression–health connection. Research on Aging, 27(2), 197–220.

Yangarber-Hicks, N. (2004). Religious coping styles and recovery from serious mental illnesses. Journal of Psychology and Theology, 32(4), 305–317.

Yoshimoto, S. M., Ghorbani, S., Baer, J. M., Cheng, K. W., Banthia, R., Malcarne, V. L., et al. (2006). Religious coping and problem-solving by couples faced with prostate cancer. European Journal of Cancer Care, 15, 481–488.

C

Resilience across the Lifespan

11

Resilience over the Lifespan
Developmental Perspectives on Resistance, Recovery, and Transformation

Ann S. Masten
Margaret O'Dougherty Wright

Ancient stories and legends about success in the face of adversity communicate a human fascination with resilience that began long before scientists took an interest in such phenomena, beginning around four decades ago (Masten, 2007). Yet it was often compelling case histories of resilience that inspired the pioneers who launched the science of resilience. These pioneering psychologists and psychiatrists included E. James Anthony, Emory Cowen, Norman Garmezy, Lois Murphy, Michael Rutter, and Emmy Werner. These investigators initially focused on groups of people thought to be at risk for developing psychiatric problems, often due to psychiatric history in the family, current symptoms (e.g., antisocial behavior), or disadvantaged environments (e.g., poverty). All of these conditions indicated elevated risk for future problems in studies designed to understand the etiology of psychopathology. When these investigators began to follow the lives of "high-risk" populations forward in time during childhood, adolescence, or adulthood, they observed dramatic variation in adjustment, including cases of unexpectedly positive development. Intrigued, these investigators set out to understand the phenomenon of resilience in development, and many other investigators soon joined this scientific quest. In this chapter, we highlight major ideas and findings from this body of work, much of which focused on the early decades of life, in the hope of guiding efforts to build a lifespan science of resilience.

Four Waves of Resilience Research

The pioneers recognized the potential significance of understanding positive development in the lives of people who seemed to overcome the odds against them, and convinced a generation of scientists to study resilience. Three waves of research on resilience in human development followed, and a fourth wave is now under way (Masten, 2007; Wright & Masten, 2005). The first wave focused on description, with considerable investment in defining and measuring resilience, and in the identification of differences between those who did well and poorly in the context of adversity or risk of various kinds. This first wave of research revealed a surprising degree of consistency in qualities of people, relationships, and resources that predicted resilience, and these potential protective factors have shown robust staying power in later waves of research. The second wave moved beyond description of the factors or variables associated with resilience to a focus on processes, the "how" questions, aiming to identify and understand specific processes that might lead to resilience. This kind of research has continued, although with increasing attention to multiple levels of analysis and neurobiological processes (Cicchetti & Curtis, 2007). The third wave began with efforts to test ideas about resilience processes through intervention, most notably in experiments to promote resilience by boosting promotive or protective processes, such as effective parenting (e.g., Forgatch & DeGarmo, 1999; Wolchik et al., 2002), school engagement (e.g., Hawkins, Catalano, Kosterman, Abbott, & Hill, 1999), and more recently, executive function skills (Diamond, Barnett, Thomas, & Munro, 2007; Rueda, Rothbart, McCandless, Saccomanno, & Posner, 2005). The fourth wave of resilience studies is integrative, seeking to encompass rapid advances in the study of genes, neurobehavioral development, and statistics for a better understanding of the complex processes that lead to resilience (Masten, 2007). Fourth-wave studies, for example, have explored the role of genetic polymorphisms as *moderators* (vulnerability or protective influences) of risk or adversity in development (Kim-Cohen & Gold, 2009) and the role of neural plasticity in resilience (Cicchetti & Curtis, 2006, 2007).

Developmental perspectives played a central role from the outset of modern resilience research. The history of resilience science is closely linked to the history of the emergence of developmental psychopathology as a framework for understanding and investigating problems of human behavior over the life course (Cicchetti, 2006; Masten, 1989, 2006a). These interrelated domains of conceptual and empirical activity share many roots and investigators, as well as a core focus on development. Scholars who were interested in the etiology of psychopathology (including those who pioneered the study of resilience) were interested in following the course of development with respect to positive and negative adaptation. Many of these studies, particularly the longitudinal investigations, began in childhood or adolescence, when there is often rapid change, and it was clear that a developmental perspective was helpful and important. Another consequence of this history is that a large proportion of the initial research on resilience focused on the earlier part of the lifespan, although some investigators always focused on positive adaptation in later life (e.g., Rowe & Kahn, 1987; Vaillant, 1977, 2002).

The Practical Goals of Resilience Research

From the outset, researchers on resilience held out the promise of informing practice and policy (Masten, 2007). Pioneers believed that understanding naturally occurring resilience would lead to knowledge with practical applications to interventions, education, and policy. Evidence-based applications certainly have emerged, and we expect this trend to continue, but we would argue that there has been a much more profound effect of resilience science on practice and policy. Resilience research, with its central focus on positive development, has had a transformative effect on practices to address problems in development, shifting goals, methods, and models away from deficit-oriented and medical disease models to approaches that focus on strengths, health, and well-being.

The Organization of this Chapter

This chapter has three sections. The first focuses on the meaning of resilience and how it has been defined in developmental research. The second section summarizes major findings on the predictors of resilience, organized in terms of the adaptive systems hypothesized to explain the most commonly found protective factors in the study of resilience. The third section briefly delineates the major components of a resilience framework for practice that emerged from this body of work. We discuss directions for a lifespan science of resilience in the Conclusion.

Defining Resilience over the Lifespan

Resilience is a broad concept that generally refers to positive adaptation in any kind of dynamic system that comes under challenge or threat (Masten & Obradović, 2008). *Human resilience* refers to the processes or patterns of positive adaptation and development in the context of significant threats to an individual's life or function. Longitudinal studies of individuals exposed to significant trauma and psychosocial adversity clearly document significant variability in both short-term and long-term outcome. The study of human resilience specifically focuses on understanding such individual differences in relation to adverse experiences.

Resilience should not be conceptualized as a static trait or characteristic of an individual. Resilience arises from many processes and interactions that extend beyond the boundaries of the individual organism, including close relationships and social support. Moreover, an individual person may be resilient with respect to some kinds of stressors and not others, or be resilient with respect to some adaptive outcomes but not

others (Rutter, 2007). Resilience itself also is dynamic: The same individual may show maladaptive function at one time and resilience later in development, or vice versa.

Different explanatory models have been explored in an effort to understand the factors and processes that promote resilience in the context of risk (Garmezy, Masten, & Tellegen, 1984; Luthar, Cicchetti, & Becker, 2000; Masten et al., 1988). These models describe patterns of association among risks and adaptive outcomes, including additional variables that may explain variations in outcome. Two of the most basic models describe compensatory and moderating influences of explanatory factors. In compensatory or "main effect" models, factors that neutralize or counterbalance exposure to risk or stress have direct, independent, and positive effects on the outcome of interest, regardless of risk level. These compensatory factors have been termed *assets*, *resources*, and *promotive factors* in the literature. In protective or "moderating effect" models, a theoretical factor or process has effects that vary depending on the level of risk. A classic "protective factor" shows stronger effects at higher levels of risk. In other words, the importance of the explanatory variable is greater when risk is higher, suggesting a buffering or ameliorative influence. A protective factor may also show a main effect (e.g., good parenting is associated with better function at all levels of risk but also provides special, "extra" protection under very high-risk conditions), but this is not necessarily the case. Analogous to an automobile airbag or antibodies, a protective factor may matter *only* in the presence of a threat.

Additional models of resilience have been delineated. Another early model, the challenge model (e.g., Garmezy et al., 1984), described the possibility of an inoculation or steeling effect, where manageable doses of exposure to the adversity prepare an organism for adversity by strengthening capacity for mobilizing an adaptive response, much like a vaccination works to boost immune function with respect to a specific infectious agent. This model has been validated in disease models examining acquisition of immunity to infections, and has been explored with respect to psychosocial adversity as well (Elder, 1974). More recently, there is great interest in models that examine the moderating influence of genes and personality on differential reactivity in the context of adversity. Models of resilience encompassing gene–environment interaction are expanding rapidly (Kim-Cohen & Gold, 2009). At the same time, models that focus on the related concepts of "differential susceptibility" and "sensitivity to context" have been advanced to explore the possibility that some children are more susceptible or sensitive to the influence of context, whether the context is adverse or beneficial (Belsky, Bakermans-Kranenburg, & IJzendoorn, 2007; Boyce & Ellis, 2005; Ellis & Boyce, 2008; Obradović, Bush, Stamperdahl, Adler, & Boyce, in press). Such children also may be differentially responsive to contextual protective factors.

In any of these models, resilience is a dynamic, interactional, and inferential concept because it refers to what happens during and following conditions that threaten the organism. Doing well in life (by whatever criteria) does not define resilience, nor does the adverse experience in and of itself. Resilience concerns the processes and outcomes of good adaptation in relation to significant threats. Thus, to study resilience requires investigators to define (and measure) "good adaptation" and "significant threat," as well as any of the processes or resources the investigator hypothesizes to explain individual differences in patterns of response or outcome. Furthermore, since adversity can occur at any point in development, with consequences that potentially alter development over the near and the far term, a lifespan developmental perspective is essential for a full understanding of resilience. In this section, we describe developmental approaches to positive adaptation and to adversity, and

highlight the methodological advances, issues, and controversies involved.

Developmental Perspectives on Positive Adaptation

Pioneers in the study of resilience recognized that "good outcomes" meant something more than "absence of problems," and turned their attention to theories and measurement of positive adjustment and normative development (Masten, Cutuli, Herbers, & Reed, 2009). *Positive adaptation* or *development* can be defined in terms of internal function (e.g., psychological well-being, maturity, health) or external function (e.g., doing well in school or work, contributing to society), or some combination of both (happy and successful). Many of the developmental scientists concerned with resilience focused particularly on the related concepts of competence and developmental tasks, which are rooted deep in the history of developmental theory and psychological science (Masten, Burt, & Coatsworth, 2006).

Competence broadly refers to effective functioning in the world, or the presumed capability for such functioning, in reference to expectations based on norms of behavior in a given context, culture, and time in history. Those expectations often are described in terms of *developmental tasks*, referring to the standards for behavior in different domains expected for people as they mature in a given society or culture (Elder, 1998; Havighurst, 1972; Masten & Coatsworth, 1998). Some of these expectations are universal developmental milestones, achieved in a small time window by all typically developing individuals, such as learning to walk or talk. Other expectations are more extended over the life course, taking on increasingly mature forms. People are expected in all cultures to form attachment relationships, initially with caregivers and later with friends, romantic partners, and eventually their own children and grandchildren, if they become parents. The expectations for the nature of friendship attachments mature as the individuals involved mature, so that adolescent friendships are expected to exhibit more intimacy and thoughtfulness than the friendships of preschoolers. Other developmental tasks are particular to a given gender, culture, or time in human evolution or history. Examples might include hunting for bison, joining a religion, or completing a high school education.

Widespread, common developmental task expectations, sometimes termed *age-salient developmental tasks*, have been used to define and measure positive adaptation in numerous studies of resilience, including the longitudinal studies initiated by Emmy Werner (Kauai Longitudinal Study; see Werner & Smith, 1982, 1992) and Norman Garmezy (Project Competence; see Masten & Powell, 2003). Criteria vary across studies, but children of school age often are viewed as resilient if they meet developmental expectations for academic success, get along with others, and behave appropriately in society. As people grow older, expectations change. In the Project Competence study for example, success in romantic relationships and work became increasingly important criteria for defining competence and resilience as children in the cohort grew up. At the same time, school success waned in significance in adulthood, although the advantages of academic attainment for success in later developmental tasks persisted (Masten et al., 2005; Obradović, Burt, & Masten, in press; Roisman, Masten, Coatsworth, & Tellegen, 2004).

A core tenet of developmental theory related to competence and developmental tasks is the idea that competence begets competence; in other words, effective engagement of developmental tasks builds the capacity that serves to facilitate future competence in that society. Stakeholders in human development presumably appreciate both the significance of developmental task achievements and failures for future prospects. Parents, societies, and, as they grow older, young people themselves often are concerned about fail-

ures in age-salient developmental tasks because these problems are assumed to signify risk for future problems. These beliefs are well-justified in some cases and probably exaggerated in others. For example, there is ample evidence in economically advanced societies that school dropout and antisocial behavior that violates norms of conduct in a community are important harbingers of worse adult success, defined in terms of financial independence, obeying the law, parenting well, and many other indicators of adult health and well-being (Masten, Burt, & Coatsworth, 2006). On the other hand, although young adolescents may believe that successful romantic relationships are crucial to their success in life, there is little evidence that romantic success in early adolescence forecasts adult romantic success (Roisman et al., 2004). Instead, it is success in the salient tasks of adolescence that forecast later adult success, most notably successes in school and in forming close friendships with prosocial peers.

In short, developmental task expectations develop over the life course. These expectations reflect the developing capacity for adaptation of individuals and age-graded changes in context or opportunity afforded by cultures and societies. For a long part of the human lifespan, capacity for adaptation broadly increases, and with aging, capacity generally declines, although there is considerable variation across domains of function, as well as individual differences in adaptive capabilities.

The tasks of midlife and aging have been delineated by Erik Erikson (1959, 1963), Robert Havighurst (1972), and lifespan psychologists (e.g., Greve & Staudinger, 2006), as well as by investigators conducting empirical studies of lifespan development and successful aging (e.g., DiRago & Valliant, 2007; Vaillant, 2002; see other examples reviewed by Depp & Jeste, 2006). Developmental tasks of midlife often include more mature forms of work attainment, committed romantic relationships, and enduring friendships, family formation, and rearing children, as well as new expectations to give back to community and others in the form of civic engagement or mentoring. Erikson described the central issue of adult development in terms of "generativity versus self-absorption." As parents age, adult children in many cultures are expected to support and care for aging parents. As adults enter later life, additional developmental tasks of "successful aging" often encompass the successful launching of children, retirement, continued active social life, life satisfaction, and acceptance of physical decline and death. Erikson viewed the central challenge of mature adulthood as "integrity versus despair."

Competence from the perspective of developmental tasks is clearly multidimensional. This means that it is possible for a person to be competent in one domain and not in another, and raises key questions for defining resilience: Does a person need to be doing well in all major developmental tasks or only some of them? How are these decisions made in studies on resilience, and how has this impacted our understanding of the phenomena?

Some studies have defined a group of resilient people in terms of doing reasonably well in multiple developmental task domains and compared that group with other groups, and particularly to people who have experienced similarly high adversity but are not doing well in the chosen domains. Examples include the Kauai Study (Werner & Smith, 1982) and Cowen's Rochester studies (Cowen, Wyman, Work, & Parker, 1990; Cowen et al., 1997). This person-focused strategy of identifying resilience is similar to diagnosing a disorder by multiple criteria and is more likely to find naturally occurring kinds of people and differences between groups that actually occur in nature. This approach also serves to highlight core protective influences for human behavior and development that are likely to matter in multiple ways across multiple domains (e.g., good parenting or general cognitive skills).

A limitation is that this approach can lead to reification of the concept and convey a static rather than dynamic picture of resilience. It also has limitations for the study of specific processes that may play a unique role for a particular domain of adaptation.

In contrast, some research on resilience has focused on a single outcome of interest (e.g., academic achievement or even learning to read) in an effort to identify specific protective processes that make a difference for a particular outcome under adverse conditions. For example, early language experience (e.g., parents talking and reading to children) may play a particularly important role in vocabulary acquisition, learning to read, on the pathway to academic resilience of disadvantaged young children (Hart & Risley, 1995). These analyses often employ a variable-focused approach with powerful multivariate statistical approaches, and they are more likely to yield clues to the role of specific risks, assets, and protective processes for a particular domain of functioning.

Finally, some studies also combine variable-focused and person-focused approaches in an effort to capitalize on the strengths of each approach. The Project Competence longitudinal study, for example, has combined both approaches (e.g., Masten et al., 1999).

Internal versus External Adaptation

Another issue for defining positive adaptation in resilience research is whether to focus on internal or external adaptation, or both (Masten, 2001). Investigators vary, for example, in their considerations of whether to include happiness versus unhappiness and related aspects of subjective well-being (including symptoms of depressed mood or anxiety) in defining adaptation for resilience research. This issue in part reflects the dual nature of all living systems that must maintain internal function (e.g., a stable temperature) at the same time they adapt to their environmental context (e.g., taking actions to stay warm in the winter). It also is related to debates in the history of psychiatric diagnosis about the significance of functional impairment for the definition of mental disorder (Masten, Burt, & Coatsworth, 2006). Some investigators include internal states in the assessments of positive adaptation, while others do not, although it is rare for investigators to focus solely on subjective well-being. No matter how happy a person may report feeling, a person who is unable to function in most of the expected ways for people of his or her approximate age in a given context is not usually identified as showing positive adaptation, mental health, or resilience (by researchers or other stakeholders in the quality of adaptation, such as parents, friends, self, or community members).

There is a need for more informative data on the issue of multiple domains of adaptation, as well as cultural similarities and differences in the identification and importance of competence domains. Existing research is limited by the extent to which multiple domains have been adequately assessed within a given context or culture, as well as across diverse contexts or cultures. These shortcomings have limited our understanding of the extent to which various aspects of adaptation are potentially influenced by various types of stressors.

Developmental Coherence and Cascades

Research on competence and developmental tasks generally supports a fundamental tenet of developmental theory (Havighurst, 1972; Sroufe, 1979) that doing adequately well in salient domains, challenges, and tasks of one period of development establishes a foundation for success in future tasks (Masten, Burt, & Coatsworth, 2006; Masten & Obradović, 2006). There is coherence in the development of competence within domains, such as peer relationships over the lifespan (i.e., earlier social competence forecasts later, more mature competence with peers). Within a broad domain such as attachment relationships, coherence has been observed over long periods of time. Positive relationships with par-

ents predict social competence with peers, which in turn predicts positive romantic relationships and effective parenting of the next generation (Shaffer, Burt, Obradović, Herbers, & Masten, 2009; Sroufe, Egeland, Carlson, & Collins, 2005). Studies of developmental tasks also suggest spreading effects of achievements or failures over time from one domain to another domain of function, a phenomenon described variously in terms of *developmental cascades*, or progressive and snowball effects (Masten et al., 2005).

Decades ago, in reviews of the research on the predictability of adult adaptation from childhood behavior, Kohlberg noted that childhood cognitive function (reflected in intellectual test performance or academic achievement) and antisocial behavior predicted adult adjustment across many different domains of outcome (Kohlberg, LaCrosse, & Ricks, 1972). Recent advances in statistical methods have made it possible to test in a more convincing fashion whether success in one domain of behavior, such as conduct according to the rules for behavior in society (rule-abiding behavior vs. aggressive, disruptive, or externalizing behavior problems), spread over time to affect other domains, as suggested early by Kohlberg and later by additional developmental scientists. In Patterson's coercion model (Patterson & Capaldi, 1990; Patterson, Reid, & Dishion, 1992), antisocial behavior that emerges from inept discipline practices in the family begins to spread to other domains of function when children go to school, leading to dual failure in peer relations and learning that eventually may contribute to feeling bad about the self and increase the risk for affiliation with deviant peers and dropping out of school. In a series of papers from the Project Competence longitudinal study, investigators have used structural equation modeling methods to demonstrate cascade effects in the adaptation of the cohort over time (Burt, Obradović, Long, & Masten, 2008; Masten et al., 2005; Obradović, Burt, & Masten, in press) and across generations (Shaffer et al., 2009).

Cascade effects have important implications for understanding and promoting competence and resilience across the lifespan. Developmental cascades offer one explanation for the high return on investment in early competence observed by economists (Heckman, 2006), and the idea of interrupting such cascades may serve to enhance the strategic timing and targeting of interventions. Cascade effects may also explain some forms of co-occurring problems and disorders observed in research on psychopathology.

Developmental Perspectives on Risk, Adversity, and Trauma

As noted earlier, evaluating positive adaptation is necessary but not sufficient for specifying or researching resilience. Resilience also requires exposure to significant risk or threats to function in a system. *Risk* generally refers to prediction of undesirable outcomes in a group. A *risk factor* is associated with a higher likelihood, though not a certainty, of manifesting one or more problems of concern. Risks include traumatic experiences and adversities of many kinds that have shown the potential to derail development or interfere substantially in adaptive function. Many kinds of adversity or risk have been examined in the literature on resilience, including war and natural disasters affecting large populations; individual traumatic experiences (e.g., rape or incidents of family violence); and chronic adversities experienced when children live in poverty or dangerous neighborhoods, grow up with discrimination, or live with a dysfunctional parent struggling with mental illness or substance abuse (Obradović, Shaffer, & Masten, in press).

Strict definitions of risk (e.g., Kraemer et al., 1997) require that a risk predictor be clearly identifiable as coming before the bad outcome of interest (e.g., high blood pressure can be measured before the heart attack occurs). In human behavior and development, however, it is often difficult to show that a chronic risk factor (e.g., family violence) occurred before any sign of problems in a child, since the risks and outcomes are ongoing in development and often do not have a readily identifiable beginning or end.

Severity and chronicity of risk or adversity are important because there often is a dose–response gradient, in which higher exposure to worse adversity is related to worse adaptive function on average among a group of exposed people. Moreover, adversities and risks often pile up in the lives of individuals. Risks tend to co-occur, and isolated risk factors are rare. As risks accumulate, particularly in a concentrated time window, problems in adaptive function often rise, though resilience research has focused attention on people who do not follow this pattern, and who manifest better than expected adaptation for the level of risk (i.e., they are "off-gradient" cases; see illustration in Masten & Obradović, 2006).

A developmental perspective is important for evaluating risk, adversity, or trauma experiences that may threaten individual adaptation. The likelihood of exposure to risks and adversities varies with development, as does the nature of the experience of an individual. Young infants, for example, are not sent into combat, nor are they likely to be kidnapped and forced into child labor, or into war as a child soldier. Infants also would not fully understand the significance of war. They do not yet form peer friendships to lose through death, and death of a parent is a very different experience for a 3-month-old and a 13-year-old for many reasons related to development. Developmental timing of adversity exposure matters. On the other hand, experiences may also be reinterpreted as individuals mature and gain new understanding or perspectives on past experiences. A person who as a young child is abandoned or sexually abused by a parent may experience greater pain and suffering at a later time in development as the meaning of the experience is reinterpreted from a more mature point of view.

Resilience Pathways and Patterns: Resistance, Recovery, Normalization, and Transformation

Resilience is manifested over time, and a variety of patterns have been described in the literature. At least four distinct patterns of resilience have been identified in reference to acute and chronic adversities (for recent illustrations of different resilience patterns, see Bonanno, 2004; Masten & Obradović, 2008). *Resistance* refers to patterns of reasonably steady and positive adaptive behavior in the presence of significant threats. An example would be children who show a steady course of good function in all age-salient developmental tasks despite growing up in a poor family in a disadvantaged neighborhood. *Recovery* refers to patterns where the individual's adaptive function declines as a result of adversity, then returns to a positive level. This pattern is normal and expected in situations of severe continuing adversity or sudden catastrophe, representing conditions so challenging that maintaining good adaptation is not expected. A child subjected to abuse or neglect is not expected to function well in age-salient developmental tasks until caregiving conditions improve. Similarly, in the case of natural disaster, recovery is expected as the threat abates and the situation improves. Recovery, of course, may be long delayed if severe adversity continues or is repeated over a long period of time. *Normalization* patterns are observed in situations where a child begins life in an adverse rearing environment (e.g., a neglecting orphanage or abusive home), then conditions improve (e.g., through adoption). In this kind of situation, a child may show accelerated development and changes that eventually put him or her back on a normal developmental trajectory (Beckett et al., 2006; Rutter and the English and Romanian Adoptees Study Team, 1998). *Transformation* patterns refer to cases where adaptive functioning improves in the aftermath of adversity. The concept of posttraumatic growth, particularly among traumatized adults, refers to transformational patterns of this kind (Linley & Joseph, 2004; Park, 2004; Tedeschi & Calhoun, 1995).

There has been some debate about the role of time in defining resilience patterns. For some scholars, recovery after trauma must occur relatively quickly or the pattern is not viewed as resilience. Bonanno (2004), for example, distinguished recovery from resilience by a time allowance following significant loss or trauma. In his view, although transient mild distress may be evident initially, resilience requires that a person return to good function and positive emotions within several weeks. If a person manifests a longer period of dysfunction followed eventually by positive adaptation, this trajectory is viewed by Bonanno as recovery rather than resilience. In contrast, we view recovery as a type of resilience, whether it occurs quickly or over a more extended time. If the evaluation of resilience occurs within a short time frame following a disaster or traumatic experience, then a later-recovering individual would not be identified as resilient at that time, but might be later, if the same cohort were followed over time. Similarly, in the case of an individual who appeared to regroup quickly and later fell apart, the identification of resilience would depend on the time frame of the assessments. Our approach focuses on understanding different pathways of resilience over time.

There is considerable interest among developmental scientists in the longer-term patterning of adaptation following adversity. In the Kauai Study, as well as Project Competence and a number of other longitudinal studies of resilience, investigators have identified and studied "late bloomers," or young people who do poorly in adolescence and turn their lives around in the transition to adulthood, when there appears to be a window of opportunity for positive change (Masten, Obradović, & Burt, 2006). There has been relatively less empirical attention to later-life turnaround cases, although anecdotal reports of such redemption exist, and there may well be developmental windows for change in middle or late life. The possibility for such a "turnaround" was particularly evident in Werner and Smith's (1992) follow-up of adolescent girls who had become teenage mothers. Overall, the teenage mothers of Kauai evidenced much better adaptation in their 30s than they had at age 18 or 26. The paths that led to improvement related to differences in subsequent educational attainment, development of a stable marriage, support from kith and kin, exposure to positive role models, and further development of personal resources. Such "turnaround" cases (Rutter, 1990) are important for identifying potential windows of opportunity for intervention.

The Challenge of Explaining Resilience

From the perspective of development, trajectories of resilience in life are assumed to reflect many processes and interactions across multiple levels of function, from cells to central nervous system, to family, school and other complex social systems (Masten, 2006a). It is assumed that adaptive behavior is influenced by many dynamic and developmental processes. This complexity is daunting for investigators who aspire to causal explanations of resilience. Nonetheless, progress can be noted from more than four decades of research on resilience in development (Luthar, 2006; Masten et al., 2009). Diverse and numerous studies of young people show striking consistency in pointing to a set of fundamental protective factors for resilience, highlighted in the next section. Though the literature is more limited, studies of adult resilience support many of the same protective factors, as is evident in many chapters of this volume. These consistencies have implications for applications to promote resilience and also point to areas where additional research is needed.

Protective Systems over the Lifespan

Research on resilience in the early decades of life implicates a short list of protective

factors with compelling consistency, leading us to conclude that resilience is powered by basic human adaptive systems shaped through processes of biological and cultural evolution (Masten, 2001; Masten & Coatsworth, 1998; Masten & Obradović, 2008; Wright & Masten, 2005). These protective systems include individual capabilities, social supports and relationships, and protections embedded in religions, community, or other cultural systems. We also have argued that nurturing the healthy development of these protective systems affords the most important preparation or "inoculation" for overcoming potential threats and adversities in human development. Similarly, damage or destruction of these systems has dire consequences for the adaptive capacity of individuals.

In this section, we focus on six examples of important protective systems and consider their changing role in resilience over the lifespan. These include attachment relationships and social support; intelligence or problem-solving skills; self-regulation skills involved in directing or inhibiting attention, emotion, and action; agency, mastery motivation and self-efficacy; *meaning making* (constructing meaning and a sense of coherence in life); and cultural traditions, particularly as engaged through religion.

Attachment Relationships

Reviewing five decades of resilience research in child development, Luthar (2006, p. 780) concluded, "Resilience rests, fundamentally, on relationships." The importance of relationships for human resilience has been noted in every major review of resilience since the pioneers first began to identify protective factors for resilience (see Masten & Obradović, 2008). A powerful biological system is implicated in this work: the attachment system originally described by John Bowlby in three classic volumes on attachment and loss (1969) and later examined in many studies of attachment in human development (Ainsworth, 1989; Bowlby, 1982,

1988; Bretherton & Munholland, 1999; Sroufe, Carlson, Levy, & Egeland, 1999; Thompson, 2000). Attachment is a universal process in human development that appears first in infancy in relationships with caregivers and later in relationships with friends, romantic partners, and one's own children. Bowlby viewed attachment as a protective system that evolved to protect vulnerable young animals from danger and to promote exploration of the environment. Once an attachment bond has formed between a young child (usually by the second half of the first year after birth) and a primary caregiver, threats perceived by either the child or the caregiver will trigger attachment behaviors in the form of seeking proximity and contact, and other forms of reassurance. These behaviors are highly motivated, as evidenced by onset of extreme anxiety, fear, or panic when the child (or parent figure) is unable to connect with the attachment partner. When conditions are nonthreatening, the presence of an attachment figure provides a "secure base" for exploring the world, and facilitates the mastery motivation system (discussed below). Loss of the attachment figure can induce profound grief, even in very young children.

As children mature, they typically form attachment relationships with other people and also with objects, such as teddy bears, pets, and blankets. Initially, they form attachment bonds with caregivers and other people in caring roles, such as teachers. The quality of these early attachment relationships is believed to influence the development of later relationships with peers and romantic partners (Sroufe, 2005; Sroufe et al., 1999). As children grow older and attachment bonds form with close friends and romantic relationships, the secure base functions of attachment include more people, and the balance shifts from caregivers to peers (Laible, Carlo, & Raffaelli, 2000; Wilkinson, 2004). Peer attachment relationships are characterized by more equal balance in the protected–protector roles compared to those in parent–child relationships, a differ-

ence widely noted in the developmental literature. When they have their own children, individuals move into the protector role.

Developmental theorists have argued that the sensitivity and general quality of early caregiving contributes to secure attachment relationships and yields internal models of good relationships that are carried forward by the child into future attachments (Sroufe, 2005; Thompson, 2000). Sensitive caregiving also has regulatory functions, serving to increase or decrease arousal levels in young children, both moderating stress and stimulating children through play.

The protective role of effective parents extends well beyond emotional security and arousal regulation, however. Parents also nurture cognitive development in many ways (e.g., talking and reading to their children), socialize children on appropriate conduct (in school, the cultural contexts of the family, and society at large), choose schools, and promote activities or the development of talents. Parents also seek help for their children, anticipate dangers that lie ahead, and in other ways function as auxiliary problem solvers until children's own capabilities mature.

Consequently, the parent–child bond is one of the most powerful of all human attachments and serves as a singularly important protective factor. What happens when this important bond is ruptured, broken, or lost due to parental maltreatment or abandonment? Longitudinal studies of children exposed to the stress of childhood abuse and neglect clearly document deleterious consequences in terms of intrapsychic, interpersonal, and occupational function. But research also documents that one-fourth to one-half of children exposed to parental abuse and neglect show positive psychosocial functioning upon follow-up (Collishaw et al., 2007; Haskett, Nears, Ward, & McPherson, 2006; McGloin & Widom, 2001). What do we know about *why*, *how*, and *for whom* such continued good functioning or later recovery is possible? In their longitudinal study of children born on the Isle of Wight, Collishaw and colleagues (2007) found that although intelligence and gender were not associated with later resilience in children who had experienced maltreatment, a number of critical interpersonal relationships were predictive of later resilience. These included having at least one parent perceived as caring, maintaining positive peer relationships from childhood to adolescence, and stability of adult love relationships. Variations in the severity, duration, and context of the abuse were associated with increased risk of later difficulty. The findings highlight the importance of positive attachment relationships across the lifespan and stress the importance of considering cumulative trauma. More needs to be learned about the processes by which children who have been abused by their parents, or who have significant disturbances in early attachment relationships, develop the needed competencies to form supportive relationships with others outside the family. Early intervention with vulnerable children may be particularly important in helping to modify internal working models of the self as worthless, other people as abusive, and the world as threatening and dangerous (Cicchetti & Toth, 2005; Toth, Cicchetti, Macfie, & Emde, 1997; Wright, 2007; Wright, Crawford, & Del Castillo, 2009). Altering such models may be an important key to facilitating positive connections with others that serve to support resilience.

Agency and the Mastery Motivation System

Another powerful system for adaptation was identified by Robert White (1959) in his classic work on competence motivation. He observed that humans (as well as closely related species, e.g., primates) are motivated to adapt to the environment and experience pleasure when they are successful, a process he termed *effectance motivation*. Perceived agency ("I did this") appears to play a substantial role in this system, with increasing importance as the sense of self develops. The joy in agency manifested in adaptive success

and competence can be observed in young children just learning to walk on their own, and in surgeons or athletes doing what they do best at the height of their skill.

Humans, more so than other species, develop the capacity to direct their own lives, to plan and manage their behavior in seeking mastery. Albert Bandura (1997) elaborated on human capabilities for agency and attendant pleasure in mastery in his concept of self-efficacy, while other scholars have emphasized the importance of intrinsic motivation (Ryan & Deci, 2000). Bandura demonstrated in his research that individuals with a more positive view of their own effectiveness exert more effort to succeed. They also are motivated to persist in the face of difficulty or failure, which makes them more likely to succeed under adverse conditions.

Teachers and employers are well-acquainted with the importance of mastery motivation for learning and performance. As people age, it is interesting to consider how pleasure in mastery may change with the ebbing of talents and skills. Erikson's concept of generativity may reflect such maturational change, in that individuals begin to experience pleasure in the mastery and accomplishments of children or others they mentor, rather than their own.

In studies of turnaround cases of resilience, mastery motivation has been implicated as a key initiating system. Some young people who are in trouble during adolescence, but who manifest resilience in adulthood, recognize first that they need to do something different, expressing motivation and goals to turn their lives in a new direction before they begin to take active steps in a new direction, often with the help of mentors (Hauser, Allen, & Golden, 2006; Masten, Obradović, & Burt, 2006).

This system probably can be damaged, shut down, or hindered by neglect and adversity that removes control or undermines agency experiences in development. The apathy observed among neglected infants in orphanages (Zeanah, Smyke, & Settles, 2006) and animals in learned helplessness experiments (e.g., Seligman & Beagley, 1975) illustrates what can happen to this powerful engine for learning and adaptation when circumstances rob individuals of control over their environments and opportunities to experience agency. Mental illness (e.g., major depression) and physical illness or decline also may undermine this system.

Intelligence

Many studies across the lifespan report that problem-solving skills, often measured by traditional "IQ" tests predict good adaptation under adversity. This is not surprising when one considers that these tests were designed to measure the cognitive skills associated with good adaptation in major developmental tasks, such as learning in school or functioning in work and in military service (Masten, Burt, & Coatsworth, 2006).

Intelligent behavior develops as the brain develops and the individual learns through experience. Healthy brain development, essential for the development of normal intelligence, requires many forms of nurturing, including nutrition, stimulation, discipline, and opportunities to learn. Education is important for learning and honing the intelligent behaviors required for success in developmental tasks of a given society. Parents, teachers, and many other adults play a role in the development of the central nervous system and the intellectual skills that afford good problem solving under normal and adverse conditions. Relationships with peers also have a role through play, stimulation, modeling, mutual encouragement, and other kinds of interactions.

Resilience does not require extraordinary intelligence in most cases, but rather the operations of a human brain in "good working order" and access to knowledge about what is happening, what to expect, and what to do. As people mature, their intellectual tools generally mature and improve. Current research on the development of executive functions in relation to brain development (Rothbart, Sheese, & Posner, 2007) is illu-

minating the processes involved in specific aspects of intelligent behavior, such as reflection, planning, and inhibiting a prepotent response. Advances in executive function skills make it increasingly possible to direct attention and action strategically, to wait in the interests of a superordinate goal, to delay gratification, and to decide what to do with longer-term objectives in mind. Executive functions are strongly implicated in the capacity of humans to control their own behavior and emotions, another key domain of adaptive skills for resilience.

Higher thinking abilities may not always be positive. Sometimes, as noted earlier, less understanding of a situation is protective, as can be seen for infants compared to adolescents in war zones (Pine, Costello, & Masten, 2005). Reports in the literature also suggest that more intelligent people may be more sensitive to certain kinds of adversity, such as pressure to be successful or existential issues that are not suffered by less cognitively sophisticated peers (Luthar, 2006). Similarly, findings have been mixed in regard to intelligence in studies examining resilience following child maltreatment. Three recent longitudinal studies (Collishaw et al., 2007; DuMont, Widom, & Czaja, 2007; Jaffee, Caspi, Moffitt, Polo-Tomas, & Taylor, 2007) reported no association between IQ and later resilience, although researchers in other areas of adversity have found positive associations. This suggests that although cognitive abilities reflect information processing (and related brain maturation) that is generally helpful for adaptation across multiple domains, better intellectual skills may not always play a protective role for all kinds of adversity, particularly for trauma that is relational in nature.

Self-Regulation

Agency requires the capacity to control one's own behavior, and the systems that make it possible to regulate attention, arousal, emotion and action in the service of voluntary goals have been widely implicated in resilience research (Masten & Coatsworth, 1998). Concepts of self-regulation in the service of adaptation have old roots in psychology, including the concept of ego functions in psychoanalytic theory (Masten, Burt, & Coatsworth, 2006). In contemporary developmental science, this group of self-regulation skills often is described by the umbrella concept of *executive functions* (EFs) that depend on neural circuitry concentrated in the frontal regions of the human brain (Rothbart et al., 2007). EFs include working memory, selective attention, inhibiting a dominant response in favor of a more adaptive response, delay of gratification, and related self-control capabilities that develop in tandem with brain maturation.

Attention and concentration skills, as well as self-control of emotions and behavior, have been linked to a wide array of indicators of both good and poor adaptation across multiple domains and diverse contexts, under low risk conditions, and particularly under high-risk conditions. EF skills are implicated for school readiness and school success, as well as social competence (Blair, 2002; Eisenberg, Champion, & Vaughn, 2007; Rueda, Posner, & Rothbart, 2004). An experiment to promote EF skills in high-risk preschoolers through the Tools of the Mind curriculum showed very promising results as a strategy for promoting resilience (Diamond et al., 2007). Stress reactivity, temperamental irritability, and the inability to regulate impulses predict many difficulties, including antisocial behavior problems (Rothbart & Bates, 2006).

Effective parenting, sensitive to individual differences in temperament and personality, is strongly implicated as an important protective influence for helping young, reactive children become well-regulated children (Kochanska & Knaack, 2003). More generally, in developmental theory on attachment, self-regulation capacity grows out of dyadic regulation provided by the caregiving/attachment system. When an attachment relationship is working well, both the relationship and the behavior of the caregiver can serve as regulatory functions for the infant until the child develops the capacity to self-regulate (Sroufe, 1996). Conversely, if caregiving is unresponsive, chaotic, and insecure, leaving an infant frequently dysregulated, the development of self-regulatory capacity in the child may be gravely affected.

Self-control of behavior in response to expectations of socializing adults, often in the form of compliance to parental directives and family routines, normally emerges early in development, during the toddler years. Eventually, children are expected to comply in the absence of the supervising adults, a form of maturation often described as *internalization*. Children's failure to develop behavioral self-regulation skills by the time they begin school can have serious and cascading repercussions for success in school and with peers, as noted by Patterson and colleagues in their pioneering work on the development of antisocial behavior and its consequences for academic and social competence, as well as internalizing problems (Patterson & Capaldi, 1990; Patterson et al., 1992). Consequently, prevention efforts directed at antisocial behavior problems now focus on helping families and children with parenting, routines, and behaviors that foster good self-control skills and compliance in young children.

The concepts of EF and self-regulation encompass a broad array of skills and behaviors that emerge and mature over the life course. Human capacities for reflection, planning, and delay of gratification show a developmental course and also individual differences. This array of skills is broadly and strongly associated with competence and resilience in childhood, adolescence, and adulthood. This is not surprising given that adaptation in general and success in overcoming adversity often require control of emotions, arousal, and impulses to evaluate information, determine a good course of action, coordinate actions, and solve problems that arise. Aging and disease may affect self-regulation capacity in ways that hinder competent function and resilience.

Developmental evidence on self-regulation capacity, particularly in relation to the development of EF that accompanies brain maturation, suggests that there are windows of opportunity for intervention. When these systems are undergoing rapid change, they show plasticity in response to experience. One such window appears to be the preschool years, when the development of EF skills needed for early school success is normally occurring. Another window of growth and change appears to occur during the transition to adulthood, when myelination of the prefrontal cortext and other advances in brain function appear to facilitate capacity for planning ahead, considering alternatives, and evaluating one's life direction, resulting in better decisions and judgment (Dahl & Spear, 2004; Masten, Obradović, & Burt, 2006).

Meaning Making

In numerous accounts, resilient individuals report that faith and hope played a key role in sustaining them through great adversity. In younger people, these beliefs are described in terms of optimism that life will improve, or trust in family or a spiritual figure to make things better again. In the classic Kauai Study, Werner and Smith (1982) noted that the resilient group expressed optimism and hope for the future, and a deeply held conviction that life has meaning. Older youth and adults under great stress have reported feelings of transcendent hope and meaning that kept them going, sometimes experienced as an epiphany. In *Man's Search for Meaning*, Victor Frankl (1946/1984) described the power of meaning for human life in the face of overwhelming suffering in his account of daily life in a Nazi concentration camp. In the harrowing and inspirational account of the life of a teenager who endured the atrocities of the Pol Pot regime, a young Cambodian woman described her sudden transformation from the depths of despair to hope as she watched a beautiful sunrise and realized that the Khmer Rouge did not control nature or the meaning of her life (Criddle & Butt Mam, 1987).

The belief that life has meaning, faith, hope for a better future or afterlife, and related convictions and attitudes appear to sustain mastery motivation and efforts to adapt or survive in the context of extreme adversity. Through the experience of coping with the aftermath of a traumatic event, many survivors report that they gain in wisdom, compassion for others, and personal strength. Survivors report a stronger religious faith, spiritual growth, and a desire to help and support others who are suffering (Tedeschi & Calhoun, 1995). Construing benefits to the self from having learned to cope with a particular trauma (e.g., "seeing the silver lining") is an important way that trauma survivors change their perspective on their traumatic experience, and it has been linked with better long-term outcomes. Other types of perceived benefits include seeing new possibilities for one's life, improvement in social relationships, learning to appreciate life, and acquiring personal strength and the ability to endure (Tedeschi & Calhoun, 1995; Wright, Crawford, & Sebastian, 2007).

However, one of the most devastating effects of traumatic experiences is the shattering of fundamental belief systems—that the world is meaningful and just, that terrible things do not happen to good people, and that individuals have control over what happens to them in their life (Janoff-Bulman, 1992). Rebuilding these shattered assumptions seems particularly difficult when the trauma involves betrayal of trust, such as sexual abuse by a parent or religious figure (Janoff-Bulman & Frantz, 1997; Wright et al., 2007). Studies of survivors of child sexual abuse reveal that many individuals are unable to find meaning in such an experience, or, if they find meaning, it is predominantly negative. While adaptation is better for those who are able to find some meaning, a prolonged and unsuccessful search for meaning has been linked with poorer adjustment (Silver, Boon, & Stones, 1983; Wright et al., 2007).

These existential beliefs and the cognitive restructuring involved in meaning making and benefit finding require considerable capacity for thinking and reflection. Therefore, they are likely to be more important as people grow older. Young children do not have the cognitive capacity to engage this kind of system. Meaning-making systems of belief are embedded in many cultures and religions (discussed in the following section), but individuals appear to be capable of generating such sustaining ideas, independent of more organized belief systems. Finally, while meaning making and benefit finding have the potential to influence adaptation following trauma in a positive way, the evidence supporting this link is limited. Research in this area (and that of posttraumatic growth more generally) also points to less adaptive potential for self-enhancing appraisals or positive illusions. Such illusory attempts to avoid the negative impact of the trauma might not foster active coping (Zoellner & Maercker, 2006). Future research needs to explore both constructive and illusory efforts to disentangle these potentially contradictory effects.

Cultural Traditions and Religion

Cultures and religions have developed and transmitted many beliefs, rituals, and practices to help people deal with expected and unexpected adversities, including rituals for loss and mourning, prayers and meditation strategies, direct assistance to those in need, and beliefs that convey the value and meaning of human life (Crawford, Wright, & Masten, 2006). The protective practices and processes embedded in cultures and religions have seen limited research with respect to resilience, although this is changing.

Crawford and colleagues (2006) proposed that cultural systems, including religions, may work by engaging the fundamental adaptive systems implicated at the individual level in resilience research, including attachment, self-regulation and meaning making. Prayer and meditation practices, for example,

may support self-regulation of arousal and emotion in protective ways, while relationships with God and other spiritual figures may provide feelings of security and comfort comparable to the secure-base functions of a positive parent–child attachment relationship. Religions also actively nourish faith and teach systems of meaning in age-sensitive ways from childhood through adulthood. Finally, religious affiliation also provides an opportunity for community engagement that can provide tremendous support during times of stress, loss, and bereavement. The potential for emotional, spiritual, and physical care embodied in a faith community can be a powerful source of protection and direct assistance in times of need.

There is growing interest in the ways that cultures may promote or protect development, in cultural similarities and differences in the nature and function of protective factors around the world, and also in deeper examination of connections between acculturation processes and resilience among immigrant groups or within multicultural societies (Masten & Motti-Stefanidi, 2009). Research in the early waves of resilience research was heavily weighted toward economically advanced nations and majority cultural or ethnic groups, although there has always been interest in resilience among cultural or ethnic minorities (Luthar, 2006; Spencer et al., 2006). Some of the classic studies of resilience highlighted cultural features of protective factors in distinct communities (e.g., the Children of Kauai; Werner & Smith, 1982, 1992). With increasingly large numbers of people around the world migrating and interacting across national and cultural boundaries, there also is growing interest in the consequences of migration and acculturation for risks and adaptation in human development. The dynamics of culture and migration are undoubtedly also changing the expectations of individuals, their parents, and their communities with respect to developmental tasks and goals, which inevitably serve to transform the definitions and assessment of resilience. Moreover, immigrant youth often face the challenge of meeting developmental task expectations of multiple cultures at the same time, with the possibility of conflicting expectations in the family, the school, and the community (Berry, Phinney, Sam, & Vedder, 2006). There is likely to be much greater attention in future research on the role of cultural processes in resilience.

Resilience-Based Frameworks for Practice

From the outset, the investigators who studied resilience had a practical goal: to improve the odds of positive outcomes and reduce the suffering among people at risk due to adverse circumstances and vulnerabilities. Experimental research on resilience-based programs and interventions is still limited, but there are clear signs of progress in realizing this overarching objective in resilience science.

Many conferences, special issues, and volumes published in recent years provide evidence that a transformation has occurred in the way goals, methods, interventions, and outcomes are conceptualized, illustrating a major shift of models and programs toward positive and strengths-based models in multiple disciplines. Examples include the Looking After Children reform movement in child welfare (Flynn, Dudding, & Barber, 2006); the Strength-Based School Counseling movement (Akos & Galassi, 2008); the positive psychology renaissance (Seligman & Csikszentmihalyi, 2000; Snyder & Lopez, 2009); the promotion of wellness, competence, and resilience in prevention science (Cicchetti, Rappaport, Sandler, & Weissberg, 2000; Greenberg, 2006); the Positive Youth Development movement (Lerner & Benson, 2003; Lerner, Dowling, & Anderson, 2003); models of resilience and recovery in psychiatry (Beardslee et al., 1997; Bonanno, 2004; Wortman & Silver, 1989); and applications of resilience models in multidisciplinary disaster planning and response (Gewirtz, Forgatch, & Weiling, 2008; Longstaff & Yang, 2008; Masten & Obradović, 2008).

Fundamental Components of a Resilience-Based Framework for Practice

Resilience-oriented models can be applied to the promotion of competence in high-risk children, the prevention of psychopathology, interventions in clinics or schools, and also in planning for disaster response. These models clearly will vary in many ways, yet there are commonalities in the broad frameworks underlying many of these efforts that appear to reflect basic components of resilience-based frameworks for practice (Luther & Cicchetti, 2000; Masten, 2006b; Masten, Herbers, Cutuli, & Lafavor, 2008; Masten & Powell, 2003; Nation et al., 2003). These fundamental components include positive missions, models, measures, and methods, or what might be viewed as the "four M's" of a resilience-based approach (Masten & Powell, 2003).

Positive Mission: Framing Positive Objectives

One of the most basic lessons gleaned from the resilience literature, and particularly from efforts to shift intervention programs to positive models, is the observation that a focus on promoting positive goals and outcomes has many benefits. These benefits include broad appeal to stakeholders, improved morale and motivation among staff, greater effectiveness in reducing problems than a goal focused narrowly on deficits or problems, and greater attention to both the measurement and achievement of positive change.

Models: Including Positive Resources, Influences, and Outcomes

One of the striking features of resilience-based interventions and programs is the nature of the explicit and implicit models underlying the design of the program or practices. In contrast to medical models of disease and deficit-based models, resilience-based models include positive predictors, processes, and outcomes. For example, models for prevention of psychopathology now often include assets or promotive factors, as well as risk factors; protective factors or processes, as well as vulnerabilities; and positive outcomes, such as competence in age-salient developmental tasks, as well as the problem or disorder targeted for prevention (Masten, Burt, & Coatsworth, 2006). The Seattle Social Development Project, which targeted improved school bonding and positive engagement in a successful effort to prevent antisocial behavior, also resulted in a number of other positive outcomes in additional domains of adaptive behavior during adolescence and early adulthood (Hawkins et al., 1999; Hawkins, Kosterman, Catalano, Hill, & Abbott, 2005). Prevention efforts for families have targeted positive parenting as a means to better outcomes in their children, including successful prevention experiments with families undergoing divorce (Forgatch & DeGarmo, 1999; Wolchik et al., 2002), families with high-risk toddlers whose mothers have a major depressive disorder (Toth, Rogosch, Cicchetti, & Manly, 2006), and efforts to reduce behavior problems in very low-income families (Dishion et al., 2008). Recent efforts to address educational achievement disparities in disadvantaged children have targeted improvements in EF skills (Diamond et al., 2007; Greenberg, 2006).

Measuring Positive Resources, Processes, and Outcomes

Positive goals and models focus considerable attention on measuring positive aspects of a person's behavior and life situation, often in addition to assessments of risks, symptoms, and disorder. Basic research on resilience required extensive development of tools to assess positive aspects of life, long-neglected in clinical fields focused on problems and risks. Concomitantly, however, scholars and practitioners in applied disciplines developed new tools, better suited to the positive goals and models emerging in various fields. In the child welfare reform effort known as

Looking After Children, initially developed in Great Britain and later adopted in dozens of other countries, it was important to assess progress in the "seven developmental dimensions of well-being" across the course of development from childhood into early adulthood. This led to development of a comprehensive set of measures known as the Assessment and Action Record (see Flynn et al., 2006).

Methods to Promote Resilience

Models of resilience typically include risk factors or conditions that threaten positive function or development, assets or resources that promote good outcomes at most levels of risk, and protective factors or processes that are particularly effective. Such models suggest that there are several basic strategies for intervention: reducing risk (e.g., prenatal care to prevent premature birth, removing landmines to prevent injuries to a population), increasing assets or resources (e.g., provision of food programs, employment counselors), and mobilizing powerful protective systems (e.g., improving the effectiveness of parents, nurturing mentor relationships, empowering the leaderships of young people in rebuilding a community after disaster or war). In addition, models of resilience have underscored the embedded nature of human life and development (Masten & Obradović, 2007). There are many interacting systems that play a role in human development and resilience during or following threatening experiences and, as a consequence, many systems and levels in which assets and protective processes can be considered and targeted to boost the odds for resilience. These systems include family, school and work, religious and other cultural contexts, community organizations, and both governmental and nongovernmental organizations. Coordinated interventions may be important. In any event, there are so many potential possibilities that strategic focus may be crucial for balancing effectiveness and cost. There is growing interest in research on strategic best practices, or knowing when to do what for whom to achieve the greatest benefit for cost.

Building a Better Evidence Base on What Works

The promise of research for improving practice and policies to foster resilience is gradually being realized, but there is much work yet to be done. Research is needed on prevention and intervention strategies that are tailored to the individual, cultural, and contextual differences. There are hints about strategic intervention windows, but there is much to be learned about timing for greatest effect and efficiency. Societies have a great stake in turning lives around toward resilience, but there is little research to guide their efforts to facilitate such change, particularly in regard to turning around the life course in adulthood. Moreover, many organizations play a role in successful development across the life course, ranging from schools to work organizations and religions, and there is much to be learned about the roles of these systems in lifelong resilience. Finally, all societies could benefit from knowledge to improve positive adaptation among individuals as the population ages, and also to prepare populations for resilience in the face of major disasters.

Conclusion

Research on resilience stands at an exciting new threshold as the fourth wave rises (Masten, 2007). Breakthroughs in methodology and knowledge are opening new horizons for understanding how resilience works, and how to nurture resilience in people of all ages and diverse cultural situations. The first three waves of research, although heavily concentrated in the early decades of the lifespan, as well as more economically advantaged groups or societies, offer a wealth of ideas, strategies, models, and findings to guide the burgeoning science about resilience across the lifespan and in diverse cultural contexts. Most importantly, the early

waves of resilience underscore the profound importance of a developmental perspective on resilience, from the beginning to the end of life.

Acknowledgments

Preparation of this chapter was supported in part by a grant to Ann S. Masten from the National Science Foundation (NSF Grant No. 0745643) and a research leave to Margaret O'Dougherty Wright from Miami University. Any opinions, conclusions, or recommendations expressed in this chapter are those of the authors and do not necessarily reflect the views of NSF.

References

Ainsworth, M. D. S. (1989). Attachments beyond infancy. *American Psychologist, 44,* 709–716.

Akos, P., & Galassi, J. P. (2008). Special issue: Strengths-Based School Counseling. *Professional School Counseling, 12.*

Bandura, A. (1997). *Self-efficacy: The exercise of control.* New York: Freeman.

Beardslee, W. R., Salt, P., Versage, E. M., Gladstone, T. R. G., Wright, E., & Rothberg, P. C. (1997). Sustained change in parents receiving preventive interventions for families with depression. *American Journal of Psychiatry, 154,* 510–515.

Beckett, C., Maughan, B., Rutter, M., Castle, J., Colvert, E., Groothues, C., et al. (2006). Do the effects of early severe deprivation on cognition persist into early adolescence?: Findings from the English and Romanian Adoptees Study. *Child Development, 77,* 696–711.

Belsky, J., & Bakermans-Kranenburg, M. J., & van IJzendoorn, M. H. (2007). For better and for worse: Differential susceptibility to environmental influences. *Current Directions in Psychological Science, 16,* 300–304.

Berry, J. W., Phinney, J. S., Sam, D. L., & Vedder, V. (2006). *Immigrant youth in cultural transition: Acculturation, identity and adaptation across national contexts.* Mahwah, NJ: Erlbaum.

Blair, C. (2002). School readiness: Integrating cognition and emotion in a neurobiological conceptualization of children's functioning at school entry. *American Psychologist, 57,* 111–127.

Bonanno, G. A. (2004). Loss, trauma, and human resilience: Have we under-estimated the human capacity to thrive after extremely aversive events? *American Psychologist, 59,* 20–28.

Bowlby, J. (1969). *Attachment and loss.* New York: Basic Books.

Bowlby, J. (1982). *Attachment and loss: Vol. 1. Attachment* (2nd ed.). New York: Basic Books.

Bowlby, J. (1988). *A secure base: Clinical applications of attachment theory.* London: Routledge.

Boyce, W. T., & Ellis, B. J. (2005). Biological sensitivity to context: A. An evolutionary-developmental theory of the origins and functions of stress reactivity. *Development and Psychopathology, 17,* 271–301.

Bretherton, I., & Munholland, K. A. (1999). Internal working models in attachment relationships: A construct revisited. In J. Cassidy & P. R. Shaver (Eds.), *Handbook of attachment: Theory, research, and clinical applications* (pp. 89–111). New York: Guilford Press.

Burt, K. B., Obradović, J., Long, J. D., & Masten, A. S. (2008). The interplay of social competence and psychopathology over 20 years: Testing transactional and cascade models. *Child Development, 79,* 359–374.

Cicchetti, D. (2006). Development and psychopathology. In D. Cicchetti & D. Cohen (Eds.), *Developmental psychopathology: Vol. 1. Theory and method* (2nd ed., pp. 1–23). Hoboken, NJ: Wiley.

Cicchetti, D., & Curtis, W. J. (2006). The developing brain and neural plasticity: Implications for normality, psychopathology, and resilience. In D. Cicchetti & D. J. Cohen (Eds.), *Developmental psychopathology: Vol. 2. Developmental neuroscience* (2nd ed., pp. 1–64). Hoboken, NJ: Wiley.

Cicchetti, D., & Curtis, W. J. (Eds.). (2007). Special issue: A multilevel approach to resilience. *Development and Psychopathology, 19*(3).

Cicchetti, D., Rappaport, J., Sandler, I., & Weissberg, R. P. (Eds.). (2000). *The promotion of wellness in children and adolescents.* Washington, DC: Child Welfare League of America Press.

Cicchetti, D., & Toth, S. L. (2005). Child mal-

treatment. *Annual Review of Clinical Psychology, 1,* 409–438.

Collishaw, S., Pickles, A., Messer, J., Rutter, M., Shearer, C., & Maugham, B. (2007). Resilience to adult psychopathology following childhood maltreatment: Evidence from a community sample. *Child Abuse and Neglect, 31,* 211–229.

Cowen, E. L., Wyman, P. A., Work, W. C., Kim, J. Y., Fagen, D. B., & Magnus, B. B. (1997). Follow-up study of young stress-affected and stress-resilient urban children. *Development and Psychopathology, 9,* 565–577.

Cowen, E. L., Wyman, P. A., Work, W. C., & Parker, G. R. (1990). The Rochester Child Resilience Project: Overview and summary of first year findings. *Development and Psychopathology, 2,* 193–212.

Crawford, E., Wright, M. O. D., & Masten, A. S. (2006). Resilience and spirituality in youth. In P. L. Benson, E. C. Roehlkepartain, P. E. King, & L. Wagener (Eds.), *The handbook of spiritual development in childhood and adolescence* (pp. 355–370). Thousand Oaks, CA: Sage.

Criddle, J. D., & Butt Mam, T. (1987). *To destroy you is no loss.* New York: Doubleday.

Dahl, R. E., & Spear, L. P. (Eds.). (2004). *Adolescent brain development: Vulnerabilities and opportunities* (Vol. 1021). New York: New York Academy of Sciences.

Depp, C. A., & Jeste, D. V. (2006). Definitions and predictors of successful aging: A comprehensive review of larger quantitative studies. *American Journal of Geriatric Psychiatry, 14,* 1064–7481.

Diamond, A., Barnett, W. S., Thomas, J., & Munro, S. (2007). Preschool program improves cognitive control. *Science, 318,* 1387–1388.

DiRago, A. C., & Vaillant, G. E. (2007). Resilience in inner city youth: Childhood predictors of occupational status across the lifespan. *Journal of Youth and Adolescence, 36,* 61–70.

Dishion, T. J., Shaw, D., Connell, A., Gardner, F., Weaver, C., & Wilson, M. (2008). The Family Check-Up with high-risk indigent families: Preventing problem behavior by increasing parents' positive behavior support in early childhood. *Child Development, 79,* 1395–1414.

DuMont, K. A., Widom, C. S., & Czaja, S. J. (2007). Predictors of resilience in abused and neglected children grown-up: The role of individual and neighborhood characteristics. *Child Abuse and Neglect, 31*, 255–274.

Eisenberg, N., Champion, C., & Vaughan, J. (2007). Effortful control and its socioemotional consequences. In J. J. Gross (Ed.), *Handbook of emotion regulation* (pp. 287–306). New York: Guilford Press.

Elder, G. H. (1974). *Children of the great depression*. Chicago: University of Chicago Press.

Elder, G. H. (1998). The life course as developmental theory. *Child Development, 69*, 1–12.

Ellis, B. J., & Boyce, W. T. (2008). Biological sensitivity to context. *Current Directions in Psychological Science, 17*, 183–187.

Erikson, E. H. (1959). Identity and the life cycle. *Psychological Issues, 1*(1).

Erikson, E. H. (1963). *Childhood and society* (2nd ed.). New York: Norton.

Flynn, R. J., Dudding, P. M., & Barber, J. G. (Eds.). (2006). *Promoting resilience in development: A general framework for systems of care*. Ottawa, ON, Canada: University of Ottawa Press.

Forgatch, M. S., & DeGarmo, D. S. (1999). Parenting through change: An effective prevention program for single mothers. *Journal of Consulting and Clinical Psychology, 67*, 711–724.

Frankl, V. E. (1984). *Man's search for meaning*. New York: Washington Square Press. (Original work published 1946)

Garmezy, N., Masten, A. S., & Tellegen, A. (1984). The study of stress and competence in children: A building block for developmental psychology. *Child Development, 55*, 97–111.

Gewirtz, A., Forgatch, M., & Weiling, E. (2008). Parenting practices as potential mechanisms for child adjustment following mass trauma. *Journal of Marital and Family Therapy, 34*, 177–192.

Greenberg, M. T. (2006). Promoting resilience in children and youth: Preventive interventions and their interface with neuroscience. *Annals of the New York Academy of Sciences, 1094*, 139–150.

Greve, W., & Staudinger, U. M. (2006). Resilience in later adulthood and old age: resources and potential for successful aging. In D. Cicchetti & D. Cohen (Eds.), *Developmental psychopathology: Vol. 3. Risk, disorder and psychopathology* (2nd ed., 796–840). New York: Wiley.

Hart, B., & Risley, T. R. (1995). *Meaningful dif-ferences in the everyday experiences of young American children*. Baltimore: Brookes.

Haskett, M. E., Nears, K., Ward, C. S., & McPherson, A. V. (2006). Diversity in adjustment of maltreated children: Factors associated with resilient functioning. *Clinical Psychology Review, 26*, 796–812.

Hauser, S. T., Allen, J. P., & Golden, E. (2006) *Out of the woods: Tales of resilient teens*. Cambridge, MA: Harvard University Press.

Havighurst, R. J. (1972). *Developmental tasks and education* (3rd ed.). New York: McKay.

Hawkins, J. D., Catalano, R. F., Kosterman, R., Abbott, R. D., & Hill, K. G. (1999). Preventing adolescent health-risk behavior by strengthening protection during childhood. *Archives of Pediatrics and Adolescent Medicine, 153*, 226–234.

Hawkins, J. D., Kosterman, R., Catalano, R. F., Hill, K. G., & Abbott, R. D. (2005). Promoting positive adult functioning through social development intervention in childhood: Long-term effects from the Seattle Social Development Project. *Archives of Pediatrics and Adolescent Medicine, 159*, 25–31.

Heckman, J. J. (2006). Skill formation and the economics of investing in disadvantaged children. *Science, 312*, 1900–1902.

Jaffee, S. R., Caspi, A., Moffitt, T. E., Polo-Tomas, M., & Taylor, A. (2007). Individual, family and neighborhood factors distinguish resilient from non-resilient maltreated children: A cumulative stressors model. *Child Abuse and Neglect, 31*, 231–253.

Janoff-Bulman, R. (1992). *Shattered assumptions*. New York: Free Press.

Janoff-Bulman, R., & Frantz, C. M. (1997). The impact of trauma on meaning: From meaningless world to meaningful life. In M. Power & C. R. Brewin (Eds.), *The transformation of meaning in psychological therapies* (pp. 75–89). New York: Wiley.

Kim-Cohen, J., & Gold, A. L. (2009). Measured gene–environment interactions and mechanisms promoting resilient development. *Current Directions in Psychological Science, 18*, 138–142.

Kochanska, G., & Knaack, A. (2003). Effortful control as a personality characteristic of young children: Antecedents, correlates, and consequences. *Journal of Personality, 71*, 1087–1112.

Kohlberg, L., LaCrosse, J., & Ricks, D. (1972). The predictability of adult mental health from childhood behavior. In B. B. Wolman (Eds.), *Manual of child psychopathology* (pp. 1217–1284). New York: McGraw-Hill.

Kraemer, H. C., Kazdin, A. E., Offord, D., Kessler, R. C., Jensen, P. S., & Kupfer, D. (1997). Coming to terms with the terms of risk. *Archives of General Psychiatry, 54*, 337–343.

Laible, D. J., Carlo, G., & Raffaelli, M. (2000). The differential relations of parent and peer attachment to adolescent adjustment. *Journal of Youth and Adolescence, 29*, 45–59.

Lerner, R. M., & Benson, P. L. (Eds.). (2003). *Developmental assets and asset-building communities: Implications for research, policy, and practice.* New York: Kluwer Academic/Plenum Press.

Lerner, R. M., Dowling, E. M., & Anderson, P. M. (2003). Positive youth development: Thriving as a basis of personal and civil society. *Applied Developmental Science, 7*, 172–180.

Linley, P. A., & Joseph, S. (2004). Positive change following trauma and adversity: A review. *Journal of Traumatic Stress, 17*, 11–21.

Longstaff, P. H., & Yang, S. (2008). Communication management and trust: Their role in building resilience to "surprises" such as natural disasters, pandemic flu, and terrorism. *Ecology and Society, 13*(1), 3. Available at *www.ecologyandsociety.org/vol13/iss1/art3.*

Luthar, S., Cicchetti, D., & Becker, B. (2000). The construct of resilience: A critical evaluation and guidelines for future work. *Child Development, 71*(3), 543–562.

Luthar, S. S. (2006). Resilience in development: A synthesis of research across five decades. In D. Cicchetti & D. J. Cohen (Eds.), *Developmental psychopathology: Vol. 3. Risk, disorder, and adaptation* (2nd ed., pp. 739–795). New York: Wiley.

Luthar, S. S., & Cicchetti, D. (2000). The construct of resilience: Implications for interventions and social policies. *Development and Psychopathology, 12*, 857–885.

Masten, A. S. (1989). Resilience in development: Implications of the study of successful adaptation for developmental psychopathology. In D. Cicchetti (Ed.), *The emergence of a discipline: Rochester Symposium on Developmental Psychopathology* (Vol. 1, pp. 261–294). Hillsdale, NJ: Erlbaum.

Masten, A. S. (2001). Ordinary magic: Resilience processes in development. *American Psychologist, 56*(3), 227–238.

Masten, A. S. (2006a). Developmental psychopathology: Pathways to the future. *International Journal of Behavioral Development, 31*, 47–54.

Masten, A. S. (2006b). Promoting resilience in development: A general framework for systems of care. In R. J. Flynn, P. M. Dudding, & J. G. Barber (Eds.), *Promoting resilience in child welfare* (pp. 3–17). Ottawa, ON, Canada: University of Ottawa Press.

Masten, A. S. (2007). Resilience in developing systems: Progress and promise as the fourth wave rises. *Development and Psychopathology, 19*, 921–930.

Masten, A. S., Burt, K. B., & Coatsworth, J. D. (2006). Competence and psychopathology in development. In D. Cicchetti & D. Cohen (Eds.), *Developmental psychopathology: Vol. 3. Risk, disorder and psychopathology* (2nd ed., pp. 696–738). New York: Wiley.

Masten, A. S., & Coatsworth, J. D. (1998). The development of competence in favorable and unfavorable environments: Lessons from research on successful children. *American Psychologist, 53*(2), 205–220.

Masten, A. S., Cutuli, J. J., Herbers, J. E., & Reed, M.-G. J. (2009). Resilience in development. In C. R. Snyder & S. J. Lopez (Eds.), *The handbook of positive psychology* (2nd ed., pp. 117–131). New York: Oxford University Press.

Masten, A. S., Garmezy, N., Tellegen, A., Pellegrini, D. S., Larkin, K., & Larsen, A. (1988). Competence and stress in school children: The moderating effects of individual and family qualities. *Journal of Child Psychology and Psychiatry, 29*(6), 745–764.

Masten, A. S., Herbers, J. E., Cutuli, J. J., & Lafavor, T. L. (2008). Promoting competence and resilience in the school context. *Professional School Counseling, 12*, 76–84.

Masten, A. S., Hubbard, J. J., Gest, S. D., Tellegen, A., Garmezy, N., & Ramirez, M. L. (1999). Competence in the context of adversity: Pathways to resilience and maladaptation from childhood to late adolescence. *Development and Psychopathology, 11*, 143–169.

Masten, A. S., & Motti-Stefanidi, F. (2009). Understanding and promoting resilience in children: Promotive and protective processes in schools. In T. B. Gutkin & C. R. Reynolds

(Eds.), *The handbook of school psychology* (4th ed., pp. 721–738). New York: Wiley.

Masten, A. S., & Obradović, J. (2006). Competence and resilience in development. *Annals of the New York Academy of Sciences, 1094,* 13–27.

Masten, A. S., & Obradović, J. (2008). Disaster preparation and recovery: Lessons from research on resilience in human development. *Ecology and Society, 13*(1), 9. Available online at *www.ecologyandsociety.org/vol13/iss1/art9.*

Masten, A. S., Obradović, J., & Burt, K. B. (2006). Resilience in emerging adulthood: Developmental perspectives on continuity and transformation. In J. J. Arnett & J. L. Tanner (Eds.), *Emerging adults in America: Coming of age in the 21st century* (pp. 173–190). Washington, DC: American Psychological Association Press.

Masten, A. S., & Powell, J. L. (2003). A resilience framework for research, policy, and practice. In S. S. Luthar (Ed.), *Resilience and vulnerabilities: Adaptation in the context of childhood adversities* (pp. 1–25). New York: Cambridge University Press.

Masten, A. S., Roisman, G. I., Long, J. D., Burt, K. B., Obradović, J., Riley, J. R., et al. (2005). Developmental cascades: Linking academic achievement, externalizing and internalizing symptoms over 20 years. *Developmental Psychology, 41,* 733–746.

McGloin, J. M., & Widom, C. S. (2001). Resilience among abused and neglected children grown up. *Development and Psychopathology, 13,* 1021–1038.

Nation, M., Crusto, C., Wandersman, A., Kumpfer, K. L., Seybolt, D., Morrissey-Kane, E., et al. (2003). What works in prevention: Principles of effective prevention programs. *American Psychologist, 58,* 449–456.

Obradović, J., Burt, K. B., & Masten, A. S. (in press). Testing a dual cascade model linking competence and symptoms over 20 years from childhood to adulthood. *Journal of Clinical Child and Adolescent Psychology.*

Obradović, J., Bush, N. R., Stamperdahl, J., Adler, N. E., & Boyce, W. T. (in press). Biological sensitivity to context: The interactive effects of stress reactivity and family adversity on socio-emotional behavior and school readiness. *Child Development.*

Obradović, J., Shaffer, A., & Masten, A. S. (in press). Risk in developmental psychopathology: Progress and future directions. In L. C. Mayes & M. Lewis (Eds.), *The environment of human development: A handbook of theory and measurement.* New York: Cambridge University Press.

Park, C. L. (2004). The notion of growth following stressful life experiences: Problems and prospects. *Psychological Inquiry, 15,* 69–76.

Patterson, G. R., & Capaldi, D. M. (1990). A meditational model for boys' depressed mood. In J. Rolf, A. S. Masten, D. Cicchetti, K. H. Nuechterlein, & S. Weintraub (Eds.), *Risk and protective factors in the development of psychopathology* (pp. 141–163). New York: Cambridge University Press.

Patterson, G. R., Reid, J. B., & Dishion, T. J. (1992). *A social interactional approach: Vol. 4. Antisocial boys.* Eugene, OR: Castalia.

Pine, D. S., Costello, J., & Masten, A. S. (2005). Trauma, proximity, and developmental psychopathology: The effects of war and terrorism on children. *Neuropsychopharmacology, 30,* 1781–1792.

Roisman, G. I., Masten, A. S., Coatsworth, J. D., & Tellegen, A. (2004). Salient and emerging developmental tasks in the transition to adulthood. *Child Development, 75*(1), 123–133.

Rothbart, M. K., & Bates, J. E. (2006). Temperament in children's development. In W. Damon, R. Lerner, & N. Eisenberg (Eds.), *Handbook of child development: Vol. 3. Social, emotional and personality development* (6th ed., pp. 99–166). Hoboken, NJ: Wiley.

Rothbart, M. K., Sheese, B. E., & Posner, M. I. (2007). Executive attention and effortful control: Linking temperament, brain networks, and genes. *Child Development Perspectives, 1,* 2–7.

Rowe, J. W., & Kahn, R. L. (1987). Human aging: Usual and successful. *Science, 237,* 143–149.

Rueda, M. R., Posner, M. I., & Rothbart, M. K. (2004). Attentional control and self-regulation. In R. F. Baumeister & K. D. Vohs (Eds.), *Handbook of self-regulation: Research, theory, and applications* (pp. 283–300). New York: Guilford Press.

Rueda, M. R., Rothbart, M. K., McCandless, B. D., Saccomanno, L., & Posner, M. I. (2005). Training, maturation, and genetic influences on the development of executive attention.

Proceedings of the National Academy of Sciences USA, 102, 14931–14936.

Rutter, M. (1990). Psychosocial resilience and protective mechanisms. In J. Rolf, A. S. Masten, D. Cicchetti, K. H. Nuechterlein, & S. Weintraub (Eds.), *Risk and protective factors in the development of psychopathology* (pp. 181–214). New York: Cambridge University Press.

Rutter, M. (2007). Resilience, competence, and coping. *Child Abuse and Neglect, 31,* 205–209.

Rutter, M., and the English and Romanian Adoptees Study Team. (1998). Developmental catch-up, and deficit, following adoption after severe global early privation. *Journal of Child Psychology and Psychiatry, 39,* 465–476.

Ryan, R. M., & Deci, E. L. (2000). Self-determination theory and the facilitation of intrinsic motivation, social development, and well-being. *American Psychologist, 55,* 68–78.

Seligman, M. E. P., & Beagley, G. (1975). Learned helplessness in the rat. *Journal of Comparative and Physiological Psychology, 88,* 534–541.

Seligman, M. E. P., & Csikszentmihalyi, M. (Eds.). (2000). Special issue: Positive psychology. *American Psychologist, 55*(1).

Shaffer, A., Burt, K. B., Obradović, J., Herbers, J. E., & Masten, A. S. (2009). Intergenerational continuity in parenting quality: The mediating role of social competence. *Developmental Psychology, 45,* 1227–1240.

Silver, R. L., Boon, C., & Stones, M. H. (1983). Searching for meaning in misfortune: Making sense of incest. *Journal of Social Issues, 39,* 81–102.

Snyder, C. R., & Lopez, S. J. (Eds.). (2009). *The handbook of positive psychology* (2nd ed.). New York: Oxford University Press.

Spencer, M. B., Harpalani, V., Cassidy, E., Jacobs, C. Y., Donde, S., Goss, T. N., et al. (2006). Understanding vulnerability and resilience from a normative developmental perspective: Implications for racially and ethnically diverse youth. In D. Cicchetti & D. J. Cohen (Eds.), *Developmental psychopathology: Vol. 1. Theory and method* (2nd ed., pp. 627–672). Hoboken, NJ: Wiley.

Sroufe, L. A. (1979). The coherence of individual development: Early care, attachment, and subsequent developmental issues. *American Psychologist, 34,* 834–841.

Sroufe, L. A. (1996). *Emotional development: The organization of emotional life in the early years.* New York: Cambridge University Press.

Sroufe, L. A. (2005). Attachment and development: A prospective, longitudinal study from birth to adulthood. *Attachment and Human Development, 7,* 349–367.

Sroufe, L. A., Carlson, E. A., Levy, A. K., & Egeland, B. (1999). Implications of attachment theory for developmental psychopathology. *Development and Psychopathology, 11,* 1–13.

Sroufe, L. A., Egeland, B., Carlson, E. A., & Collins, B. E. (2005). *The development of the person: The Minnesota Study of Risk and Adaptation from Birth to Adulthood.* New York: Guilford Press.

Tedeschi, R. G., & Calhoun, L. G. (1995). *Trauma and transformation: Growing in the aftermath of suffering.* Thousand Oaks, CA: Sage.

Thompson, R. A. (2000). The legacy of early attachments. *Child Development, 71,* 145–152.

Toth, S. L., Cicchetti, D., Macfie, J., & Emde, R. N. (1997). Representations of self and other in the narratives of neglected, physically abused, and sexually abused preschoolers. *Development and Psychopathology, 9,* 781–796.

Toth, S. L., Rogosch, F. A., Cicchetti, D., & Manly, J. T. (2006). The efficacy of toddler-parent psychotherapy to reorganize attachment in the young offspring of mothers with major depressive disorder: A randomized preventive trial. *Journal of Consulting and Clinical Psychology, 74,* 1006–1016.

Vaillant, G. (1977). *Adaptation to life: How the best and the brightest came of age.* Boston: Little, Brown.

Vaillant, G. (2002). *Aging well.* Boston: Little, Brown.

Werner, E. E., & Smith, R. S. (1982). *Vulnerable but invincible: A study of resilient children.* New York: McGraw-Hill.

Werner, E. E., & Smith, R. S. (1992). *Overcoming the odds: High risk children from birth to adulthood.* Ithaca, NY: Cornell University Press.

White, R. W. (1959). Motivation reconsidered: The concept of competence. *Psychological Review, 66,* 297–333.

Wilkinson, R. B. (2004). The role of parental and peer attachment in the psychological health and self-esteem of adolescents. *Journal of Youth and Adolescence, 33,* 479–493.

Wolchik, S. A., Sandler, I. N., Millsap, R. E., Plummer, B. A., Greene, S. M., Anderson, E. R., et al. (2002). Six-year follow-up of preventive interventions for children of divorce: A randomized controlled trial. *Journal of the American Medical Association, 288,* 1874–1881.

Wortman, C. B., & Silver, R. C. (1989). The myths of coping with loss. *Journal of Consulting and Clinical Psychology, 57,* 349–357.

Wright, M. O. (2007). *Childhood emotional abuse: Mediating and moderating processes affecting long-term impact.* Binghamton, NY: Haworth Press.

Wright, M. O., Crawford, E., & Del Castillo, D. (2009). Childhood emotional maltreatment and later psychological distress among college students: The mediating role of maladaptive schemas. *Child Abuse and Neglect, 33,* 59–68.

Wright, M. O., Crawford, E., & Sebastian, K. (2007). Positive resolution of childhood sexual abuse experiences: The role of coping, benefit-finding, and meaning-making. *Journal of Family Violence, 22,* 597–608.

Wright, M. O., & Masten, A. S. (2005). Resilience processes in development: Fostering positive adaptation in the context of adversity. In S. Goldstein & R. Brooks (Eds.), *Handbook of resilience in children* (pp. 17–37). New York: Kluwer Academic/Plenum Press.

Zeanah, C. H., Smyke, A. T., & Settles, L. D. (2006). Orphanages as a developmental context for early childhood. In K. McCartney & D. Phillips (Eds.), *Blackwell handbook of early childhood development* (pp. 424–454). Malden, MA: Blackwell.

Zoellner, T., & Maercker, A. (2006). Posttraumatic growth in clinical psychology: A critical review and introduction of a two component model. *Clinical Psychology Review, 26,* 626–653.

12

Early Adversity and Resilience in Emerging Adulthood

Linda J. Luecken
Jenna L. Gress

Although the world is full of suffering,
it is full also of the overcoming of it.
—HELEN KELLER

It is a sad fact that exposure to significant adversity during childhood and adolescence is surprisingly common. An expansive research literature links adverse childhood experiences to the development of a variety of mental, physical, and behavioral problems in childhood, adolescence, and adulthood, representing a substantial public health problem (Kessler, Davis, & Kendler, 1997). Although these problems often resolve over time, many studies have found that early life trauma results in an increased risk of psychological and physical disorders over the lifespan.

The majority of research to date has focused on identifying predictors of poor mental and physical health outcomes following childhood adversity. However, studies of adaptation failures alone cannot tell the full story of long-term adjustment following stressful early life experiences. Despite exposure to potentially severe forms of ad-

versity, many children demonstrate remarkable resilience, managing to avoid negative health consequences and develop into competent and well-adjusted adults (Masten et al., 2004; Werner & Smith, 1982). These children pose a unique opportunity for researchers and practitioners to identify the factors that promote resilience following traumatic childhood experiences.

Our purpose in this chapter is to review existing research relating early life experiences to long-term mental and physical health outcomes, and explore the potential mechanisms by which protective social, psychological, and biological factors promote resilience in adulthood following exposure to adverse situations or environments in childhood. In doing so, we focus attention on resilience during an understudied developmental period termed *emerging adulthood* (Arnett, 2000), in which myriad new risks and opportunities provide an important context in which to evaluate the process of resilience following adverse childhood experiences.

Prevalence of Childhood Adversity

Population prevalence rates of childhood adversity vary widely, reflecting the wide range of adverse experiences that children may encounter in a variety of settings (e.g., chronic poverty, war, natural disasters, disabling illness, child abuse, parental death), as well as differences in definitions and methods of data acquisition. Perhaps one of the most startling and large-scale recent news reports of childhood adversity is seen with the Lost Boys of Sudan, more than 27,000 orphaned children (mostly boys) who were forced to flee their homes during the Sudanese civil wars to avoid persecution by government troops that invaded their villages (see *www. lostboysfilm.com*). Thousands died as they faced severe hardship crossing hundreds of miles of desert on foot, including starvation, lion attacks, disease, and gunfire. Since 2001, more than 4,000 Lost Boys have been given refugee status and were resettled in foster homes in the United States, although many have experienced severely limited resources and continuing adversity in their new environments.

Several longitudinal research studies have documented prevalence rates of more "common" adversities. In the Kauai Longitudinal Study, begun in 1955, researchers identified about one-third of children as being at "high risk" due to birth complications, chronic poverty, parental mental illness, or family discord (Werner & Smith, 1982, 1992). Several notable, large-scale studies have specifically focused on adverse aspects of the childhood family environment, including physical, sexual, or emotional abuse; parental death or prolonged separation from a parent; parental separation/divorce; witnessing domestic violence; parental mental illness or substance abuse; or parental criminal behavior. Epidemiological estimates suggest that

these types of experiences are common in the United States. Anda and colleagues (2006) found that 64% of respondents (ages 19–92) in a large national survey (the Adverse Childhood Experiences [ACE] study) reported at least one adverse childhood family experience (emotional abuse: 10.6%; physical abuse: 28.3%; sexual abuse: 20.7%; parental substance abuse: 26.9%; parental mental illness: 19.4%; witnessing violence toward one's mother: 12.7%). Childhood sexual and physical abuse rates of 11–30% have been reported (Felitti et al., 1998; Kendall-Tackett, Williams, & Finkelhor, 1993). Walker and colleagues (1999) found child abuse and/or neglect histories in 43% of women (ages 18–65) recruited from a health management organization (HMO). Approximately 3.5% of children under age 18 experience the death of a parent (Social Security Administration, 2000). Not surprisingly, parental divorce or separation is even more common. Although estimates of the number of divorces that involve children vary widely, most suggest that 18–23% of children experience parental divorce (Amato & Sobolewski, 2001; Anda et al., 2006; Kessler et al., 1997). Including children whose parents are cohabiting, approximately one-third of children under age 16 will experience parental separation or divorce (Bumpass & Lu, 2000).

The prevalence of exposure to other types of adversity is less well documented. However, the U.S. National Comorbidity Survey, a representative survey of over 8,000 U.S. households, conducted between 1990 and 1992 (participant ages 18–54), reported prevalence of childhood exposure to natural or manmade disasters (9.3%), accidents (6.6%), witnessing a traumatic episode (9.3%), and being mugged or kidnapped (3.8%) (Kessler et al., 1997). In combination with family-related adversities, it was estimated that 74.4% of the sample experienced at least one significant childhood adversity. Further, both the U.S. National Comorbidity Survey and the ACE study found strong evidence of clustering among family adversities (Dong, Anda, Dube, Giles, & Felitti,

2003; Kessler et al., 1997), reinforcing the importance of assessing multiple forms of childhood adversity.

Psychological and Physical Health Outcomes Associated with Childhood Adversity

A large research literature documents that adverse childhood events markedly increase the risk for negative psychological and physical health outcomes over the lifespan. Adverse childhood experiences have been most consistently linked to the development of psychiatric disorders in adulthood, including major depression, suicidal behavior, anxiety disorders, substance use and abuse, and disorders involving aggression (Afifi et al., 2008; Anda et al., 2006; Kessler et al., 1997; MacMillan et al., 2001). Consistent findings that link childhood adversity to poor mental health outcomes have been demonstrated in late adolescents/young adults (ages 18–22) and may be particularly evident in socioeconomically disadvantaged samples (Schilling, Aseltine, & Gore, 2007).

A series of articles emanating from the ACE study have linked childhood adversity to a wide range of behavioral and physical health–related outcomes as well, including sleep disturbances, severe obesity, alcoholism, smoking initiation and prevalence, sexual disorders, somatic symptoms, chronic obstructive pulmonary disease, chronic bronchitis and emphysema, ischemic heart disease, and use of prescription drugs (Anda et al., 2006, 2008; Dong et al., 2004; Dube, Anda, Felitti, Edwards, & Croft, 2002; Felitti et al., 1998). The ACE study is notable for clearly demonstrating the dose–response relation of family-related childhood adversities to long-term mental and physical health outcomes. In each case, the risk of a negative outcome increased in a graded fashion as the extent of adverse exposure increased. Others have similarly linked exposure to childhood adversity to chronic fatigue syndrome and chronic pain in adulthood (Davis, Luecken, & Zautra, 2005; Heim et al., 2006).

Anda and colleagues (2006) outlined a strong case for the causal nature of childhood adversity in the long-term development of disorder, articulating plausible neurobiological pathways for the relation, including experience-dependent alterations in brain structure and function, neuroendocrine activity, and gene × environment interactions. These researchers evaluate current evidence with respect to Sir Bradford Hill's nine criteria (van Reekum, Striner, & Conn, 2001) for establishing an argument for causation (specificity, temporal sequence, etc.), and conclude that there is "striking convergence of evidence from neurosciences" (Anda et al., 2006, p. 183) and epidemiological studies supporting a causal relation between childhood adversity and enduring mental and physical health problems. A number of animal studies have shown that early life stress causes lasting changes in the structure and function of the hippocampus and frontal cortex, and evidence suggests comparable brain effects on abused children and adults with posttraumatic stress disorder (PTSD) (Bremner, 2003). A growing research literature consistently supports the assertion that adverse early life experiences exert a powerful influence on the development of physiological stress response systems (Boyce & Ellis, 2005; Bremner, 2003; Luecken & Lemery, 2004; McEwen, 2003; Nemeroff, 2004). Williams and colleagues (2008) report new evidence that both low childhood socioeconomic status (SES; independent of current SES) and a long allele of the serotonin transporter gene promoter (5-HTTLPR) are associated with exaggerated cardiovascular reactivity to mental distress in adulthood. Direct, enduring effects of adverse early life experiences are associated with the development of dysregulated neurobiological stress response systems (DeBellis, 2002; Elzinga et al., 2008; Meaney, Brake, & Gratton, 2002), contributing over time to the etiology of a wide range of physical and psychological illnesses (Bauer, Quas, & Boyce, 2002; McEwen, 2003). Childhood parental death has been associated with higher blood pressure

(BP) and elevated daily stress hormones in adulthood (Luecken, 1998; Nicolson, 2004). In severely maltreated children, diverse patterns of neurohormonal activity have been noted, including significantly increased or decreased daily cortisol and diminished cortisol stress responses (Cicchetti & Rogosch, 2007; DeBellis et al., 1999; Teicher, Andersen, Polcari, Anderson, & Navalta, 2002), and growing evidence suggests that physiological dysregulations associated with childhood abuse can persist into adulthood (Carpenter et al., 2007; Heim et al., 2000; Heim, Newport, Bonsall, Miller, & Nemeroff, 2001).

The Transition to Adulthood

A growing number of retrospective and longitudinal studies now demonstrate that the relation between childhood adversity and health outcomes extends across the lifespan. Typically, these studies include any person over the age of 18 in the category of "adulthood" and do not distinguish between different phases of adulthood. For example, the ACE study included participants across ages 19–92 (mean age 56). Few studies have incorporated a developmental perspective into describing and understanding the relation between childhood adversity and health outcomes.

The focus of the current chapter is on the developmental stage between adolescence and adulthood, when individuals are typically transitioning from dependence on parents to full autonomy. The term *emerging adulthood* has appeared relatively recently in the literature and is typically used to describe this developmental period, roughly 18–25 years of age (Arnett, 2000). This time period is distinguished from *young adulthood* (typically the late 20s through the 30s), which assumes that adulthood has been achieved (i.e., most people have completed their education and settled into marriages, families, and careers). As described by Arnett (2000), emerging adulthood is a period of profound change, during which time individuals typically explore the variety of life options available to them and eventually make decisions that will lay the foundation for their adult romantic and work lives. Although the process of beginning to develop a coherent identity is typical of adolescence, emerging adulthood is a particularly intense time of identify formation. Emerging adults experience a relative independence from social norms and roles that will be more restrictive later in adulthood, and typically feel more freedom than at any other point in their lives to explore a wide range of life alternatives. Although the cultural context must be considered, in American society there are generally fewer societal rules and structures imposed on emerging adults but also less external guidance. Indeed, emerging adults spend considerably more time alone than at any other point so far in their lives (Arnett, 2000).

Although many theorists assume that this transition period in development is generally a time of stress and fear, evidence suggests that most emerging adults are highly contented, experience increasing well-being, and feel optimistic about their futures (Arnett, 2007). However, leaving home, reaching legal age for many behaviors, and entering higher education, the military, or the workplace means that emerging adulthood involves increased risks, as well as increased opportunities. There is growing clinical and research interest in this developmental period as a time when individual trajectories related to both competence and psychopathology become more firmly established, and psychological problems are increasingly likely to appear (Arnett & Tanner, 2006; Masten et al., 2004; Romer & Walker, 2007). It is a time period with the highest rates of risk behavior (e.g., binge drinking, unprotected sex) and spikes in the occurrence of major depression (Arnett, 2000, 2007). These risks may be compounded by reduced external structure and guidance, and increased solitary time. In short, not all emerging adults will easily navigate this challenging time period.

Some emerging adults appear well prepared to make their way into the roles and responsibilities of adulthood, bolstered with more stable, coherent, and commitment-based identities, whereas others may require external help (e.g., intervention) to transition into adult roles and responsibilities. (Schwartz, Côté, & Arnett, 2005, p. 224)

Little is known about specific developmental experiences that influence the ability to transition successfully into young adulthood, and few studies have focused on transition into adulthood following childhood adversity. However, significant adversity can "push" children into non-normative early transitions into adulthood (e.g., early sexual activity, teenage pregnancy, leaving home early, assuming adult responsibilities during childhood) that are typically associated with poor outcomes (Wickrama, Conger, & Abraham, 2005). Adverse childhood experiences may also inhibit the development of adaptive self-regulatory abilities (e.g., coping skills) and personal resources (e.g., self-esteem, social skills) that can promote positive experiences during the transition into adulthood, in essence leaving youth less "prepared" to face the challenges of autonomy (Luecken & Lemery, 2004; Repetti, Taylor, & Seeman, 2002).

Conversely, the emerging adult period may provide relief for some from a chronic stressful or overcontrolling home environment, and the opportunity to choose healthier contexts and more supportive relationships, which may prove to be beneficial to long-term mental and physical health. The significance of emerging adulthood as a unique developmental period is supported by the common appearance during this time period of opportunities for altering the direction of one's life trajectory. A number of theorists have noted that emerging adulthood can be a time period that offers "turning points," "second chances," or opportunities for disadvantaged youth to redirect their lives onto healthier, more resilient (or more destructive) paths (Masten et al., 2004; Rutter, 2006; Werner, 2005).

Resilience

Despite the widespread nature of childhood adversity, the majority of children successfully transition into competent and well-adjusted adults, demonstrating the powerful human potential for resilience. The term *resilience* has been used in a variety of contexts and has existed in the literature for several decades. However, its definition has evolved over time. Broadly, the term *resilience* refers to positive or successful adaptation following adversity. In studies of child resilience, this has commonly been measured as an outcome marked by competence in age-appropriate tasks (e.g., school achievement) or an absence of pathology, or it has been equated to a personality trait. More current research has recommended that the concept of resilience move away from variables and be conceptualized as a process (Rutter, 2007). As a result, current terminology related to resilience research becomes quite confusing, particularly from a developmental perspective, because it is often conceptualized and discussed as a process but largely measured as an outcome. As will be apparent, most of the studies referenced in this chapter evaluate resilience as an outcome.

Furthermore, it has been stressed that resilience is relative and should be thought of as a function of risk exposure. In other words, both the severity and frequency of adversity need to be considered in assessing resilience (Rutter, 2006). Many of the Lost Boys of Sudan, who were resettled in the United States with limited resources, faced continuing difficulties and did not fare well, suffering violent deaths or severe depression. Conversely, some achieved a level of success that few from even the most advantageous backgrounds ever reach, such as the 2008 Olympic athlete who carried the U.S. torch in the 2008 Opening Ceremonies (Lopez Lomong, a 23-year-old 1,500-meter track runner). But the true stories of resilience during emerging adulthood come from those who finished their high school educations, attended college, found full-time employment, and established families in the United States, and in this sense their stories of resilience are remarkable. The interested reader is referred to the recent documentary *The Lost Boys of Sudan*, which highlights the stories of two of these resilient refugees, who are now in their early 20s and attending colleges in the United States (*www.lost-boysfilm.com*).

A broad assortment of terms is used in the literature on resilience theory and the factors that comprise or predict resilience. Indeed one limitation in resilience research is the amount of overlapping terminology used. This confusing array of terminology is apparent in studies evaluating person-level factors associated with resilience. Early studies referred to person-level variables as protective factors, which are not simply the opposite of risk factors, as the name may imply. *Protective factors* have been defined as processes that ameliorate the negative effects of adversity, but only if the risk factor is experienced; with little or no exposure to the risk factor, protective factors do not manifest, implying a necessary interaction (Rutter, 1985). Recent literature has used different terms that share common ground with Rutter's (1985) protective factors but also have marked differences. Masten and colleagues (2004) use the term *core resources*, which can be thought of as resources that are evident in childhood and provide a foundation for resilience (e.g., intelligence, SES). In other words, core resources function as early predictors of resilience. However, core resources differ from protective factors in that an interaction with risk is not necessary (i.e., they are beneficial for all children, independent of risk exposure). *Promotive factors* and *adaptive resources* are also commonly used terms that characterize another person-level aspect of resilience. These terms refer to internal factors that are utilized during stress (e.g., self-esteem), similar to *adaptive capacity*, as suggested by Olsson, Bond, Burns, Vella-Brodrick, and Sawyer (2003). Together, protective factors (e.g., core resources) and adaptive resources (e.g., internal processes) constitute a more complete concept of individual-level factors in resilience.

Resilience has been described as a continuing developmental process that builds from childhood into adulthood, as children and adolescents are able to identify and utilize internal and external resources in the face of adversity (Yates, Egeland, & Sroufe, 2003). All of these aspects of resilience highlight the complexity of resilience theory as an interaction among environment, person, and stressor. As Rutter (2006) points out, it is necessary to understand what happens *after* exposure to adversity to understand resilience, emphasizing why resilience needs to be viewed through a lifespan lens; that is, we cannot fully understand how resilience progresses without examining it within and throughout specific developmental periods.

Resilience in Emerging Adulthood

Most studies of resilience following early life stress have focused on psychosocial health during childhood or adolescence or have considered adulthood as comprising a homogenous group. Several books and hundreds of research articles have been written about childhood resilience. An extensive body of literature examines a long list of moderators and mediators of childhood resilience and adaptation. Among these, the powerful influence of parenting and parent–child relationships (for a review, see Seifer, 2003) has received special attention. Resilience theory has also been examined during adolescence in conjunction with the specific stressors of that developmental time period (Compas, Hinden, & Gerhardt, 1995; Fergus & Zimmerman, 2005; Olsson et al., 2003), and during adulthood and older adulthood. Less commonly examined is the continuity of resilience through emerging adulthood.

As a result, little is known about the long-term *process* of resilience, and its unique presentation and predictors during emerging adulthood. This is an important distinction because existing literature typically evaluates the accomplishment of age-appropriate developmental competencies as evidence of resilience, thereby necessitating different measurement strategies at different ages. Furthermore, the factors that promote or reflect resilience in childhood or later adulthood may not function similarly in emerging adulthood. Whether or not the factors identified as resilience-promoting in children who have experienced childhood adversity carry through into adulthood, as other unique stressors are experienced, is less understood. Available resilience resources likely must go through a developmental process alongside the individual's development. For these and additional reasons, the need for this lifespan perspective on resilience has been emphasized (Rutter, 2006, 2007).

Research in adolescent resilience has begun to incorporate some of these points and can lend itself to the advancement of theories regarding resilience in emerging adulthood. In particular it has been noted that resilience should be placed in a more ecological context that involves assets (internal factors, e.g., coping skills) and resources (external factors, e.g., parental and community support) (Fergus & Zimmerman, 2005). This is further discussed by Olsson and colleagues (2003), who underscore resilience as a process and multifactorial concept that should include individual-, social-, and societal-level factors. Olsson and colleagues posit that resilience should be assessed by means of an "adaptive capacity" that involves factors from each of the three levels.

These and other important factors mentioned previously need to be incorporated into a resilience framework that is specifically applied to emerging adults. During adolescence, higher levels of independence and autonomy, and a shift in social support from parents to peers, are normative developmental experiences (Petersen, 1988). These changes are even more prominent in emerging adulthood, as individual-, social-, and societal-level resources may be in flux. In emerging adulthood, a unique set of individual-level resilience resources may be central to handling problems and challenges of adult life. These resources include a sense of control, self-efficacy, and self-responsibility; the ability to plan and pursue goals; social skills to negotiate jobs and develop new social networks; and self-regulatory and coping skills (Hines, Merdinger, & Wyatt, 2005; Masten et al., 2004). These individual-level variables take on a greater meaning during emerging adulthood and may occur in a new or different context than that of adolescence. Thus, a comprehensive framework that includes both individual factors and the context (or environment) must be taken into special consideration when examining emerging adulthood resilience.

This concept of context as a part of resilience theory has been discussed (Masten, 2007; Riley & Masten, 2005) but rarely applied directly to emerging adulthood. By assessing the context of the individual, a greater understanding and organization of a resilience framework can be obtained. Furthermore, by looking at several contexts in which an individual interacts (e.g., job, family, romantic relationships) positive outcomes can be seen and measured in various areas or levels (Riley & Masten, 2005). It is common practice for research to examine resilience in a singular context, however; taking multiple contexts into account would be advantageous, leading to a greater understanding of resilience and its unique manifestations across different contexts. The repercussions of not taking context into account have also been discussed: "Underestimating the importance of context can result in misplaced blame, ineffective interventions, findings that fail to replicate, and theory that does not generate useful ideas" (Riley & Masten, 2005, p. 22). Context is a particularly salient factor during emerging adulthood, which typically involves frequent changes in living and social situations (Arnett, 2000). Changes in context can be either positive or negative. Leaving a resource-rich home environment may be a risky move for an emerging adult who does not have the resources to provide adequately for him- or herself. Alternatively, an abused child who has the opportunity to leave a negative home environment may be able to become embedded in a positive environment, where resilient resources can accumulate.

These theoretical components are well linked in a contextual model of adaptation to a childhood stressor, proposed by Sandler, Wolchik, and Ayers (2008). Although this model was conceived for children who suffered the early death of a parent, it can be broadly applied to other childhood adversities and across different developmental periods, including emerging adulthood. This theoretical model focuses on adaptation following adversity. The model comprises three main parts that constitute the transactions between individuals and their environments as they acclimate following adversity. First, a stressor is experienced, which has the potential to endanger a person's well-being or become a barrier to developmental capability. The second part of the model includes *adaptation processes*, which broadly refer to the adjustments a person makes over time to cope with the trauma. The adaptation processes comprise both environmental processes (e.g., parenting) and individual processes (e.g., self-efficacy) that interact to help meet the basic needs and developmental competencies necessary to overcome adversity. The final part of the model includes the outcomes, or *resilience trajectories*, which can be negative or positive. For example, if a person successfully adapts to a stressor, then the outcomes or resilience trajectories may include well-being, developmental competence, and overall life satisfaction. On the other hand, if a person fails to adjust, poor outcomes and negative trajectories, such as poor mental health or substance use, may follow. The major strengths of this contextual resilience model are that it takes into account person-level factors and contexts, and helps to explain the possible multiple paths and outcomes following childhood adversity.

Longitudinal Studies of Resilience

Although considerably less common than cross-sectional or retrospective studies, a number of large-scale longitudinal studies have examined the process of resilience from birth to adulthood, and provide some of the best indications of the process of resilience during emerging adulthood following exposure to childhood adversity. An excellent summary of significant longitudinal studies is provided by Werner (2005). Few of these studies have focused specifically on resilience during the transition from adolescence to emerging adulthood. Two representative longitudinal studies of resilience are discussed here: the Kauai Longitudinal Study (Werner & Smith, 1992) and Project Competence (Garmezy, Masten, & Tellegen, 1984).

One of the earliest studies to include a focus on resilience, the Kauai Longitudinal Study, began in 1955 and followed all 698 babies born that year in Kauai, with a goal of evaluating long-term outcomes associated with exposure to adverse rearing conditions (Werner & Smith, 1992). Participants were followed from birth through age 40 (Werner & Smith, 2001). About one-third were designated as high risk due to factors including chronic poverty, parental mental illness, perinatal complications, or chronic family discord. Of these, the researchers noted that about one-third grew into competent, caring young adults despite considerable childhood adversity (Werner, 1993). Three main types of protective factors were identified: *core resources*, such as sociability, average intelligence, communication skills, having an internal locus of control, and attachment to parents; *adaptive resources*, such as emotional support from parents, siblings, spouse, or mate; and *external support* through an outside source, such as school, work, or religious affiliation.

In separate analyses with the same sample, participants were evaluated as they faced the beginning of emerging adulthood (age 18) and after the transition to young adulthood (age 32). A number of important findings are evident regarding the factors that promoted a successful transition to adulthood (Werner, 1993). First, core resources established in childhood and associated with resilient outcomes in adulthood (defined as high levels of life satisfaction and functioning via self-report, lack of criminal record, and absence of psychiatric disorder) included better social skills, more positive parenting experiences, the presence of supportive adults other than the parents, better cognitive skills, higher self-esteem, and a more developed sense of personal control. A pathway of cascading resilience resources was apparent. For example, an "easy" temperament at birth predicted more positive parental interactions at age 1–2, which predicted scholastic competence and support from teachers and peers at age 10, which were linked to higher self-esteem and sense of control at age 18, which were linked to better mental health at age 32. Second, there was a clear continuity, in that most participants who showed signs of resilience in adolescence remained resilient into adulthood, suggesting that core resources formed during childhood continue to promote resilience through various types of adversity into adulthood (Werner, 1991). Third, although most people demonstrated relatively stable resilience, Werner (2005) noted that the transition from adolescence to adulthood was a turning point during which some resilient adolescents began to experience degraded mental health, whereas some nonresilient adolescents rebounded into resilient adults. The availability of new opportunities (e.g., work, marriage, military service) provided by emerging adulthood was identified as a key factor that enabled such "second chances."

Project Competence, a longitudinal study of competence and resilience, followed 205 Minneapolis schoolchildren from ages 10 to 30 (Garmezy et al., 1984), including emerging adulthood (ages 17–23) and young adulthood (ages 28–36). Adverse experiences were widely assessed through structured life events interviews and questionnaires, and were rated on a 7-point scale closely related to the Severity of Psychosocial Stressors Scale for Axis IV of the DSM (American Psychiatric Association, 1987). Approximately 37% of participants were rated as having experienced high levels of adversity during childhood and/or adolescence (Masten et al., 1999). Participants were classified as high or low in adversity. *Competence* was defined as a record of successful functioning in age-salient developmental tasks (Masten et al., 1995, 1999, 2004), including education, work, romantic relationships, and parenting. Similar to results from the Kauai Longitudinal Study, striking evidence of continuity in resilience from adolescence to emerging adulthood to young adulthood was found, although the researchers did identify a minority of participants who demonstrated radical changes in life course in the transition to adulthood suggestive of emergent resilience (Masten et al., 2004). Consistent with other studies of resilience, parenting quality during childhood was the most potent predictor of resilience in emerging adulthood in those who had experienced significant childhood adversity (Masten et al., 1999). Masten and colleagues (1999) concluded that even in the presence of severe or chronic adversity, the potential for resilience in emerging adulthood is high for children with core resources of strong parent–child relationships and cognitive skills. Competence and the availability of adaptive resources (planfulness, future motivation, autonomy, adult support, and coping) in emerging adulthood were strongly predictive of a successful transition to adulthood. These adaptive resources were particularly strong predictors of emergent resilience in young adults previously identified as maladaptive.

Werner (2005) suggests a number of lessons that can be drawn from existing large-scale longitudinal studies of resilience. The importance of secure attachment and positive parent–child relationships early in life is a recurring theme among studies of long-term resilience. Children exhibiting early signs of competence are also more likely to continue on a path of resilience during adolescence and the transition to adulthood. However, longitudinal studies also demonstrate that resilience can be late-emerging, reinforcing the importance of a lifespan developmental approach to the study of resilience. Most often, individuals who demonstrated a shift toward resilience in emerging adulthood were able to take advantage of new opportunities that became available to them (e.g., adult education, military service, religious participation). Werner also noted that longitudinal studies reveal the interconnectedness of protective resources over time; that is, the presence of resilience resources increases the availability of more resilience resources, which accumulate over time and increase the likelihood of a resilient life trajectory.

An additional body of literature has examined childhood abuse and neglect, and the relation to resilience in emerging adulthood. These studies provide insight into the proportion of abused children who nonetheless develop into resilient young adults, as well as some additional support for protective factors associated with resilience that extend from childhood into young adulthood. Du-Mont, Widom, and Czaja (2007) conducted a long-term evaluation of children with court-documented abuse/neglect before the age of 11. In young adulthood (mean age 29) 30% were categorized as resilient, as defined by success in six of eight domains, including high school graduation, psychiatric disorder, substance abuse, arrests, violent behavior, employment, homelessness, and social activity. Lending support to the common finding that females are more resilient (Masten et al., 2004; Werner, 1991), abused or neglected females were more likely than males to be resilient both in adolescence and young adulthood. The number of stressful life events was negatively correlated with resilience, and having a highly supportive spouse or partner was positively related to resilience in young adulthood. Also, positive neighborhood conditions and cognitive ability were not independently linked to resilience, but there was a significant interaction between the two in young adulthood. Having higher cognitive ability and coming from a more favorable neighborhood were strongly predictive of increasing resilience. Interestingly, race and household stability were related to resilience in adolescence but lost significance in young adulthood.

The Continuity of Resilience

Taken together, these studies suggest the importance of understanding the continuity of resilience through emerging adulthood. Resilience clearly forms a firm base during childhood through individual, family, and environmental factors. However, it is also suggested that this foundation is movable. For example, the development of supportive relationships in emerging adulthood (most commonly a spouse or partner) allows the experience of emotional support in a new context and can promote resilience later in life.

A powerful argument for the importance of a lifespan developmental approach to the study of resilience following childhood adversity comes from the common finding that although considerable stability in resilience from childhood to adulthood is the norm, shifts are also evident (Masten et al., 2004; Rutter, 2006; Werner, 2005); that is, some children who initially demonstrate considerable resilience may become more vulnerable in adulthood, whereas others who initially are quite vulnerable can develop a capacity for resilience in adulthood given the right context, capabilities, and opportunities. DuMont and colleagues (2007) found that whereas 48% of abused/neglected children were resilient in adolescence, only 30% were resilient in young adulthood. However, 11% of abused/neglected children who were nonresilient as adolescents became resilient in young adulthood. Similarly, in the Kauai Longitudinal Study, approximately one-third of high-risk children who showed maladjustment in adolescence grew up to be conscientious adults, partners, and parents (Werner, 1993). Transitions in resilience also occurred in children of alcoholics, victims of abuse, and through life transitions (e.g., marriage, transition into high school or the work force) (Werner, 2001, 2005). In some cases, experiences during emerging adulthood may be necessary to "activate" resilience (Rutter, 2006). Late-emerging transitions toward resilience highlight resilience as a process and resource base rather than a personality trait with a linear trajectory across developmental periods. Furthermore, the potential for shifts later in life confirm the fluid nature of resilience into adulthood and the importance of measuring resilience during periods of life transition, including emerging adulthood.

The transactional and dynamic nature of resilience suggests that it is malleable across different developmental periods. Unfortunately, many of the core resources identified as resilience-promoting cannot be easily modified (e.g., temperament, gender, IQ, SES) and are of little help in identifying pathways for intervention or increasing resilience later in life. A better understanding of malleable, adaptive resources may be more helpful in designing interventions to promote resilience in emerging adulthood. Adaptive resources, or promotive factors of resilience, include patterns or resources that can be built upon and used during periods of stress. In a study we already discussed, Masten and colleagues (2004) studied the relative permanence of resilience through the transition into adulthood, and examined unique resources in emerging adulthood that were predictive of resilience in young adulthood. These included skills and characteristics such as future motivation and planfulness, autonomy, support from an adult, and coping skills. Coping flexibility may also be an important promotive factor. In a sample of Chinese young adults (mean age 21), those who utilized more coping strategies reported lower levels of depression during stress (Bun Lam & McBride-Chang, 2007). In a separate study, several individual factors were

found to be characteristic of resilient college students (ages 19–35; resilience marked by academic achievement) who were in the foster system during childhood (Hines et al., 2005). Through in-depth interviews, factors such as hopes and plans for the future, sense of social responsibility, desire for family, assertiveness, independence, being goal oriented, being determined to be different from abusers, able to accept and request help, and having a flexible self-image were identified. Additionally, results from this study suggested that factors that were evident in more than one domain (individual, family, and community) were important characteristics of resilient young adults. Taken together, these results offer a considerable contribution to our knowledge of resilience resources with the potential to be modified, and suggest ways to increase resilience in emerging adulthood, thus increasing the possibility of a more resilient young adulthood.

Methodological Considerations

Although existing studies of resilience in emerging adulthood provide exciting glimpses into the process and potential for resilience, a number of methodological concerns are worth noting. First, greater consideration needs to be taken in assessing context and "age-salient developmental tasks" (Masten et al., 2004). Many of the studies described here are laudable for their measurement of resilience across multiple domains. For example, McGloin and Widom (2001) conceptualized resilience as functioning across eight domains, and each person was given a score of 0 (*unsuccessful*) or 1 (*successful*) for each of the eight domains. Scores were then added, and individuals scoring above 6 were labeled as being resilient. In a similar vein, Masten and colleagues (2004) and Fergusson and Horwood (2003) also measured resilience as a function of competence across several domains, but only Masten and colleagues specifically selected domains that were thought to be developmentally appropriate. Furthermore, despite the common view that resilience should be thought of as a process, all of the studies measured resilience as an outcome.

A number of studies have found that the level of resilience is predicted by the level of severity of childhood adversity (Collishaw et al., 2007; DuMont et al., 2007). Although intuitive, these findings necessarily raise concerns about "resilience" being an artifact of risk (Rutter, 2006). In other words, studies should be careful to control for the magnitude of risk before identifying individuals who appear resilient (i.e., they just may have had lesser exposure to risk). For example, the extent of hardship experienced by the Lost Boys of Sudan varied widely, and their level of resilience should be considered within the context of their level of traumatic exposure. In addition, studies often define *resilience* as the absence of psychopathology, despite common acknowledgment that lacking a psychological disorder does not equate to having a satisfying or well-adjusted life. This practice also ignores one's potential for resilience *despite* having a psychiatric disorder. That is, what resilience resources promote recovery from major depression or an addictive disorder? What factors allow one with schizophrenia to live a relatively resilient life? Research developing theoretically sound tools of measurement is especially needed. We cannot fully understand the intricacies of resilience and its multiple pathways without consensus on how to measure it. Improper measurement may possibly lead to improper results and interpretations, and a lack of theory advancement.

Another measurement issue concerns the extremely common method of dichotomously categorizing individuals as either resilient or nonresilient, even after what sometimes are quite sophisticated analyses of a number of domains of functioning. Although dichotomization has the advantage of simplifying statistical analyses and interpretation, resilience is clearly not an either–or phenomenon. A number of theorists have noted that individuals may demonstrate resilience in some domains but not others, or at some time periods but not others, yet it is surprising how little attention is paid to the full range of resilience. For many years quantitative psychologists have strongly discouraged dichotomization of continuous variables because of the tremendous potential for loss of power and precision, and the risk of misleading results (Cohen, 1983; MacCallum, Zhang, Preacher, & Rucker, 2002). The practice is particularly risky when individual domains are dichotomized into "competent" or not, then summed to create a dichotomous resilient category. Furthermore, important information is lost when seemingly arbitrary cutoffs (e.g., more than three moves in the last year, history of psychiatric disorder, marital breakup) are used to categorize outcomes. Frequent job changes, for example, can mark one as "nonresilient" (e.g., DuMont et al., 2007), although they may indicate advancing education or rapid development of job skills. It is our hope that future studies will consider the full range of resilience.

In addition to fine-tuning our understanding of the relative impact of predictors, evaluating resilience as a continuous variable will also enable more sophisticated analyses of nonlinear and dynamic processes. As a number of researchers have noted, exposure to adversity may not exert a linear effect on risk. Moderate exposure to adversity under the right conditions (e.g., strong parental support) may increase the potential to develop resilience-promoting skills and self-regulatory abilities that promote long-term resilient outcomes, often referred to as a *steeling* or *inoculation* effect (Fergus & Zimmerman, 2005; Rutter, 2006). Although framed within a "risk" format, Boyce and Ellis (2005) similarly theorize that either highly adverse or highly protective childhood conditions promote elevated stress reactivity (i.e., sensitization) assumed to underlie vulnerability to psychological and physical disorder, whereas moderate stress exposure promotes the development of adaptive stress reactivity.

Rutter (2006) suggests that "controlled exposure" to early adversity can in some cases strengthen resistance to later stress, potentially as a result of successful coping with the earlier event. Adverse events in childhood can provide a powerful context for a caring parent to shape the child's development of strong emotion regulation skills, resulting in stress inoculation. For example, recent data from our lab find that for parentally bereaved emerging adults, higher caring from the surviving parent was associated with fewer reports of minor stress in daily life and less stress-related negative emotion than that of nonbereaved participants with highly caring parents (Luecken, Kraft, Appelhans, & Enders, 2009). Similarly, Luecken (2000a) found that emerging adults who experienced early parental death in the presence of strong family-of-origin relationships reported fewer depressive symptoms and higher social support than nonbereaved participants with strong family relationships.

The previous discussion of the methodological limitations of most current studies of resilience argues for more complex modeling of the process of resilience, including thorough measures of context, multiple potential promotive pathways, components of resilience that may have additive or interactive influences, multiple levels of analysis, longitudinal measures of the development of competencies over time, and outcomes that do not require dichotomous categorization. It is recognized that such modeling requires sophisticated study designs and complicated statistical techniques that represent a considerable challenge for future research, but it offers considerable potential to move the field toward a much more mature understanding of the potential for resilience in at-risk populations.

Theoretical and Empirical Challenges for Future Research

The study of resilience has had an enormous impact on theories of adjustment following childhood adversity, yet a number of theoretical and empirical challenges remain. A critical challenge for resilience research is to begin to define the underlying processes that contribute to long-term adaptive capacities in individuals affected by early adversity (Sandler, Wolchik, Davis, Haine, & Ayers, 2003; Wyman, Sandler, Wolchik, & Nelson, 2000). Analyses of mediation, attending to the underlying causal mechanisms and processes by which psychosocial factors influence resilience, will be helpful in this regard. In addition to the theoretical interest inherent in understanding causal pathways, analyses of mediation are essential for the development of efficient and effective interventions by identifying crucial program components (MacKinnon & Luecken, 2008). Consistent research demonstrates, for example, the power of positive parenting experiences to promote resilience, but *how* positive parenting promotes resilience (e.g., via improved self-esteem?) is not fully understood (Luthar, Sawyer, & Brown, 2006) yet is a critical piece of knowledge for designing the most effective parenting programs. A good example of this approach is seen in analyses of the New Beginnings Program, a family-focused intervention that has taken a prospective, process-oriented approach to uncovering the pathways to resilience in youth who experience parental divorce (Wolchik et al., 2000; Wolchik, Sandler, Weiss, & Winslow, 2007). Program development was guided by "small theory," by first identifying potentially modifiable risk factors and resilience resources associated with positive postdivorce adaptation, then developing program components that targeted the processes most likely to impact adaptation positively. Because of their consistent association in the literature with resilient outcomes, key targets for intervention were the mother–child relationship, effective discipline, interparental conflict, and contact with the noncustodial parent (Wolchik, Schenck, & Sandler, in press). Participation in the intervention enhanced the mother–child relationship, which was associated with improved youth adaptation

6 years after the intervention. Mediational analyses further suggested that child coping efficacy mediated the effects of mother–child relationship quality on mental health outcomes (Wolchik et al., in press).

A second challenge for research on resilience is to move beyond static evaluations of resilience. Most studies evaluate resilience through the use of self-report measures assessed at a single point in time (e.g., a score on a scale rating externalizing problems). In emerging adulthood, these measures generally rely on participants to rate globally how they are doing overall (e.g., life satisfaction, presence or absence of psychological illness). Often, measures focus on major life achievements (e.g., stable career, marriage, children). What these measures can miss are the more subtle aspects of how nonclinically affected individuals are functioning in their daily lives. How happy is the marriage? How satisfied are they in their jobs? How well do they manage the normal, daily challenges of adult life (e.g., conflict with their children, traffic jams, job demands)? Few, if any, studies have evaluated a dynamic model of the *process* of resilience in individuals' day-to-day interactions with their environment. To do so involves considerable methodological challenges, but would be worth the investment for the rich data such a study would provide.

A third critical challenge for the study of resilience is to examine the process from multiple, integrated levels of analysis. It is clear that early adversity can significantly impact physiological systems associated with mental and physical health, yet little is known about how resilience resources can mitigate the impact of adversity, or how preexisting biological or genetic factors can promote or inhibit the process of resilience. The bulk of existing research on resilience has focused on behavioral or psychological factors. Integration of biological perspectives into the theoretical framework of resilience, along with empirical examination of biological foundations, is imperative for research on resilience to move forward (Curtis & Cicchetti, 2003).

As stated by Curtis and Cicchetti, "The goal of future research on resilience should be to increasingly incorporate multiple biological measures as part of a multiple levels of analysis approach to resilience research" (2003, p. 775). Models of the negative long-term effects of childhood stress typically focus on dysregulated biological stress responses, known to contribute over time to the etiology of physical and psychological illnesses, including heart disease, depression, anxiety, and infectious illnesses (McEwen, 1998, 2003). Less has been theorized regarding resilient physiological responses; however, it is critical for an organism to be able to react quickly and flexibly, such that internal physiological systems meet but do not exceed environmental demands, and terminate when no longer needed (see Charney, Westphal, & Feder, Chapter 2, this volume).

The potential for protective factors to promote resilient physiological responses in those who experience early adversity remains a critical direction for research. Although less studied than psychosocial resilience, emerging evidence shows the potential for parenting to influence physiological resilience as well. An intriguing series of animal studies demonstrates that high-quality parenting can promote the development of highly adaptive physiological stress responses and improve lifespan health (Liu et al., 1997). Studies with children demonstrate that a responsive primary caregiver plays a critical role in regulation of stress responses by modulating arousal as the child explores his or her environment, and soothing an upset child (Streeck-Fisher & van der Kolk, 2000). Although it has been theorized that positive childhood relationships can improve physiological stress responses into adulthood (see, e.g., Repetti et al., 2002), few empirical studies have been reported. As an initial foray into the long-term resilience-promoting potential of positive family relationships, Luecken (2000b) found that the physiological impact of early parental death in emerging adults (ages 18–27) was moderated by the quality of the parent–child relationship, such that early parental death was associated with more adaptive cortisol reactivity to later stress if participants reported higher perceived caring from the surviving parent. Luecken, Rodriquez, and Appelhans (2005) found that emerging adults (ages 18–29) who experienced early parental death and reported more positive family relationships showed more adaptive cardiovascular responses to a stressful speech task than those reporting poorer relationships. The combination of parental death and positive parenting may uniquely shape adaptive self-regulatory ability, contributing to resilience in the face of later stress.

Also of considerable interest is the potential for early focused interventions to promote the process of physiological resilience following childhood adversity. Several studies have shown short-term biological benefits of early intervention. Fisher, Stoolmiller, Gunnar, and Burraston (2007) found that children in foster care who were randomly assigned to a family-based therapeutic intervention began to exhibit cortisol activity similar to that of nonmaltreated children after 1 year. In contrast, children in the regular foster care condition exhibited an increasingly flattened diurnal pattern of cortisol activity. Because neuroendocrine dysregulations are associated with mental health and physical health problems for adults who have experienced childhood adversities, these findings have significant implications for the long-term resilience-promoting potential of early, targeted preventive interventions for at-risk children.

An exciting new area of research on resilience focuses on genetic factors and gene × environment (GE) interactions. Generally thought of within a risk format, wherein the presence of a particular genotype increases the negative impact of an adverse childhood experience, GE interactions can also be thought of as a potential resilience process (Kim-Cohen, Moffitt, Caspi, & Taylor, 2004; Rutter, 2003). For example, now classic findings by Caspi and colleagues (2002) show that maltreated children with

a genotype conferring high levels of monoamine oxidase A (MAO-A) expression were less likely to develop conduct disorder than those with a low-activity MAO-A genotype. Because Lemery-Chalfant (Chapter 3, this volume) discusses genetic influences on resilience, it is not covered in detail here. However, it is important to note that the childhood developmental period is a prime time for salient life experiences, including both adverse and positive life events, to exert phenotypic influence. Furthermore, the consequences of GE interactions associated with childhood adversity may first become apparent during the period of emerging adulthood.

Finally, it is important to note the need for future studies that take cultural context into greater consideration. There is still much to be learned about cultural context and its connection to resilience; this is especially true in young or emerging adulthood. Cultural influences and traditions are an essential aspect of a comprehensive resilience framework and can impact resilience through various pathways. O'Dougherty Wright and Masten (2005) point out that current factors associated with resilience (e.g., self-esteem, self-efficacy, coping flexibility) are widely influenced by culture. Culture can impact resilience through large contexts, such as individualism or collectivism in cultures, or through smaller systems, such as family networks. In a study that examined past child abuse and cultural factors, Ferrari (2002) found that cultural values significantly impacted parenting actions of fathers but not those of mothers. Furthermore, it is suggested that measuring resilience within cultures and replicating findings across cultures would provide insight into how the same or different resilience factors manifest in various cultural contexts (O'Dougherty Wright & Masten, 2005). Factors that promote resilience in one culture may not do so in another. For example, although self-mastery may be a source of resilience in individualistic societies, it may be less beneficial or even have detrimental effects for individuals from collectivist societies, where factors reflective of cultural values of family and social networks are more valued and may play a more significant role in health outcomes. Purdom, Stevenson, Lemery-Chalfant, Howe, and Luecken (2008) report preliminary findings that for low-acculturated Mexican American women, a higher sense of self-mastery predicted lower self-rated health 5 months after childbirth. Although their study did not evaluate childhood adversity, the findings nonetheless illustrate the importance of considering cultural factors in studies of resilience.

Conclusions

Given the alarming prevalence of childhood adversity, studies that focus on the potential for lifespan resilience despite traumatic early life experiences are a welcome addition to the research literature. Although most studies focus on the dramatic psychological and physical health risks associated with childhood adversity, it is clear that many children beat the odds and develop into competent, well-adjusted adults. These resilient children and adults demonstrate the incredible buoyancy of the human spirit to overcome tremendous adversity.

Studies of the potential for psychological, social, behavioral, and physiological resilience following adverse childhood experiences demonstrate recurring promotive aspects of resilience that are formulated during childhood, including internal qualities (self-esteem, control beliefs) and positive, supportive relationships. However, the end point cannot be determined in childhood or adolescence. The challenges and opportunities for dramatic alterations in life course that define the transition from adolescence to adulthood provide an important context for the continuing development of resilience processes. The pathways of resilience through emerging adulthood remain to be revealed, making this developmental period an exciting area for theory growth, psychometric research, and intervention development.

References

Afifi, T. O., Enns, M. W., Cox, B. J., Asmundson, J. G., Stein, M. B., & Sareen, J. (2008). Population attributable fractions of psychiatric disorders and suicide ideation and attempts associated with adverse childhood experiences. *American Journal of Public Health*, 98(5), 946–952.

Amato, P. R., & Sobolewski, J. M. (2001). The effects of divorce and marital discord on adult children's psychological well-being. *American Sociological Review*, 66(6), 900–921.

American Psychiatric Association. (1987). *Diagnostic and statistical manual of mental disorders* (3rd ed.). Washington, DC: Author.

Anda, R. F., Brown, D. W., Dube, S. R., Bremner, J. D., Felitti, V. J., & Giles, W. H. (2008). Adverse childhood experiences and chronic obstructive pulmonary disease in adults. *American Journal of Preventive Medicine*, 34(5), 396–403.

Anda, R. F., Felitti, V. J., Bremner, J. D., Walker, J. D., Whitfield, C., Perry, B. D., et al. (2006). The enduring effects of abuse and related adverse experiences in childhood: A convergence of evidence from neurobiology and epidemiology. *European Archives of Psychiatry and Clinical Neuroscience*, 256, 174–186.

Arnett, J. J. (2000). Emerging adulthood: A theory of development from the late teens through the twenties. *American Psychologist*, 55(5), 469–480.

Arnett, J. J. (2007). Suffering, selfish, slackers?: Myths and reality about emerging adults. *Journal of Youth and Adolescence*, 36, 23–29.

Arnett, J. J., & Tanner, J. L. (Eds.). (2006). *Emerging adults in America: Coming of age in the 21st century*. Washington, DC: American Psychological Association.

Bauer, A. M., Quas, J. A., & Boyce, W. T. (2002). Associations between physiological reactivity and children's behavior: Advantages of a multisystem approach. *Developmental and Behavioral Pediatrics*, 23(2), 102–113.

Boyce, W. T., & Ellis, B. J. (2005). Biological sensitivity to context: I. An evolutionary–developmental theory of the origins and functions of stress reactivity. *Development and Psychopathology*, 17, 271–301.

Bremner, J. D. (2003). Long-term effects of childhood abuse on brain and neurobiology. *Child and Adolescent Psychiatric Clinics of North America*, 12(2), 271–292.

Bumpass, L., & Lu, H. H. (2000). Trends in cohabitation and implications for children's family contexts in the United States. *Population Studies, 54* 29–41.

Bun Lam, C., & McBride-Chang, C. A. (2007). Resilience in young adulthood: The moderating influences of gender-related personality traits and coping flexibility. *Sex Roles, 56,* 159–172.

Carpenter, L. L., Carbalho, J. P., Tyrka, A. R., Wier, L. M., Mello, A. F., Mello, M. F., et al. (2007). Decreased adrenocorticotropic hormone and cortisol responses to stress in healthy adults reporting significant childhood maltreatment. *Biological Psychiatry, 62,* 1080–1087.

Caspi, A., McClay, J., Moffitt, T. E., Mill, J., Martin, J., Craig, I. W., et al. (2002). Role of genotype in the cycle of violence in maltreated children. *Science, 297,* 851–853.

Cicchetti, D., & Rogosch, F. A. (2007). Personality, adrenal steroid hormones, and resilience in maltreated children: A multilevel perspective. *Development and Psychopathology, 19,* 787–809.

Cohen, J. (1983). The cost of dichotomization. *Applied Psychological Measurement, 7*(3), 249–253.

Collishaw, S., Pickles, A., Messer, J., Rutter, M., Shearer, C., & Maughan, B. (2007). Resilience to adult psychopathology following childhood maltreatment: Evidence from a community sample. *Child Abuse and Neglect, 31,* 211–229.

Compas, B. E., Hinden, B. R., & Gerhardt, C. A. (1995). Adolescent development: Pathways and processes of risk and resilience. *Annual Review of Psychology, 46,* 265–293.

Curtis, W. J., & Cicchetti, D. (2003). Moving research on resilience into the 21st century: Theoretical and methodological considerations in examining the biological contributors to resilience. *Development and Psychopathology, 15,* 773–810.

Davis, D., Luecken, L. J., & Zautra, A. (2005). Are reports of childhood maltreatment related to the development of chronic pain in adulthood?: A meta-analytic review of the literature. *Clinical Journal of Pain, 21,* 398–405.

DeBellis, M. D. (2002). Developmental traumatology: A contributory mechanism for alcohol and substance use disorders. *Psychoneuroendocrinology, 27,* 155–170.

Dong, M., Anda, R. F., Dube, S. R., Giles, W. H., & Felitti, V. J. (2003). The relationship of exposure to childhood sexual abuse to other forms of abuse, neglect, and household dysfunction during childhood. *Child Abuse and Neglect, 27,* 625–639.

Dong, M., Giles, W. H., Felitti, V. J., Dube, S. R., Williams, J. E., Chapman, D. P., et al. (2004). Insights into causal pathways for ischemic heart disease: Adverse childhood experiences study. *Circulation, 110*(13), 1761–1766.

Dube, S. R., Anda, R. F., Felitti, V. J., Edwards, V. J., & Croft, J. B. (2002). Adverse childhood experiences and personal alcohol abuse as an adult. *Addictive Behaviors, 27,* 713–725.

DuMont, K. A., Widom, C. S., & Czaja, S. J. (2007). Predictors of resilience in abused and neglected children grown-up: The role of individuals and neighborhood characteristics. *Child Abuse and Neglect, 31,* 255–274.

Elzinga, B. M., Roelofs, K., Tollenaar, M. S., Bakvis, P., van Pelt, J., & Spinhoven, P. (2008). Diminished cortisol responses to psychosocial stress associated with lifetime adverse events: A study among healthy young subjects. *Psychoneuroendocrinology, 33*(2), 227–237.

Felitti, V. J., Anda, R. F., Nordenberg, D., Williamson, D. F., Spitz, A. M., Edwards, V., et al. (1998). Relationship of childhood abuse and household dysfunction to many of the leading causes of death in adults. *American Journal of Preventive Medicine, 14,* 245–258.

Fergus, S., & Zimmerman, M. A. (2005). Adolescent resilience: A framework for understanding healthy development in the face of risk. *Annual Review of Public Health, 26,* 399–419.

Fergusson, D. M., & Horwood, L. J. (2003). Resilience to childhood adversity: Results of a 12-year study. In S. S. Luthar (Ed.), *Resilience and vulnerability: Adaptation in the context of childhood adversities* (pp. 130–155). New York: Cambridge University Press.

Ferrari, A. M. (2002). The impact of culture upon child rearing practices and definitions of maltreatment. *Child Abuse and Neglect, 26,* 793–813.

Fisher, P. A., Stoolmiller, M., Gunnar, M. R., & Burraston, B. O. (2007). Effects of a therapeutic intervention for foster preschoolers on diurnal cortisol activity. *Psychoneuroendocrinology, 32,* 892–905.

Garmezy, N., Masten, A. S., & Tellegen, A. (1984). The study of stress and competence in children: A building block for developmental psychopathology. *Child Development, 55,* 97–111.

Heim, C., Newport, D. J., Bonsall, R., Miller, A. H., & Nemeroff, C. B. (2001). Altered pituitary–adrenal axis responses to provocative challenge tests in adult survivors of childhood abuse. *American Journal of Psychiatry, 158*(4), 575–581.

Heim, C., Newport, D. J., Heit, S., Graham, Y. P., Wilcox, M., Bonsall, R., et al. (2000). Pituitary-adrenal and autonomic responses to stress in women after sexual and physical abuse in childhood. *Journal of the American Medical Association, 284*(5), 592–597.

Heim, C., Wagner, D., Maloney, E., Papanicolaou, D. A., Solomon, L., Jones, J. F., et al. (2006). Early adverse experience and risk for chronic fatigue syndrome: Results from a population-based study. *Archives of General Psychiatry, 63(11), 1258–1266.*

Hines, A. M., Merdinger, J., & Wyatt, P. (2005). Former foster youth attending college: Resilience and the transition into young adulthood. *American Journal of Orthopsychiatry, 75,* 381–394.

Kendall-Tackett, K. A., Williams, L. M., & Finkelhor, D. (1993). Impact of sexual abuse on children: A review and synthesis of recent empirical studies. *Psychological Bulletin, 113,* 164–180.

Kessler, R. C., Davis, C. G., & Kendler, K. S. (1997). Childhood adversity and adult psychiatric disorder in the U.S. National Comorbidity Survey. *Psychological Medicine, 27,* 1101–1119.

Kim-Cohen, J., Moffitt, T. E., Caspi, A., & Taylor, A. (2004). Genetic and environmental processes in young children's resilience and vulnerability to socioeconomic deprivation. *Child Development, 75,* 651–668.

Liu, D., Diorio, J., Tannenbaum, B., Caldji, C., Francis, D., Freedman, A., et al. (1997). Maternal care, hippocampal glucocorticoid receptors, and hypothalamic–pituitary–adrenal responses to stress. *Science, 12,* 1659–1662.

Luecken, L. J. (1998). Childhood attachment and loss experiences affect adult cardiovascular and cortisol function. *Psychosomatic Medicine, 60,* 765–772.

Luecken, L. J. (2000a). Attachment and loss experiences during childhood are associated with adult hostility, depression, and social support. *Journal of Psychosomatic Research, 49,* 85–91.

Luecken, L. J. (2000b). Parental caring and loss during childhood and adult cortisol responses to stress. *Psychology and Health, 15,* 841–851.

Luecken, L. J., Appelhans, B. A., Kraft, A. J., & Enders, C. (2009). Emotional and cardiovascular sensitization to daily stress following childhood parental loss. *Developmental Psychology, 45*(1), 296–302.

Luecken, L. J., & Lemery, K. (2004). Early caregiving and adult physiological stress responses. *Clinical Psychology Review, 24,* 171–191.

Luecken, L. J., Rodriquez, A., & Appelhans, B. M. (2005). Cardiovascular stress responses in young adulthood associated with family-of-origin relationships. *Psychosomatic Medicine, 67,* 514–521.

Luthar, S. S., Sawyer, J. A., & Brown, P. J. (2006). Conceptual issues in studies of resilience. *Annals of the New York Academy of Science, 1094,* 105–115.

MacCallum, R. C., Zhang, S., Preacher, K. J., & Rucker, D. D. (2002). On the practice of dichotomization of quantitative variables. *Psychological Methods, 7*(1), 19–40.

MacKinnon, D. P., & Luecken, L. J. (2008). How and for whom?: Mediation and moderation in health psychology. *Health Psychology, 27,* 99–100.

MacMillan, H. L., Fleming, J. E., Streiner, D. L., Lin, E., Boyle, M. H., Jamieson, E., et al. (2001). Childhood abuse and lifetime psychopathology in a community sample. *American Journal of Psychiatry, 158*(11), 1878–83

Masten, A. S. (2007). Resilience in developing systems: Progress and promise as the fourth wave rises. *Development and Psychopathology, 19,* 921–930.

Masten, A. S., Burt, K. B., Roisman, G. I., Obradovic, J., Long, J. D., & Tellegen, A. (2004). Resources and resilience in the transition to adulthood: Continuity and change. *Development and Psychopathology, 16,* 1071–1094.

Masten, A. S., Coatsworth, J. D., Neeman, J., Gest, S. D., Tellegen, A., & Garmezy, N. (1995). The structure and coherence of competence from childhood through adolescence. *Child Development, 66,* 1635–1659.

Masten, A. S., Hubbard, J. J., Gest, S. D., Tellegen, A., Garmezy, N., & Ramirez, M. (1999). Competence in the context of adversity: Pathways to resilience and maladaptation from childhood to late adolescence. *Development and Psychopathology, 11*, 143–169.

McEwen, B. S. (1998). Stress, adaptation, and disease: Allostasis and allostatic load. *Annals of the New York Academy of Science, 840*, 33–34.

McEwen, B. S. (2003). Early life influences on life-long patterns of behavior and health. *Mental Retardation and Developmental Disabilities Research Reviews, 9*, 149–154.

McGloin, J. M., & Widom, C. S. (2001). Resilience among abused and neglected children grown up. *Development and Psychopathology, 13*, 1021–1038.

Meaney, M. J., Brake, W., & Gratton, A. (2002). Environmental regulation of the development of mesolimbic dopamine systems: A neurobiological mechanism for vulnerability to drug abuse? *Psychoneuroendocrinology, 27*, 127–138.

Nemeroff, C. B. (2004). Neurobiological consequences of childhood trauma. *Journal of Clinical Psychiatry, 65*, 18–28.

Nicolson, N. (2004). Childhood parental loss and adult cortisol levels. *Psychoneuroendocrinology, 29*, 1012–1018.

O'Dougherty Wright, M., & Masten, A. S. (2005). Resilience processes in development? In S. Goldstein & R. B. Brooks (Eds.), *Handbook of resilience in children* (pp. 17–37). New York: Kluwer Academic/Plenum Press.

Olsson, C. A., Bond, L., Burns, J. M., Vella-Brodrick, D. A., & Sawyer, S. M. (2003). Adolescent resilience: A concept analysis. *Journal of Adolescence, 26*, 1–11.

Petersen, A. C. (1988). Adolescent development. *Annual Review of Psychology, 39*, 583–607.

Purdom, C. L., Stevenson, M. M., Lemery-Chalfant, K., Howe, R., & Luecken, L. J. (2008). *Acculturation moderates the effect of self-mastery on self-rated health in Hispanic women*. Presentation at the annual meeting of the Society of Behavioral Medicine Abstracts, San Diego, CA.

Repetti, R. L., Taylor, S. E., & Seeman, T. E. (2002). Risky families: Family social environments and the mental and physical health of offspring. *Psychological Bulletin, 128*(2), 330–366.

Riley, J. R., & Masten, A. S. (2005). Resilience in context. In R. D. Peters, B. Leadbeater, & R. J. McMahon (Eds.), *Resilience in children, families, and communities: Linking context to practice and policy* (pp. 13–25). New York: Kluwer Academic/Plenum Press.

Romer, D., & Walker, E. F. (Eds.). (2007). *Adolescent psychopathology and the developing brain*. New York: Oxford University Press.

Rutter, M. (1985). Resilience in the face of adversity, protective factors and resistance to psychiatric disorder. *British Journal of Psychiatry, 147*, 598–611.

Rutter, M. (2003). Genetic influences on risk and protection: implications for understanding resilience. In S. S. Luthar (Ed.), *Resilience and vulnerability: Adaptation in the context of childhood adversities* (pp. 489–509). New York: Cambridge University Press.

Rutter, M. (2006). Implications of resilience concepts for scientific understanding. *Annals of the New York Academy of Science, 1094*, 1–12.

Rutter, M. (2007). Resilience, competence, and coping. *Child Abuse and Neglect, 31*, 205–209.

Sandler, I. N. (2001). Quality and ecology of adversity as common mechanisms of risk and resilience. *American Journal of Community Psychology, 29*, 19–61.

Sandler, I. N., Wolchik, S. A., & Ayers, T. S. (2008). Resilience rather than recovery: A contextual framework on adaptation following bereavement. *Death Studies, 32*, 59–73.

Sandler, I. N., Wolchik, S. A., Davis, C. H., Haine, R. A., & Ayers, T. A. (2003). Correlational and experimental study of resilience for children of divorce and parentally-bereaved children. In S. S. Luthar (Ed.), *Resilience and vulnerability: Adaptation in the context of childhood adversities* (pp. 213–240). New York: Cambridge University Press.

Schilling, E. A., Aseltine, R. H., & Gore, S. (2007). Adverse childhood experiences and mental health in young adults: A longitudinal study. *BMC Public Health, 7*, 30.

Schwartz, S. J., Côté, J. E., & Arnett, J. J. (2005). Identity and agency in emerging adulthood: Two developmental routes in the individualization process. *Youth and Society, 37*(2), 201–229.

Seifer, R. (2003). Young children with mentally ill parents: Resilient developmental systems. In S. S. Luthar (Ed.), *Resilience and vulnerabili-*

ty: *Adaptation in the context of childhood adversities* (pp. 29–49). New York: Cambridge University Press.

Social Security Administration. (2000). *Intermediate assumptions of the 2000 Trustees Report*. Washington, DC: Office of the Chief Actuary of the Social Security Administration.

Streeck-Fisher, A., & van der Kolk, B. A. (2000). Down will come baby, cradle and all: Diagnostic and therapeutic implications of chronic trauma on child development. *Australian and New Zealand Journal of Psychiatry, 34*, 903–918.

Teicher, M. H., Andersen, S. L., Polcari, A., Anderson, C. M., & Navalta, C. P. (2002). Developmental neurobiology of childhood stress and trauma. *Psychiatric Clinics of North America, 25*(2), 397–426.

van Reekum, R., Striner, D. L., & Conn, D. K. (2001). Applying Bradford Hill's criteria for causation to neuropsychiatry: Challenges and opportunities. *Journal of Neuropsychiatry and Clinical Neurosciences, 13*, 318–325.

Walker, E. A., Gefland, A., Katon, W. J., Koss, M. P., Von Korff, M., Bernstein, D., et al. (1999). Adult health status of women with histories of childhood abuse and neglect. *American Journal of Medicine, 107*, 332–339.

Werner, E. E. (1991). High-risk children in young adulthood: A longitudinal study from birth to 32 years. In S. Chess & M. E. Hertzig (Eds.), *Annual progress in child psychiatry and child development, 1990* (pp. 180–193). Philadelphia: Brunner/Mazel.

Werner, E. E. (1993). Risk, resilience, and recovery: Perspectives from the Kauai Longitudinal Study. *Development and Psychopathology, 5*, 503–575.

Werner, E. E. (2005). What can we learn about resilience from large-scale longitudinal studies?. In S. Goldstein & R.B. Brooks (Eds.), *Handbook of resilience in children* (pp. 91–105). New York: Kluwer Academic/Plenum Press.

Werner, E. E., & Smith, R. S. (1992). *Overcoming the odds: High risk children from birth to adulthood*. Ithaca, NY: Cornell University Press

Werner, E. E., & Smith, R. S. (1982). *Vulnerable but not invincible: A study of resilient children*. New York: McGraw-Hill.

Werner, E. E., & Smith, R. S. (2001). *Journeys from childhood to midlife: Risk, resilience, and recovery*. Ithaca, NY: Cornell University Press.

Wickrama, K. A. S., Conger, R. D., & Abraham, W. T. (2005). Early adversity and later health: The intergenerational transmission of adversity through mental disorder and physical illness. *Journals of Gerontology: Psychological Sciences and Social Sciences, 60*B, 125–129.

Williams, R. B., Marchuk, D. A., Siegler, I. C., Barefoot, J. C., Helms, M. J., Brummett, B. H., et al. (2008). Childhood socioeconomic status and serotonin transporter gene polymorphism enhance cardiovascular reactivity to mental stress. *Psychosomatic Medicine, 70*(1), 32–39.

Wolchik, S. A., Sandler, I. N., Weiss, L., & Winslow, E. (2007). New beginnings: An empirically based intervention program for divorced mothers to promote resilience in their children. In J. M. Briesmeister & C. E. Schaefer (Eds.), *Handbook of parent training: Helping parents prevent and solve problem behaviors* (pp. 25–62). New York: Wiley.

Wolchik, S. A., Schenck, C. E., & Sandler, I. N. (in press). Promoting resilience in youth from divorced families: Lessons learned from experimental trials of the New Beginnings Program. *Journal of Personality.*

Wolchik, S. A., West, S. G., Sandler, I. N., Tein, J.-Y., Coatsworth, D., Lengua, L., et al. (2000). An experimental evaluation of theory-based mother and mother–child programs for children of divorce. *Journal of Consulting and Clinical Psychology, 68*, 843–856.

Wyman, P. A., Sandler, I. N., Wolchik, S. A., & Nelson, K. (2000). Resilience as cumulative competence promotion and stress protection: Theory and intervention. In D. Cicchetti, J. Rappaport, I. Sandler, & R. P. Weissberg (Eds.), *The promotion of wellness in children and adolescents* (pp. 133–184). Washington, DC: Child Welfare League of America.

Yates, T. M., Egeland, B., & Sroufe, L. A. (2003). Rethinking resilience: A developmental process perspective. In S. S. Luthar (Ed.), *Resilience and vulnerability: Adaptation in the context of childhood adversities* (pp. 243–266). New York: Cambridge University Press.

13

Resilience to Potential Trauma
Toward a Lifespan Approach

Anthony D. Mancini
George A. Bonanno

It is an undeniable truism: Bad things happen. Natural disaster, the loss of friends and relatives, accidental harm, or even senseless violence from others, all can befall us. Indeed, at every stage of life we are vulnerable to these events. Epidemiological studies indicate that most adults experience at least one potentially traumatic event during the course of their lives (Kessler, Sonnega, Bromet, Hughes, & Nelson, 1995), and that most children are also exposed to such experiences (Copeland, Keeler, Angold, & Costello, 2007). It has long been commonplace that acutely aversive events almost always cause some form of lasting emotional damage, likely because they are so dreaded. However, this is, in fact, wrong. There are measurable and important individual differences in how people respond to such events (Bonanno, 2004, 2005). To emphasize these individual differences, we use the phrase *potentially traumatic* to describe such events. In other words, highly aversive events that fall outside the range of normal experience are "potentially" traumatic for the simple reason that not everyone experiences them as traumatic. Indeed, a growing body of research on various potentially traumatic events has consistently revealed a wide range of reactions. Although a small subset of people may suffer extreme distress following exposure to a potentially traumatic event, most people cope with such events extremely well (Bonanno, 2004, 2005).

In this chapter, we briefly trace the history of the construct of psychological trauma, then describe recent empirical research on response to potentially traumatic events. We consider how resilience is defined in the context of research on adults and on children, and argue for the necessity of defining resilience as an outcome following exposure to extreme adversity, as opposed to a trait inherent in the person. We consider the most common or prototypical outcomes people exhibit after exposure to potentially traumatic events, including not only pathological reactions but also adaptive ones. We then address the growing evidence for the human capacity to thrive even after the most difficult of experiences. We enumerate individual differences and contextual factors associated with a resilient outcome among children and adults. Finally, we consider the implications of resilience across the lifespan for therapeutic intervention.

Resilience: Trait, Process, or Outcome?

How should resilience be conceptualized? Researchers and theorists have offered various answers to this question and, indeed, the field has suffered from a lack of conceptual and terminological clarity as a result. This definitional ambiguity is perhaps most clearly illustrated in the development of trait measures of "resilience." For example, two commonly used measures of resilience are the Connor–Davidson Resilience Scale (CD-RISC; Connor & Davidson, 2003) and the Ego Resiliency Scale (Block & Block, 1980). The CD-RISC posits that resilience can be measured as a congeries of personality traits, views of the self, perceived support from others, and behavioral responses to stress (Connor & Davidson, 2003). Quite apart from the sheer heterogeneity of this specific measure, which raises the question of what it assesses, is the broader question of what it means to posit resilience as a trait. In relation to this question, it is worth noting that Block and Block's Ego Resiliency Scale (Block & Block, 1980, p. 351) measures "motivational control and resourceful adaptation as relatively enduring, structural aspects of personality." In other words, the Ego Resiliency Scale is intended explicitly to measure a personality construct, whereas the CD-RISC obfuscates, in our view, the conceptual distinction between a personality trait that may (or may not) promote resilience and the unfolding adaptive response to adversity that constitutes resilience.

We and others have argued (Bonanno & Mancini, 2008; Luthar, Cicchetti, & Becker, 2000; Masten, 1994) that it is critical to maintain this distinction. Indeed, it can be argued that it is meaningless to assess resilience in the absence of adversity. Moreover, positing resilience as an enduring component of personality carries with it some untoward implications. Is someone who reports low levels of trait resilience condemned to dysfunction when confronted with an acute stressor? Although that appears absurd, we think it is important to consider the implicit logic of resilience, which mandates that we consider human functioning not in the abstract but in response to extreme adversity. Only under such conditions can we define someone as resilient (Bonanno, 2004). It is for these and other reasons that Masten (1994) has argued that we should use the term *resiliency* when referring to a personality construct and *resilience* when describing the ability to sustain equilibrium and adaptive functioning under stressful circumstances. We would emphasize that this perspective does not gainsay the relevance of enduring person-centered traits in achieving resilience. Indeed, the Ego Resiliency Scale has generated an influential body of literature that has enhanced our understanding of personality factors in stress responding. The point here is that the concept of resilience loses a large portion of its meaning when it is conflated with personality characteristics.

One other point is whether the term is best conceptualized as a process or an outcome. Developmental researchers and theorists who study the impact of corrosive environments on child development typically characterize resilience as a dynamic *process* of adaptive functioning that unfolds in the context of substantial and enduring adversity (Luthar et al., 2000). By contrast, researchers studying adults exposed to acutely adverse but time-limited stressors have argued that resilience should be characterized as an *outcome* reflecting adaptive functioning in the face of adversity (e.g., Bonanno, 2004). As these descriptions imply, whether resilience is described as a process or an outcome is largely dependent on the nature of the stressor and the population being studied. Because developmental resilience researchers usually study enduring stressors, such as socioeconomic disadvantage, parental mental illness, neglect, and maltreatment, it is conceptually coherent to consider resilience as a process unfolding across chronological and developmental time. On the other hand, when considering the impact of acute stressors in adulthood, it makes sense to consider adaptation as an outcome determined by a person's response to a specific event, usually of brief duration. Based on these considerations, we would suggest that, as a conceptual matter, these different literatures reflect no meaningful differences in their underlying operational understanding of resilience. Rather, these different usages (process vs. outcome) primarily reflect the different questions being asked, populations being studied, and duration of the stressors under study.

Historical Conceptions of Psychological Trauma

Well before its formal definition as a psychological disorder, researchers, theorists, and practitioners viewed violent or life-threatening events as in some way causally related to psychological and physiological dysfunction (Ellenberger, 1970; Lamprecht & Sack, 2002). However, the primary source of dysfunction, even in the cases of extreme stressor events, was generally situated within the individual, as for example in Kardiner's (1941) concept of "traumatic neuroses." The great wars of the 20th century, and in particular World War II, brought increasing awareness to the caustic impact of extreme stress on human functioning (Keegan, 1976). Nevertheless, not until late in the 20th century did consensus begin to emerge that extremely aversive events by themselves could be the primary source of trauma-related dysfunction. In 1980, the American Psychiatric Association (1980) first formalized posttraumatic stress disorder (PTSD) as a legitimate diagnostic category, filling an enormous gap in public health knowledge about the impact

of trauma. At the same time, the PTSD category also helped consolidate and promote a surge of new research on traumatic stress (McNally, 2003). As a result, our understanding of the neurobiology, etiology, and treatment of PTSD has advanced considerably (Dalgleish, 2004; Foa & Rothbaum, 1998; Ozer, Best, Lipsey, & Weiss, 2003).

However, there has also been a downside to this nearly exclusive emphasis on PTSD in relation to extreme stress. When viewed from the perspective of the lay and professional literatures, this emphasis has tended to obscure the diversity in people's responses to potentially traumatic events. Indeed, the impact of potentially traumatic events is still commonly seen in relatively simplistic, binary terms of pathology versus the absence of pathology. And this simplistic view has resonated with lingering controversies about the sometimes elusive distinction between genuine psychological trauma and malingering. This issue has had particular relevance to war-related PTSD. Throughout the 20th century, warfare had been plagued by an enduring tension about the proper time and place for diagnosis or treatment (Lamprecht & Sack, 2002; Shepard, 2001). During the most recent Iraq War, these issues have once again flared into the open. For example, a recent study of returning Army and Marine Corps soldiers involved in combat operations in Iraq and Afghanistan found that many soldiers wanted but did not seek treatment because of the stigma still associated with treatment for psychological difficulties in the armed forces (Hoge et al., 2004).

In the case of bereavement, there has been a similar historical confusion among grief, healthy functioning, and denial. As with reactions to trauma, bereavement researchers tended to view acute and chronic grief reactions as normative, while offering little insight about possible resilience to loss. This emphasis on dysfunction has perhaps grown out of widespread assumptions about the appropriate way to grieve. For example, a report summarizing the views of bereavement experts in the 1980s stated that it was commonly assumed, particularly by clinicians, "that the absence of grieving phenomena following bereavement represents some form of personality pathology" (Osterweis, Solomon, & Green, 1984, p. 18). In similar fashion, Bowlby (1980a) considered the "prolonged absence of conscious grieving" (p. 138) as a type of disordered mourning, whereas, according to Rando (1993), bereaved individuals who do not experience intense distress following a loss are in a state of denial and have "a powerful ability to block out reality" (p. 158). Indeed, the failure to grieve in response to bereavement was thought to reflect underlying psychopathology because it suggested that the person was inhibiting or dissociating from negative feelings (Middleton, Moylan, Raphael, Burnett, & Martinek, 1993) or lacked a strong attachment to the deceased (Fraley & Shaver, 1999). When a person does not display overt distress, he or she may be presumed to be avoiding the "tasks" of grieving (Worden, 1991). Only recently has the lack of pronounced distress following the experience of loss been seen as resilience (Bonanno, 2004). Next we take up the different patterns of response to potentially traumatic events, including delayed reactions.

Trajectories of Response to Potentially Traumatic Events

In stark contrast to the binary view of traumatic stress, empirical studies of individual variation in response to potentially traumatic events have revealed a number of unique patterns or trajectories. It is generally thought that most of the variability in outcome can be captured by four prototypical types: chronic dysfunction, delayed reactions, recovery, and resilience (Bonanno, 2004). These trajectories are graphically represented in Figure 13.1; we elaborate on each trajectory below.

Chronic Dysfunction

It is increasingly apparent that only a relatively small subset of those exposed to potentially traumatic events will eventually develop chronic pathological reactions. Although the type and degree of exposure to a potentially

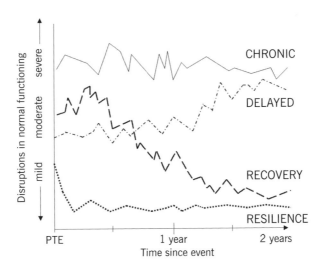

FIGURE 13.1. Prototypical patterns of disruption in normal functioning across time following potentially traumatic events (PTE). From Bonanno (2004). Copyright 2004 by the American Psychological Association. Adapted by permission.

traumatic event is a critical factor in stress reactions, PTSD (American Psychiatric Association, 2000) is typically observed in only 5–10% of exposed individuals (Kessler et al., 1995). In cases of prolonged exposure or exceptionally aversive events, the proportion of full-blown PTSD reactions may reach higher levels, sometimes as high as one-third of the sample. This was evident in a study of 2,752 individuals drawn by probability sampling from the New York metropolitan area during the weeks and months following the 9/11 terrorist attacks. Overall, the prevalence of PTSD for this sample was estimated at 6% (Bonanno, Galea, Bucciarelli, & Vlahov, 2006). However, among those physically injured in the attacks, PTSD prevalence rose to 26%. In another study reanalyzing the National Vietnam Veterans Readjustment data, a representative sample of 1,200 veterans, chronic PTSD was estimated at 9% overall, but among veterans with the highest levels of combat exposure the estimate was 28% (Dohrenwend et al., 2006).

In studies of bereavement, the proportion of persons who display more severe and chronic reactions to loss is similar. Although estimates vary somewhat, it is typically thought that 10–15% of bereaved people will develop chronically elevated grief reactions (Bonanno & Kaltman, 2001). As was the case for potentially traumatic events in general, however, chronic grief reactions tend to be more prevalent following more extreme losses, such as loss from a violent cause (Kaltman & Bonanno, 2003; Zisook, Chentsova-Dutton, & Shuchter, 1998) or when the lost loved one was a child (Bonanno, Papa, Lalande, Zhang, & Noll, 2005).

Delayed Reactions

What about delayed reactions? A long-held assumption in the bereavement literature is that the absence of overt signs of grieving, by virtue of its assumed link with denial, will eventually manifest in delayed grief reactions (Bowlby, 1980a; Deutsch, 1937; Osterweis et al., 1984; Parkes & Weiss, 1980; Rando, 1993; Sanders, 1993). Despite the strength of this belief, however, empirical evidence for delayed grief has never been reported (Bonanno & Kaltman, 1999; Wortman & Silver, 1989), even in longitudinal studies explicitly designed to measure the phenomenon (Bonanno & Field, 2001; Middleton, Burnett, Raphael, & Martinek, 1996). By contrast, there is some evidence for delayed PTSD reactions following potentially traumatic events, occurring in approximately 5–10% of exposed individuals (Bonanno, Rennicke, & Dekel, 2005; Buckley, Blanchard, & Hickling, 1996). It is crucial to note, however, that this pattern does not conform to the traditional idea of denial manifesting in delayed reactions. Rather, exposed individuals who eventually manifest delayed PTSD tend to have had relatively high levels of symptoms in the aftermath of the stressor event (Bonanno, Rennicke, et al., 2005; Buckley et al., 1996). Thus, the delayed pattern is more appropriately conceptualized as subthreshold psychopathology that gradually grew worse over time (Bonanno, 2004; Buckley et al., 1996).

Recovery and Resilience

Until recently, it was widely assumed that the enduring absence of trauma symptoms following exposure to a potentially traumatic event was rare and would occur only in people with exceptional emotional strength (Casella & Motta, 1990; McFarlane & Yehuda, 1996; Tucker et al., 2002). And, as noted earlier, bereavement theorists have persistently regarded the relative absence of grief as a form of denial or hidden psychopathology (Middleton et al., 1993). There is now compelling evidence, however, that a genuine and enduring resilience is not rare but is common and neither a sign of exceptional strength or psychopathology, but a fundamental feature of normal coping skills (Bonanno, 2004). Moreover, there is growing evidence that resilience and recovery can be mapped as discrete and empirically separable outcome trajectories. Distinctions between resilience and recovery have been identified, for example, following loss (Bonanno et al., 2002), major illness (Deshields, Tibbs, Fan, & Taylor, 2006), disease epidemic (Bonanno et al., 2008), and terrorist attack (Bonanno, Rennicke, et al., 2005). We consider these distinctions in more detail below.

Development of the Construct of Psychological Resilience

Much of the original theorizing on resilience came from developmental psychologists and psychiatrists during the 1970s. These pioneering researchers documented the large number of children who despite growing up in caustic socioeconomic circumstances (e.g., poverty) nonetheless evidenced healthy developmental trajectories (Garmezy, 1991; Murphy & Moriarty, 1976; Rutter, 1979; Werner, 1995). A surprising feature was that this work showed resilience in at-risk children to be common (Masten, 2001). Whereas traditional deficit-focused models of development had assumed that only children with remarkable coping ability could thrive in such adverse contexts, a growing body of evidence began to suggest that resilience is a result of normal human adaptational mechanisms (Masten, 2001). As noted earlier, however, most of this research focused on enduring aversive contexts rather than isolated, potentially traumatic events.

Although, at the time of these studies, the construct of resilience had not yet "trickled up" to the adult literature, there were sporadic reports of widespread resilience among adults exposed to isolated, potentially traumatic events (Bonanno, 2004; Rachman, 1978). More recently, however, as the resilience construct has gained currency among trauma researchers, the differences between resilience outcomes in adults and children have become apparent (Bonanno, 2004,

2005; Bonanno & Mancini, 2008). Some of the key differences seem to hinge on the temporal and sociocontextual characteristics of stress and adaptation at different points in the lifespan. For developing children, the definition of healthy adaptation is a complex issue (Luthar, Cicchetti, & Becker, 2000; Masten, 2001). For example, children at risk may evidence competence in one domain but fail to meet long-term developmental challenges in other domains (Luthar, Doernberger, & Zigler, 1993). By contrast, for adults exposed to a potentially traumatic event, this situation is arguably more straightforward (Bonanno, 2004, 2005). Most, but certainly not all, of the potentially traumatic events that adults may confront can be classified as isolated stressor events (e.g., an automobile accident) that occur in a broader context of otherwise normative (i.e., low stress) circumstances. Concomitant stressors may accompany or extend the potentially traumatic event (e.g., enduring health problems or change in financial situation), but this level of variability is usually straightforward and can be measured with a reasonable degree of reliability (Bonanno et al., 2006; Bonanno, Moskowitz, Papa, & Folkman, 2005). Finally, because developmental considerations are less pronounced in adults, responses to potentially traumatic events can usually be assessed in terms of deviation from or return to normative (baseline) functioning (Carver, 1998).

Based on these considerations, Bonanno (2004) defined *resilience* as "the ability of adults in otherwise normal circumstances who are exposed to an isolated and potentially highly disruptive event such as the death of a close relation or a violent or life-threatening situation to maintain relatively stable, healthy levels of psychological and physical functioning … as well as the capacity for generative experiences and positive emotions" (pp. 20–21). This definition contrasts resilience with a more traditional *recovery* pathway characterized by readily observable elevations in psychological symptoms that endure for at least several months before gradually returning to baseline, pretrauma levels.

A key point is that even resilient individuals may experience at least some form of transient stress reaction. However, these reactions are usually mild to moderate in degree, relatively short term, and do not significantly interfere with their ability to continue functioning (Bisconti, Bergeman, & Boker, 2006; Bonanno, Moskowitz, et al., 2005; Bonanno et al., 2002; Ong, Bergeman, Bisconti, & Wallace, 2006). For example, resilient individuals may have difficulty sleeping, or experience intrusive thoughts or memories of the event for several days or even weeks, but most can still manage to perform adequately the tasks of their daily life or career, or care for others. This is not to say, of course, that people showing resilient outcomes were not upset, disturbed, or unhappy about the occurrence of the event. Our point is merely that as undesirable as potentially traumatic events might be, many people cope with such events extremely well and are able to continue meeting the normal daily demands of their lives.

Until recently, most of the evidence that might support such a definition of *resilience* has been indirect. The earliest observations of resilience in response to an isolated but potentially devastating stressor event came from retrospective and unsystematic accounts (Janis, 1951; Rachman, 1978). More recently, a number of studies have demonstrated widespread resilience among people confronted with the untimely death of a spouse or child (Bonanno, Moskowitz, et al., 2005; Bonanno et al., 2002). Although these studies used a variety of different measures of adaptation, a resilient trajectory was consistently observed in about half the bereaved participants.

Several studies have also demonstrated widespread resilience among survivors of the 9/11 terrorist attacks in New York City. In one study using a sample of people in or near the World Trade Center at the time of the attacks, resilient individuals showed little

or no symptoms of PTSD or depression and were also described as *resilient* in anonymous ratings made by their close friends and relatives (Bonanno, Rennicke, et al., 2005). Another more encompassing study examined the prevalence of resilient outcomes using data from a large probability sample ($N = 2752$) that closely matched more recent New York census data (Bonanno et al., 2006). Of particular importance, because the sample varied in both geographic location and experiences during and after the attacks, it was possible to compare directly the prevalence of resilient outcomes across different levels of potential trauma exposure. Resilience in this study was defined as one or zero PTSD symptoms during the first 6 months after the attacks, and an absence of depression and substance use. Consistent with previous studies, across most exposure groups, the proportion with resilient outcomes was at or above 50% of the sample. Even among the groups with the most pernicious levels of exposure and highest probable PTSD, the proportion that was resilient never dropped below one-third of the sample.

Similar findings have also begun to emerge following serious health-related stressors. Deshields and colleagues (2006) mapped the same outcome trajectories depicted in Figure 13.1 using depression scores obtained from women immediately following radiation treatment for breast cancer, and again 3 and 6 months after treatment. Although 21% of the sample evidenced clinically significant levels of depression at 6 months, the majority (61%) had extremely low levels of depression throughout the study. A comparable pattern was recently observed in a large sample of hospitalized survivors of the 2003 severe acute respiratory syndrome (SARS) epidemic in Hong Kong. In keeping with the frightening nature of the epidemic, latent class analyses revealed that an unusually large proportion of the sample (42%) had chronically low levels of psychological functioning across the first 18 months after hospitalization. Nonetheless, despite the epidemic's impact, there were still almost as many individuals (35%) with consistently high levels of psychological functioning across the same time period (Bonanno et al., 2008).

Resilience across the Lifespan

How strongly do lifespan developmental factors influence resilience? Is resilience to potentially traumatic events observed to a similar degree in children and in older adults? Somewhat surprisingly, there are relatively few data on trauma and grief reactions among children, and results have provided somewhat mixed conclusions. In their study of children's reactions to Hurricane Andrew, a Category 4 storm, La Greca, Silverman, Vernberg, and Prinstein (1996) found that 55.8% fell into the categories of moderate to very severe PTSD 3 months after the storm, declining to 33.5% at 10 months. On the other hand, 44.2% of the sample showed minimal to absent symptoms at 3 months, indicating that a substantial proportion most likely showed resilience. Consistent with the adult literature, the most robust predictor of PTSD scores at 3 months was an exposure variable, accounting for 15% of the variance. These findings would seem to suggest that children, when compared to adults, are equally and perhaps more vulnerable to PTSD. However, this study used a self-report measure that does not map directly onto a PTSD diagnosis. The researchers also employed a convenience sample. By contrast, studies using representative samples and diagnostic interviews have suggested PTSD prevalence rates for children that are equal to or substantially lower than those of adults. For example, another investigation of Hurricane Andrew found that among children ages 12–17 only 2.9% of males and 9.0% of females met criteria for a PTSD diagnosis (Garrison et al., 1995). Interestingly, increased age was associated with higher rates of PTSD, underlining the role of developmental factors. A similar prevalence of PTSD was observed (4.5%) in a study of child and adolescent survivors of the 1999 earthquake

in Ano Liosia, Greece (Roussos et al., 2005). Moreover, a recent epidemiological investigation of PTSD among children and teenagers, ages 9–16, found even lower prevalence rates using a diagnostic interview measure and a representative sample (Copeland et al., 2007). In a longitudinal design spanning 8 years, less than 0.5% of children met criteria for a PTSD diagnosis, despite being exposed to a variety of extreme stressors (violence, interpersonal loss, sexual trauma). Together, these findings suggest that children cope well with isolated potentially traumatic events and only rarely develop full-blown PTSD. Nevertheless, a remaining question is whether the phenomenology of PTSD in children is different from that in adults (Perrin, Smith, & Yule, 2000). In contrast to PTSD, studies of children's bereavement reactions report levels of complicated grief similar to those of adults (Christ, 2000). As we discuss below, however, it is important to keep in mind that the question of adjustment to loss and to other extremely aversive experiences is in many ways more complex among children; therefore, these proportions should be considered with caution.

What about PTSD and grief in older adults? Investigations have generally suggested that increased age protects against dysfunction related to loss or to other potentially traumatic events. For example, Phifer (1990) found that older adults with high exposure to a severe flood were less vulnerable to psychological distress than were middle-aged adults with similar exposure. Although a comparison of younger and older adults' reactions to the 1988 earthquake in Armenia failed to reveal differences in overall PTSD symptoms (Goenjian et al., 1994), other studies have also suggested that older adults experience fewer symptoms than do younger adults in response to various natural disasters, including a tornado (Bell, 1978) and the Buffalo Creek dam collapse (Green et al., 1990). Moreover, in their meta-analysis of PTSD risk factors, Brewin, Andrews, and Valentine (2000) reported that older age is modestly associated with less PTSD, though this effect showed heterogeneity across samples.

Research also indicates that older adults' grief reactions are generally less intense than those of younger adults (Nolen-Hoeksema & Ahrens, 2002; Sanders, 1993; Sherbourne, Meredith, Rogers, & Ware, 1992), perhaps because loss is viewed as a normative experience of late life (Neugarten, 1979). Indeed, other common stressors of late life, such as disability, may have more long-lasting and deleterious effects than bereavement (Reich, Zautra, & Guarnaccia, 1989). Older bereaved persons are more likely to have provided high levels of care to a disabled spouse, and the strain of caregiving may have represented an acute stressor in itself. Schulz and colleagues (2001) found that bereaved older adults who experienced stressful caregiving reported *declines* in psychological distress following the death of a loved one. However, spousal illness by itself, even in the absence of caregiver strain, may be enough to produce this pattern. In the Bonanno and colleagues (2002) prospective study of spousally bereaved older adults, mentioned earlier, 10% of the sample evidenced a similar trajectory of elevated depression in the years prior to bereavement, then improved functioning following the spouse's death. Although individuals showing the improved pattern did not report greater caregiving strain relative to bereaved individuals, their spouses were nonetheless markedly more likely to have been ill in the years prior to their death.

The depression improvement pattern was also observed in a recent study of bereavement among HIV-positive gay men who had been caregivers for partners who died of AIDS (Bonanno, Moskowitz, et al., 2005). Again, the improvement pattern was associated with spousal illness but not caregiver burden per se. We recently found important additional confirmation for this pattern using a latent growth mixture modeling approach in a large representative sample of German citizens, including both pre- and postloss data (Mancini, Bonanno, & Clark,

2009). In this study, an improved pattern was evidenced in approximately 5% of the population. As these studies show, bereavement may not always represent an acutely stressful event and can sometimes result in improved psychological functioning, further demonstrating that adaptation to loss often is not accompanied by significant disruptions in functioning in old age.

What other more general factors might be relevant to resilience to potentially traumatic events in old age? One pertinent factor is that the ratio of positive to negative affect appears to increase linearly with age (Charles, Reynolds, & Gatz, 2001; Mroczek & Kolarz, 1998). In addition, older adults also generally show a superior capacity to regulate their own emotional experience (Lawton, Kleban, Rajagopal, & Dean, 1992) and report more complex or mixed emotional states (Labouvie-Vief, DeVoe, & Bulka, 1989). These age differences in the regulation and complexity of emotion suggest that older persons may be particularly competent managers of their emotional states. These abilities likely assist in managing the distress related to loss and other potentially traumatic events. Taken together, findings largely support the view that older age is associated with more resilient responses to potentially traumatic events than is younger age.

How does age interact with other factors to contribute to or detract from a resilient outcome? Although this question poses substantial methodological difficulties because large-scale longitudinal datasets on adaptation to acute stress are rare and cross-sectional age differences are confounded with cohort effects, Thompson, Norris, and Hanacek (1993) have proposed some intriguing answers to this question using a dataset on survivors of Hurricane Hugo, a devastating storm that caused widespread damage and injury. Specifically, they confirmed that the oldest adults did indeed enjoy protective benefits and show lower levels of symptoms than did younger or middle-aged adults. However, they also observed an unusual curvilinear pattern whereby middle-aged persons, when compared to younger and older adults, showed the highest level of symptoms under conditions of high exposure to the storm. Why would this be the case? The researchers found some evidence to support what has been described as the *burden perspective* on stress responding in middle age. Specifically, this perspective maintains that symptoms in response to acute stress are partly a function of the degree to which the acute event disrupts one's life and interferes with key role obligations. Because middle-age adults are likely to be more responsible for providing care to older parents or paying tuition for children, they are more likely to experience the most disturbance when their ability to meet these obligations is impaired. This explanation further comports with Hobfoll's (1989) conservation of resources model of stress responding, in which the retention of resources is a critical variable in understanding the relationship between stress and dysfunction.

Heterogeneous Factors Contribute to Resilience

A critical question is why some people are more or less likely to be resilient following exposure to a potentially traumatic event. A wide variety of factors influence whether a person will display resilience. Initial pioneering research into the nature of resilience in children suggested that there are multiple buffers against adversity. These include person-centered variables (e.g., temperament of the child) and sociocontextual factors (e.g., supportive relations, community resources) (Cowen, 1991; Rutter, 1999; Werner, 1995). Researchers on resilience in adults have researched a similar conclusion (Bonanno, 2005; Hobfoll, 2002): Resilience does not result from any single, dominant factor or set of factors. Instead, multiple independent risk and protective factors may contribute to or subtract from the overall likelihood of a resilient outcome. Consider, for example, the enduring but mistaken notion that resilience depends on trait-like characteristics of the person. As we review below, a variety of person-centered factors are associated with resilience. Indeed, personality undoubtedly plays a role in resilience to trauma but, as Mischel (1969) famously observed, personality rarely explains more than 10% of the actual variance in people's behavior across situations. We maintain, therefore, that it is more accurate to conceive of personality as just one of many potential sources of resilient outcomes.

Demographic Variables

A prosaic category of predictors is found in simple demographic variation. Resilience to trauma has been associated with male gender, older age, and greater education (Bonanno, Galea, Bucciarelli, & Vlahov, 2007). Racial/ethnic minority status is often considered as a risk factor for PTSD. However, these effects usually disappear when socioeconomic status is statistically controlled. A recent exception, however, was a finding that among New Yorkers, ethnic Chinese were considerably more likely to be resilient following the 9/11 attacks (Bonanno et al., 2007). Additionally, people with children were less likely to be resilient after hospitalization for SARS (Bonanno et al., 2008).

Personal and Social Resources

Numerous theorists have delineated a crucial role for social and personal resources in the ways adults cope with stress (Hobfoll, 2002; Holahan & Moos, 1991; Murrell & Norris, 1983). There is also considerable research linking resources, or change in resources, with adjustment following potentially traumatic events (Freedy, Shaw, Jarrell, & Masters, 1992; Ironson et al., 1997; Kaniasty & Norris, 1993; Norris & Kaniasty, 1996). Recent research on resilience to trauma has highlighted the particular importance of maintaining full-time employment and social resources (e.g., social support) (Bonanno, Galea, et al., 2007; Bonanno et al., 2008).

Additional Life Stress

There is strong evidence linking PTSD with increased life stress prior to and following the marker traumatic event (Brewin et al., 2000; Kubiak, 2005). Recent evidence suggests an even stronger relationship between the relative absence of current and prior life stress, and resilience to trauma (Bonanno, Galea, et al., 2007).

Flexible and Pragmatic Coping

A number of different personality-based coping behaviors have been associated with resilient outcomes. In previous work, we have parsed these behaviors into two broad categories labeled *flexible adaptation* and *pragmatic coping* (Bonanno, 2005; Bonanno & Mancini, 2008; Mancini & Bonanno, 2006). The idea of pragmatic coping stems from the fact that highly stressful life events often pose very specific coping demands. Successfully meeting these demands may require a highly *pragmatic*, or "whatever it takes," approach that is single-minded and goal-directed. Although pragmatic coping can arise in response to the situational demands, it has also been observed as a consequence of relatively rigid personality characteristics, such as repressive coping and the habitual use of self-enhancing attributions and biases. A compelling finding is that although these pragmatic styles have been associated with some negative features (e.g., narcissism, health consequences), they consistently predict superior adjustment to loss and other potentially traumatic life events.

We stress, however, that most people who are capable of resilience to adversity are genuinely healthy and appear to possess a capacity for behavioral elasticity, or *flexible adaptation*, to impinging challenges. A more genuinely health personality dimension is suggested by the concept of *adaptive flexibility*. A core aspect of flexibility is the capacity to shape and modify one's behavior to meet the demands of a given stressor event. This capacity for flexibility has been observed very early in development, yet it can change over time as a result of the dynamic interplay of personality and social interactions with key attachment figures (Block & Block, 2006). Practically speaking, then, flexibility is a personality resource that helps bolster resilience to aversive events, such as childhood maltreatment (Flores, Cicchetti, & Rogosch, 2005), but it may also be enhanced or reduced by developmental experiences (Shonk & Cicchetti, 2001). Preliminary research on flexibility in adults suggests that the construct does eventually become stable and predicts resilience to potentially traumatic events (Bonanno, Papa, Lalande, Westphal, & Coifman, 2004; Fredrickson, Tugade, Waugh, & Larkin, 2003). Flexible adaptation may also be facilitated by individual-difference factors, including more favorable preexisting beliefs (Lazarus & Folkman, 1984; Tomaka & Blascovich, 1994) and positive emotions (Bonanno & Keltner, 1997; Fredrickson et al., 2003). Next we consider, in turn, individual-difference variables, demographics, and contextual factors that predict resilience to potentially traumatic events in adults.

Repressive Coping

A perhaps unlikely source of resilience to potentially traumatic events is found among people who habitually employ coping mechanisms designed to minimize negative affects. Repressive coping is marked by simultaneous avoidance of threatening or negative stimuli and increased physiological arousal in response to those stimuli (Bonanno & Singer, 1990; Hock & Krohne, 2004; Tomarken & Davidson, 1994). For example, under stressful circumstances, repressive copers tend to report minimal or no feelings of distress, but physiological measures reveal marked autonomic arousal (Weinberger, Schwartz, & Davidson, 1979). This kind of dissociation from one's emotions or internal states has historically been seen as maladaptive (Bowlby, 1980b; Osterweis et al., 1984) and may be associated with long-term health costs (Bonanno & Singer, 1990; King, Taylor, Albright, & Haskell, 1990). However, a growing literature has linked these same tendencies to adaptation to loss and other forms of adversity. For example, repressors tend to show relatively little grief or distress at any point across 5 years of bereavement, a pattern consistent with resilience (Bonanno & Field, 2001; Bonanno, Keltner, Holen, & Horowitz, 1995). The benefits of repressive coping also emerged in a study of young women with documented histories of childhood sexual abuse. Although repressors were less likely to disclose their abuse voluntarily when provided the opportunity to do so, they also showed better adjustment than other survivors (Bonanno, Noll, Putnam, O'Neill, & Trickett, 2003). More recent work has shown that repressive coping in bereaved persons is associated with not only fewer symptoms but also fewer reported health problems and higher ratings of adjustment by close friends (Coifman, Bonanno, Ray, & Gross, 2007). Furthermore, the benefits of repressive coping are also apparent among nonbereaved controls, suggesting a general adaptive advantage for repressors.

Why would repressive coping facilitate adaptive coping with extremely aversive events? One important point is that repressive coping is largely an automatic process in which the person effortlessly orients away from threatening stimuli (Bonanno, Davis, Singer, & Schwartz, 1991). Thus, repressive coping is distinct from more conscious and effortful strategies to manage aversive thoughts and feelings, such as thought suppression or deliberate cognitive avoidance (Bonanno & Singer, 1990; Bonanno et al., 1995). Largely because it requires significant cognitive resources, suppression has been associated with a variety of untoward consequences in interpersonal, physiological, and emotional functioning (Gross & John, 2003; Gross & Levenson, 1993, 1997). By contrast, repressive coping appears to mitigate the potentially overwhelming and threatening nature of aversive experiences, without

exacting a cost in cognitive resources. By easing the threatening nature of their experience, repressors may be more likely to employ active, problem-focused coping rather than passive, emotion-focused coping (Lazarus & Folkman, 1984; Olff, Langeland, & Gersons, 2005), which would be particularly ineffective in the context of bereavement. Indeed, when confronted with highly threatening stimuli, repressors report more active rather than passive coping strategies (Langens & Moerth, 2003).

Self-Enhancing Biases

Another factor that has been shown to contribute to the likelihood of resilience is a dispositional tendency to view the self in highly favorable and even unrealistic terms (Taylor & Brown, 1988, 1994), a characteristic often described as *trait self-enhancement*. Historically, a positive view of the self has been considered highly beneficial, but only when coupled with a realistic appreciation of personal limitations and negative characteristics (Allport, 1937; Erikson, 1950; Maslow, 1950; Vaillant, 1977). Although there is also evidence that self-enhancement is associated with real costs in relationships with others (Paulhus, 1998), self-enhancers appear to cope unusually well with extreme adversity (Taylor & Armor, 1996). These benefits have been revealed in a number of studies examining different types of events. For example, in a study of survivors of the 9/11 terrorist attacks, self-enhancement was associated with a resilient outcome, ratings of better adjustment prior to 9/11, greater positive affect, and reduced perceptions of social constraints (Bonanno, Rennicke, et al., 2005). Similar findings were observed among survivors of the civil war in Bosnia and persons who suffered a premature spousal loss (Bonanno, Field, Kovacevic, & Kaltman, 2002). Among both samples, self-enhancement predicted lower grief symptoms at multiple intervals across bereavement and with different assessments of symptoms.

How does self-enhancement facilitate coping and promote resilience? Because the aversive experience of loss represents a potential threat to the self and may induce feelings of vulnerability and weakness, bereaved persons are likely motivated to restore their sense of control over the event and their sense of optimism about the future (Taylor & Armor, 1996). Self-enhancing cognitions could facilitate this process through downward social comparisons to others who are less fortunate (Helgeson & Taylor, 1993), or through reframing the aversive experience as providing unexpected benefits (Taylor, Wood, & Lichtman, 1983). Moreover, although self-enhancement can entail social liabilities, it also may play a role in whether the bereaved person draws effectively on social supports and has opportunities to disclose thoughts and feelings related to the event. An ample literature has shown the beneficial effects of self-disclosure after experiencing an acute stressor (Lepore, Silver, Wortman, & Wayment, 1996). Consistent with this notion, the study of high-exposure survivors of the 9/11 attacks revealed that self-enhancement's beneficial effects on coping are mediated by perceived constraints against disclosing distressing experiences (Bonanno, Rennicke, et al., 2005). Indeed, the beneficial effects of self-disclosure appear to depend on the degree to which others are perceived as willing or available to listen to one's concerns. In the absence of that belief, the beneficial effects of self-disclosure are typically negated (Lepore, Ragan, & Jones, 2000). Perhaps unsurprisingly, self-enhancers are particularly likely to view their friends as willing to listen to their deepest worries and concerns, even if this perception is at odds with friends' actual behavior (Goorin & Bonanno, 2009).

Worldviews (A Priori Beliefs)

A broadly beneficial component of resilience is favorable a priori beliefs, or *worldviews*, that comprise our most abstract and generalized conceptions of whether life is just, fair,

predictable, and benevolent (Janoff-Bulman, 1992; Park & Folkman, 1997; Rubin & Peplau, 1975). Because worldviews are widely thought to be influenced by extremely stressful events (Janoff-Bulman, 1992; Schwartzberg & Janoff-Bulman, 1991) it has historically been difficult to untangle their direct effects on coping. The only methodological solution to this confound is to employ a design in which worldview is assessed before the potentially traumatic event occurs. For obvious reasons, this poses practical and methodological difficulties. Indeed, to our knowledge, only a few studies have managed to meet this condition. In one study of spousal loss, researchers collected baseline data from a representative sample of older couples and married individuals, then invited persons who subsequently suffered a loss to participate in follow-up interviews at 6 and 18 months of bereavement. Using these data to map trajectories of bereavement outcome, Bonanno and colleagues (2002) identified four primary trajectories (resilience, recovery, chronic grief, and chronic depression), each of which was associated with unique predictors. Among the preloss predictors of resilience were stronger beliefs in the world's justice and more accepting attitudes toward death. We recently provided additional confirmation for the role of a priori beliefs by showing that favorable worldviews were related to adjustment over time only among bereaved persons and not among nonbereaved controls (Mancini & Bonanno, 2008). In one of the few investigations of PTSD to use preevent data, Bryant and Guthrie (2007) assessed firefighters during their training, then collected a second wave of data 4 years later. Similar to the findings on bereavement, more negative preevent beliefs, particularly about the self, were associated with elevated PTSD symptoms 4 years later, accounting for 20% of the variance in those symptoms.

Positive Emotions

It is widely acknowledged that positive emotional experiences provide an array of adaptive benefits, both for everyday life and in response to stressful events (Bonanno, Colak, et al., 2007; Fredrickson & Losada, 2005; Tugade & Fredrickson, 2004; but see also Bonanno, Colak, et al., 2007). However, the link between positive emotion and adjustment is especially prominent in aversive contexts. In a recent experimental study (Papa & Bonanno, 2008), for example, the expression of positive emotion following exposure to a sad film predicted better psychological adjustment 2 years later. By contrast, positive emotional expressions following an amusing film were unrelated to long-term adjustment. Not surprisingly, then, the expression of positive emotions consistently has been shown to be a critical pathway to resilience (Bonanno & Keltner, 1997; Keltner & Bonanno, 1997). For example, bereaved individuals who exhibited genuine laughs and smiles when speaking about a recent loss had better adjustment over several years of bereavement (Bonanno & Keltner, 1997), and also evoked more favorable responses in observers (Keltner & Bonanno, 1997). Moreover, resilient bereaved people also reported the fewest regrets about their behavior with the spouse, or about things they might have done, or failed to do, when he or she was still alive. Finally, resilient individuals are less likely to search to make sense of or find meaning in the spouse's death, suggesting that they are less likely to engage in rumination, which has negative consequences for adjustment to loss (Nolen-Hoeksema, McBride, & Larson, 1997).

Positive emotions also serve a critical function in adapting to more extreme and acute events. In a prospective study on reactions to the 9/11 terrorist attacks among college students, for example, Fredrickson and colleagues (2003) found that positive emotions, such as love, interest, and gratitude, fully mediated the relation between preevent ego resilience, a trait-like personality characteristic, and postevent depression and growth experiences. In the Bonanno, Renneke, and colleagues (2005) study of high-exposure survivors of the 9/11 attacks, the trait self-

enhancers who had coped so effectively in that study were also more likely to have experienced positive affect when talking about the event.

These findings have highlighted the salutary effects of positive emotion under extreme stress. But how do positive emotions facilitate coping? One way is through quieting or undoing negative emotions, which thereby reduces levels of distress following a potentially traumatic event (Keltner & Bonanno, 1997; Papa & Bonanno, 2008; Tugade & Fredrickson, 2004). Furthermore, positive emotions can facilitate coping by increasing the availability of social supports (Bonanno & Keltner, 1997; Papa & Bonanno, 2008). Positive emotional expression also indicates to close others one's willingness to maintain prosocial contact (Malatesta, 1990), which can lead to beneficial interactions with others. Indeed, an earlier study found that positive emotional expression was most prevalent among bereaved individuals with higher scores on the socially oriented personality characteristics of extraversion, agreeableness, and conscientiousness (Keltner, 1996). Continued contact with important others in the bereaved person's social environment can have a variety of salutary consequences (Lepore et al., 1996), especially when one considers that social isolation and loneliness are basic components of more complicated grief reactions (Horowitz, Siegel, Holen, & Bonanno, 1997), and that talking about a stressful event often has positive effects (Lepore et al., 2000).

Resilience Factors in Childhood

Given the paucity of research on resilience to potentially traumatic events in childhood, it is more difficult to identify factors specific to childhood that predict adult resilience. In many cases, it may be possible to identify resilience factors as the inverse of identified risk factors (Bonanno, 2004). Indeed, as Masten (2001) has pointed out, risk and resilience factors often index a bipolar characteristic that can be either positive or negative, such as parenting (good or poor) or emotional stability (high or low). Although research on resilience in adults does not always conform to this simple bipolar scheme (e.g., Bonanno, Galea, et al., 2007), such a scheme may be more plausible in predicting childhood outcomes due to the longer-term developmental considerations. Proceeding in this way, we can identify some characteristics of children that are associated with better outcomes, though we are again confronted with the difficulty of finding studies that obtain measures before the acute event occurred. One study that met this criterion examined children's responses to Hurricane Andrew. The researchers collected data 15 months in advance of the hurricane and then at 3 and 7 months after the hurricane (La Greca, Silverman, & Wasserstein, 1998). Among the findings that emerged in this study, levels of anxiety and better school performance were associated with significantly lower levels of PTSD symptoms, suggesting that emotional stability and academic achievement are resilience factors. A somewhat surprising finding was that black children were more vulnerable to PTSD symptoms than were white and Hispanic youth.

The Role of Culture in Resilience

These last findings raise the important question of cultural variations in resilience. Western, independence-oriented countries tend to focus more heavily than do collectivist countries on the personal experience of grief (Bonanno, Papa, Lalande, Zhang, & Noll, 2005). Cushman (1990) has described a pervasive assumption in the West of a "bounded, interior self," in which autonomy and self-reliance are primary values, that stands in opposition to Eastern notions of a collectivist self. What are the implications of such cultural beliefs for coping with extreme adversity? Although we cannot take up this issue in detail, preliminary evidence suggests that coping strategies do have different consequences for adjustment in dif-

ferent cultures. For example, bereaved people in China recover more quickly from loss than do bereaved Americans, and for the Chinese, coping is enhanced by a continuing psychological bond with the deceased (Bonanno, Papa, et al., 2005), perhaps because the self is construed in connection to the broader community. By contrast, American bereaved persons who report a continuing bond to the deceased tend to do quite poorly (Bonanno, Papa, et al., 2005), underlining the cultural imperative of a more individualistic society.

These findings are consistent with the notion that adaptation may be linked to normative cultural values regarding appropriate grieving and views of the self. Moreover, these data raise the intriguing question of whether resilience has different meanings in different cultural contexts or, perhaps even more intriguing, whether different cultures may learn from each other about effective and not so effective ways of coping with extreme adversity (Bonanno, 2005). A further question that has not been studied is whether these cultural variations are also related to lifespan issues. For example, it may be more appropriate in some cultures for parents to sustain a continued bond with a child but not a spouse who has passed away. Unfortunately, data about cultural variation are quite sparse in grief and trauma research, and much remains to be known about the impact of cultural factors in adaptation to extreme adversity.

Implications of Resilience across the Lifespan for Treatment

The burgeoning literature on resilience has important implications for how mental health professionals and close others respond to persons exposed to potentially traumatic events. Although, in many ways, a deeply ingrained cultural assumption that psychotherapeutic intervention for potentially traumatic events is invariably beneficial, the study of resilience suggests that this assumption is misguided and could even lead to harm. For most persons, intrinsic recovery processes will restore equilibrium relatively soon after exposure. Early interventions, such as critical incident stress debriefing, targeted indiscriminately at persons immediately after exposure to a potentially traumatic event, are not only ineffective but also may exacerbate trauma reactions by interfering with natural recovery processes (Litz, Gray, Bryant, & Adler, 2002). Although research on early interventions up to now has been confined to adults, we see no reason to think that children are more likely to benefit from such early interventions. Indeed, because children are more suggestible, it appears likely that processes that give rise to deterioration effects from early interventions may indeed be more, and not less, salient for children.

With regard to grief counseling, although opinion is somewhat mixed (e.g., Larson & Hoyt, 2007), we maintain that the balance of evidence has not been favorable to traditional models of grief counseling (Bonanno & Lilienfeld, 2008). Meta-analyses have consistently indicated that grief counseling has small and often nonsignificant effects that are substantially less than effects observed in traditional psychotherapies (Allumbaugh & Hoyt, 1999; Jordan & Neimeyer, 2003; Kato & Mann, 1999). Moreover, no long-term benefits were found for grief counseling in a recent authoritative meta-analysis (Currier, Neimeyer, & Berman, 2008). Previously we have argued that given increasing awareness that resilience is the modal response to loss, grief counseling should only target those who genuinely need help and show significant dysfunction (Bonanno & Mancini, 2006; Mancini & Bonanno, 2006). Indeed, recent studies of grief interventions that adopted just such a targeted approach (e.g., Boelen, de Keijser, van den Hout, & van den Bout, 2007; Shear, Frank, Houck, & Reynolds, 2005) have seen more promising results than were previously observed. We suggest that similar guidelines should be applied when considering treatment for bereaved children. Rather than assume that all children will benefit, it seems to be the wiser course to reserve treatment for those children experiencing genuine and persistent difficulties, and not just an expectable reaction to loss.

Although the story is somewhat more complicated for adults and children who have experienced other types of acutely aversive experiences, the study of resilience makes clear that PTSD afflicts only a small minority of those exposed. This appears to be the case in childhood, adulthood, and old age. For this reason, we again argue that only those persons who evidence genuine dysfunction in the face of potentially traumatic events, as defined by recurring symptoms and interference with social roles and obligations, should be candidates for treatment. It is inarguable that there are effective treatments for PTSD, particularly with respect to exposure treatment (Institute of Medicine, 2007). However, this does not preclude the possibility of iatrogenic effects, as witnessed in blanket early interventions following potentially traumatic events. This cautionary note only underscores how important it is to see resilient responses to potentially traumatic events as a basic human capabilities that are neither rare nor extraordinary.

References

Allport, G. W. (1937). *Personality: A psychological interpretation*. New York: Holt, Rinehart & Winston.

Allumbaugh, D. L., & Hoyt, W. T. (1999). Effectiveness of grief therapy: A meta-analysis. *Journal of Counseling Psychology, 46*, 370–380.

American Psychiatric Association. (1980). *Diagnostic and statistical manual of mental disorders* (3rd ed.). Washington, DC: Author.

American Psychiatric Association. (2000). *Diagnostic and statistical manual* (4th ed., text revision). Washington, DC: American Psychiatric Association.

Bell, B. D. (1978). Disaster impact and response: Overcoming the thousand natural shocks. *Gerontologist, 18*, 531–540.

Bisconti, T. L., Bergeman, C. S., & Boker, S. M.

(2006). Social support as a predictor of variability: An examination of the adjustment trajectories of recent widows. *Psychology and Aging, 21,* 590–599.

Block, J., & Block, J. H. (2006). Venturing a 30-year longitudinal study. *American Psychologist, 61,* 315–327.

Block, J., & Kremen, A. M. (1996). IQ and ego-resiliency: Conceptual and empirical connections and separateness. *Journal of Personality and Social Psychology, 70,* 349–361.

Boelen, P. A., de Keijser, J., van den Hout, M. A., & van den Bout, J. (2007). Treatment of complicated grief: A comparison between cognitive-behavioral therapy and supportive counseling. *Journal of Consulting and Clinical Psychology, 75,* 277–284.

Bonanno, G. A. (2004). Loss, trauma, and human resilience: Have we underestimated the human capacity to thrive after extremely aversive events? *American Psychologist, 59,* 20–28.

Bonanno, G. A. (2005). Resilience in the face of loss and potential trauma. *Current Directions in Psychological Science, 14,* 135–138.

Bonanno, G. A., Colak, D. M., Keltner, D., Shiota, M. N., Papa, A., Noll, J. G., et al. (2007). Context matters: The benefits and costs of expressing positive emotion among survivors of childhood sexual abuse. *Emotion, 7,* 824–837.

Bonanno, G. A., Davis, P. J., Singer, J. L., & Schwartz, G. E. (1991). The repressor personality and avoidant information processing: A dichotic listening study. *Journal of Research in Personality, 25,* 386–401.

Bonanno, G. A., & Field, N. P. (2001). Examining the delayed grief hypothesis across 5 years of bereavement. *American Behavioral Scientist, 44,* 798–816.

Bonanno, G. A., Field, N. P., Kovacevic, A., & Kaltman, S. (2002). Self-enhancement as a buffer against extreme adversity: Civil war in Bosnia and traumatic loss in the United States. *Personality and Social Psychology Bulletin, 28,* 184–196.

Bonanno, G. A., Galea, S., Bucciarelli, A., & Vlahov, D. (2006). Psychological resilience after disaster: New York City in the aftermath of the September 11th terrorist attack. *Psychological Science, 17,* 181–186.

Bonanno, G. A., Galea, S., Bucciarelli, A., & Vlahov, D. (2007). What predicts psychological resilience after disaster?: The role of demographics, resources, and life stress. *Journal of Consulting and Clinical Psychology, 75,* 671–682.

Bonanno, G. A., Ho, S. M. Y., Chan, J., Kwong, R. S. Y., Yick, M., Shung, E., et al. (2008). Psychological resilience and dysfunction following SARS: The mental health of hospitalized survivors after the 2003 epidemic in Hong Kong. *Health Psychology, 27,* 659–667.

Bonanno, G. A., & Kaltman, S. (1999). Toward an integrative perspective on bereavement. *Psychological Bulletin, 125,* 760–776.

Bonanno, G. A., & Kaltman, S. (2001). The varieties of grief experience. *Clinical Psychology Review, 21,* 705–734.

Bonanno, G. A., & Keltner, D. (1997). Facial expressions of emotion and the course of conjugal bereavement. *Journal of Abnormal Psychology, 106,* 126–137.

Bonanno, G. A., Keltner, D., Holen, A., & Horowitz, M. J. (1995). When avoiding unpleasant emotions might not be such a bad thing: Verbal–autonomic response dissociation and midlife conjugal bereavement. *Journal of Personality and Social Psychology, 69,* 975–989.

Bonanno, G. A., & Lilienfeld, S. O. (2008). Let's be realistic: When grief counseling is effective and when it's not. *Professional Psychology: Research and Practice, 39,* 377–378.

Bonanno, G. A., & Mancini, A. D. (2006). Bereavement-related depression and PTSD: Evaluating interventions. In L. Barbanel & R. J. Sternberg (Eds.), *Psychological interventions in times of crisis* (pp. 37–55). New York: Springer.

Bonanno, G. A., & Mancini, A. D. (2008). The human capacity to thrive in the face of potential trauma. *Pediatrics, 121,* 369–375.

Bonanno, G. A., Moskowitz, J. T., Papa, A., & Folkman, S. (2005). Resilience to loss in bereaved spouses, bereaved parents, and bereaved gay men. *Journal of Personality and Social Psychology, 88,* 827–843.

Bonanno, G. A., Noll, J. G., Putnam, F. W., O'Neill, M., & Trickett, P. K. (2003). Predicting the willingness to disclose childhood sexual abuse from measures of repressive coping and dissociative tendencies. *Child Maltreatment, 8,* 302–318.

Bonanno, G. A., Papa, A., Lalande, K., Westphal, M., & Coifman, K. (2004). The importance of being flexible: The ability to both enhance and suppress emotional expression predicts long-term adjustment. *Psychological Science, 15,* 482–487.

Bonanno, G. A., Papa, A., Lalande, K., Zhang, N., & Noll, J. G. (2005). Grief processing and deliberate grief avoidance: A prospective comparison of bereaved spouses and parents in the United States and the People's Republic of China. *Journal of Consulting and Clinical Psychology, 73,* 86–98.

Bonanno, G. A., Rennicke, C., & Dekel, S. (2005). Self-enhancement among high-exposure survivors of the September 11th terrorist attack: Resilience or social maladjustment? *Journal of Personality and Social Psychology, 88,* 984–998.

Bonanno, G. A., & Singer, J. L. (1990). Repressor personality style: Theoretical and methodological implications for health and pathology. In J. L. Singer (Ed.), *Repression and dissociation* (pp. 435–470). Chicago: University of Chicago Press.

Bonanno, G. A., Wortman, C. B., Lehman, D. R., Tweed, R. G., Haring, M., Sonnega, J., et al. (2002). Resilience to loss and chronic grief: A prospective study from preloss to 18-months postloss. *Journal of Personality and Social Psychology, 83,* 1150–1164.

Bowlby, J. (1980a). *Attachment and loss.* New York: Basic Books

Bowlby, J. (1980b). *Attachment and loss: Vol. 3. Loss: Sadness and depression.* New York: Basic Books.

Brewin, C. R., Andrews, B., & Valentine, J. D. (2000). Meta-analysis of risk factors for posttraumatic stress disorder in trauma-exposed adults. *Journal of Consulting and Clinical Psychology, 68,* 748–766.

Bryant, R. A., & Guthrie, R. M. (2007). Maladaptive self-appraisals before trauma exposure predict posttraumatic stress disorder. *Journal of Consulting and Clinical Psychology, 75,* 812–815.

Buckley, T. C., Blanchard, E. B., & Hickling, E. J. (1996). A prospective examination of delayed onset PTSD secondary to motor vehicle accidents. *Journal of Abnormal Psychology, 105,* 617–625.

Carver, C. S. (1998). Resilience and thriving: Issues, models, and linkages. *Journal of Social Issues, 54,* 245–266.

Casella, L., & Motta, R. W. (1990). Comparison of characteristics of Vietnam veterans with and without posttraumatic stress disorder. *Psychological Reports, 67,* 595–605.

Charles, S. T., Reynolds, C. A., & Gatz, M. (2001). Age-related differences and change in positive and negative affect over 23 years. *Journal of Personality and Social Psychology, 80,* 136–151.

Christ, G. H. (2000). *Healing children's grief: Surviving a parent's death from cancer.* New York: Oxford University Press.

Coifman, K. G., Bonanno, G. A., Ray, R. D., & Gross, J. J. (2007). Does repressive coping promote resilience?: Affective–autonomic response discrepancy during bereavement. *Journal of Personality and Social Psychology, 92,* 745–758.

Connor, K. M., & Davidson, R. T. (2003). Development of a new resilience scale: The Connor–Davidson Resilience Scale (CD-RISC). *Depression and Anxiety, 18,* 76–82.

Copeland, W. E., Keeler, G., Angold, A., & Costello, E. J. (2007). Traumatic events and posttraumatic stress in childhood. *Archives of General Psychiatry, 64,* 577–584.

Cowen, E. L. (1991). In pursuit of wellness. *American Psychologist, 46,* 404–408.

Currier, J. M., Neimeyer, R. A., & Berman, J. S. (2008). The effectiveness of psychotherapeutic interventions for bereaved persons: A comprehensive quantitative review. *Psychological Bulletin, 134,* 648–661.

Cushman, P. (1990). Why the self is empty: Toward a historically situated psychology. *American Psychologist, 45,* 599–611.

Dalgleish, T. (2004). Cognitive approaches to posttraumatic stress disorder: The evolution of multirepresentational theorizing. *Psychological Bulletin, 130,* 228–260.

Deshields, T., Tibbs, T., Fan, M. Y., & Taylor, M. (2006). Differences in patterns of depression after treatment for breast cancer. *Psycho-Oncology, 15,* 398–406.

Deutsch, H. (1937). Absence of grief. *Psychoanalytic Quarterly, 6,* 12–22.

Dohrenwend, B. P., Turner, J. B., Turse, N. A., Adams, B. G., Koenen, K. C., & Marshall, R. D. (2006). The psychological risks of Vietnam for U.S. veterans: A revisit with new data and methods. *Science, 313,* 979–982.

Ellenberger, H. F. (1970). *The discovery of the unconscious: History and evolution of dynamic psychiatry.* New York: Basic Books.

Erikson, E. H. (1950). *Childhood and society* (2nd ed.). New York: Norton.

Flores, E., Cicchetti, D., & Rogosch, F. A. (2005). Predictors of resilience in maltreated and non-maltreated Latino children. *Developmental Psychology, 41*, 338–351.

Foa, E. B., & Rothbaum, B. O. (1998). *Treating the trauma of rape: Cognitive behavioral therapy for PTSD.* New York: Guilford Press.

Fraley, R. C., & Shaver, P. R. (1999). Loss and bereavement: Attachment theory and recent controversies concerning "grief work" and the nature of detachment. In J. Cassidy & P. R. Shaver (Eds.), *Handbook of attachment: Theory, research, and clinical applications* (pp. 735–759). New York: Guilford Press.

Fredrickson, B. L., & Losada, M. F. (2005). Positive affect and the complex dynamics of human flourishing. *American Psychologist, 60*, 678–686.

Fredrickson, B. L., Tugade, M. M., Waugh, C. E., & Larkin, G. R. (2003). What good are positive emotions in crisis?: A prospective study of resilience and emotions following the terrorist attacks on the United States on September 11th, 2001. *Journal of Personality and Social Psychology, 84*, 365–376.

Freedy, J. R., Shaw, D. L., Jarrell, M. P., & Masters, C. R. (1992). Towards an understanding of the psychological impact of natural disasters: An application of the conservation resources stress model. *Journal of Traumatic Stress, 5*, 441–454.

Garmezy, N. (1991). Resilience and vulnerability to adverse developmental outcomes associated with poverty. *American Behavioral Scientist, 34*, 416–430.

Garrison, C. Z., Bryant, E. S., Addy, C. L., Spurrier, P. G., Freedy, J. R., & Kilpatrick, D. G. (1995). Posttraumatic stress disorder in adolescents after Hurricane Andrew. *Journal of the American Academy of Child and Adolescent Psychiatry, 34*, 1193–1201.

Goenjian, A. K., Najarian, L. M., Pynoos, R. S., Steinberg, A. M., Manoukian, G., Tavosian, A., et al. (1994). Posttraumatic stress disorder in elderly and younger adults after the 1988 earthquake in Armenia. *American Journal of Psychiatry, 151*, 895–901.

Goorin, L., & Bonanno, G. A. (2009). Would you buy a used car from a self-enhancer?: Social benefits and illusions in trait self-enhancement. *Self and Identity, 8*, 162–175.

Green, B. L., Lindy, J. D., Grace, M. C., Gleser, G. C., Leonard, A. C., Korol, M., et al. (1990). Buffalo Creek survivors in the second decade: Stability of stress symptoms. *American Journal of Orthopsychiatry, 60*, 43–54.

Gross, J. J., & John, O. P. (2003). Individual differences in two emotion regulation processes: Implications for affect, relationships, and well-being. *Journal of Personality and Social Psychology, 85*, 348–362.

Gross, J. J., & Levenson, R. W. (1993). Emotional suppression: Physiology, self-report, and expressive behavior. *Journal of Personality and Social Psychology, 64*, 970–986.

Gross, J. J., & Levenson, R. W. (1997). Hiding feelings: The acute effects of inhibiting negative and positive emotion. *Journal of Abnormal Psychology, 106*, 95–103.

Helgeson, V. S., & Taylor, S. E. (1993). Social comparisons and adjustment among cardiac patients. *Journal of Applied Social Psychology, 23*, 1171–1195.

Hobfoll, S. E. (1989). Conservation of resources: A new attempt at conceptualizing stress. *American Psychologist, 44*, 513–524.

Hobfoll, S. E. (2002). Social and psychological resources and adaptation. *Review of General Psychology, 6*, 307–324.

Hock, M., & Krohne, H. W. (2004). Coping with threat and memory for ambiguous information: Testing the repressive discontinuity hypothesis. *Emotion, 4*, 65–86.

Hoge, C. W., Castro, C. A., Messer, S. C., McGurk, D., Cotting, D. I., Koffman, R. L., et al. (2004). Combat duty in Iraq and Afghanistan, mental health problems, and barriers to care. *New England Journal of Medicine, 351*, 13–22.

Holahan, C. J., & Moos, R. H. (1991). Life stressors, personal and social resources, and depression: A 4-year structural model. *Journal of Abnormal Psychology, 100*, 31–38.

Horowitz, M. J., Siegel, B., Holen, A., & Bonanno, G. A. (1997). Diagnostic criteria for complicated grief disorder. *American Journal of Psychiatry, 154*, 904–910.

Institute of Medicine. (2007). *Treatment of posttraumatic stress disorder: An assessment of the evidence.* Washington, DC: National Academies Press.

Ironson, G., Wynings, C., Schneiderman, N., Baum, A., Rodriguez, M., Greenwood, D., et al. (1997). Posttraumatic stress symptoms, intrusive thoughts, loss, and immune function after Hurricane Andrew. *Psychosomatic Medicine, 59,* 128–141.

Janis, I. L. (1951). *Air war and emotional stress.* New York: McGraw-Hill.

Janoff-Bulman, R. (1992). *Shattered assumptions: Towards a new psychology of trauma.* New York: Free Press.

Jordan, J. R., & Neimeyer, R. A. (2003). Does grief counseling work? *Death Studies, 27,* 765–786.

Kaltman, S., & Bonanno, G. A. (2003). Trauma and bereavement: Examining the impact of sudden and violent deaths. *Journal of Anxiety Disorders, 17,* 131–147.

Kaniasty, K., & Norris, F. H. (1993). A test of the social support deterioration model in the context of natural disaster. *Journal of Personality and Social Psychology, 64,* 395–408.

Kardiner, A. (1941). *The traumatic neuroses of war.* New York: Hoeber.

Kato, P. M., & Mann, T. (1999). A synthesis of psychological interventions for the bereaved. *Clinical Psychology Review, 19,* 275–296.

Keegan, J. (1976). *The face of battle.* Harmondsworth, UK: Chaucer Press.

Keltner, D. (1996). Facial expressions of emotion and personality. In C. Magai & S. H. McFadden (Eds.), *Handbook of emotion, adult development, and aging* (pp. 385–401). San Diego, CA: Academic Press.

Keltner, D., & Bonanno, G. A. (1997). A study of laughter and dissociation: Distinct correlates of laughter and smiling during bereavement. *Journal of Personality and Social Psychology, 73,* 687–702.

Kessler, R. C., Sonnega, A., Bromet, E., Hughes, M., & Nelson, C. B. (1995). Posttraumatic stress disorder in the National Comorbidity Survey. *Archives of General Psychiatry, 52,* 1048–1060.

King, A. C., Taylor, C., Albright, C. A., & Haskell, W. L. (1990). The relationship between repressive and defensive coping styles and blood pressure responses in healthy, middle-aged men and women. *Journal of Psychosomatic Research, 34,* 461–471.

Kubiak, S. P. (2005). Trauma and cumulative adversity in women of a disadvantaged social location. *American Journal of Orthopsychiatry, 75,* 451–465.

Labouvie-Vief, G., DeVoe, M., & Bulka, D. (1989). Speaking about feelings: Conceptions of emotion across the life span. *Psychology and Aging, 4,* 425–437.

La Greca, A. M., Silverman, W. K., Vernberg, E. M., & Prinstein, M. J. (1996). Symptoms of posttraumatic stress in children after Hurricane Andrew: A prospective study. *Journal of Consulting and Clinical Psychology, 64,* 712–723.

La Greca, A. M., Silverman, W. K., & Wasserstein, S. B. (1998). Children's predisaster functioning as a predictor of posttraumatic stress following Hurricane Andrew. *Journal of Consulting and Clinical Psychology, 66,* 883–892.

Lamprecht, F., & Sack, M. (2002). Posttraumatic stress disorder revisited. *Psychosomatic Medicine, 64,* 222–237.

Langens, T. A., & Moerth, S. (2003). Repressive coping and the use of passive and active coping strategies. *Personality and Individual Differences, 35,* 461–473.

Larson, D. G., & Hoyt, W. T. (2007). What has become of grief counseling?: An evaluation of the empirical foundations of the new pessimism. *Professional Psychology: Research and Practice, 38,* 347–355.

Lawton, M., Kleban, M. H., Rajagopal, D., & Dean, J. (1992). Dimensions of affective experience in three age groups. *Psychology and Aging, 7,* 171–184.

Lazarus, R. S., & Folkman, S. (1984). *Stress, appraisal, and coping.* New York: Springer.

Lepore, S. J., Ragan, J. D., & Jones, S. (2000). Talking facilitates cognitive–emotional processes of adaptation to an acute stressor. *Journal of Personality and Social Psychology, 78,* 499–508.

Lepore, S. J., Silver, R. C., Wortman, C. B., & Wayment, H. A. (1996). Social constraints, intrusive thoughts, and depressive symptoms among bereaved mothers. *Journal of Personality and Social Psychology, 70,* 271–282.

Litz, B. T., Gray, M. J., Bryant, R. A., & Adler, A. B. (2002). Early intervention for trauma: Current status and future directions. *Clinical Psychology: Science and Practice, 9,* 112–134.

Luthar, S. S., Cicchetti, D., & Becker, B. (2000). The construct of resilience: A critical evaluation and guidelines for future work. *Child Development, 71,* 543–562.

Luthar, S. S., Doernberger, C. H., & Zigler, E. (1993). Resilience is not a unidimensional construct: Insights from a prospective study of inner-city adolescents. *Development and Psychopathology, 5,* 703–717.

Malatesta, C. Z. (1990). The role of emotions in the development and organization of personality. In R. A. Thompson (Ed.), *Nebraska Symposium on Motivation* (Vol. 36, pp. 1–56). Lincoln: University of Nebraska Press.

Mancini, A. D., & Bonanno, G. A. (2006). Resilience in the face of potential trauma: Clinical practices and illustrations. *Journal of Clinical Psychology, 62,* 971–985.

Mancini, A. D., & Bonanno, G. A. (2009). *The role of worldviews in grief reactions: Prospective and longitudinal analyses.* Manuscript submitted for publication.

Mancini, A. D., Bonanno, G. A., & Clark, A. (2009). *Stepping off the hedonic treadmill: Latent class analyses of individual differences in response to major life events.* Manuscript submitted for publication.

Maslow, A. H. (1950). Self-actualizing people: A study of psychological health. *Personality: Symposium, 1,* 11–34.

Masten, A. S. (1994). Resilience in individual development: Successful adaptation despite risk and adversity. In M. C. Wang & E. W. Gordon (Eds.), *Educational resilience in inner-city America: Challenges and prospects* (pp. 3–25). Hillsdale, NJ: Erlbaum.

Masten, A. S. (2001). Ordinary magic: Resilience processes in development. *American Psychologist, 56,* 227–238.

McFarlane, A. C., & Yehuda, R. (1996). Resilience, vulnerability, and the course of posttraumatic reactions. In B. A. van der Kolk, A. C. McFarlane, & L. Weisaeth (Ed.), *Traumatic stress* (pp. 155–181). New York: Guilford Press.

McNally, R. J. (2003). Progress and controversy in the study of posttraumatic stress disorder. *Annual Review of Psychology, 54,* 229–252.

Middleton, W., Burnett, P., Raphael, B., & Martinek, N. (1996). The bereavement response: A cluster analysis. *British Journal of Psychiatry, 169,* 167–171.

Middleton, W., Moylan, A., Raphael, B., Burnett, P., & Martinek, N. (1993). An international perspective on bereavement related concepts. *Australian and New Zealand Journal of Psychiatry, 27,* 457–463.

Mischel, W. (1969). Continuity and change

in personality. *American Psychologist, 24,* 1012–1018.

Mroczek, D. K., & Kolarz, C. M. (1998). The effect of age on positive and negative affect: A developmental perspective on happiness. *Journal of Personality and Social Psychology, 75,* 1333–1349.

Murphy, L. B., & Moriarty, A. E. (1976). *Vulnerability, coping, and growth.* New Haven, CT: Yale University Press.

Murrell, S. A., & Norris, F. H. (1983). Resources, life events, and changes in psychological states: A prospective framework. *American Journal of Community Psychology, 11,* 473–491.

Neugarten, B. L. (1979). Time, age, and the life cycle. *American Journal of Psychiatry, 136,* 887–894.

Nolen-Hoeksema, S., & Ahrens, C. (2002). Age differences and similarities in the correlates of depressive symptoms. *Psychology and Aging, 17,* 116–124.

Nolen-Hoeksema, S., McBride, A., & Larson, J. (1997). Rumination and psychological distress among bereaved partners. *Journal of Personality and Social Psychology, 45,* 855–862.

Norris, F. H., & Kaniasty, K. (1996). Received and perceived social support in times of stress: A test of the social support deterrence deterrence model. *Journal of Personality and Social Psychology, 71,* 498–511.

Olff, M., Langeland, W., & Gersons, B. P. R. (2005). Effects of appraisal and coping on the neuroendocrine response to extreme stress. *Neuroscience and Biobehavioral Reviews, 29,* 457–467.

Osterweis, M., Solomon, F., & Green, F. (1984). *Bereavement: Reactions, consequences, and care.* Washington, DC: National Academies Press.

Ozer, E. J., Best, S. R., Lipsey, T. L., & Weiss, D. S. (2003). Predictors of posttraumatic stress disorder and symptoms in adults: A meta-analysis. *Psychological Bulletin, 129,* 52–73.

Papa, A., & Bonanno, G. A. (2008). Smiling in the face of adversity: The interpersonal and intrapersonal functions of smiling. *Emotion, 8,* 1–12.

Park, C. L., & Folkman, S. (1997). Meaning in the context of stress and coping. *Review of General Psychology, 1,* 115–144.

Parkes, C. M., & Weiss, R. S. (1980). *Recovery from bereavement* New York: Basic Books.

Paulhus, D. L. (1998). Interpersonal and intrapsychic adaptiveness of trait self-enhancement: A mixed blessing? *Journal of Personality and Social Psychology, 74*, 1197–1208

Perrin, S., Smith, P., & Yule, W. (2000). Assessment and treatment of PTSD in children and adolescents. *Journal of Child Psychiatry and Psychology, 41*, 277–289.

Phifer, J. F. (1990). Psychological distress and somatic symptoms after natural disaster: Differential vulnerability among older adults. *Psychology and Aging, 5*, 412–420.

Rachman, S. J. (1978). *Fear and courage.* New York: Freeman.

Rando, T. A. (1993). *Treatment of complicated mourning.* Champaign, IL: Research Press.

Reich, J. W., Zautra, A. J., & Guarnaccia, C. A. (1989). Effects of disability and bereavement on the mental health and recovery of older adults. *Psychology and Aging, 4*, 57–65.

Roussos, A., Goenjian, A. K., Steinberg, A. M., Sotiropoulou, C., Kakaki, M., Kabakos, C., et al. (2005). Posttraumatic stress and depressive reactions among children and adolescents after the 1999 earthquake in Ano Liosia, Greece. *American Journal of Psychiatry, 162*, 530–537.

Rubin, Z., & Peplau, L. A. (1975). Who believes in a just world? *Journal of Social Issues, 31*, 65–89.

Rutter, M. (1979). Protective factors in children's responses to stress and disadvantage. In M. W. Kent & J. E. Rolf (Eds.), *Primary prevention of psychopathology: Social competence in children* (Vol. 3, pp. 49–74). Hanover, NH: University Press of New England.

Rutter, M. (1999). Resilience concepts and findings: Implications for family therapy. *Journal of Family Therapy, 21*, 119–144.

Sanders, C. M. (1993). Risk factors in bereavement outcome. In M. S. Stroebe, W. Stroebe, & R. O. Hansson (Eds.), *Handbook of bereavement: Theory, research, and intervention* (pp. 255–267). Cambridge, UK: Cambridge University Press.

Schulz, R., Beach, S. R., Lind, B., Martire, L. M., Zdaniuk, B., Hirsch, C., et al. (2001). Involvement in caregiving and adjustment to death of a spouse: Findings from the Caregiver Health Effects Study. *Journal of the American Medical Association, 285*, 3123–3129.

Schwartzberg, S. S., & Janoff-Bulman, R. (1991). Grief and the search for meaning: Exploring the assumptive worlds of bereaved college students. *Journal of Social and Clinical Psychology, 10*, 270–288.

Shear, K., Frank, E., Houck, P. R., & Reynolds, C. F. (2005). Treatment of complicated grief: A randomized controlled trial. *Journal of the American Medical Association, 293*, 2601–2608.

Shepard, B. (2001). *A war of nerves: Soldiers and psychiatrists in the twentieth century.* Cambridge, MA: Harvard University Press.

Sherbourne, C., Meredith, L., Rogers, W., & Ware, J. (1992). Social support and stressful life events: Age differences in their effects on health-related quality of life among the chronically ill. *Quality of Life Research, 1*, 235–246.

Shonk, S. M., & Cicchetti, D. (2001). Maltreatment, competency deficits, and risk for academic and behavioral maladjustment. *Developmental Psychology, 37*, 3–17.

Taylor, S. E., & Armor, D. A. (1996). Positive illusions and coping with adversity. *Journal of Personality, 64*, 873–898.

Taylor, S. E., & Brown, J. D. (1988). Illusion and well-being: A social psychological perspective on mental health. *Psychological Bulletin, 103*, 193–210.

Taylor, S. E., & Brown, J. D. (1994). "Illusion" of mental health does not explain positive illusions. *American Psychologist, 49*, 972–973.

Taylor, S. E., Wood, J. V., & Lichtman, R. R. (1983). It could be worse: Selective evaluation as a response to victimization. *Journal of Social Issues, 39*, 19–40.

Thompson, M. P., Norris, F. H., & Hanacek, B. (1993). Age differences in the psychological consequences of Hurricane Hugo. *Psychology and Aging, 8*, 606–616.

Tomaka, J., & Blascovich, J. (1994). Effects of justice beliefs on cognitive appraisal of and subjective physiological, and behavioral responses to potential stress. *Journal of Personality and Social Psychology, 67*, 732–740.

Tomarken, A. J., & Davidson, R. J. (1994). Frontal brain activation in repressors and nonrepressors. *Journal of Abnormal Psychology, 103*, 339–349.

Tucker, P., Pfefferbaum, B., Doughty, D. E., Jones, D. E., Jordan, F. B., & Nixon, S. J. (2002). Body handlers after terrorism in Oklahoma City: Predictors of posttraumatic stress and other symptoms. *American Journal of Orthopsychiatry, 72*, 469–475.

Tugade, M. M., & Fredrickson, B. L. (2004). Resilient individuals use positive emotions to bounce back from negative emotional experiences. *Journal of Personality and Social Psychology, 86*, 320–333.

Vaillant, G. (1977). *Adaptation to life.* Boston: Little, Brown.

Weinberger, D. A., Schwartz, G. E., & Davidson, R. J. (1979). Low-anxious, high-anxious, and repressive coping styles: Psychometric patterns and behavioral and physiological responses to stress. *Journal of Abnormal Psychology, 88*, 369–380.

Werner, E. E. (1995). Resilience in development. *Current Directions in Psychological Science, 4*, 81–85.

Worden, J. W. (1991). *Grief counseling and grief therapy: A handbook for the mental health practitioner* (2nd ed.). New York: Springer.

Wortman, C. B., & Silver, R. C. (1989). The myths of coping with loss. *Journal of Consulting and Clinical Psychology, 57*, 349–357.

Zisook, S., Chentsova-Dutton, Y., & Shuchter, S. R. (1998). PTSD following bereavement. *Annals of Clinical Psychiatry, 10*, 157–163.

D

Social Dimensions of Resilience

14

Resilience in Adolescence
Overcoming Neighborhood Disadvantage

Marc A. Zimmerman
Allison B. Brenner

Resilience in adolescents is very similar to that of adults. It is the idea of successful coping in the face of adversity, which Anne Masten (2001) refers to as *ordinary magic*. Examination of resilience processes during adolescence may be vital for informing adult resiliency. Although adolescents confront different challenges than adults, these challenges help to shape their adult lives: Adolescents may be more influenced by peers (both inside and outside of school) than adults; many adolescent outcomes that are studied may be age-specific (e.g., school failure, alcohol use, delinquency); and the stressors relevant to adolescents may differ from those of adults, but the resilience process is expected to operate in a similar fashion. In addition to distinctions between the two populations, risk and resilience in adolescence is related directly to potential health and behavioral outcomes in adulthood. Consequently, this chapter focuses on resilience during adolescence and provides a foundation for research on adult resilience.

Research on adolescent resilience spans several decades, and consistently suggests that even high-risk youth often beat the odds. In fact, even under extreme circumstances and "glaring adversities" (p. 598) it is not uncommon for over half of the children to avoid problems associated with risk (Rutter, 1985). Though the term *resilience* became more commonly used in the mid- to late 1980s (Rutter, 1987), the concept dates back to the early 1970s with studies on invulnerability and stress resistance in children at risk for psychopathology (Anthony, 1974; Garmezy, 1970, 1971, 1974).

Despite this history, researchers continue to debate terminology. Luthar, Cicchetti, and Becker (2000), for example, favor the term *resilience* over *resiliency* to distinguish processes that help youth overcome the odds (resilience) from a personal trait conception (resiliency) of the construct. We agree with Luthar and colleagues that it is vital to distinguish process from traits, and we also prefer a process-oriented approach. Yet we use *resilience* and *resiliency* interchangeably because it is simply more appropriate grammatically to use one term or the other depending on the context in which it appears. It is imperative, however, that *resilience/resiliency* be conceptualized as a process (and not a trait) to help focus attention on context, resources and assets, and the developmental (dynamic) nature of the construct (Cicchetti & Garmezy, 1993; Rutter, 1987).

We begin this chapter with a discussion of terminology and resiliency models. We follow this overview with a history of the construct as it relates to adolescents, and a model-focused review of the literature. We conclude the chapter with a brief review of resiliency interventions, a critical analysis of resiliency research, and suggestions for future directions.

Adolescent Resiliency

Norman Garmezy, Emmy Werner, Anne Masten, and Sir Michael Rutter pioneered the field of adolescent resiliency. Although this resulted in a rich and diverse history, it also raised questions about terminology and definitions. Most current work recognizes a form of Masten, Best, and Garmezy's (1990) definition of *resilience*: "adaptation in the face of some type of stress, threat or adversity" (p. 426). Masten and others specifically refer to *resilience* as a process, capacity, or outcome, and not a trait of the child (Cicchetti & Garmezy, 1993; Luthar et al., 2000; Masten et al., 1990). Luthar and colleagues (2000) recognize *resilience* as a "dynamic process encompassing positive adaptation within the context of a significant adversity" (p. 543). Resilience theory, as related to adolescents, focuses on resources and positive adaptation applied to achieve healthy development despite risk (Fergus & Zimmerman, 2005). Common to all populations and definitions are two necessary and sufficient causes: an experience of adversity and utilization of promotive factors after risks arise

(Fergus & Zimmerman, 2005; Luthar et al., 2000; Rutter, 1985, 1987).

Researchers conceptualize risk, vulnerability, protection, competence and resilience differently. They also debate whether differences between risk and vulnerability, and between protection, competence, and resilience, are semantic or actual conceptual differences (Cicchetti & Garmezy, 1993; Luthar et al., 2000; Rutter, 1987). Though these distinctions are important, they are often blurred in the research on adolescent resilience and require clarification to maintain consistency across studies, improve communication and understanding across researchers, and help to develop a program of research to inform resilience theory.

Most generally, *risk* can be defined as any factor or situation that increases a youth's chance of developing negative health or behavioral outcomes (Grizenko & Fisher, 1992). Turbin and colleagues (2006) offer a unique perspective of risk by defining risk factors as variables that

> decrease the likelihood of engaging in health-enhancing behavior by providing models for health-compromising behaviors or for problem behaviors that are incompatible with health enhancing behaviors, by providing greater opportunity for engaging in health-compromising behavior or problem behavior, and by constituting greater personal vulnerability to health-compromising or problem behavior involvement. (p. 446)

Vulnerability is defined by Rutter (1987) as "intensification ... of the reaction to a factor that in ordinary circumstances leads to a maladaptive outcome" (p. 317). Like protection, vulnerability is dependent on exposure to a risk factor; youth who succumb to the risk may be more vulnerable to the particular exposure than less vulnerable youth (Rutter, 1987). From these definitions the distinction between risk and vulnerability becomes more apparent. Risk and vulnerability function in concert; multiple risk factors increase a youth's vulnerability for developing unfavorable health and behavioral outcomes (Grizenko & Fisher, 1992; Rutter, 1987).

Most research on adolescent health and development has taken a risk or disease-specific approach (Cicchetti & Garmezy, 1993). The popularity of a risk model may be the result of the extensive adolescent storm and stress literature that identifies adolescence as a tumultuous time of transition (Eccles et al., 1993). Though the period of adolescence contains many significant transitions (e.g., school, puberty, cognitive development), researchers have found that most youth escape this period without significant problems (Eccles et al., 1993).

The burgeoning field of adolescent resiliency has helped to develop a program of research that focuses on factors that help youth cope successfully with life's challenges. Resiliency, however, is not simply the absence of, or the positive counterpart of risk (Jessor, 1991; Rutter, 1985, 1987). Rather, it is a distinct and active process in which adolescents avoid the negative consequences of risk exposure, increase positive health behaviors, and promote healthy development (Jessor, 1991; Rink & Tricker, 2005). Rutter (1987) noted that resiliency processes operate by redirecting the life trajectory away from the negative outcomes associated with risk and toward healthy adaptation. Notably, however, resiliency refers to reduction of risk effects, and not necessarily their elimination. Thus, resiliency does not suggest extraordinary achievement. Resilient youth may not even achieve as successfully as non-at-risk youth, but they will have better outcomes than their at-risk counterparts. Youth exposed to risk may be resilient in a number of ways. We describe below three basic models of resiliency.

Models of Adolescence Resiliency

When confronted with risk, youth rely on promotive factors to maintain stability, overcome adversity, and occasionally increase competence (Fergus & Zimmerman, 2005; Luthar et al., 2000). *Promotive factors* are resources and assets that represent positive aspects in youth's lives. They are, however, not necessarily the opposite end of the continuum from a risk factor (i.e., low score on a risk is not necessarily indicative of a promotive factor). *Resources* refer to factors external to the individual, and *assets* refer to factors that reside within individual youth. Thus, resources include social support (familial or nonfamilial), youth programs in the community, and adult mentors. Assets include factors such as competence, intelligence, and motivation (Masten et al., 1990). Researchers identified three main models of resiliency (Figure 14.1) to explain how promotive factors alter the trajectory from risk exposure to negative outcome: (1) compensatory, (2) protective, and (3) challenge (Fergus & Zimmerman, 2005; Garmezy & Masten, 1986; Luthar et al., 2000). These models guide research questions and the data-analytic approach.

The *compensatory model* is a main effects (or direct effect) model, in which the adverse consequences of stress exposure are counteracted by one ore more promotive factors (Fergus & Zimmerman, 2005; Garmezy, Masten, & Taylor, 1984). Conceptually, this model demonstrates two main effects: the direct effect of the risk (stressor), and the direct effect of the compensatory factor. Typically, the effects of the risk and compensatory factors are in the opposite direction. Hence, the promotive factor compensates for, or counteracts, the negative effects of a risk. These main effects are completely independent and are tested mathematically in regression equations where the risk is entered first, followed by the compensatory factor (Fergus & Zimmerman, 2005; Garmezy et al., 1984). Consequently, the compensatory model is simply a linear model that contains terms for the risk and promotive factor(s), which are tested separately. Findings from a study of urban African American youth

Model 1: Compensatory   Model 2: Protective

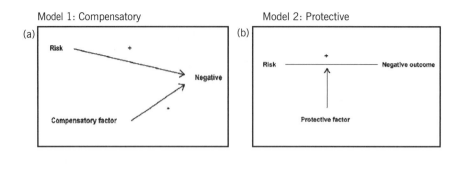

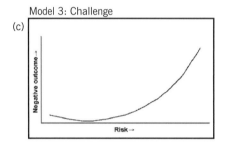

Model 3: Challenge

FIGURE 14.1. Resiliency models. From Fergus and Zimmerman (2005). Copyright 2005 by Annual Reviews. Reprinted by permission.

in Michigan, for example, indicate that parental support compensates for the risks associated with having violent friends, being around violent adults, and fighting (Zimmerman, Steinman, & Rowe, 1998). The positive effect of parental support is independent of the negative relationship between the risk factors and violent adolescent behavior, and therefore counteracts the risk trajectory, helping youth become resilient in the face of exposure to violence (Zimmerman et al., 1998). The compensatory model is represented in Figure 14.1a.

A second resiliency model, the *protective model*, suggests that promotive factors may buffer adolescents from harm, and that adolescents who demonstrate high levels of these factors have a lower risk of negative outcomes than adolescents with low levels of protection (Garmezy et al., 1984). Statistically, the protective model is a moderation model, in which the interaction term contains both the risk and the promotive fac-

tor. Thus, the protective model is a third step in the regression equation described earlier, whereby the interaction term (risk multiplied by promotive factor) is entered after the main effects for the risk and promotive factor. McLoyd (1998) found, for example, that parental monitoring (a resource) protects youth against the negative effects of living in poverty for poor academic outcomes. Figure 14.1b depicts the protective factor model.

Researchers have described different types of risk-protective models. Luthar and colleagues (2000), for example, posit protective–stabilizing, protective–reactive, and protective–protective models. These models differ only in their risk-negative outcome trajectories. In the protective–stabilizing model, for example, the likelihood of a negative outcome does not increase as risk increases in the presence of a promotive factor. If the promotive factor is absent, then negative consequence increases with higher levels of risk (Fergus & Zimmerman, 2005).

Conversely, in a protective–reactive model, the level of negative outcomes increases as risk increases for adolescents with and without the promotive factor, but the overall level of the negative consequences remains lower for adolescents who possess the promotive factor across all levels of risk (Fergus & Zimmerman, 2005).

Brook, Gordon, Whiteman, and Cohen (1986, 1989) also suggest that protective–protective mechanisms are possible. In this kind of model, two promotive factors (either two assets, two resources, or an asset and a resource) interact with each other to enhance outcomes. Thus, one promotive factor amplifies the positive effects of the other promotive factor. Zimmerman, Ramírez, Washienko, Walter, and Dyer (1995), for example, found that the effects of high self-esteem and cultural identity resulted in the lowest levels of substance use for Native American youth. Although high self-esteem compensated for the negative effects of perceived family drug problems on adolescent substance use, cultural identity further enhanced (i.e., interacted with) the effect of self-esteem (Zimmerman et al., 1995). Thus, cultural identity had a protective–protective effect on the relationship between self-esteem and substance use.

A third resiliency model is the *challenge model* (Garmezy et al., 1984). Conceptually, the challenge model suggests that low levels of risk help to inoculate youth, so that later exposure to higher levels of risk is less deleterious (Fergus & Zimmerman, 2005). Too little risk may not prepare youth adequately for the inevitable risk exposure they are likely to encounter as they develop into young adults, and too much risk may just be too difficult to overcome (see Figure 14.1c). Moderate risk exposure, however, may be associated with less negative outcomes for adolescents (Garmezy et al., 1984). When adolescents are able to cope successfully with moderate levels of risk exposure, it helps prepare them to overcome greater risks in the future (Fergus & Zimmerman, 2005). If the risk is too great, however, inoculation

may be ineffective, and the youth may succumb to negative health or behavioral outcomes (Luthar, 2004). Mathematically, the challenge model indicates the presence of a second-order term in a multiple regression equation, which accounts for the nonlinear relationship between risk and the adolescent outcome (Garmezy et al., 1984).

Although these three resiliency models are analytically different, conceptually they are not mutually exclusive. Garmezy and colleagues (1984) suggest that more than one model can be used to describe adolescent resiliency processes, and that the models are best used as a guide in the analysis. Protective processes during adolescence often involve both direct and indirect effects, which complicate issues of causality. To examine carefully these factors in resiliency theory it is essential to consider longitudinal research for testing hypotheses (Rutter, 1985). Researchers also recommend focusing on transitional periods in adolescence, which shortens the study, while capturing critical, developmentally sensitive information (Rutter, 1985).

Early Work in Adolescent Resilience

Most early work on adolescent resiliency focused on youth who were considered to be at risk based on maternal psychopathology (Garmezy, 1971, 1987; Garmezy et al., 1984; Garmezy & Masten, 1986; Rutter, 1979a). Garmezy and Masten (1986; Garmezy et al., 1984) studied children of mothers with schizophrenia and found that many vulnerable children escaped psychological distress and incompetence despite extreme adversity. These findings were similar to those of Bleuler (1978), and though this work was not characterized as studies of resiliency, it reinforced the idea that children can succeed despite great odds, and set the stage for investigations of stress resistance.

Research on *stress resistance* (competence despite exposure to stress) in the face of adversity set the foundation for Project Competence—a study of risk, competence, and adaptation initiated by Garmezy and Masten in 1977 (Garmezy, 1987; Garmezy et al., 1984; Garmezy & Masten, 1986), who followed a cohort of 205 school-age children in Minneapolis through early adulthood, focusing on aspects of competence and resilience. Though additional studies under Project Competence concentrated on at-risk youth, the core sample included a normative and diverse group of children. Risk factors included death of a parent, and marital separation and divorce, among others. Competence was measured using school and home-based measures, as well as peer ratings of social reputation (Garmezy, 1987; Garmezy et al., 1984; Garmezy & Masten, 1986).

Garmezy and colleagues (1984) found evidence that both high family socioeconomic status (SES) and intellectual ability (IQ) are independently associated with engagement in school. Children from wealthy families fared better under stress than low-SES children in terms of the disruptive dimension of academic competence, which suggests the presence of a compensatory process (Garmezy, 1987; Garmezy et al., 1984; Garmezy & Masten, 1986). Garmezy and colleagues did not find support for a challenge model, in which a certain level of stress actually enhances a child's competence, resulting in a curvilinear relationship between stress and competence. They did, however, find evidence of a protective relationship between stress and academic achievement, based on the level of the child's IQ. High levels of stress had a greater effect on achievement (lowering achievement scores) for children with low IQ than for those with high IQ. In fact, for children judged to have a high IQ, the effect of stress was virtually flat across levels (Garmezy et al., 1984).

Sir Michael Rutter's (1979a) early research focused on identifying family factors that were related to psychiatric disorders in young children. He identified six family factors based on data collected as a part of the Isle of Wight and Inner London studies (Rutter, 1976; Rutter et al., 1974), including (1) severe marital discord, (2) low social status, (3) overcrowding/large family, (4) paternal criminality, (5) maternal psychiatric disorder, and (6) admission into the care of a local authority. Rutter found that the presence of any single family risk did not necessarily increase a child's risk for disorder. The presences of multiple risk factors, however, increased risk at least fourfold (Rutter, 1979a).

Although much of Rutter's (1979b) early work focused on risk and vulnerability to psychiatric illness, he also dedicated substantial research to invulnerability and stress because, as he noted, "There is a regrettable tendency to focus gloomily on the ills of mankind and on all that can and does go wrong" (p. 49). Despite the extreme poverty endured by one in six British children (in 1979), Rutter found that nearly half were well adjusted, and that one in seven demonstrated outstanding ability. Amazed by the invulnerability he witnessed, Rutter hypothesized that the identification of competence factors and protective influences could help to determine why some children survive and even prosper despite extreme deprivation.

Although early research (Anthony, 1974; Garmezy, 1971) initially labeled children who succeeded despite living in extreme poverty as *invulnerable*, this term has been replaced by *resilient* (Rutter, 1993). Invulnerability implies something of a superhero—children who are unbreakable, invincible, and indestructible under even the most noxious stressors. Rutter notes the impossibility of being completely resistant to stressful or traumatic situations. Researchers have come to realize, however, that even youth who avoid negative outcomes are achieving something important, particularly in the case of extreme risk. Invulnerability suggests something extraordinary and does not recognize the success, or ordinary magic, in simply avoiding problems (Masten, 2001; Rutter, 1993). The term *resilience* was adopted to reflect more accurately what was observed in children who bounced back from adversity but may not have been indestructible (they suffered some, but not as much as less resilient children).

In his search for promotive factors, Rutter (1979a) discovered that temperamentally balanced children were more likely to escape the negative effects of discordant homes and depressive and irritable parents, and were less likely to draw criticism from parents. Based on results from the Isle of Wight study, Rutter and colleagues (Rutter, 1976, 1979a; Rutter, Tizard, & Whitmore, 1970) also found that children of high intelligence were less likely to be deviant than were children of average intelligence. In addition, children from disadvantaged homes appeared to be buffered from behavioral deviance by high scholastic achievement. Though the mechanism for the findings was uncertain, Rutter hypothesized that self-esteem played a mediating role. This research indicated that children with above average intelligence and academic achievement were protected from deviance despite living in economically and socially disadvantaged homes. Rutter's early work helped to mold initial studies of risk and invulnerability into the current conceptualization of resilience; he identified several common risk factors for children, and the assets and resources that enable them to avoid negative outcomes.

Werner, Bierman, and French (1971) focused on SES as a risk factor for problems in adolescence and studied the lives of children growing up in poverty on the island of Kauai, Hawaii. Results for the outcomes during adolescence and the transition into early adulthood are presented in the book *Overcoming the Odds* (Werner & Smith, 1992). Werner followed a 1955 birth cohort in Kauai, which featured unique cultural influences on childrearing and childbearing. Assessments were conducted during each trimester of pregnancy and at 1-, 2-, 10-, and 18-year follow-up. The final follow-up assessment occurred when the children were 31 and 32 years old. Despite the various levels of poverty children experienced, most of them thrived. Almost all of the youth graduated from high school, and 88% of men

and 80% of women received at least some post–high school education. At the final follow-up, most of the men and 88% of the women were employed and happy with their careers; for men, these numbers are higher than the rates of employed American men. Werner and Smith also found that most of the Kauai cohort were considered low risk as adults (despite their high-risk status as adolescents) and had normal coping capacities. Of the youth who exhibited delinquent behaviors, who had criminal records and mental health problems in adolescence, only half or less experienced problems in adulthood. In fact, many of the high-risk toddlers (four or more risk factors) entered childhood and adolescence problem free. This process of recovery continued into early adulthood; as young adults, the children of Kauai told their tales "without rancor, with a sense of compassion—and above all, with optimism and hopefulness" (Werner & Smith, 1992, p. 74).

Werner attributed the successful development of children from Kauai to several personal, environmental, and social assets and resources. She found that resilient children had more education and more skilled jobs on average. These children tended to rely on their competence and determination to cope with stressors, and often relied on themselves instead of peers for support (Werner, 1989; Werner & Smith, 1992). Resilient youth tended to benefit from living in smaller families and typically had close relationships with their mothers. Many children who had less access to their caregivers developed close relationships with other family members and adult mentors outside the family, including neighbors, teachers and church officials (Werner, 1989).

As adults, the children Werner labeled as *resilient* based on their positive adolescent development were more likely to rely on their spouses for emotional support. They were more committed to being supportive parents than their lower-risk peers, and they reported more religious faith than these lower-risk peers (Werner & Smith, 1992). In general,

Werner described the children of Kauai as ordinary people who succeeded based on their own determination, as well as the hopes of their immigrant families (Werner & Smith, 1992). Thus, Werner documented several factors associated with helping high-risk youth overcome the odds.

Early studies of resilience provide a solid framework on which to build. Results from these studies suggest that high-risk adolescents can withstand trauma and chronic stressors; and that assets and resources can play significant roles in avoidance of problems and successful coping during adolescence and beyond. Researchers have identified individual-level assets and resources (e.g., high IQ, academic achievement), interpersonal-level resources (e.g., social support), and social- or community-level resources (e.g., neighborhood monitoring and cohesion, opportunities for prosocial involvement) on which youth rely to overcome risk (Elder, Nguyen, & Caspi, 1985; Garmezy & Masten, 1986; Rutter, 1985; Werner, 1989; Werner & Smith, 1992).

Social Context and Adolescent Resiliency

Although early research in adolescent resiliency identified a variety of assets and resources that help youth successfully navigate the social contexts in which they function, most have focused on the peer and family context. Ecological models are favored by developmental researchers because they consider many of the contextual factors that are relevant to youth: peers, family, neighborhood, and school. It is in these contexts that youth develop the assets they need to adapt and function in the face of risks. Adolescents also draw necessary resources from these social contexts. These resources often include social support, the school environment, and opportunities for prosocial participation.

Many researchers have studied peer and family influences on youth (Beam, Gil-Rivas, Greenberger, & Chen, 2002; Belsky, 1984;

Davis-Kearn, 2005; Elder, Foster, Ardelt, & Conger, 1992; Elder et al., 1985; McLoyd, 1990; Prelow, Loukas, & Jordan-Green, 2007; Turbin et al., 2006) and how families and peers function within an adolescent resiliency framework (Bryant & Zimmerman, 2003; Fagan, Van Horn, Hawkins, & Arthur, 2007; Jenkins & Smith, 1990; Kempton, Armistead, Wierson, & Forehand, 1991; Prevatt, 2003; Rodgers & Rose, 2002; Tiet et al., 2001; Zimmerman et al., 1995). The research on family risks and adolescent health and behavior outcomes suggests that youth can overcome parental divorce, instability, parental conflict, parental substance use, and maternal psychopathology with the aid of promotive factors.

Current findings suggest that assets such as high IQ and having educational goals appear to benefit youth exposed to family risk (Tiet et al., 2001). Additional resources that protect adolescents from risks in the family include peer, parental, sibling, friend, and other adult support; school and parental attachment; relationship with parents; involvement in activities; and rewards for prosocial involvement (Fagan et al., 2007; Kempton et al., 1991; Rodgers & Rose, 2002; Tiet et al., 2001; Wills, Sandy, Yaeger, & Shinar, 2001). Bryant and Zimmerman (2003) found that youth who identified their parents as role models showed less psychological distress, higher self-acceptance, and better coping than youth without a parental role model.

Additional factors may reduce adolescent externalizing behavior due to family risk. Findings suggest that youth with an easy temperament, high self-esteem, and a strong sense of cultural identity experience fewer externalizing problems than do youth without these promotive factors (Wills et al., 2001; Zimmerman et al., 1995). In addition, the presence of siblings in the context of parental divorce proved beneficial to youth in protection against externalizing symptoms (Kempton et al., 1991).

Research that focuses on neighborhood effects and adolescent development often includes aspects of the peer and family context (Brooks-Gunn, Duncan, Klevanov, & Sealand, 1993; Duncan & Raudenbush, 1999; Gutman, McLoyd, & Tokoyawa, 2005; Leventhal & Brooks-Gunn, 2000; Mayer & Jencks, 1989). The neighborhood is the larger social context in which youth, families, and peers interact, and it is virtually impossible to study neighborhoods without considering these subcontexts. Many researchers in fact examine conceptual models in which peer and family influences mediate the indirect effects of the neighborhood on adolescent outcomes (Gutman et al., 2005; Jackson, 2003; Leventhal & Brooks-Gunn, 2004). Neighborhood disadvantage, for instance, is considered a *distal risk* because it threatens the health of adolescents indirectly through parental factors, peer factors, or access to resources (Brooks-Gunn et al., 1993; Masten et al., 1990). Families living in these communities are likely to experience chronic stress, and parents under stress are more likely to express less warmth to their children, to monitor less, and to provide poorer discipline than parents living in less stressful environments (McLoyd, 1990; Pinderhughes, Nix, Foster, & Jones, 2001). In addition, youth living in disadvantaged neighborhoods are more likely to be exposed to and to associate with deviant peers, which may increase their risk and decrease their protective resources (Elliott et al., 1996; Wills et al., 2001).

Indirect pathways (i.e., mediating models) may complicate studies of resiliency because it can become difficult to determine whether promotive factors are compensating for or protecting against the distal effect of neighborhood or more proximal effects, such as parents or peers (Masten et al., 1990). Yet the use of multigroup structural equation modeling provides a useful analytic tool to examine whether the hypothesized path model differs depending on values of a promotive factor (this would be test of a protective model). If the mediating model tested reduces or eliminates the direct effects of a risk factor, and the media-

tor has a counteracting (opposite) effect on the risk factor, a compensatory model may be supported.

We focus our attention on the neighborhood as a primary risk factor for several reasons. First, neighborhoods are particularly relevant for adult resiliency because they set life trajectories and are persistent in their influence across the lifespan. An adolescent who lives in a neighborhood with more poverty and crime, and fewer resources will frequently remain low SES, and live in disadvantaged neighborhoods as an adult (Garmezy, 1991). Second, although neighborhood risks are persistent and may extend into adulthood, they may also be more amenable to change than other risks, and may therefore be a vital focus for intervention. Third, neighborhood influence and resiliency theory have not been widely integrated by researchers. This connection may be a critical area for future research and prevention because it could provide important insights into the way neighborhoods can influence youth problem behavior.

Neighborhood Context as Risk

Neighborhoods present youth with a variety of risks that can negatively influence behavior and development (Brooks-Gunn et al., 1993). High-risk neighborhoods are characterized by crime and violence, crowding and noise, and high levels of unemployment (Elliott et al., 1996; Wilson, 1987). These communities are often referred to as being *disadvantaged*. Disadvantaged neighborhoods can increase adolescent risk for mental health and behavioral problems in several ways. The environmental stress model, for instance, posits that neighborhood characteristics directly influence resident stress levels, resulting in inadequate coping, mental health problems, and problem behavior (Wandersman & Nation, 1998).

Families that live in disadvantaged communities are more likely to be poor, and stress due to poverty fosters living environments with high levels of violence, drug and alcohol abuse, environmental hazards, poor school systems, and inadequate health care (Landis et al., 2007; Sampson, 1999). Factors in the community and in the family are linked to increased experiences of adolescent stress, anxiety, and depression (Gutman et al., 2005). In addition, because youth living in disadvantaged communities are exposed to multiple sources of stress, they are more likely to experience risk accumulation. Researchers suggest that the number of risks to which youth are exposed is a better predictor of well-being that the type of risks (Meyers & Miller, 2004; Rutter, 1979). Therefore, adolescents who live in disadvantaged neighborhoods are likely to experience higher

rates of risk exposure and worse outcomes than those youth who live in more advantaged neighborhoods.

We review research that examines the negative effects of neighborhood disadvantage on two specific adolescent outcomes that are also significant in adulthood: internalizing (anxiety, depression) and externalizing problems (substance use, problem behavior, and violent behavior). Table 14.1 displays the assets, resources, and outcomes related to neighborhood risk for youth according to the compensatory model, based on literature published over the past 15 years. Table 14.2 is organized in the same manner, and represents a sample of recent research on the protective resiliency model.

TABLE 14.1. Compensatory Resiliency Model for Neighborhood Disadvantage

Resiliency model tested	Risk factor	Asset	Resource	Outcome
Compensatory				
Kliewer et al. (2004)	Neighborhood disadvantage	Emotional regulation	Relationship with caregivers, felt acceptance from caregiver, caregiver emotional regulation of sadness, caregiver emotional regulation of anger, neighborhood cohesion	Depression, anxiety, aggressive, delinquent and hostile behavior
Ozer & Weinstein (2004)	Exposure to neighborhood violence		Mother helpfulness, sibling helpfulness, school safety	Depression, PTSD
Dubow et al. (1997)	Neighborhood disadvantage and stress	Self-worth	Family and peer support	Antisocial behavior, substance use
Xue et al. (2007)	Neighborhood disadvantage		Prosocial participation	Substance use
Fagan et al. (2007)	Neighborhood risk		Prosocial involvement, attachment to parents, opportunities for prosocial involvement, rewards for prosocial involvement	Substance use
Taylor & Kliewer (2006)	Exposure to neighborhood violence		Felt acceptance from caregiver	Substance use
Brookmeyer et al. (2005)	Neighborhood disadvantage and violence		Parent support	Violence

TABLE 14.2. Protective Resiliency Model for Neighborhood Disadvantage

Resiliency model tested	Risk factor	Asset	Resource	Outcome
Protective				
Kliewer et al. (2004)	Neighborhood violence	Emotional regulation	Felt acceptance from caregiver, caregiver regulation of anger	Depression, anxiety, aggression, delinquent and hostile behavior
Ozer & Weinstein (2004)	Exposure to neighborhood violence		Mother support, father support, sibling support	Depression, PTSD
Hammack et al. (2004)	Exposure to neighborhood violence		Maternal closeness, social support, time spent with family	Depressive symptoms, anxiety
Dubow et al. (2007)	Neighborhood stressors		Peer support	Substance use, antisocial behavior
Brookmeyer et al. (2005)	Neighborhood disadvantage and violence exposure		Parent support	Violence perpetration
Gorman-Smith et al. (2004)	Exposure to neighborhood violence		Exceptional family functioning	Violence perpetration
Xue et al. (2007)	Neighborhood disadvantage		Prosocial participation (school activities, community activities)	Substance use

Neighborhoods and Internalizing Problems

Neighborhood disorder (defined by high crime rates, vandalism, and drug use; and the presence of abandoned buildings, graffiti, garbage, and noise) and exposure to neighborhood violence has been found to be associated with higher rates of resident stress, internalizing behavior, depression, fear, and anxiety for adults and adolescents (Aisenberg & Herrenkohl, 2008; Hill, Ross, & Angel, 2005; McLoyd, 1990, 1994; Sampson, 1999; Steptoe, Brydon, & Kunz-Ebrecht, 2005). McLoyd (1990) posits that the elevated mental health problems among poor African Americans are primarily due to stressful life events and chronic, uncontrollable stressors that result from disadvantaged neighborhoods.

Many researchers have examined promotive factors that mitigate or buffer adolescents from psychological distress caused by a variety of risks. Research indicates that strong parent–child relationships, prosocial activities, good sibling relationships, family cohesion, family support, and self-perception of popularity, attractiveness, and intelligence compensate for risk or protect youth from risks and mental health problems (Grizenko & Fisher, 1992; Jenkins & Smith, 1990; Rutter, 1985; Werner & Smith, 1992).

Few researchers have examined factors that help youth overcome neighborhood risks that lead to internalizing problems. Based on these studies, compensatory and protective assets and resources were identified that help adolescents avoid internalizing problems despite living in disadvantaged and violent communities. Only emotional regulation emerged as an asset that mitigated and protected youth against risks due to neighborhood disadvantage (Kliewer et al., 2004). Several resources, however, were found to benefit youth living in high-risk contexts. Family support from caregivers and siblings, peer support, maternal closeness, relationship with caregivers, time spent with family, perceived safety of the school, and neighborhood cohesion were promotive factors for adolescents who witnessed or experienced violence (Hammack, Richards, Luo, Edlynn, & Roy, 2004; Kliewer et al., 2004; Ozer & Weinstein, 2004). These results are consistent with past findings that cite the family as a critical resource for high-risk youth (Rutter, 1979, 1987; Werner, 1989). Details of the studies are given below.

Compensatory Model

Several studies tested compensatory models of resilience related to neighborhoods and adolescent internalizing problems (see Table 14.1; protective models were often simultaneously examined and results are presented separately in Table 14.2). One mechanism by which living in a disadvantaged neighborhood affects adolescents' internalizing problems is through exposure to community violence (Hill et al., 2005; Kliewer et al., 2004; Sampson, Raudenbush, & Earls, 1997). Kliewer and colleagues (2004) examined the effects of violence on adolescents' internalizing problems and the promotive factors that help youth avoid these negative outcomes (they also examined protective models, which we discuss in the following section). They considered various environmental contexts (child, caregiver, child–caregiver relationship, and neighborhood), and tested the compensatory model using both cross-sectional and longitudinal designs.

Kliewer and colleagues (2004) found that felt acceptance from a caregiver and caregiver regulation of sadness compensated for the negative association between exposure to violence and internalizing problems. This research indicates the vital role that family plays as a resource for youth living in impoverished, high-crime, violent communities.

Ozer and Weinstein (2004) also investigated the ways in which promotive resources could help youth avoid negative mental health consequences associated with living in a violent neighborhood. Most of the youth in their sample had either witnessed violence or had been victimized at some point in the past 6 months. They found that support from a mother and perceived safety of the school environment reduced the negative effects of community violence exposure and experiencing violence on adolescent depressive symptoms. The support of a sibling reduced symptoms of posttraumatic stress disorder (PTSD) in the context of a violent community (Ozer & Weinstein, 2004). These findings suggest that supportive environments in the home and school alleviate certain internalizing symptoms associated with living in a violent neighborhood.

Protective Model

Kliewer and colleagues (2004) and others (see Table 14.2) have also considered protective resiliency models to explain the relationship between living in a disadvantaged neighborhood and adolescent mental health. These models consider the modifying effects of assets and resources on neighborhood risk and internalizing problems among adolescents.

Kliewer and colleagues (2004) utilized the four protective models proposed by Luthar and colleagues (2000) (protective, protective–stabilizing, protective–reactive, and protective–protective) to test adolescent resiliency in the face of community violence. They found that the adolescent's emotion regulation skills and felt acceptance from a caregiver attenuated the effect of exposure to violence on symptoms of depression and anxiety. These protective effects supported the protective–reactive model proposed by Luthar and colleagues; high emotion regulation skills and high felt acceptance were only useful under low levels of violence. This suggests that when youth are exposed to very high levels of community violence, even strong felt acceptance from a caregiver or positive emotion regulation skills cannot fully protect against mental health problems. Kliewer and colleagues noted, however, that high violence exposure was rare, and that at lower levels of risk, even moderate felt acceptance from a caregiver and emotion regulation successfully protected against mental health problems.

In their research on the effects of living in violent communities on adolescent depressive and PTSD symptoms, Ozer and Weinstein (2004) discovered protective effects for family social support. They found that both mother and father support buffered the negative relationship between violent neighborhoods and PTSD symptoms. Sibling and mother support also protected adolescents against risk for depression (Ozer & Weinstein, 2004). In general, for youth with supportive families, living in violent communities, and being victimized within these communities, did not have a negative effect on their mental health. For youth with less parent and sibling support, however, experiences of violence had a detrimental effect on their psychological well-being.

Hammack and colleagues (2004) also examined the effects of community violence (exposure and victimization) on adolescents' internalizing symptoms. They considered social support, maternal closeness, and time spent with family as resources to protect youth from increased internalizing problems, and examined these relationships at the time of exposure and longitudinally. They studied 196 African American sixth-grade students from schools in high-crime neighborhoods. Almost half of their mainly low SES sample was comprised of single-parent families and included parents with only a high school education.

Hammack and colleagues (2004) found that adolescents who witnessed violence in their neighborhood, and who reported closeness to their mothers, experienced less anxiety and depression than their peers who were not close to their mother. Hammack and colleagues found that two types

of protective models emerged from the findings: protective–reactive and protective–stabilizing. For youth who witnessed neighborhood violence, maternal closeness had a protective-stabilizing effect on anxiety; under high levels of maternal closeness, even those adolescents who reported witnessing frequent violence had lower anxiety levels than youth who were not close to their mothers. Similar patterns emerged for the protective effect of family time (Hammack et al., 2004). For girls who experienced the highest levels of victimization, however, high social support did not sufficiently buffer them from increasing depressive symptoms. This protective–reactive effect suggests that social support alone is not sufficient for youth to overcome this great trauma. It is possible that, in combination with social support, other resources and assets may allow adolescents to be resilient despite victimization.

Neighborhoods and Externalizing Problems

Living in disadvantaged neighborhoods is also believed to lead to greater adolescent risk-taking behavior, delinquency, antisocial behavior, violence, and alcohol and substance use (Leventhal & Brooks-Gunn, 2000; Seidman et al., 1998). These externalizing problem behaviors are of concern to researchers because they put youth on a deleterious developmental trajectory. Youth who are involved in problem behaviors are also at greater risk for aggression, academic problems, social problems, and future alcohol and drug use. Research has shown that early problem behavior is associated with continued participation in crime and deviance across the life course (Kaplow, Curran, Angold, & Costello, 2001; Patchin, 2006; Seidman et al., 1998).

Researchers have reported an association between living in disadvantaged neighborhoods and adolescent problem behavior (Brooks-Gunn et al., 1993; Seidman et al., 1998; Taylor & Kliewer, 2006). Research on promotive factors that help youth overcome the negative effects of violent and disadvantaged neighborhoods on externalizing behavior, however, is less common. The studies reviewed identified compensatory and protective factors that reduce risk for externalizing problems for youth who live in violent and disadvantaged neighborhoods.

Researchers identified a variety of family factors that help youth avoid neighborhood risks. Specifically, felt acceptance from a caregiver, parental support, attachment to parents, and family functioning emerged as compensatory or protective factors in the relationship between neighborhood risk and externalizing behaviors (Brookmeyer, Henrich, & Schwab-Stone, 2005; Dubow, Edwards, & Ippolito, 1997; Fagan et al., 2007; Gorman-Smith, Henry, & Tolan, 2004; Taylor & Kliewer, 2006). Another resource that protects adolescents from harm is *prosocial participation* (Xue, Zimmerman, & Caldwell, 2007). Participation in school, community, and church activities may be particularly vital for youth with limited parental support because it may compensate for the absence of parental promotive resources. Details of studies that examined adolescent resiliency to externalizing problems despite neighborhood risk are given in Tables 14.1 (compensatory models) and 14.2 (protective models). Many researchers examined compensatory and protective models, and the results are listed separately in the following two sections.

Compensatory Model

Kliewer and colleagues (2004) examined externalizing problem behavior in addition to internalizing problems. They found evidence for compensatory effects of felt acceptance from a caregiver and observed caregiver–child interactions on their externalizing behavior scale. Although both resources compensated for the detrimental effects of neighborhood violence, caregiver felt acceptance completely mitigated the effects of violence on externalizing behaviors (Kliewer et al., 2004).

Dubow and colleagues (1997) examined neighborhood risk due to disadvantage, and how family and peer support, as well as self-worth, counteract the effects of risk on adolescent drug use. They studied 315 adolescents living in urban areas in three Midwestern cities. Although youth from more disadvantaged neighborhoods were more likely to use drugs than youth from less disadvantaged areas, Dubow and colleagues found that perceived family support compensated for the detrimental effects of neighborhood disadvantage. Adolescents' self-worth and their perceived peer support also reduced the negative effects of stress from neighborhood risk on youth antisocial behavior (Dubow et al., 1997).

Xue and colleagues (2007) examined neighborhood effects on adolescents' cigarette use and considered the ameliorative effects of prosocial participation. *Prosocial participation* is defined as participation in organized community, school, or church activities (Xue et al., 2007). Researchers have documented the positive effects of youth prosocial participation (Elder, Leaver-Dunn, Wang, Nagy, & Green, 2000; Luthar et al., 2000; Zimmerman & Arunkumar, 1994), but findings for its effect on disadvantaged neighborhoods and substance use are mixed (Xue et al., 2007).

Xue and colleagues (2007) used hierarchical linear modeling (HLM) to examine adolescent outcomes nested within neighborhoods. They found that living in a disadvantaged neighborhood did account for a portion of the variance in adolescent smoking behavior. Participation in prosocial activities, however, reduced the detrimental neighborhood effects on youth cigarette use. More specifically, participation in school and church activities reduced cigarette use among adolescents and mitigated the harmful effects of living in disadvantaged neighborhoods (Xue et al., 2007). This research suggests that youth living in disadvantaged neighborhoods who participate in school and church activities are less at risk for smoking cigarettes that youth who do not participate in prosocial activities.

Fagan and colleagues (2007) were also interested in prosocial involvement as a compensatory resource for youth. They examined how prosocial involvement and attachment to parents helped adolescents avoid substance use despite community risk. This was the only study that used aggregate community-level risk factors to predict adolescent outcomes 2 years later. Fagan and colleagues considered a variety of neighborhood risks, including low neighborhood attachment, neighborhood disadvantage, residential mobility, norms and laws surrounding drug use, and perceived availability of drugs. Neighborhood attachment and disadvantage are measures that gauge the closeness of residents and the amount of crime in the area. Fagan and colleagues also examined the compensatory effect of several aspects of prosocial involvement, including community and family rewards for prosocial involvement, and family opportunities for prosocial involvement, on monthly and lifetime alcohol, cigarette, and marijuana use, as well as on binge drinking.

Fagan and colleagues (2007) found evidence for the compensatory effect of all aspects of prosocial involvement on substance use outcomes except monthly marijuana use. In general, rewards and opportunities for prosocial involvement in the family and community counteracted risks for substance use due to living in disadvantaged communities. These results are consistent with those of Xue and colleagues (2007) and substantiate the idea that prosocial engagement can have positive effects on youth development. Fagan and colleagues also found that attachment to parents compensated for the negative effect of community risk on all substance use outcomes except binge drinking.

Taylor and Kliewer (2006) examined adolescents' felt acceptance from a caregiver and its effect on mitigating risk of adolescent alcohol use due to community violence exposure. They studied 101 African Ameri-

can families living in moderate- and high-violence neighborhoods, and examined adolescent exposure to violence and alcohol use over a 6-month period. The researchers found that felt acceptance from a caregiver was related inversely to adolescent alcohol use, thus compensating for the detrimental effects of being victimized and hearing about violence in the community. Like the work of Kliewer and colleagues (2004), findings supported the positive effect of a supportive family on adolescent outcomes.

Brookmeyer and colleagues (2005) examined the relationship between witnessing violence and perpetrating violence for adolescents living in disadvantaged communities. They studied a large, diverse sample of sixth- and eighth-grade students from disadvantaged neighborhoods to determine whether parental support would have a direct and opposite effect on the relationship between witnessing violence and committing violence. Brookmeyer and colleagues found that parental support—as measured by the parent–child relationship, parent–child communication, and parental involvement in adolescents' activities—had a negative direct effect on violent behavior. Relative to youth violent behavior, this compensatory factor almost completely eliminated the harmful effects of living in a violent community (Brookmeyer et al., 2005).

Protective Model

Kliewer and colleagues (2004) found that only caregiver regulation of anger protected youth from the harmful effects of exposure to violence in the community. Similar to their results for violence and internalizing problems, Kliewer and colleagues discovered a protective–reactive effect for violence exposure and caregiver regulation of anger; for youth with low violence exposure, strong caregiver regulation of anger fully protects against externalizing behavior. For youth who experience high levels of violence exposure, however, even high levels of caregiver regulation of anger did not buffer the harmful effects of violence exposure (Kliewer et al., 2004).

Dubow and colleagues (1997) also examined a protective resiliency model for neighborhood disadvantage, antisocial behavior, and drug use. They found that social support from peers helped to protect adolescents from the stress of living in disadvantaged communities. Youth who had high levels of peer support were less likely to use drugs or to engage in antisocial behavior than youth with lower levels of peer support (Dubow et al., 2007). Peers may serve as a buffer against problem behavior for youth who live in high-risk neighborhoods.

Brookmeyer and colleagues (2005) found evidence for the protective effect of parental support on youth exposed to community violence. Adolescents who witnessed community violence but reported high levels of parental support were less likely to be involved in violence than were youth with low parental support. Gorman-Smith and colleagues (2004) examined the same relationship and found that exceptional family functioning moderated the association between exposure to violence and youth violence perpetration. Youth from families with the highest level of functioning were protected from the deleterious effects of violent neighborhoods, while adolescents from families with moderate or poor levels of functioning were at greater risk for violence perpetration due to neighborhood violence exposure (Gorman-Smith et al., 2004).

Xue and colleagues (2007) also examined a protective model in which prosocial participation may buffer youth from the negative effects of living in a poor neighborhood. They found evidence for protective effects of participation in prosocial activities, noting that greater participation was associated with fewer cigarettes smoked per day for all youth. Examination of each activity separately revealed that school and community activities were particularly important for adolescents living in the highest-risk neighborhoods, and that participation in church activities was most protective for youth living in neighborhoods with a high proportion of black residents (Xue et al., 2007). In addition, participation in one or more activities was related to lower rates of smoking for youth living in disadvantaged neighborhoods than for their counterparts involved in only one activity (Xue et al., 2007).

Cross-Cultural Considerations

Ungar (2006) has raised a question about an ethnocentric focus of research in adolescent resiliency. Resiliency theory was originally developed from studies of children and adolescents in Western cultures (Anthony, 1974; Garmezy, 1970, 1971, 1974), but resiliency is not necessarily culturally dependent because it is the process of overcoming adversity despite risk. The conceptual foundation of resiliency theory can be applicable across cultures; the extent to which resources and assets are applied by youth in their experiences of adversity, however, may not be consistent across all contexts. As a theory, resiliency and the idea of relying on assets and resources to alleviate or protect against risk may be stable across cultural contexts. It is likely that cultural differences may shape differences in risks, resources, and assets. Yet adolescents may face similar risks across cultures (e.g., low SES, violence, family adversity, deviant peers, traumas), and may rely on many similar promotive factors to alleviate the negative results of risk (i.e., social support, coping, future orientation).

One reason why some researchers believe that resiliency has not adequately considered cultural diversity may emerge from confusion over how resiliency is conceptualized. Clauss-Ehlers (2008) and Ungar (2006) criticize current measures of resiliency for their lack of cultural specificity. The measures, however, are inconsistent with the models of resiliency discussed in this chapter because they treat resiliency as a trait instead of a process. We agree with others (Garmezy et al., 1984; Luthar et al., 2000; Masten et al., 1990) who assert that research on adolescent resiliency requires studies of processes based on the models of risk, promotive factors, and developmental or behavioral outcomes (as noted earlier), but these considerations may require attention to the unique circumstances of different cultural contexts. Although particular assets and resources may be culturally specific, the way they operate and compensate for, protect against, or inoculate youth from the negative effects of risk exposure is expected to be consistent across cultures.

Notably, though much of the recent research on resilience focuses mainly on samples from the United States, Werner and Rutter both examined resilience in culturally diverse populations (Rutter, 1976, 1985; Werner et al., 1971). As noted previously, Werner's study of youth in Kauai identified promotive factors in a native Hawaiian population comparable to those found by researchers in Western populations (Werner, 1989; Werner & Smith, 1992). Similar to results in recent research in Western populations, Werner found that social support, academic achievement, and competence helped youth to overcome the negative effects of socioeconomic risk (Brookmeyer et al., 2005; Dubow et al., 1997; Kliewer et al., 2004). Rutter's work with resilient British youth living in poverty also suggests that protective factors may be similar across countries. Although this British sample has many similarities to U.S. samples, it is also operating in different cultural and social contexts than studies of youth in the United States.

More recently, Jessor and colleagues (2003) examined the detrimental effects of individual risk (e.g., depression, low self-esteem), and family, peer, school and neighborhood risk for adolescent problem behavior in American and Chinese youth. Problem behavior included alcohol use, delinquency, and cigarette smoking. They studied the ways in which contextually dependent resources, such as parental and peer values, support, and sanctions on behavior, protect against youth risk and problem behavior. Jessor and colleagues found that despite cul-

tural differences in parental, peer, school, and community protection, and differences in the average levels of problem behavior, the resiliency models accounted for almost an identical percentage of outcome variance in both cultures. Model coefficients for risk by protective resource interactions were similar in Chinese and American youth, and buffered adolescents against increased involvement in deviant and externalizing behavior. These results "provide support for the generality of the explanatory model across these samples of adolescents from two very different societies" (p. 352). Although Jessor and colleagues found differences in the types of social support that protected American and Chinese youth from risk, their findings suggest that social support is a critical resource for youth regardless of context.

Similar to Werner's work with children of Kauai, Carlton and colleagues (2006) also studied resilience in native Hawaiian youth. They examined internalizing problems among native and non-native Hawaiian youth who experienced adversity in the family (e.g., family discord, low SES, family health problems), and the types of compensatory factors that mitigated family risks. Carlton and colleagues found that the assets and resources that attenuated the relationship between risk and mental health problems were very similar among native and non-native Hawaiian youth. Family support, academic achievement, and physical activity, for instance, helped to compensate for the detrimental effects of family risk. Some promotive factors differed across the two groups: Optimism and speaking a Hawaiian language were useful for native Hawaiian adolescents, and relationship formation was useful for non-native youth (Carlton et al., 2007). This study suggests that although youth rely on many similar assets (achievement) and resources (social support), it is also important to consider cultural differences (language).

In the International Resilience Project (IRP), a study of youth from 11 countries, Ungar (2006) argued that the choice of measures and outcomes has a Eurocentric bias. He provided an example of two children to demonstrate how non-culturally-sensitive measures can contribute to incorrect interpretations of how promotive factors might benefit youth. Sasha, a Canadian youth, related her success to her teacher and school, whereas Akili, a Tanzanian youth, related her resilience to support from her mother in finding employment and starting a business (Ungar, 2006). Ungar argues that a stay-in-school program might benefit youth like Sasha, but not youth like Akili. Although it is vital to design interventions that focus on a particular population on which the descriptive study is based, Ungar ultimately determined that social support appears to be a protective resource for youth regardless of culture. This suggests that resiliency theory is operating in a similar manner for Akili and Sasha, despite their reliance on different sources of support.

Although we posit that resiliency theory can be generalized to non-Western cultures, we are not suggesting that these cultural and historical differences should be ignored. Differences between cultures need to be considered as they relate to experiences of risk, promotive factors, and measures of developmental and behavioral outcomes. Culture and background, for instance, influence experiences of adversity (i.e., through discrimination, immigration experiences, family stressors) and cannot be ignored as potential sources of stress. Cultural issues may also affect differences in assets and resources available to youth. A greater reliance on the extended family may be a more relevant resource in one cultural context than in another, and social identity may be a more vital asset for youth from one cultural background than those from another.

Critique of Adolescent Resiliency

Literature searches for articles on adolescent resiliency result in numerous articles on this topic, but many of the studies do not test models of resiliency theory described in this chapter. Many of the studies, for instance, compare promotive factors between two groups of youth that are prelabeled as resilient or nonresilient based on cutoffs of an outcome of interest (i.e., competence scores, academic achievement, or psychological symptoms). These labels, however, are somewhat arbitrary because they are predetermined by the researcher and based on a dichotomous (resilient vs. not resilient) outcome (Buckner, Mezzacappa, & Beardslee, 2003; Neighbors, Forehand, & McVicar, 1993). The researcher then pursues a search for promotive factors to explain why some children are resilient and others are not, instead of testing a model of risk, promotive factors, and adolescent outcomes.

This method is problematic because it does not test a priori theory-based resiliency models. In addition, a search for promotive factors that differ between resilient and non-resilient youth essentially turns the research question upside down. Instead of examining how predetermined promotive factors can affect the relationship between risk and outcome, this method simply identifies promotive factors in the at-risk group of adolescents and determines whether they are associated with group membership. This method, however, may be useful in identifying promotive factors to be tested in the resiliency models discussed earlier.

Another criticism of resiliency theory is that much of the research considers avoiding problems as a positive outcome. Although this is true, it needs to be considered in context. For high-risk youth, simply avoiding negative outcomes may be a critical first step in achieving more positive outcomes (Masten, 2001). *Resiliency*, as described by Masten (2001), is overcoming adversity, and not necessarily exceeding expectations. This may also raise questions about the need to asses the level of exposure. Although most researchers measure risk using a continuous variable (i.e., average of scores from high to low), few examine a cut point at which risk becomes deleterious. Sameroff, Seifer, Barocas, Zax, and Greenspan (1987) studied multiple risk factors and suggested that too much risk may be nearly impossible to overcome. Yet, Ostaszewski and Zimmerman (2006) noted that multiple promotive factors may help youth overcome the negative effects posed by multiple risk factors, both cross-sectionally and longitudinally.

Conceptual ambiguity among similar constructs raises problems as well. Masten and colleagues (1990), for example, discussed the difference between resilience and coping. *Coping*, they point out, is an immediate response to a stressor, with an immediate or short-term outcome, while *resilience* develops over time. Coping can be an integral part of the resilience process in which youth overcome adversity and potentially even exceed expectations. Adolescent resilience, however, is distinct, in that it accounts for the process of overcoming or avoiding negative outcomes, recovering from trauma, or exceeding the odds despite risk (Fergus & Zimmerman, 2005).

Positive adjustment is also occasionally confused with resilience. It refers to a possible resilient outcome, but is distinct from resilience because it does not account for the process of overcoming risk. Positive adjustment is an outcome that can be achieved by low-risk adolescents and does not require an experience of adversity (Fergus & Zimmerman, 2005). *Competence* is another term that is often conflated with *resilience*. Competence, an asset that has been found to help youth overcome risk (Fergus & Zimmerman, 2005), is thus related to resilience, but it is only one of many assets that benefit adolescents. Youth who are not exposed to risk can exhibit competence (e.g., perform well in school) but would not be considered resilient because there is no prior risk exposure. Zimmerman, Ramírez-Valles, and Maton (1999), for example, examined a measure of competence in the sociopolitical area, and how it protected youth from feelings of helplessness.

Despite these limitations, resiliency theory provides a useful conceptual framework for understanding why risk exposure only predicts negative outcomes half the time (at best). Another benefit of applying resiliency theory to the study of adolescent development is that it uses a strengths-based approach (Fergus & Zimmerman, 2005; Luthar et al., 2000; Masten, 2001; Masten et al., 1990). This is particularly beneficial for designing prevention methods and interventions for youth. Interventions designed using resiliency theory focus on helping youth develop promotive factors in their lives. Helping youth build and strengthen their assets and resources will benefit them across risk contexts and throughout development.

Strengths-Based Interventions

Like the research focused on adolescent health and development, most youth interventions also take a deficit-based approach. These programs tend to focus on ameliorating problems or helping youth avoid risks associated with negative outcomes (Brendtro, Brokenleg, & Van Bockern, 2005; Catalano et al., 2004; Mills, Dunham, Aber, & Alpert, 1988). Overall, risk-based interventions have not sustained changes for improved adolescent outcomes (Cairns & Cairns, 1994; Mills et al., 1988; Weissberg & O'Brien, 2004; Wilson, Gottfredson, & Najaka, 2001). Although much time and money are dedicated to youth substance use prevention, current programs in the United States have strong initial effects that quickly dissipate (Cairns & Cairns, 1994). Research on adolescent resilience, however, has helped to identify positive factors to enhance contexts in which practitioners can intervene.

Yet theory based intervention programs designed to build and increase promotive factors in at-risk youth are limited. Garmezy (1971) noted over 30 years ago the importance of interventions that focus on promotive factors, but this approach has been slow to develop. This may partially be the result of changes in the definition and conceptualization of resilience (e.g., from invulnerable and invincible to the current idea of resilience), and the slow transition from prevention of negative outcomes and a focus on risk factors, to promotion of health and a focus on promotive factors (Masten, 2001).

Initial strength-based intervention efforts have focused on life skills (Catalano et al., 2004; LaFromboise & Rowe, 1983; Perry, Kelder, Murray, & Klepp, 1992). These programs concentrate on enhancing self-efficacy and outcome expectations (LaFromboise & Rowe, 1983). Although life skills training embraces the idea of improving assets, thus resembling some of the resiliency framework, it also assumes a deficit model. The Class of 1989 Study, for instance, was a school-based smoking intervention that taught adolescents skills for resisting peer and other social influences to smoking (Perry et al., 1992). Though it focused on building the ability to resist social pressure, this framework also assumed that the adolescents were lacking this asset, and therefore did not address their strengths.

Several school-based interventions focus on promoting resiliency in adolescents. A meta-analysis of 165 school-based programs suggests that programs directed at increasing social competency and self-control, as well as changing the school environment, are more successful than traditional instructional and behavior modification methods for preventing adolescent problem behavior (Perry et al., 1992; Wilson et al., 2001). Schools that embraced environmental changes (establishing norms and expectations and reorganizing classes), and schools that employed self-control or competency interventions were most successful in reducing alcohol and drug use. These interventions promote positive youth development by focusing on strengthening personal assets and school resources. Researchers have consistently found that positive school environments can buffer adolescents from risk (Garmezy, 1991; Rutter, 1979; Werner & Smith, 1992). Self-control and competency interventions, on the other hand, are designed to increase or strengthen assets that

can help mitigate risk or protect youth from risks. Wilson and colleagues' (2001) analysis concluded that school-based prevention programs that focus on enhancing strengths (i.e., applied principles of resiliency theory) are more successful than the traditional problem-focused approach.

Caplan and colleagues (1992) conducted a school-based competency intervention for sixth- and seventh-grade students in an urban and in a suburban school (control group). The goal of their program was to promote general competency and prevent substance use by improving stress management and problem solving; increasing self-esteem, assertiveness, and substance use knowledge; and strengthening social networks. Postintervention, adolescents in the urban school demonstrated gains in coping, conflict resolution, impulse control, popularity (a measure of social network) and problem solving that were not found for the control group (Caplan et al., 1992). They found that excessive alcohol use decreased for the intervention group but not for the control group.

Another point of intervention for youth resiliency interventions is the family. The Iowa Strengthening Families Program (ISFP), a parent training intervention, was designed to increase family competency and reduce risk by improving family protective factors (Spoth, Redmond, & Shin, 1998). The intervention included separate parent, child, and family components, and focused on parent training, adolescent social interaction and drug refusal skills, family communication and conflict resolution, and family cohesion. Spoth and colleagues (1998) found improvements for general child management skills (discipline, parental monitoring), specific intervention behaviors (supportive communication, anger management, communication surrounding substance use expectations and involvement of adolescent in family decisions), and parent–child interaction (positive affect). Compared to the control group, participants in the ISFP improved in all promotive factors between pretest and posttest, suggesting that even a five-session family intervention can improve assets and resources available to youth (Spoth et al., 1998).

The Fathers and Sons Program is another family-based intervention designed to improve communication and closeness among nonresidential African American fathers and their 8- to 12-year-old sons. The goals of the program were to reduce substance use, violence, and early sexual debut among the youth, and improve parenting skills among the fathers (Caldwell et al., 2004). The intervention components were designed to strengthen resources (e.g., social networks, social support, father–son relationships, parenting skills) and assets (e.g., racial identity and self-efficacy in substance refusal skills). Results indicated that the intervention was effective in improving fathers' ability to monitor their sons, to communicate about risky behaviors, and to enhance their communication intentions (Caldwell, Rafferty, Reischl, De Loney & Brooks, in press). They also found that the youth reported improved efficacy for communicating about risky behavior with their fathers and increased intentions to use alternative strategies to deal with violence.

The Youth Empowerment Solutions for Peaceful Communities (YES) program was designed to involved youth in community change activities to prevent and reduce youth violence. YES gives youth the opportunity to design community change projects (e.g., murals, community gardens) and addresses neighborhood violence via three main intervention components: youth empowerment, adult capacity building, and community development. Youth were connected with supportive adults (neighborhood advocates) to help them develop citizenship skills; ethnic identity and pride; and program development and implementation experience. The final evaluation results have not yet been reported, but initial findings suggest that the geographic areas around the intervention sites have shown improved property conditions (Franzen, Morrel-Samuels, Reischl, & Zimmerman, 2009).

Future Directions

Although substantial gains in adolescent resiliency research have been made since the early work of Garmezy, Rutter, and Werner, future research could include more diverse populations of youth (Fergus & Zimmerman, 2005). In addition, although recent studies have included African American and Latino adolescents (Dubow et al., 1997; Hammack et al., 2004; Kliewer et al., 2004; Wills et al., 2001; Xue et al., 2007), few have studied Asian American and Native American youth (Dubow et al., 1997; Landis et al., 2007; Wills et al., 2001; Zimmerman et al., 1995). Research could also focus on a greater diversity of at-risk youth, including homeless youth; lesbian, gay, bisexual, transgendered and transexual (LGBTT) youth; youth with physical and intellectual disabilities; and recently immigrated youth. Sampling these groups, however, can be challenging because it is difficult to obtain representative samples and locate participants.

Another area for future research is to examine the challenge or inoculation model. Few researchers have explicitly studied inoculation. This requires both longitudinal data and information on risk and promotive factors, but it could be explored using growth curve modeling approaches. The difficulty in testing the challenge model is to determine which risk exposures may have beneficial effects at moderate levels (e.g., a friend's alcohol use), then to compare their trajectories with the trajectories of detrimental outcomes (e.g., marijuana use). Similarly, longitudinal data can be used to explore further how developmental transitions may be successfully navigated, and to juxtapose these trajectories on the pattern of change in promotive factors.

Despite the challenging transitions experienced during adolescence, most youth develop into successful adults. Youth exposed to trauma and significant risk are able to overcome adversity and achieve positive outcomes, even though they do not necessarily become rich or famous. Yet by relying on personal assets and external resources in their families, schools, and communities, these youth can overcome adversity and develop into healthy adults.

Acknowledgments

This research was funded by the National Institute on Drug Abuse, Grant No. DA07474-09. The research here does not necessarily represent the views or policies of the National Institute on Drug Abuse.

References

Aisenberg, E., & Herrenkohl, T. (2008). Community violence in context: Risk and resilience in children and families. *Journal of Interpersonal Violence*, 23(3), 296–315.

Anthony, E. J. (Ed.). (1974). *The child in his family: Children at psychiatric risk*. New York: Wiley.

Beam, M. R., Gil-Rivas, B., Greenberger, E., & Chen, C. (2002). Adolescent problem behavior and depressed mood: Risk and protection with and across social contexts. *Journal of Youth and Adolescence*, 31(5), 343–357.

Belsky, J. (1984). The determinants of parenting: A process model. *Child Development*, 55(1), 83–96.

Bleuler, M. (1978). *The schizophrenic disorders: Long-term patient and family studies*. New Haven, CT: Yale University Press.

Brendtro, L. K., Brokenleg, M., & Van Bockern, S. (2005). The circle of courage and positive psychology. *Reclaiming Children and Youth*, 14(3), 130–136.

Brook, J. S., Gordon, A. S., Whiteman, M., & Cohen, P. (1986). Dynamics of childhood and adolescent personality traits and adolescent drug use. *Developmental Psychology*, 22, 403–414.

Brook, J. S., Whiteman, M., Gordon, A. S., & Cohen, P. (1989). Changes in drug involvement: A longitudinal study of childhood and adolescent determinants. *Psychological Reports*, 65, 707–726.

Brookmeyer, K. A., Henrich, C. C., & Schwab-Stone, M. (2005). Adolescents who witness community violence: Can parent support and prosocial cognitions protect them from committing violence? *Child Development*, 76(4), 917–929.

Brooks-Gunn, J., Duncan, G. J., Klevanov, P., & Sealand, N. (1993). Do neighborhoods influence child and adolescent development? *American Journal of Sociology*, 99(2), 353–395.

Bryant, A. L., & Zimmerman, M. A. (2003). Role models and psychosocial outcomes among African American adolescents. *Journal of Adolescent Research*, 18(1), 36–67.

Buckner, J. C., Mezzacappa, E., & Beardslee, W. R. (2003). Characteristics of resilient youths living in poverty: The role of self-regulatory processes. *Development and Psychopathology*, 15, 139–162.

Cairns, R. B., & Cairns, B. D. (1994). *Lifelines and risks: Pathways of youth in our time*. Cambridge, UK: Cambridge University Press.

Caldwell, C. H., Rafferty, J., Reischl, T. M., De Loney, E. H., & Brooks, C. L. (2008). *Enhancing parenting skills among nonresident African American fathers as a strategy for preventing youth risk behavior*. Manuscript submitted for publication.

Caldwell, C. H., Wright, J. C., Zimmerman, M. A., Walsemann, K. M., Williams, D., & Isichei, P. A. (2004). Enhancing adolescent health behaviors through strengthening nonresident father–son relationships: A model for intervention with African-American families. *Health Education Research*, 19(6), 644–656.

Caplan, M., Weissberg, R. P., Grober, J. S., Sivo, P. J., Grady, K., & Jacoby, C. (1992). Social competence promotion with inner-city and suburban young adolescents: Effects on social adjustment and alcohol use. *Journal of Consulting and Clinical Psychology*, 60(1), 56–63.

Carlton, B. (2006). Resilience, family adversity and well-being among Hawaiian and non-Hawaiian adolescents. *International Journal of Social Psychiatry*, 52(4), 291–308.

Catalano, R. F., Berglund, M. L., Ryan, J. A. M., Lonczak, H. S., & Hawkins, D. (2004). Positive youth development in the United States: Research findings on evaluations of positive youth development programs. *Annals of the American Academy of Political and Social Science*, 591(1), 98–124.

Cicchetti, D., & Garmezy, N. (1993). Prospects and promises in the study of resilience. *Development and Psychopathology*, 5, 497–502.

Clauss-Ehlers, C. S. (2008). Sociocultural factors, resilience, and coping: Support for a culturally sensitive measure of resilience. *Journal of Applied Developmental Psychology*, 29, 197–212.

Davis-Kearn, P. E. (2005). The influence of parent education and family income on child achievement: The indirect role of parental expectations and the home environment. *Journal of Family Psychology*, 19(2), 294–304.

Dubow, E. F., Edwards, S., & Ippolito, M. (1997). Life stressors, neighborhood disadvantage, and resources: A focus on inner-city children's adjustment. *Journal of Clinical Child Psychology*, 26(2), 130–144.

Duncan, G. J., & Raudenbush, S. (1999). Assessing the effects of context in studies of child and youth development. *Educational Psychologist*, 34, 29–41.

Eccles, J. S., Midgley, C., Wigfield, A., Buchanan, C. M., Reuman, D., Flanagan, C., et al. (1993). Development during adolescence: The impact of stage–environment fit on young adolescents' experiences in schools and in families. *American Psychologist*, 48(2), 90–101.

Elder, C., Leaver-Dunn, D., Wang, M. Q., Nagy, S., & Green, L. (2000). Organized group activity as a protective factor against adolescent substance use. *American Journal of Health Behavior*, 24, 108–113.

Elder, G., Conger, R. D., Foster, M., & Ardelt, M. (1992). Families under economic pressure. *Journal of Family Issues*, 13(1), 5–37.

Elder, G. H., Jr., Nguyen, T. V., & Caspi, A. (1985). Linking family hardship to children's lives. *Child Development*, 56(2), 361–375.

Elliott, D., Wilson, W., Huizinga, D., Sampson, R., Elliott, A., & Rankin, B. (1996). The effects of neighborhood disadvantage on adolescent development. *Journal of Research in Crime and Delinquency*, 33, 389–426.

Fagan, A. A., Van Horn, M. L., Hawkins, D., & Arthur, M. (2007). Using community and family risk and protective factors for community-based prevention planning. *Journal of Community Psychology*, 35(4), 535–555.

Fergus, S., & Zimmerman, M. A. (2005). Adolescent resilience: A framework for understanding healthy development in the face of risk. *Annual Review of Public Health*, 26, 399–419.

Franzen, S., Morrel-Samuels, S., Reischl, T., & Zimmerman, M. A. (in press). Using process evaluation to strengthen intergenerational partnerships in the Youth Empowerment Solutions program. *Journal of Prevention and Intervention in the Community.*

Garmezy, N. (1970). Process and reactive schizophrenia: Some conceptions and issues. *Schizophrenia Bulletin*, 2, 30–73.

Garmezy, N. (1971). Vulnerability research and the issue of primary prevention. *American Journal of Orthopsychiatry*, 41(1), 101–116.

Garmezy, N. (1974). The study of competence in children at risk for severe psychopathology. In E. J. Anthony & C. Koupernik (Eds.), *The child in his family: Children at psychiatric risk* (Vol. III, 3rd ed., pp. 77–97). New York: Wiley.

Garmezy, N. (1987). Stress, competence and development: Continuities in the study of schizophrenic adults, children vulnerable to psychopathology, and the search for stress-resistant children. *American Journal of Orthopsychiatry*, 57(2), 159–174.

Garmezy, N. (1991). Resiliency and vulnerability to adverse developmental outcomes associated with poverty. *American Behavioral Scientist*, 34(4), 416–430.

Garmezy, N., & Masten, A. S. (1986). Stress, competence and resilience: Common frontiers for therapist and psychopathologist. *Behavior Therapy*, 17, 500–521.

Garmezy, N., Masten, A. S., & Taylor, R. (1984). The study of stress and competence in children: A building block for developmental psychopathology. *Child Development*, 55(1), 97–111.

Gorman-Smith, D., Henry, D. B., & Tolan, P. (2004). Exposure to community violence and violence perpetration: The protective effects of family functioning. *Journal of Clinical Child and Adolescent Psychology*, 33(3), 439–449.

Grizenko, N., & Fisher, C. (1992). Review of studies of risk and protective factors for psychopathology in children. *Canadian Journal of Psychiatry*, 37, 711–721.

Gutman, L. M., McLoyd, V. C., & Tokoyawa, T. (2005). Financial strain, neighborhood stress, parenting behaviors, and adolescent adjustment in urban African American families. *Journal of Research on Adolescence*, 15(4), 425–449.

Hammack, P. L., Richards, M. H., Luo, M., Edlynn, E. S., & Roy, K. (2004). Social support factors as moderators of community violence exposure among inner-city African American young adolescents. *Journal of Clinical Child and Adolescent Psychology, 33*(3), 450–462.

Hill, T. D., Ross, C. E., & Angel, R. J. (2005). Neighborhood disorder, psychophysiological distress, and health. *Journal of Health Social Behavior, 46*(2), 170–186.

Jackson, A. (2003). Mothers' employment and poor and near-poor African American children's development: A longitudinal study. *Social Services Review, 77*(1), 93–109.

Jenkins, J. M., & Smith, M. A. (1990). Factors protecting children living in disharmonious homes: Maternal reports. *Journal of the American Academy of Child and Adolescent Psychiatry, 29*, 60–69.

Jessor, R. (1991). Risk behavior in adolescence: A psychosocial framework for understanding and action. *Journal of Adolescent Health, 12*, 597–605.

Jessor, R., Turbin, M. S., Costa, F. M., Dong, Q., Zhang, H., & Wang, C. (2003). Adolescent problem behavior in China and the United States: A cross-national study of psychosocial protective factors. *Journal of Research on Adolescence, 13*(3), 329–360.

Kaplow, J. B., Curran, P. J., Angold, A., & Costello, E. J. (2001). The prospective relation between dimensions of anxiety and the initiation of adolescent alcohol use. *Journal of Clinical Child Psychology, 30*, 316–326.

Kempton, T., Armistead, L., Wierson, M., & Forehand, R. (1991). Presence of a sibling as a potential buffer following parental divorce: An examination of young adolescents. *Journal of Clinical Child and Adolescent Psychology, 20*(4), 434–438.

Kliewer, W., Cunningham, J. N., Diehl, R., Parish, K. A., Walker, J. M., Atiyeh, C., et al. (2004). Violence exposure and adjustment in inner-city youth: Child and caregiver emotion regulation skill, caregiver–child relationship quality, and neighborhood cohesion as protective factor. *Journal of Clinical Child and Adolescent Psychology, 33*(3), 477–487.

LaFromboise, T., & Rowe, W. (1983). Skills training for bicultural competence: Rationale and application. *Journal of Counseling Psychology, 30*(4), 589–595.

Landis, D., Gaylord-Harden, N. K., Malinowski, S. L., Grant, K. E., Carleton, R. A., & Ford, R. E. (2007). Urban adolescent stress and hopelessness. *Journal of Adolescence, 30*(6), 1051–1070.

Leventhal, T., & Brooks-Gunn, J. (2000). The neighborhoods they live in: The effects of neighborhood residence on child and adolescent outcomes. *Psychological Bulletin, 126*(2), 309–337.

Leventhal, T., & Brooks-Gunn, J. (2004). A randomized study of neighborhood effects on low-income children's educational outcomes. *Developmental Psychology, 40*(4), 488–507.

Luthar, S. S. (2004). Children's exposure to community violence: Implications for understanding risk and resilience. *Journal of Clinical Child and Adolescent Psychology, 33*(3), 499–505.

Luthar, S. S., Cicchetti, D., & Becker, B. (2000). The construct of resilience: A critical evaluation and guidelines for future work. *Child Development, 71*(3), 543–562.

Masten, A. S. (2001). Ordinary magic: Resilience processes in development. *American Psychologist, 56*, 227–238.

Masten, A. S., Best, K. M., & Garmezy, N. (1990). Resilience and development: Contributions from the study of children who overcome adversity. *Development and Psychopathology, 2*, 425–444.

Mayer, S., & Jencks, C. (1989). Growing up in poor neighborhoods: How much does it matter? *Science, 243*, 1441–1445.

McLoyd, V. (1990). The impact of economic hardship on black families and children: Psychological distress, parenting and socioemotional development. *Child Development, 61*, 311–346.

McLoyd, V. (1994). Unemployment and work interruption among African American single mothers: Effects on parenting and adolescent socioemotional functioning. *Child Development, 65*, 562–589.

McLoyd, V. (1998). Socioeconomic disadvantage and child development. *American Psychologist, 53*(2), 185–204.

Meyers, S. A., & Miller, C. (2004). Direct, mediated, moderated, and cumulative relations between neighborhood characteristics and adolescent outcomes. *Adolescence, 39*, 121–144.

Mills, R. C., Dunham, R. G., Aber, J. L., & Alpert, G. P. (1988). Working with high-risk youth in prevention and early intervention programs: Towards a comprehensive wellness model. *Adolescence*, 23, 643–660.

Neighbors, B., Forehand, R., & McVicar, D. (1993). Resilient adolescents and interparental conflict. *American Journal of Orthopsychiatry*, 63(3), 462–471.

Ostaszewski, K., & Zimmerman, M. A. (2006). The effects of cumulative risks and promotive factors on urban adolescent alcohol and other drug use: A longitudinal study of resiliency. *American Journal of Community Psychology*, 38, 237–249.

Ozer, E. J., & Weinstein, R. S. (2004). Urban adolescent's exposure to community violence: The role of support, school safety and social constraints in a school-based sample of boys and girls. *Journal of Clinical Child and Adolescent Psychology*, 33(3), 463–476.

Patchin, J. W. (2006). Exposure to community violence and childhood delinquency. *Crime and Delinquency*, 52(2), 307–332.

Perry, C., Kelder, S., Murray, D., & Klepp, K. (1992). Communitywide smoking prevention: Long-term outcomes of the Minnesota Heart Health Program and the Class of 1989 Study. *American Journal of Public Health*, 82(9), 1210–1216.

Pinderhughes, E., Nix, R., Foster, M., & Jones, D. (2001). Parenting in context: Impact of neighborhood poverty, residential stability, public services, social networks and danger on parental behaviors. *Journal of Marriage and Family*, 63(4), 941–953.

Prelow, H. M., Loukas, A., & Jordan-Green, L. (2007). Socioenvironmental risk and adjustment in Latino youth: The mediating effects of family processes and social competence. *Journal of Youth and Adolescence*, 36(4), 465–476.

Prevatt, F. (2003). The contribution of parenting practices in a risk and resiliency model of children's adjustment. *British Journal of Developmental Psychology*, 21, 469–480.

Rink, E., & Tricker, R. (2005). Promoting healthy behaviors among adolescents: A review of the resiliency literature. *American Journal of Health Studies*, 20(1/2), 39–46.

Rodgers, K. B., & Rose, H. A. (2002). Risk and resiliency factors among adolescents who experience marital transitions. *Journal of Marriage and Family*, 64(4), 1024–1037.

Rutter, M. (1976). Research report: Isle of Wight studies. *Psychological Medicine*, 6, 313–332.

Rutter, M. (1979a). Maternal deprivation, 1972–1978: New findings, new concepts, new approaches. *Child Development*, 50(2), 283–305.

Rutter, M. (1979b). Protective factors in children's responses to stress and disadvantage. In M. Kent & J. Rolf (Eds.), *Primary prevention of psychopathology* (Vol. 3, pp. 49–74). Hanover, NH: University Press of New England.

Rutter, M. (1985). Resilience in the face of adversity: Protective factors and resistance to psychiatric disorder. *British Journal of Psychiatry*, 147, 598–611.

Rutter, M. (1987). Psychosocial resilience and protective mechanisms. *American Journal of Orthopsychiatry*, 57(3), 316–331.

Rutter, M. (1993). Resilience: Some conceptual considerations. *Journal of Adolescent Health*, 14, 626–631.

Rutter, M., Tizard, J., & Whitmore, K. (Eds.). (1970). *Education, health and behavior*. London: Longmans.

Rutter, M., Yule, B., Quinton, D., Rowlands, O., Yule, W., & Berger, M. (1974). Attainment and adjustment in two geographical areas: III. Some factors accounting for area differences. *British Journal of Psychiatry*, 125, 520–533.

Sameroff, A. J., Seifer, R., Barocas, R., Zax, M., & Greenspan, S. (1987). Intelligence quotient scores of 4-year old children: Social–environmental risk factors. *Pediatrics*, 79, 343–350.

Sampson, R., Raudenbush, S., & Earls, F. (1997). Neighborhoods and violent crime: A multilevel study of collective efficacy. *Science*, 277, 918–924.

Sampson, R. J. (1999). Systematic social observation of public spaces: A new look at disorder in urban neighborhoods. *American Journal of Sociology*, 105(3), 603–651.

Seidman, E., Yoshikawa, H., Roberts, A., Chesir-Teran, D., Allen, L., Friedman, J. L., et al. (1998). Structural and experiential neighborhood contexts, developmental stage, and antisocial behavior among urban adolescents in poverty. *Development and Psychopathology*, 10(2), 259–281.

Spoth, R., Redmond, C., & Shin, C. (1998). Direct and indirect latent-variable parenting outcomes of two universal family-focused preventive interventions: Extending a public health-oriented research base. *Journal of Consulting and Clinical Psychology, 66*(2), 385–399.

Steptoe, A., Brydon, L., & Kunz-Ebrecht, S. (2005). Changes in financial strain over three years, ambulatory blood pressure, and cortisol responses to awakening. *Psychosomatic Medicine, 67*, 281–287.

Taylor, K. W., & Kliewer, W. (2006). Violence exposure and early adolescent alcohol use: An exploratory study of family risk and protective factors. *Journal of Child and Family Studies, 15*(2), 207–221.

Tiet, Q. Q., Bird, H. R., Hoven, C. W., Wu, P., Moore, R., & Davies, M. (2001). Resilience in the face of maternal psychopathology and adverse life events. *Journal of Child and Family Studies, 10*(3), 347–365.

Turbin, M. S., Jessor, R., Costa, F. M., Dong, Q. I., Zhang, H., & Wang, C. (2006). Protective and risk factors in health-enhancing behavior among adolescents in china and the United States: Does social context matter? *Health Psychology, 25*(4), 445–454.

Ungar, M. (2006). Nurturing hidden resilience in at-risk youth in different cultures. *Journal of the Canadian Academy of Child and Adolescent Psychiatry, 15*(2), 53–58.

Wandersman, A., & Nation, M. (1998). Urban neighborhoods and mental health: Psychological contributions to understanding toxicity, resilience and interventions. *American Psychologist, 53*(6), 647–656.

Weissberg, R. P., & O'Brien, M. U. (2004). What works in school-based social and emotional learning programs for positive youth development. *Annals of the American Academy of Political and Social Science, 591*(1), 86–97.

Werner, E. E. (1989). High-risk children in young adulthood: A longitudinal study from birth to 32 years. *American Journal of Orthopsychiatry, 59*(1), 72–81.

Werner, E. E., Bierman, J. M., & French, F. E. (1971). *The children of Kauai: A longitudinal study from the prenatal period to age ten.* Honolulu: University of Hawaii Press.

Werner, E. E., & Smith, R. S. (1992). *Overcoming the odds.* Ithaca, NY: Cornell University Press.

Wills, T. A., Sandy, J. M., Yaeger, A., & Shinar, O. (2001). Family risk factors and adolescent substance use: Moderation effects for temperament dimensions. *Developmental Psychology, 37*(3), 283–297.

Wilson, D., Gottfredson, D., & Najaka, S. S. (2001). School-based prevention of problem behaviors: A meta-analysis. *Journal of Quantitative Criminology, 17*(3), 247–272.

Wilson, W. (1987). *The truly disadvantaged: The inner city, the underclass and public policy.* Chicago: University of Chicago Press.

Xue, Y., Zimmerman, M. A., & Caldwell, C. H. (2007). Neighborhood residence and cigarette smoking among urban youths: The protective role of prosocial activities. *American Journal of Public Health, 97*, 1865–1872.

Zimmerman, M. A., & Arunkumar, R. (1994). Resiliency research: Implications for schools and policy. *Social Policy Report, 8*, 1–18.

Zimmerman, M. A., Ramírez, J., Washienko, K. M., Walter, B., & Dyer, S. (1995). Enculturation hypothesis: Exploring direct and protective effects among Native American youth. In H. I. McCubbin, E. A. Thompson, & A. I. Thompson (Eds.), *Resiliency in ethnic minority families: Vol. 1. Native and immigrant American families* (pp. 199–220). Madison: University of Wisconsin Press.

Zimmerman, M. A., Ramírez-Valles, J., & Maton, K.I. (1999). Resilience among urban African American adolescents: A study of the protective effects of sociopolitical control on their mental health. *American Journal of Community Psychology, 27*(6), 733–751.

Zimmerman, M. A., Steinman, K. J., & Rowe, K. J. (1998). Violence among urban African American adolescents: The protective effects of parental support. In X. B. Arriaga & S. Oskamp (Eds.), *Addressing community problems: Psychological research and interventions* (pp. 78–103). Thousand Oaks, CA: Sage.

15

Social Support and Growth Following Adversity

Vicki S. Helgeson
Lindsey Lopez

The truth is that cancer was the best thing that ever happened to me. I don't know why
I got the illness, but it did wonders for me, and I wouldn't want to walk away from it.
Why would I want to change, even for a day, the most important and shaping event in
my life? ... People have asked me what I mean when I say that given a choice between
cancer and winning the Tour de France, I'd choose cancer. What I mean is that I wouldn't
have learned all I did if I hadn't had to contend with cancer. I couldn't have won even
one Tour without my fight, because of what it taught me. I truly believe that. I had a deep
sense of illness, and not only wasn't I ashamed of it, I valued it above everything.
—ARMSTRONG (2000, pp. 4, 283–284)

For decades researchers have focused on the negative psychological and physical consequences of stressful life events. Although researchers have noted the potential for people to experience positive consequences early on (i.e., Taylor, 1983), it is only in the last 10–20 years that this possibility has been taken seriously. It is not uncommon for people to make the kinds of remarks that Lance Armstrong made in response to having a life-threatening illness, in this case, testicular cancer. Today, there are a variety of theories having to do with how people benefit from adversity, most often referred to as *posttraumatic growth*, *stress-related growth*, or *benefit finding*. Common areas of positive change (i.e., domains of growth) include an enhanced appreciation of life, closer relationships, increased spirituality, a shift in priorities, and increased personal

strength (Stanton, Bower, & Low, 2006; Tedeschi & Calhoun, 1996).

Although all theories have at their core the potential for a positive outcome following adversity, the theories differ in terms of the magnitude and nature of those positive outcomes. One issue is whether the positive consequences following adversity simply reflect a return to one's situation before the stressful life event (i.e., return to baseline or recovery) or an improvement over one's situation before the stressful life event. In their theory of posttraumatic growth, Tedeschi and Calhoun (2004) are very clear in stating that "posttraumatic growth is not simply a return to baseline—it is an experience of improvement that for some persons is deeply profound" (p. 4). In this case, growth may differ conceptually from the way that resilience has been traditionally defined. *Resil-*

ience is a term that has been used to describe good outcomes in the face of trauma, competence during times of stress, and recovery from trauma (Werner, 1995, 2000). Others have defined *resilience* as a way to weather or endure a trauma that reflects no more than a return to baseline (Carver, 1998; Luthar, Cicchetti, & Becker, 2000; O'Leary & Ickovics, 1995). Yet Kahn (1991, cited in O'Leary & Ickovics, 1995) suggested that the return to baseline is simply recovery, and that thriving represents exceeding baseline. In this chapter, we focus on the kind of resilience that represents *thriving*—the improvement that occurs following a stressful event that did not exist prior to the trauma. We use the term *growth* to refer to the variety of ways that people's lives are enhanced following a traumatic or stressful life event.

Much has been written about the prevalence of growth following adversity, and the implications of growth for psychological and physical well-being (e.g., Helgeson, Reynolds, & Tomich, 2006; Park & Helgeson, 2006). Much less has been written about the origins of growth. Our goal in this chapter is to examine whether the social environment contributes to resilience or growth following trauma, and, if so, to articulate the nature of that contribution. A wealth of research shows that social support facilitates *adjustment* to trauma and *adaptation* to disease (Revenson, 2003; Uchino, 2004), but that is not the same as linking the social environment to thriving or growth. Researchers have alluded to the possibility that people are more likely to construe benefits and to experience growth in the presence of a supportive network, but little research has directly tested this assumption.

We begin by making some conceptual distinctions with respect to the social environment. Then we review how theories of growth conceptualize the role of the social environment in promoting growth. Next, we integrate the ideas from existing theorists with our own to develop a theoretical model outlining the processes by which the social environment might contribute to growth.

Then we review the literature that has examined the relation of the social environment to growth to determine the extent to which our theoretical model is upheld. Only a few of these studies set out explicitly to test this relation; more often, a support measure and a growth measure are included in a study that is focused on a different topic and the correlation (or lack thereof) between support and growth is reported. We also present some of our own data that we collected for the sole purpose of exploring the relation of the social environment to growth. Finally, we conclude the chapter by outlining a set of directions for future research.

The Social Environment: Important Distinctions

When considering how the social environment might contribute to growth, a number of important distinctions within the social environment need to be made. First, there are quantitative and qualitative measures of the social environment. *Quantitative measures* include the number of social ties, frequency of contact with network members, or the amount of social support received. *Qualitative measures* refer to the nature or functions of social relations. Three commonly assessed support functions of the social environment are emotional, instrumental, and informational (House & Kahn, 1985). *Emotional support* comprises of understanding, expressions of love, caring, empathy, and concern. *Instrumental support* reflects concrete actions that network members may perform, such as running errands, lifting heavy furniture, and lending money. *Informational support* reflects guidance or advice. For each of these three support functions, a distinction can be made between perceived and received support. *Perceived support* refers to the subjective perception that network members are available to help, if needed. An example of a perceived support question is "To what extent can you turn to family or friends for advice?" *Received support* refers to actual behaviors that network members have performed. An example of a received support question is "Did family and friends provide advice?" As we review the theories of growth, we try to determine whether predictions can be made about how growth is related to the amount of social contact, the kind of support, and perceived versus received support.

Theories of Growth: What Do They Say about the Social Environment?

According to Janoff-Bulman (1992), traumatic life events threaten one's assumptions about the self and the world. People successfully adjust to trauma by restoring these assumptions. Janoff-Bulman states that the rebuilding of assumptions takes place in an *interpersonal context*; that is, others play a role in the reconstruction of the self and world assumptions. However, she does not explicitly outline that role. Others seem to be involved to the extent that one discloses to and discusses the traumatic event with network members. There are two effects of this disclosure. First, the disclosure has an effect on others' behavior. Others' responses can be either supportive or unsupportive—although it is not clear from Janoff-Bulman's theory how this is tied to the construal of benefits or growth. Second, regardless of others' responses, disclosing provides opportunities for cognitive and emotional processing of the event, which may facilitate growth. We elaborate on this idea in the next paragraph. Thus, according to Janoff-Bulman, self-disclosure to network members and received emotional support should be associated with growth.

In their theory of posttraumatic growth, Tedeschi and Calhoun (1995, 2004) articulate some of Janoff-Bulman's ideas in more detail. They argue that growth occurs when traumatic events lead to changed schemas about the self and the world. Tedeschi and Calhoun suggest that growth is influenced by three factors: personality, schema revision, and social resources. Social resources stem

from the social environment. The authors suggest several ways in which the social environment might contribute to growth. First, the mere act of disclosing the trauma to network members is likely to promote cognitive processing that can facilitate growth; that is, disclosure provides the opportunity for reflection and contemplation, which allows the individual time to develop, plan, and implement life changes. This pathway to growth, however, does not necessarily require the presence of other people. Indeed, Pennebaker (2002) has an entire program of research that demonstrates self-disclosure through expressive writing is associated with health benefits, in part due to cognitive processing. Two studies have linked vocal and written expression of feelings about a trauma to growth (Murray & Segal, 1994; Ullrich & Lutgendorf, 2002). These effects appeared to be mediated by cognitive processing. Thus, there is some evidence that self-disclosure is related to growth via cognitive processing, but the response of the support provider seems to have been left out of this equation. Tedeschi and Calhoun (1995, 2004) argue that self-disclosure is especially likely to lead to cognitive processing and growth when one self-discloses to a supportive other. When network members respond to disclosure by withdrawing from the interaction, changing the subject, criticizing, or minimizing the trauma, cognitive processing is inhibited (Lepore & Revenson, 2007). One study showed that these kinds of social constraints were related to less cognitive processing, which was ultimately related to less growth (Cordova, Cunningham, Carlson, & Andrykowski, 2001).

Tedeschi and Calhoun (1995, 2004) also suggest that supportive others can facilitate growth by offering new ways of understanding or reconceptualizing the trauma. Therapists may be especially skilled in helping victims to experience growth through this means. However, network members also can suggest ways in which a person has grown from a trauma or might be able to experience growth. Tedeschi and Calhoun suggest that this is more likely to occur when network members have undergone the same trauma. When people who have not experienced the trauma suggest that one might be a stronger person for having weathered the trauma or note some other potential for growth, it can be viewed as disingenuous. Observing similar others who have undergone the trauma and grown from it can be a source of growth possibilities. Taken collectively, like Janoff-Bulman, Tedeschi and Calhoun hypothesize relations of both self-disclosure and received support to growth.

Whereas the previous theorists have emphasized the role that the social environment plays in revising schemas and facilitating cognitive processing, McMillen (1999, 2004) argues that the link between the social environment and growth may be more direct. The receipt of support during times of stress demonstrates that other people are good, helpful, and can be counted on when needed. Receiving support also can make one aware of the importance of relationships. These effects are directly linked to growth, in that one of the most common domains of growth is interpersonal—specifically, improved social relations, greater appreciation of social relationships, and a more positive view of other people. In this sense, the social network's response to one's traumatic life event becomes the domain of growth. Thus, like Tedeschi and Calhoun (1995, 2004), McMillen would hypothesize a relation between received support and growth.

Schaefer and Moos (1992) applied the stress and coping framework to understand how people derive benefits from trauma. In their model, both personal and environmental factors influence growth. The social environment contributes to growth by providing resources (emotional or instrumental) that enable the individual to perceive the event as less threatening, allowing energies to be redirected from minimizing stress to focusing on opportunities for growth. Therefore, Schaefer and Moos would predict that received emotional or instrumental support leads to growth.

Joseph and Linley's (2005) organismic valuing process theory suggests that there are three possible outcomes from exposure to trauma: assimilation or return to baseline; negative accommodation or psychopathology; and positive accommodation or growth. Although they assume that human beings are naturally inclined toward growth, they argue that the social environment's response to trauma can impede or facilitate growth. Positive accommodation occurs when the social environment meets individuals' needs for autonomy, competence, and relatedness. Individual differences in response to trauma are a function of whether the social environment has satisfied these needs in the past, and whether the social environment satisfies these needs in the presence of trauma. Having had needs met in the past provides people with a sense of resilience, so that they can accommodate to future traumas. The history of support receipt would seem to lead to perceived support, whereas having current needs met would seem to reflect received support. Thus, it appears that Joseph and Linley would argue that both perceived and received support are associated with growth.

Taken collectively, the major theorists in the area have suggested that the social environment contributes to growth, emphasizing the role of received support and self-disclosure. A key tenet of all the theories is that growth follows a major stressful life event or trauma. Theorists differ in the extent to which they believe that this event must be cataclysmic—threatening one's core beliefs in the self and the world. This is one reason that Tedeschi and Calhoun (2004) use the term *posttraumatic growth*, whereas others have used the term *stress-related growth* (Park, Cohen, & Murch, 1996). Indeed, some studies have examined growth following a major trauma (e.g., natural disaster or diagnosis of cancer), and others have focused on growth following more common stressful life events (e.g., relationship breakup). We maintain that individual differences in perception and response to both traumatic events and stressful life events make it difficult to identify the category of stressor that leads to growth. Therefore, we do not take a position on the issue of the degree of stress required to elicit growth, but regard this issue to be a subject of future research. However, we maintain that some level of stress is required to spark the growth process. Indeed, a meta-analytic review of the growth literature showed that greater perceived stress or threat was related to more growth (Helgeson et al., 2006). Below, we integrate the ideas of the major theorists in the area with some of our own to develop a theoretical model of how the social environment might influence growth. Then, we review the literature in the area to evaluate how it fits with this theoretical model.

Theoretical Model of the Social Environment and Growth

The theoretical model that outlines the pathways by which different aspects of the social environment might influence growth is shown in Figure 15.1, in which we identify the most common domains of growth: new possibilities (e.g., a change in career), personal strength (e.g., better able to cope with stress), spirituality (e.g., become closer to God), appreciation of life (e.g., live each day one at a time), and improved relationships (e.g., closer to one's spouse). These are the domains that map onto the Posttraumatic Growth Inventory (PTGI; Tedeschi & Calhoun, 1996), one of the most widely used measures of growth. The three aspects

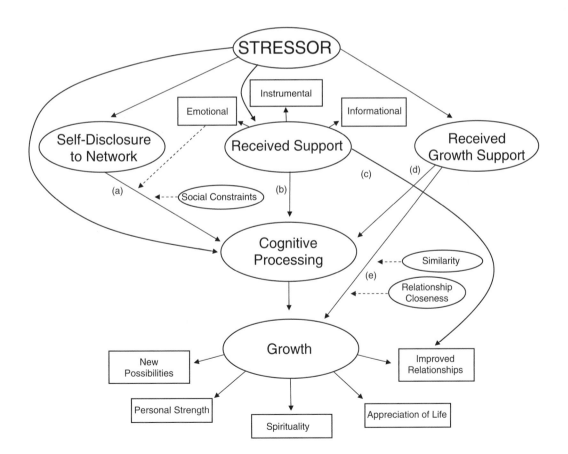

FIGURE 15.1. Model of the relation of the social environment to growth.

of the social environment upon which we focus are self-disclosure to network members, received support, and received growth support. We focus on self-disclosure and received support, which, we believe, contain the strongest conceptual rationale for relations to growth. We also included a third aspect of the social environment, received growth support, which reflects network members' direct remarks about ways in which one has grown or could grow because of a stressful life event. We recognize that received growth support is a new construct that has not received much attention in the literature. In a previous study investigating received growth support from parents in a study of adolescents with diabetes, we found that received growth support was strongly related to adolescents' reports of growth as a result of having diabetes (Helgeson, Lopez, & Mennella, 2009).

As can be seen from Figure 15.1, the entire growth process is activated by a stressful life event. These stressful life events can span a variety of domains—social, health, or achievement. There are both direct and indirect pathways by which the social environment leads to growth. There also is a series of moderator variables that influence whether or how strongly an aspect of the social environment is related to growth (depicted by the dashed lines in Figure 15.1). Below we describe each of the pathways by which the social environment contributes to growth:

(a) Self-disclosing to network members indirectly contributes to growth by providing opportunities for personal reflection and contemplation, or cognitive processing. Self-disclosure is most likely to lead to cognitive processing when network members convey understanding, caring, and concern (i.e., received emotional support), and least likely to lead to cognitive processing when network members constrain or inhibit the disclosure.

(b) Received support also may indirectly lead to growth via cognitive processing. When people provide support in times of stress, some of the burden that requires one's time and attention is reduced, making attentional resources available for cognitive processing. Emotional, instrumental, and informational support each reduce distress in different ways, so that one is able to move beyond coping with the distress to process and assimilate the traumatic life event and accommodate one's life to the traumatic life event in positive ways.

(c) Network members also can affect growth directly by providing support and demonstrating that people are good, helpful, and that they can be counted on in times of stress. The effect on growth here is limited to the specific domain of interpersonal growth, which is characterized by the realization that people are good, that one's own relationships have improved, or that relationships are important. Here the support provided by others is the source of a specific kind of growth.

(d) Received growth support indirectly affects growth via cognitive processing. This pathway is similar to (b) except that network members are providing specific suggestions of potential benefits upon which one then reflects. The opportunity to reflect (i.e., cognitive processing) then leads one to pursue areas of growth.

(e) Network members directly affect growth by sharing their observations about the way one has grown (e.g., personal strengths gained, improved relationships) or the ways one could grow from an event. Exposure to these suggestions of growth, or *received growth support*, may lead one to recognize growth or seek those opportunities for growth. This is more likely to occur when those network members have had experience with the stressor, and/or when the relationship with the network member is closer, so that such suggestions are regarded positively.

The one aspect of the social environment that is not included in this model is perceived support. Support perceptions are based on a multitude of factors, including perceived similarity to network members, personality factors, relationship quality, and, to some extent, past experiences of support receipt (Kaul & Lakey, 2003; Lakey, Lutz, & Scoboria, 2004). We do not hypothesize a relation between perceived support and growth that is independent of received support. Therefore, we did not include perceived support in this model. Perceived support is unlikely to influence growth directly; rather, it is likely to influence the appraisal of an event. In contrast, received support is likely to influence an individual's ability to cope with the event. Received support can encourage and support individuals in their attempt to understand the event. In this way, received support can influence cognitive processing of the event. However, many of the studies that examine the relation between the social environment and growth focus on perceived support, as we described below. Unfortunately, none of the studies includes both perceived and received support.

Studies of the Social Environment and Growth

In a fairly recent review of the cancer literature, Stanton and colleagues (2006) concluded that neither the amount of social support nor support satisfaction was consistently linked to growth outcomes. However, at that time, only six studies of people with cancer addressed these relations. Not limiting our review to people with cancer and including studies published through 2007, we located 33 studies that examined relations between the social environment and growth. Each of these studies is listed in Table 15.1. Some studies are listed more than once because they examined more than one aspect of the social environment. Five different aspects of the social environment have been examined: perceived support, received support, support satisfaction, self-disclosure, and amount of social contact. Table 15.1 identifies whether the study is cross-sectional (C) or longitudinal (L), provides characteristics of the sample, identifies the support and growth

measures used, and indicates the findings in the last two columns. Below, we describe the results of the studies in Table 15.1, then evaluate how those studies support or fail to support the model shown in Figure 15.1.

Perceived Support

Of the 11 studies that examine the relation of perceived support to growth, eight are cross-sectional and three are longitudinal. Five of the eight cross-sectional studies revealed a positive relation between perceived support and growth, one revealed no relation, and two provided mixed evidence for a relation. Of the two equivocal studies, one found that perceived support from friends was associated with more growth, but perceived support from family was not (Lev-Wiesel & Amir, 2003). The other found relations of perceived emotional support to four of seven areas of growth—areas that were largely interpersonal—but did not find a relation between instrumental support and any of the seven areas of growth (McMillen & Cook, 2003). The study that obtained a null relation was the only one of the 11 studies to measure growth with a single, open-ended interview item rather than a well-established scale (McCausland & Pakenham, 2003). Thus, there appears to be strong support for a cross-sectional relation between perceived support and growth. This relation extends across a variety of populations.

None of the three longitudinal studies detected a relation of perceived support to growth. Each used the PTGI (Tedeschi & Calhoun, 1996). In one study, a measure of perceived support was administered to prisoners of war, who were then followed for 5 years (Erbes et al., 2005). Perceived support did not predict growth. Perceived support following treatment for breast cancer did not predict growth 12 months later (Sears, Stanton, & Danoff-Burg, 2003), nor did perceived support prior to bone marrow transplant predict growth 6 months following hospital discharge (Widows, Jacobsen, Booth-Jones, & Fields, 2005). These studies

TABLE 15.1. Studies of the Relation of the Social Environment to Growth

Authors of study	Design	Sample	N	Age	% Female	% White	Support scale	Growth scale	Relation	Results
Perceived										
Erbes et al. (2005)	L	Prisoners of war	95	M = 80, 70–91	0%	100%	18 items	PTGI	Null	r = .15, n.s.
Karanci & Erkam (2007)	C	Breast cancer	90	M = 43, 23–67	100%	Turkey	12 items	SRGS	Positive	pr = .22**
Kinsinger et al. (2006)	C	Prostate cancer	250	M = 65, —	0%	41%	ESSI (emotional and instrumental)	BFS	Total positive; emotional positive; instrumental positive	Total: r = .17**; Emotional: r = .16**; Instrumental: r = .10*
Lev-Wiesel & Amir (2003)	C	Holocaust survivors	97	M = 68, —	52%	Israel	PSS	PTGI	Friends positive; family null	Friends: r = .24*; Family: r = .14, n.s.
Littlewood et al. (2008)	C	HIV/AIDS	221	M = 40, 22–59	44%	46%	15 items	BFS	Positive	r = .31**
McCausland & Pakenham (2003)	C	HIV/AIDS caregivers	64	M = 43, 19–70	41%	89%	8 items	Open-ended interview question	Null	r = –.29, n.s.
McMillen & Cook (2003)	C	Spinal cord injury	42	M = 43, —	19%	71%	ISEL (emotional and instrumental)	PBS	Emotional positive (4 of 7); instrumental null	Emotional self-efficacy: r = .28; community closeness: r = .47**; faith in people: r = .54***; spirituality: r = .39**; compassion: r = .43**; family closeness: r = .22; material gain: r = .07 Instrumental self-efficacy: r = .19; community closeness: r = .19; faith in people: r = .16; spirituality: r = –.06; compassion: r = .19; family closeness: r = .02; material gain: r = .00
Sears et al. (2003)	L	Breast cancer	60	M = 52, 28–76	100%	87%	3 items (emotional)	PTGI	Null	r = .15, n.s.

316

Study	Design	Population	N	Age	%	%	Support measure	PTG measure	Result	Correlation
Siegel et al. (2005)	C	HIV/AIDS	138	M = 38, 22–48	100%	28%	6 items (emotional and instrumental)	PTS	Emotional positive; instrumental positive	Emotional: r = .54* Practical: r = .40*
Siegel & Schrimshaw (2007)	C	HIV/AIDS	138	M = 38, 22–48	100%	28%	7 items	PTS	Positive	r = .50**
Widows et al. (2005)	L	Bone marrow transplant	72	M = 48, 25–66	74%	85%	ISEL	PTGI	Null	r = .05, n.s.

Received

Study	Design	Population	N	Age	%	%	Support measure	PTG measure	Result	Correlation
Abraido-Lanza et al. (1998)	L	Chronic illness	66	M = 51, 19–86	100%	Hispanic	8 items (emotional)	PTS	Null	T1: r = .00, n.s. T2: r = .08, n.s.
Karanci & Acarturk (2005)	C	Earthquake	200	M = 32, 18–60	34%	Turkey	2 items	SRGS	Positive	r = .21, p < .05
Linley & Joseph (2006)	L	Disaster workers	31	M = 45, 24–71	36%	96%	CSS	PTGI & CiOQ	Null	PTGI T1: r = -.03, n.s. T2: r = -.06, n.s. CiOQ T1: r = -.06, n.s. T2: r = -.01, n.s.
Luszczynska et al. (2005)	L	Cancer	97	M = 63, 24–86	38%	Germany	BSSS (emotional, instrumental, informational)	BFS	Positive (2 of 4)	Life imperfection: r = .16, n.s. Personal growth: r = .19, n.s. Changes in family: r = .31** Increased sensitivity to others: r = .26*
Schulz & Mohamed (2004)	L	Gastrointestinal cancer	105	M = 62, 27–86	39%	Germany	BSSS (emotional & instrumental)	BFS	Positive; positive	Emotional: r = .41** Instrumental: r = .38**
Schwarzer et al. (2006)	L	Cancer	117	M = 63, —	38%	Germany	BSSS (emotional)	7 items (Author)	T1 positive; T2 null; T3 positive	T1: r = .27** T2: r = .12, n.s. T3: r = .20*

(cont.)

TABLE 15.1. (cont.)

Authors of study	Design	Sample	N	Age	% Female	% White	Support scale	Growth scale	Relation	Results
Support satisfaction										
Cordova et al. (2001)	C	Breast cancer	70	M = 55, 27–87	100%	90%	DUKE-SSQ	PTGI	Null	r = .13, n.s.
Linley & Joseph (2006)	L	Disaster workers	31	M = 45, 24–71	36%	96%	CSS	PTG and CiOQ	Null	PTGI T1: r = −.05, n.s. T2: r = −.05, n.s. CiOQ T1: r = −.04, n.s. T2: r = .21, n.s.
McCausland & Pakenham (2003)	C	HIV/AIDS caregivers	64	M = 43, 19–70	41%	89%	Caregiver social support	Open-ended interview question	Null	r = −.10, n.s.
Pakenham et al. (2004)	C	Parents of child with Asperger syndrome	59	M = 43, 39–46	80%	Australia	Brief SSQ	Open-ended and 1 item (author)	Null (3 of 3)	Benefits (yes, no): r = .10, n.s. No. of benefits: r = .17, n.s. Anticipated benefits: r = .22, n.s.
Pakenham & Bursnall (2006)	C	Children of parents with MS	48	M=16, 10–24	56%	—	Brief SSQ	18 items (author)	Null	r = .24, n.s.
Park et al. (1996), Study 3	L	Self-reported negative event	147	College freshmen	68%	> 90%	SSQ	SRGS	Positive	T1: r = .23* T2: r = .35**
Porter et al. (2006)	C	Breast cancer	524	M = 65, 50 and up	100%	70%	SSQ	Growth Through Uncertainty Scale	Positive	*
Sheikh (2004)	C	Heart disease	110	M = 64, 36–81	21%	89%	SSQ	PTGI	Positive	r = .19*

Weiss (2004)	C	Husbands of wives with breast cancer	72	M = 57, 35–84	0%	Primarily European American	SSQ	PTGI	Null	r = .14, n.s.
Amount of social contact										
Erbes et al. (2005)	L	Prisoners of war	95	M = 80, 70–91	0%	100%	18 items	PTGI	Positive	r = .24*
Pakenham et al. (2004)	C	Parents of child with Asperger syndrome	59	M = 43, 39–46	80%	Australia	Brief SSQ	8 items (author)	Positive (2 of 3)	Benefits (yes, no): r = .41***; No. of benefits: r = .24, n.s.; Anticipated benefits: r = .29*
Pakenham & Bursnall (2006)	C	Children of parents with MS	48	M = 16, 10–24	56%	—	Brief SSQ	18 items (author)	Null	r = .23, n.s.
Park et al. (1996), Study 3	L	Self-reported negative event	147	College freshmen	68%	> 90%	SSQ	SRGS	T1 null; T2 positive	T1: r = .09, n.s.; T2: r = .29**
Weiss (2004)	C	Husbands of wives with breast cancer	67	M = 57, 35–84	0%	Primarily European American	Brief SSQ	PTGI	Positive	r = .28**
Self-disclosure										
Cordova et al. (2001)	C	Breast cancer	70	M = 55, 27–87	100%	90%	1 item	PTGI	Positive	r = .25*
Henderson et al. (2002)	C	Breast cancer	299	M = 59, —	100%	97.1%	Patient Profile Questionnaire	SRGS	Positive	beta = .12*
Milam et al. (2005)	C	War/terrorism	514	M = 14, 8th graders	63%	16%	1 item	PTGI	Positive	r = .13**

(cont.)

TABLE 15.1. *(cont.)*

Authors of study	Design	Sample	N	Age	% Female	% White	Support scale	Growth scale	Relation	Results
Mixed										
Cadell et al. (2003)	C	Bereavement	174	M = 41, 19–79	46%	Canada	Perceived support, social integration	SRGS	Positive	t = 3.17*
Frazier et al. (2004)	L	Assault victims	92	M = 27, 16–52	100%	77%	1 satisfaction item and 1 received item	Positive Life Changes (author)	Positive	**
Joseph et al. (1993)	C	Disaster	35	M = 48, 23–75	77%	United Kingdom	CSS (6 received and 1 satisfaction item)	CiOQ	Null	r = –.13, n.s.
Linley & Joseph (2005)	C	Bereavement	78	M = 50, 19–72	10%	100%	CSS (6 received and 1 satisfaction item)	CiOQ	Mixed	r = .14, n.s, beta = .40**
Linley & Joseph (2007)	C	Personal trauma history	156	M = 54, 27–85	78%	97%	CSS (6 received and 1 satisfaction item)	PTGI and CiOQ	Null; positive	PTGI: beta = .07, n.s. CiOQ: beta = .18, t = 2.22*
Luszczynska et al. (2007)	C	HIV/AIDS	104	M=35, 18–54	64%	India	BSSS (received support and support satisfaction)	BFS	Positive	r = .54***
Updegraff et al. (2002)	C	HIV/AIDS	189	M = 37, 19–62	100%	33%	SSQ (received and 1 satisfaction item)	Positive and Negative HIV-Related Changes	Null	r = .09, n.s.

Note. C, cross-sectional; L, longitudinal; BFS, Benefit-Finding Scale (Tomich & Helgeson, 2004); Brief-SSQ, Brief Social Support Questionnaire (Siegert et al., 1987); BSSS, Berlin Social Support Scale (Schulz & Schwarzer, 2003); CiOQ, Changes In Outlook Questionnaire (Joseph et al., 1993); CSS, Crisis Support Scale (Joseph et al., 1992); DUKE-SSQ, Duke–UNC Functional Social Support Questionnaire (Broadhead et al., 1989); ESSI, ENRICHD Social Support Instrument (ENRICHD Investigators, 2001); ISEL, Interpersonal Support Evaluation List (Cohen et al., 1985); ISSB, Inventory of Socially Supportive Behaviors (Barrera et al., 1981); PBS, Perceived Benefits Scale (McMillen & Fisher, 1998); PSS, Perceived Social Support (Procidano & Heller, 1983); PTS, Psychological Thriving Scale (Abraido-Lanza et al., 1998); PTGI, Posttraumatic Growth Inventory (Tedeschi & Calhoun, 1996); SRGS, Stress-Related Growth Scale (Park et al., 1996); SSQ, Social Support Questionnaire (Sarason et al., 1983).
*p < .05; **p < .01; ***p < .001.

suggest that the relation of perceived support to growth does not hold up over time. Although all three studies measured growth months or years after perceived support was measured, none of the studies controlled for baseline levels of growth; that is, although the studies were longitudinal, they did not attempt to predict *changes* in growth over time.

Received Support

Six studies examined the relation of received support to growth, five of which were longitudinal. The one cross-sectional study, survivors of the Marmara earthquake in Turkey, showed that received support was related to more growth (Karanci & Acarturk, 2005). Of the five longitudinal studies, three involved people with cancer, and all three showed a positive relation of received support to growth. A study of people with gastrointestinal cancer assessed received support and growth at three times: before surgery, 1 month after surgery, and 12 months after surgery (Schwarzer, Luszczynska, Boehmer, Taubert, & Knoll, 2006). Cross-sectional relations of received support to growth appeared for two of the three waves—after surgery and at 12 months, but not at 1 month. In addition, received support before surgery was related to growth 1 month and 12 months later. However, previous levels of growth were not statistically controlled in these analyses. The other longitudinal study found relations between received emotional support and received instrumental support 1 month after surgery, and growth 12 months later (Schulz & Mohamed, 2004). The third longitudinal study of people with cancer revealed a relation of received support to two of the four domains of growth—the two interpersonal domains: changes in family relationships and increased sensitivity to others (Luszczynska, Mohamed, & Schwarzer, 2005). There were no controls for previous levels of growth in either of these studies.

Two longitudinal studies found no relations of received support to growth. In a study of disaster workers, received support was not related to either of two growth measures cross-sectionally or longitudinally 6 months later (Linley & Joseph, 2006). In a study of people with chronic illness (mostly arthritis), neither received support at baseline nor received support 3 years later predicted growth 3 years later (Abraído-Lanza, Guier, & Colon, 1998). Neither of the longitudinal analyses controlled for earlier measures of growth.

Support Satisfaction

Ten studies examined the relation between support satisfaction and growth, typically measuring support satisfaction with the subscale from the Social Support Questionnaire (SSQ; Sarason, Levine, Basham, & Sarason, 1983). Of the eight cross-sectional studies, five revealed no relation of support satisfaction to growth, and three revealed a relation of support satisfaction to more growth. Of the two longitudinal studies, one found a relation of support satisfaction to growth and the other did not. The one that found a relation employed a longitudinal design but only examined cross-sectional relations (Park et al., 1996, Study 3). Support satisfaction was cross-sectionally associated with more growth both at baseline and 6 months later among college students who were asked to recall a stressful life event. In the one study that conducted longitudinal analyses, support satisfaction among disaster workers was not related to either of two measures of growth 6 months later (Linley & Joseph, 2006).

Amount of Social Contact

Five studies examined the relation between the amount of social contact and growth, four of which used the Number of Support Providers subscale from the SSQ (Sarason et al., 1983). Of the three cross-sectional studies, two found that the number of support providers was positively related to growth, and one found no relation. One of the two longitudinal studies only examined cross-sectional relations and found mixed evidence for the relation between number of supporters and growth. A study of college students who were asked to recall a stressful life event found that the number of support providers was cross-sectionally associated with growth at 6 months but not at baseline (Park et al., 1996, Study 3). The other longitudinal study found that structural support predicted greater growth 5 years later among prisoners of war (Erbes et al., 2005), but earlier growth was not statistically controlled in the analysis.

Self-Disclosure

We were only able to locate three studies that measured self-disclosure to network members and growth. Each was cross-sectional and showed positive relations to growth.

Mixed Social Environment

Seven studies measured aspects of the social environment that included two or more of the support distinctions we have made, making it difficult for us to disentangle the relations to growth. Six of the seven studies used a measure of support that combined received support with an assessment of satisfaction with that support. The seventh used a measure that combined two measures of perceived support with social integration. Thus, we were unable to classify those studies into a social environment category. Three studies revealed positive relations of the support measure to growth, two revealed mixed evidence, and two revealed no relations to growth. Three of the studies used the same 7-item support measure, the Crisis Support Scale (Joseph, Andrews, Williams, & Yule, 1992), which contains six received support items and one satisfaction item. Even among those three studies, the findings of a relation to growth were inconsistent: One found mixed evidence, another found no relation to growth, and still another found no zero-order correlation to growth but a positive re-lation that emerged in a regression analysis that included other variables.

The one longitudinal study in this area found a positive relation between a support measure (satisfaction and received support) and growth using hierarchical linear modeling (Frazier, Tashiro, Berman, Steger, & Long, 2004). Support and positive life changes were assessed two to four times over a 1-year period. Although an overall positive relation emerged, lagged analyses were not conducted to tease out the direction of causality. Taken collectively, these mixed studies do not shed light on the issue of whether the social environment is related to growth, or which component might be implicated in growth.

Summary

Among the social environment categories that we examined, there was fairly consistent evidence that perceived support was cross-sectionally associated with more growth, despite the fact that we did not include perceived support in our model, shown in Figure 15.1. However, none of the longitudinal studies found evidence for such a relation—even without controls for earlier growth. The meaning of a cross-sectional relation between perceived support and growth is unclear because perceived support reflects so many other features of the person and of the relationship, aside from specific support interactions (Kaul & Lakey, 2003; Lakey et al., 2004). There were fewer studies of received support. Yet it is impressive that most of those studies were longitudinal and suggested a positive relation of received support to growth that held over time, supporting our model in Figure 5.1. It would have been helpful if studies had measured both perceived and received support to determine whether received support accounted for the relation of perceived support to growth. There was only weak evidence for a relation of support satisfaction with growth. Self-disclosure was only examined by three studies, but all three showed a positive relation with growth, again, consistent with our model. The evidence for the relation of amount of social contact to growth was mixed. Taken collectively, the evidence for the relation of the social environment to growth is mixed, with slightly more than half of the studies finding a positive relation between an aspect of the social environment and more growth. There is not enough research in the area to determine whether the aspects of support shown in Figure 15.1 are the definitive aspects of the social environment linked to growth.

Three other points can be made from this review. First, most studies employed generic measures of support that did not distinguish among the support functions. The few studies that did distinguish between emotional and instrumental support seemed to find similar positive relations for both (Kinsinger et al., 2006; Schulz & Mohamed, 2004; Siegel, Schrimshaw, & Pretter, 2005; but for an exception, see McMillen & Cook, 2003).

Second, the vast majority of studies were cross-sectional. Even when longitudinal studies were conducted, often only cross-sectional relations were examined. When longitudinal relations were examined, there were no statistical controls for earlier levels of growth. Thus, when positive longitudinal relations did emerge, the social environment predicted one's perception of a life change over time (i.e., perceived growth) but not necessarily actual life change over time.

Third, among the studies that examined distinct areas of growth, the social environment seemed to be most strongly linked to interpersonal domains of growth, as indicated by the two studies shown in Table 15.1 (Luszczynska et al., 2005; McMillen & Cook, 2003). Two other studies examined not only the overall PTGI growth score, which is reported in Table 15.1, but also the five growth subscales not shown in Table 15.1. One found evidence consistent with the idea that support is more strongly related to the interpersonal domain of growth. A study of prisoners of war found that structural support (i.e., amount of social contact) was related to the total PTGI score and to the

individual domains of Relationships with Others and Spirituality, but not to New Possibilities, Personal Strength, or Appreciation of Life (Erbes et al., 2005). In addition, perceived support was related to the same two domains (Relationships with Others, Spirituality), but not to the overall PTGI score. However, a study of Holocaust survivors did not support our conclusion (Lev-Wiesel & Amir, 2003). Perceived Support from Family was not related to the total PTGI score or to any of the five subscales; Perceived Support from Friends was related to the overall score, but only to the New Possibilities subscale. Thus, there was some modest support for the idea that there would be stronger links between the social environment and interpersonal growth, a finding that we hypothesized (shown in Figure 15.1).

Support and Growth: A Study of College Students

To test aspects of the model shown in Figure 15.1 and to address some of the unanswered questions in regard to the relation of the social environment to growth, we conducted a study of college students who had experienced a stressful event in the past 6 months. In this study, we measured multiple aspects of the social environment to help disentangle the aspects most strongly related to growth. We also measured both received and perceived support, and hypothesized that received support would show stronger relations to growth than would perceived support. Again, we argue that support perceptions are based on a multitude of factors, only one of which is actual support receipt. In understanding how the social environment might facilitate growth, people must actually receive some kind of resources from the social environment—emotional, tangible, or informational. These resources either directly result in growth, as in the case of improved relationships, or indirectly promote growth by encouraging the individual to contemplate and evaluate the event (i.e., cognitive processing). In this study, we also examined whether cognitive processing mediated the relation between received support and growth.

Participants and Method

Participants were 107 college students (41 males, 66 females), mostly between the ages of 18 and 20 years (84%). Just over half of participants were white (52%), with most others classifying themselves as Asian (45%). To be eligible, participants had to have indicated that they had experienced one of 11 stressful events during the past 6 months: death of a friend, family member, or pet; romantic relationship difficulties; major conflict with someone; trauma; major illness; major illness of a loved one; problems with parents; physical abuse; major academic stress; public humiliation; or another major stressful event. Participants most frequently indicated that they had experienced romantic relationship difficulties (29%) or major academic stressors (22%). All questionnaires were completed online at participants' leisure and preferred location.

For all support questions, the support provider that we chose to examine was a parent of the participant's choice. Participants' disclosure of the event to their identified parent was assessed with a 4-item scale that we created to assess depth and frequency of disclosure (e.g., "I have discussed this event in great detail with my parent"; alpha = .96). We used the Social Support Behaviors Scale (SS-B; Vaux, Riedel, & Stewart, 1987) to measure perceived support, then adapted the Emotional Support and Guidance subscales to measure received support from the selected parent. We also developed a measure of received growth support, which focused on how frequently the selected parent had made suggestions for different areas of possible growth (alpha = .94). Because received emotional support, received instrumental support, and received growth support were highly intercorrelated (r's = .50 to .68, p's < .001), they were combined into a single index of received support.

Included was a 10-item cognitive processing measure that we developed for this study (alpha = .86), incorporating items from the Emotional Processing Scale (Stanton, Kirk, Cameron, & Danoff-Burg, 2000) and the Planning and Acceptance scales of the COPE (Carver, Scheier, & Weintraub, 1989). We measured growth with the PTGI (Tedeschi & Calhoun, 1996).

Results

First, we examined the relation of self-disclosure, received support, and perceived support to growth. All three social environment variables were associated with more growth: self-disclosure ($r = .27$, $p < .01$); received support ($r = .48$, $p < .01$); and perceived support ($r = .34$, $p < .01$).

Second, we examined whether perceived support could account for the relations of received support to growth. As expected, received support was related to perceived support ($r = .36$, $p < .01$). We used multiple regression analysis to address this question. Received support was entered in the first step, and the measure of perceived support was added in the second step to predict growth. Results are shown in Table 15.2. Perceived support emerged as a significant predictor of posttraumatic growth (PTG) but received support remained significant, with the beta coefficient largely unchanged. Perceived support did not account for the effect of received support, as indicated by the

TABLE 15.2. Beta Coefficients from Regression Analyses Testing Whether Perceived Support Accounts for the Relation of Received Support to Growth

	PTG
Equation 1	
Received support	.48***
Equation 2	
Received support	.42***
Perceived support	.18*

*$p < .05$; **$p < .01$; ***$p < .0001$.

Sobel (1982) test. In the final equation, the beta coefficient for perceived support was modest in comparison to that for received support.

Third, we determined whether the relations between self-disclosure and growth, and between received support and growth could be explained by cognitive processing. We used the procedures outlined by Baron and Kenny (1986) to test mediation. We already had demonstrated that self-disclosure and received support were related to growth. Received support was related to cognitive processing ($r = .31$, $p < .01$), but self-disclosure was not. Therefore, we could only test whether cognitive processing mediated the relation of received support to growth. Cognitive processing was related to PTG ($r = .48$, $p < .01$). As shown in Table 15.3, when both received support and cognitive processing were entered into the regression to predict PTG, the relation between received support and PTG was still significant (beta $= .36$, $p < .01$) but was significantly lower. Using the procedures outlined by Sobel (1982), we found that cognitive processing accounted for 23% of the effect of received support on PTG ($t = 2.82$, $p < .01$).

Summary

Although each of the social environment variables that we examined was related to growth, the relation between received support and growth seemed to be strongest,

TABLE 15.3. Beta Coefficients from Regression Analysis: Testing Cognitive Processing as a Mediator of the Relation between Received Support and Growth

	PTG
Equation 1	
Received support	.48***
Equation 2	
Received support	.37***
Cognitive processing	.36***

***$p < .0001$.

supporting our model in Figure 15.1. This relation held even when perceived support was statistically controlled. We also found some evidence that the relation between received support and growth was mediated by cognitive processing, as hypothesized in our model in Figure 15.1.

Conclusion and Future Research Directions

In conclusion, both theory and empirical data suggest that the social environment may play a significant role in the development of growth following adversity. The aspects of the social environment that might be most directly involved in the development of growth are self-disclosure to network members and received support. Although theorists in the area of PTG have not fully integrated the social environment into their models, suggestions have been made that self-disclosing to and receiving support from network members have both direct and indirect effects on growth. Given that we located 33 studies examining the relation between the social environment and growth, we cannot conclude that empirical data in this area are lacking. However, few of these studies were designed to examine the relation of the social environment to growth, which explains why most only included a single measure of the social environment. More often, the study focused on adjustment to trauma, and included growth and a support measure among the battery of instruments. The fact that theory is underdeveloped in this area, and that strong empirical studies are lacking leads to several directions for future research.

First, researchers should examine multiple aspects of the social environment, carefully distinguishing among dimensions, such as perceived and received support, to determine which aspect is most strongly related to growth. Researchers also should distinguish among the functions of support (emotional, instrumental, and informational) because understanding the function most strongly implicated in growth will shed light on the process by which the social environment influences growth. Second, researchers should examine distinct domains of growth. When different domains of growth were distinguished, it appeared that the social environment was more strongly related to the interpersonal domains. To the extent that this is the case, one needs to be sure that this relation is not artifactual, in that people's satisfaction with network members is not scored as both social support and interpersonal growth.

Understanding more about which aspect of the social environment is related to which aspects of growth will help to shed light on the second research direction, which is to understand more about the processes by which the social environment contributes to growth. Both longitudinal field studies and experimental laboratory studies can help to address this issue. Field studies that employ multiple waves of follow-up can test in a more naturalistic way how the relation of the social environment to growth unfolds, whereas laboratory studies can more definitively test the causal sequence between the social environment and growth. Laboratory studies could manipulate the provision of emotional support or growth support, and examine whether this manipulation influences cognitive processing and growth.

Third, another distinction that can help to shed light on the relation between the social environment and growth has to do with the nature of the stressor. Although growth has been found to occur across a wide array of stressors (see Helgeson et al., 2006, for a review), researchers have not examined whether certain classes of stressors are more likely to lead to growth. It is possible that certain kinds of stressors are linked to certain kinds of growth. For example, health-related stressors may be more strongly linked to the growth domain of "appreciation of life" or "increased spirituality." Relationship-related stressors may be more strongly linked to "interpersonal growth." The question that remains is whether the role of the social en-

vironment in shaping growth is dependent on the nature of the stressor.

Fourth, given the inconsistent relations found between aspects of the social environment and growth, researchers need to learn more about the circumstances under which the social environment could affect growth. Characteristics of the support provider, the support receiver, or the stressor are all candidates for moderator variables. One of the reasons that the effect sizes for many of the studies reviewed in Table 15.1 are small might be that there are conditions under which the relations between support and growth would be stronger. However, it also is the case that the majority of these studies did not aim to evaluate the relation between support and growth. Note that the effect size in the study presented in this article was larger. Thus, another reason for small effect sizes might have to do with the failure to develop measures explicitly aimed at evaluating the relation between the social environment and growth. Researchers also should examine the social environment from both persons' perspectives—the person who has sustained the traumatic life event and the support provider.

Finally, to understand how the social environment contributes to growth, researchers need to find alternative ways of measuring growth. We noted earlier that there is a dearth of longitudinal studies in this area. However, even longitudinal designs are limited in helping us to examine change over time because our measures of growth have change embedded in them. Participants are asked to report their subjective perception of change in a positive direction, or growth. Longitudinal studies often assess social support soon after the trauma, and growth months or years later. There are no growth measures administered at baseline for which one could statistically control. Growth measures do not make sense shortly after trauma. In fact, people might be insulted if you ask them about benefits before enough time has passed for benefits to be realized or opportunities for benefits have presented themselves.

Yet without some kind of controls at baseline, it is difficult to know whether support is leading to growth or growth is leading to support. In fact, there is reason to believe that growth could lead to support because people are attracted more to those who are coping well than those who are distressed. One study that examined the prospective relation between growth and support found that growth did affect support receipt 18 months later (Cheng, Wong, & Tsang, 2006). There are two potential solutions to this problem. First, multiple follow-up assessments would provide for multiple measures of growth. Second, rather than measuring growth directly at baseline, one could measure the current status of variables for which one expected change. For example, if a common domain of growth is interpersonal, one could measure the condition of one's current relationships and see whether that condition actually changes over time rather than (or in addition to) a growth measure that asks people to report change. Understanding the relation of the social environment to growth rests on the validity of measures of growth.

Acknowledgment

We are grateful to Meredith Moersch for helping to identify and code the articles contained in this review.

References

Abraído-Lanza, A. F., Guier, C., & Colon, R. M. (1998). Psychological thriving among Latinas with chronic illness. *Journal of Social Issues, 54,* 405–424.

Armstrong, L. (2000). *It's not about the bike: My journey back to life.* New York: Berkley Books.

Baron, R. M., & Kenny, D. A. (1986). The moderator–mediator variable distinction in social psychological research: Conceptual, strategic, and statistical considerations. *Journal of Personality and Social Psychology, 51*(6), 1173–1182.

Barrera, M., Jr., Sandler, I. N., & Ramsay, T. B. (1981). Preliminary development of a scale of social support: Studies on college students. *American Journal of Community Psychology, 9,* 435–447.

Broadhead, W. E., Gehlbach, S. H., De Gruy, F. V., & Kaplan, B. H. (1989). The Duke–UNC Functional Social Support Questionnaire: Measurement of social support in family medicine patients. *Medical Care, 26,* 709–723.

Cadell, S., Regehr, C., & Hemsworth, D. (2003). Factors contributing to posttraumatic growth: A proposed structural equation model. *American Journal of Orthopsychiatry, 73,* 279–287.

Carver, C. S. (1998). Resilience and thriving: Issues, models, and linkages. *Journal of Social Issues, 54,* 245–266.

Carver, C. S., Scheier, M. F., & Weintraub, J. K. (1989). Assessing coping strategies: A theoretically based approach. *Journal of Personality and Social Psychology, 56*(2), 267–283.

Cheng, C., Wong, W., & Tsang, K. W. (2006). Perception of benefits and costs during SARS outbreak: An 18-month prospective study. *Journal of Consulting and Clinical Psychology, 74,* 870–879.

Cohen, S., Memelstein, R., Karmack, T., & Hoberman, H. M. (1985). Measuring the functional components of social support. In I. G. Sarason & B. R. Sarason (Eds.), *Social support: Theory, research and application* (pp. 73–94). Boston: Martinus Nijhoff.

Cordova, M. J., Cunningham, L. L. C., Carlson, C. R., & Andrykowski, M. A. (2001). Posttraumatic growth following breast cancer: A controlled comparison study. *Health Psychology, 20,* 176–185.

ENRICHD Investigators. (2001). Enhancing recovery in coronary heart disease (ENRICHD) study intervention: Rationale and design. *Psychosomatic Medicine, 63*(5), 747–755.

Erbes, C., Eberly, R., Dikel, T., Johnsen, E., Harris, I., & Engdahl, B. (2005). Posttraumatic growth among American former prisoners of war. *Traumatology, 11,* 285–295.

Frazier, P., Tashiro, T., Berman, M., Steger, M., & Long, J. (2004). Correlates of levels and patterns of positive life changes following sexual assault. *Journal of Consulting and Clinical Psychology, 72,* 19–30.

Helgeson, V. S., Lopez, L., & Mennella, C. (2009). Benefit-finding among adolescents with chronic illness. In C. Park, S. Lechner, A.

Stanton, & M. Antoni (Eds.), *Medical illness and positive life change* (pp. 65–86). Washington, DC: American Psychological Association.

Helgeson, V. S., Reynolds, K. A., & Tomich, P. L. (2006). A meta-analytic review of benefit finding and growth. *Journal of Consulting and Clinical Psychology, 74,* 797–816.

Henderson, B. N., Davison, K. P., Pennebaker, J. W., Gatchel, R. J., & Baum, A. (2002). Disease disclosure patterns among breast cancer patients. *Psychology and Health, 17,* 51–62.

House, J. S., & Kahn, R. L. (1985). Measures and concepts of social support. In S. Cohen & L. Syme (Eds.), *Social support and health* (pp. 83–108). Orlando, FL: Academic Press.

Janoff-Bulman, R. (1992). *Shattered assumptions: Towards a new psychology of trauma.* New York: Free Press.

Joseph, S., Andrews, B., Williams, R., & Yule, W. (1992). Crisis support and psychiatric symptomatology in adult survivors of the Jupiter cruise ship disaster. *British Journal of Clinical Psychology, 31,* 63–73.

Joseph, S., & Linley, P. A. (2005). Positive adjustment to threatening events: An organismic valuing theory of growth adversity. *Review of General Psychology, 9*(3), 262–280.

Joseph, S., Williams, R., & Yule, W. (1993). Changes in outlook following disaster: The preliminary development of a measure to assess positive and negative responses. *Journal of Traumatic Stress, 6,* 271–279.

Karanci, N. A., & Acarturk, C. (2005). Posttraumatic growth among Marmara earthquake survivors involved in disaster preparedness as volunteers. *Traumatology, 11,* 307–323.

Karanci, N. A., & Erkam, A. (2007). Variables related to stress-related growth among Turkish breast cancer patients. *Stress and Health, 23,* 315–322.

Kaul, M., & Lakey, B. (2003). Where is the support in perceived support?: The role of generic relationship satisfaction and enacted support in perceived support's relation to low distress. *Journal of Social and Clinical Psychology, 22,* 59–78.

Kinsinger, D. P., Panedo, F. J., Antoni, M. H., Dahn, J. R., Lechner, S., & Schneiderman, N. (2006). Psychosocial and sociodemographic correlates of benefit-finding in men treated for localized prostate cancer. *Psycho-Oncology, 15,* 954–961.

Lakey, B., Lutz, C. J., & Scoboria, A. (2004). The information used to judge supportiveness depends on whether the judgment reflects the personality of perceivers, the objective characteristics of targets, or their unique relationships. *Journal of Social and Clinical Psychology, 23,* 817–835.

Lepore, S. J., & Revenson, T. A. (2007). Social constraints on disclosure and adjustment to cancer. *Social and Personality Psychology Compass, 1,* 1–19.

Lev-Wiesel, R., & Amir, M. (2003). Posttraumatic growth among Holocaust child survivors. *Journal of Loss and Trauma, 8,* 229–237.

Linley, P. A., & Joseph, S. (2005). Positive and negative changes following occupational death exposure. *Journal of Traumatic Stress, 18,* 751–758.

Linley, P. A., & Joseph, S. (2006). The positive and negative effects of disaster work: A preliminary investigation. *Journal of Loss and Trauma, 11,* 229–245.

Linley, P. A., & Joseph, S. (2007). Therapy work and therapists' positive and negative well-being. *Journal of Social and Clinical Psychology, 26,* 385–403.

Littlewood, R. A., Vanable, P. A., Carey, M. P., & Blair, D. C. (2008). The association of benefit finding to psychosocial and health behavior adaptation among HIV+ men and women. *Journal of Behavioral Medicine, 31,* 145–155.

Luszczynska, A., Mohamed, N. E., & Schwarzer, R. (2005). Self-efficacy and social support predict benefit finding 12 months after cancer surgery: The mediating role of coping strategies. *Psychology, Health and Medicine, 10,* 365–375.

Luszczynska, A., Sarkar, Y., & Knoll, N. (2007). Received social support, self-efficacy, and finding benefits in disease as predictors of physical functioning and adherence to antiretroviral therapy. *Patient Education and Counseling, 66,* 37–42.

Luthar, S. S., Cicchetti, D., & Becker, B. (2000). The construct of resilience: A critical evaluation and guidelines for future work. *Child Development, 71,* 543–562.

McCausland, J., & Pakenham, K. I. (2003). Investigation of the benefits of HIV/AIDS caregiving and relations among caregiving adjustment, benefit finding, and stress and coping variables. *AIDS Care, 15,* 853–869.

McMillen, J. C. (1999). Better for it: How people

benefit from adversity. *Social Work*, *44*(5), 455–467.

McMillen, J. C. (2004). Posttraumatic growth: What's it all about? *Psychological Inquiry*, *15*, 48–52.

McMillen, J. C., & Cook, C. L. (2003). The positive by-products of spinal cord injury and their correlates. *Rehabilitation Psychology*, *48*, 77–85.

McMillen, J. C., & Fisher, R. (1998). The Perceived Benefit Scales: Measuring perceived positive life changes following negative life events. *Social Work Research*, *22*, 173–187.

Milam, J., Ritt-Olson, A., Tan, S., Unger, J., & Nezami, E. (2005). The September 11th 2001 terrorist attacks and reports of posttraumatic growth among a multi-ethnic sample of adolescents. *Traumatology*, *11*, 233–246.

Murray, E. J., & Segal, D. L. (1994). Emotional processing in vocal and written expression of feelings about traumatic experiences. *Journal of Traumatic Stress*, *7*, 391–405.

O'Leary, V. E., & Ickovics, J. R. (1995). Resilience and thriving in response to challenge: An opportunity for a paradigm shift in women's health. *Women's Health: Research on Gender, Behavior, and Policy*, *1*, 121–142.

Pakenham, K., & Bursnall, S. (2006). Relations between social support, appraisal and coping and both positive and negative outcomes for children of a parent with multiple sclerosis and comparisons with children of healthy parents. *Clinical Rehabilitation*, *20*, 709–723.

Pakenham, K. I., Sofronoff, K., & Samios, C. (2004). Finding meaning in parenting a child with Asperger syndrome: Correlates of sense making and benefit finding. *Research in Developmental Disabilities*, *25*, 245–264.

Park, C. L., Cohen, L. H., & Murch, R. L. (1996). Assessment and prediction of stress-related growth. *Journal of Personality*, *64*, 71–105.

Park, C. L., & Helgeson, V. S. (2006). Growth following highly stressful life events: Current status and future directions. *Journal of Consulting and Clinical Psychology*, *74*, 791–796.

Pennebaker, J. W. (2002). Writing, social processes, and psychotherapy: From past to future. In S. J. Lepore & J. M. Smyth (Eds.), *The writing cure: How expressive writing promotes health and emotional well-being* (pp. 279–292). Washington, DC: American Psychological Association.

Porter, L. S., Clayton, M. F., Belyea, M., Mishel, M., Gil, K. M., & Germino, B. B. (2006). Predicting negative mood state and personal growth in African American and White long-term breast cancer survivors. *Annals of Behavioral Medicine*, *31*(3), 195–204.

Procidano, M. E., & Heller, K. (1983). Measures of perceived social support from friends and from family: Three validation studies. *American Journal of Community Psychology*, *11*, 1–25.

Revenson, T. A. (2003). Scenes from a marriage: Examining support, coping, and gender within the context of chronic illness. In J. Suls & K. A. Wallston (Eds.), *Social psychological foundations of health and illness* (pp. 530–559). Malden, MA: Blackwell.

Sarason, I. G., Levine, H. M., Basham, R. B., & Sarason, B. R. (1983). Assessing social support: The Social Support Questionnaire. *Journal of Personality and Social Psychology*, *44*, 127–139.

Schaefer, J. A., & Moos, R. H. (1992). Life crises and personal growth. In B. N. Carpenter (Ed.), *Personal coping: Theory, research, and application* (pp. 149–170). Westport, CT: Praeger/Greenwood.

Schulz, U., & Mohamed, N. E. (2004). Turning the tide: Benefit finding after cancer surgery. *Social Science and Medicine*, *59*, 653–662.

Schulz, U., & Schwarzer, R. (2003). Soziale Unterstützung bei der Krankheitsbewältigung: Die Berliner Social Support Skalen (BSSS) [Social support and coping with illness: The Berlin Social Support Scales (BSSS)]. *Diagnostica*, *49*, 73–82.

Schwarzer, R., Luszczynska, A., Boehmer, S., Taubert, S., & Knoll, N. (2006). Changes in finding benefit after cancer surgery and the prediction of well-being one year later. *Social Science and Medicine*, *63*, 1614–1624.

Sears, S. R., Stanton, A. L., & Danoff-Burg, S. (2003). The Yellow Brick Road and the Emerald City: Benefit finding, positive reappraisal coping, and posttraumatic growth in women with early-stage breast cancer. *Health Psychology*, *22*, 487–497.

Sheikh, A. I. (2004). Posttraumatic growth in the context of heart disease. *Journal of Clinical Psychology in Medical Settings*, *11*, 265–273.

Siegel, K., & Schrimshaw, E. W. (2007). The stress moderating role of benefit finding on psychological distress and well-being among women living with HIV/AIDS. *AIDS Behavior*, *11*, 421–433.

Siegel, K., Schrimshaw, E. W., & Pretter, S. (2005). Stress-related growth among women living with HIV/AIDS: Examination of an explanatory model. *Journal of Behavioral Medicine*, *28*, 403–414.

Siegert, R. J., Patten, M. D., & Walkey, F. H. (1987). Development of a brief Social Support Questionnaire. *New Zealand Journal of Psychology*, *16*(2), 79–83.

Sobel, M. E. (1982). Asymptotic intervals for indirect effects in structural equations models. In S. Leinhart (Ed.), *Sociological methodology 1982* (pp. 290–312). San Francisco: Jossey-Bass.

Stanton, A. L., Bower, J. E., & Low, C. A. (2006). Posttraumatic growth after cancer. In L. G. Calhoun & R. G. Tedeschi (Eds.), *Handbook of posttraumatic growth: Research and practice* (pp. 138–175). Mahwah, NJ: Erlbaum.

Stanton, A. L., Kirk, S. B., Cameron, C. L., & Danoff-Burg, S. (2000). Coping through emotional approach: Scale construction and validation. *Journal of Personality and Social Psychology*, *78*(6), 1150–1169.

Taylor, S. E. (1983). Adjustment to threatening events: A theory of cognitive adaptation. *American Psychologist*, *38*, 1161–1173.

Tedeschi, R. G., & Calhoun, L. G. (1995). *Trauma and transformation: Growth in the aftermath of suffering*. Thousand Oaks, CA: Sage.

Tedeschi, R. G., & Calhoun, L. G. (1996). The Posttraumatic Growth Inventory: Measuring the positive legacy of trauma. *Journal of Traumatic Stress*, *9*(3), 455–472.

Tedeschi, R. G., & Calhoun, L. G. (2004). Target article: "Posttraumatic growth: Conceptual foundations and empirical evidence." *Psychological Inquiry*, *15*(1), 1–18.

Tomich, P. L., & Helgeson, V. S. (2004). Is finding something good in the bad always good?: Benefit finding among women with breast cancer. *Health Psychology*, *23*, 16–23.

Uchino, B. N. (2004). *Social support and physical health: Understanding the health consequences of our relationships*. New Haven, CT: Yale University Press.

Ullrich, P. M., & Lutgendorf, S. K. (2002). Journaling about stressful events: Effects of cognitive processing and emotional expression. *Annals of Behavioral Medicine*, *24*(3), 244–250.

Updegraff, J. A., Taylor, S. E., Kemeny, M. E., & Wyatt, G. E. (2002). Positive and negative effects of HIV infection in women with low socioeconomic resources. *Personality and Social Psychology Bulletin*, *28*, 382–394.

Vaux, A., Riedel, S., & Stewart, D. (1987). Modes of social support: The social support behaviors scale. *American Journal of Community Psychology*, *15*(2), 209–232.

Weiss, T. (2004). Correlates of posttraumatic growth in husbands of breast cancer survivors. *Psycho-Oncology*, *13*, 260–268.

Werner, E. E. (2000). Protective factors and individual resilience. In J. P. Shonkoff & S. J. Meisels (Eds.), *Handbook of early childhood intervention* (2nd ed., pp. 115–132). New York: Cambridge University Press.

Widows, M. R., Jacobsen, P. B., Booth-Jones, M., & Fields, K. K. (2005). Predictors of posttraumatic growth following bone marrow transplantation for cancer. *Health Psychology*, *24*, 266–273.

E

Organizational and Public Policy Dimensions of Resilience

16

Building Organizational Resilience and Adaptive Management

Janet Denhardt
Robert Denhardt

There has been growing interest in the concept of resilience as a device for understanding organizational change, responsiveness, innovation, and flexibility. In the wake of the 9/11 attacks, Hurricane Katrina, and other natural and man-made disasters, no one needs to be reminded of the need for resilient organizations and the sometimes tragic consequences of a lack of resilience. Organizations stretched to the breaking point need the capacity to bounce back and to recover. For this reason, much of the existing work that focuses on resilience in organizations emphasizes corporate survival and adaptive management under dire circumstances.

While this is important, it is also useful to think about resilience in a different way. In our view, organizational resilience speaks to more than simply the time-specific response to a particular disaster; it brings into focus much larger issues of organizational capacity and adaptability. If *organizational resilience* is defined as the ability to bounce back, or to recover from challenges in a manner that

leaves the organization more flexible and better able to adapt to future challenges, then organizational resilience is a quality that leaders and managers in all organizations should seek to foster at all times.

Resilience involves the ability to adapt creatively and constructively to change, and change is the one constant in organizational life today. Virtually all organizations are buffeted with the forces of globalization, shifts in the economy, and a changing workforce. Public organizations, for example, can experience a sharp change in public policy or public opinion, or a loss of revenue. Private organizations can go through mergers and acquisitions, sharp competition, and market downturns. Organizations can have instances of personal violence in the workplace, a lapse of ethics by a previously respected leader, a major reorganization, threats to their belief system and culture, dramatic changes in management, or even natural disasters. But organizational stressors can come in all shapes and sizes. There are also smaller stressors, such as personnel turnover, power struggles, looming deadlines and intergroup conflict. All of these, and other challenges, can be experienced as both threats or stressors, and opportunities to change and build adaptive capacity. For our purposes here, it matters less what the stress is, and more how the organization responds to a variety of stressors over time.

What we argue here is that although the focus is frequently on catastrophic events, it is actually the practice of everyday resilience in responding to those thousands of daily stresses and disjunctures that may best equip organizations to also handle catastrophic and unexpected challenges to their health and survival. How can we foster resilience and adaptability in organizations and, in so doing, build organizations that can be not only resilient to more potentially devastating events but also more adaptive under daily conditions of change and discontinuity? And rather than just considering resilience retrospectively (when it is already too late to do anything about it), how can we approach resilience prospectively by purposively instilling it in organizations over time?

In this chapter, we explore the way the notion of resilience has been treated in the traditional and more contemporary literature on organization and management, then explore contemporary conceptions of organizational resilience. First, we briefly examine the meaning of resilience as it relates to individuals, ecological systems, and organizations. Second, we consider some of the key characteristics of resilient organizations. Third, we look at traditional constructs of organization and management theory, and examine how these views can actually impede the development of resilience. Fourth, we look at more contemporary expressions of organizational theory that begin to open the door to the possibilities of creating more resilient organizations. Fifth, we explore an emerging, resilience-based framework for organizational and management theory. We conclude with some implications for organizational leadership and management.

Resilience in Individuals and Systems

The meaning and importance of resilience, and the manner that it can be developed and maintained, differs according to the level of analysis being studied. Resilience can be understood as characteristic of objects, individuals, organizations, and systems. Some scholars do not clearly distinguish between differing types. For example, Horne and Orr (1998) define *resilience* as

> a fundamental quality of individuals, groups, organizations, and systems as a whole to respond productively to significant change that disrupts the expected pattern of events without engaging in an extended period of regressive behavior. This robust response capability is a direct reflection of the richness of internal/external connections for physical, emotional and resource support in learning alternative adaptive behavior. (p. 31)

While this definition may seem to encompass resilience in all its forms, a careful reading points to its reliance on behavior and, most particularly, individual behavior. We think it is useful and important to unbundle how the concept has evolved "upward" from individual psychology and "downward" from natural systems and ecology to expand our understanding of resilience at a level of analysis that falls between: that of organizations.

The term *resilience* originally was used in the material sciences to refer to the ability of certain materials, like rubber, to withstand compression or expansion and return to their original shape or position. We take this property of resilience for granted in many everyday objects, ranging from the bumpers of our cars to tennis rackets, from the gaskets in our faucets to the weather stripping on our doors. Psychologists and ecologists adopted the concept of resilience to describe how individual human beings and ecosystems can "bounce back" when challenged. But there are distinct differences between how these fields have translated, defined, and used the concept of resilience.

In psychology, the term *resilience* was first used to describe qualities possessed by certain children, who, despite a number of serious risk factors that would otherwise have predicted significant problems, instead thrived and prospered. Studies of how to foster resilience in children emphasize the importance of *social competence*, including the ability to elicit positive responses from others, flexibility, empathy, communications skills, and a sense of humor; *problem-solving skills*, including the ability to plan, to be resourceful in seeking help, and to think critically, creatively, and reflectively, and *development of a critical consciousness* of sources of oppression and strategies for overcoming them (Benard, 1995). Similarly, Sybil and Steven Wolin (1993) describe resilience in children and adolescents as involving insight, independence, relationships, initiative, humor, creativity, and morality.

Resilience has also been used to describe the characteristics of certain adults in work settings. Here, *resilience* is defined as "the skill and capacity to be robust under conditions of enormous stress and change" (Coutu, 2002, p. 52). Resilient individuals, according to Coutu (2002), face reality rather than having misguided optimism, have strong value systems, and are skilled in making do with what is on hand, or *bricolage* and improvisation. Key to psychological resilience is the idea that individuals do not simply survive by returning to their previous state (like a rubber ball) but can actually adapt, learn, and change, and as a result become more resilient over time.

Resilience in ecological terms refers to the capacity of natural systems to recover from environmental stresses in a way that leads to system sustainability, that is, "the use of environment and resources to meet the needs of the present without compromising the ability of future generations to meet their own needs" (Berkes, Colding, & Folke, 2003, p. 2). In natural systems, such as coastal wetlands, feedback processes often lead to effective adaptation to environmental stresses. Feedback loops work to a point. But at a certain level of change in conditions, the system can change very rapidly and even catastrophically. Of special interest is the way in which human interventions affect natural systems, sometimes in quite damaging ways—when resource management "aims to reduce natural variation in an effort to make an ecosystem more productive, predictable, economically efficient, and controllable. But the reduction in the range of natural variation is the very process that may lead to a loss of resilience in a system, leaving it more susceptible to resource and environmental crisis" (Holling, in Berkes et al., 2003, p. xv). As we will see, both the individual and socioecological systems approaches have influenced discussions of organizational resilience.

Characteristics of Resilient Organizations

It is important to recognize that understanding organizational resilience requires us to parse out what conceptions of resilience are most useful in relationship to organizations and what conceptions are less useful. As Lance Gunderson (2000) points out, there are distinct differences between the desired outcomes of engineering resilience (return to a stable state), ecological resilience (move to different stable state), and adaptive capacity (to deal with long-term change). What we argue here is that organizational resilience needs to focus on adaptive capacity. It should take into account both the psychological resilience of individuals and systems resilience, with one important caveat. As Westley, Carpenter, Brock, Holling, and Gunderson (2002) note, "In contrast to ecological systems, social systems are structured by the human ability to construct and manipulate symbols, the most obvious being words" (p. 104). In other words, organizations are socially constructed, based on elements such as power relationships, resources, patterns of authority, rules, and procedures. The ability to construct meaning permits human organizations to "flip from one kind of organization into another and back again … by shifting the system configuration, in the same way that a soccer team will flip from offensive to defensive alignments" (p. 104). In addition to this systems orientation, it is also the case that organizations are made up of human actors whose individual and collective behavior can contribute to or impede organizational resilience. However, organizations, unlike individuals, are not born with more or less innate capacity for resilience. The capacity for resilience must be instilled and practiced in organizations, if it is to develop at all. So, when looking at the somewhat less developed literature on organizational resilience, it is useful to consider when and how the authors are drawing from psychological resilience, ecological resilience, or both. Some seem to view resilience as a by-product of individual behavior, while others focus on the organization adapting to the external environment as a system. It is also important to examine whether they are focusing on a reaction to a dire circumstance or longer-term adaptive capacity, or what we might call "everyday" resilience.

For example, Horne (1997) is clearly relying on a systems metaphor in his view of resilience. In fact, he explicitly states that organizations should be metaphorically understood as natural ecosystems rather than machines, and that the focus is on survival. He defines *resilience* as "the ability of a system to withstand the stresses of environmental 'loading' based on the combination/composition of the system pieces, their structural interlinkages, and the way environmental change is transmitted and spread throughout the entire system" (p. 27). Note that the object is to "withstand" stresses, not to improve overall organizational capacity.

Mallack (1998), on the other hand, builds from an individual psychological perspective and emphasizes the importance of fostering individual self-efficacy. He suggests that *resilience* involves perceiving experiences constructively, performing positive adaptive behaviors, ensuring adequate external re-

sources, expanding decision making boundaries, practicing *bricolage*, developing tolerance for uncertainty, and building virtual role systems as an advanced form of work–team relationships.

Lengnick-Hall and Beck (2003) also rely on a psychological model to explain *organizational resilience*, which they define as "a composite pattern of cognitive, behavioral, and contextual characteristics that promotes advantageous organizational transformation when confronted with a discontinuous disruption" (p. 8). With regard to the question of whether organizational resilience and psychological resilience are different, they state, "We will not assume that the factors are identical across the two levels of analysis" but that it is "individual capabilities used collectively" that enable organizational resilience (p. 8). What we argue here is that organizational resilience is not only based on individual capabilities used collectively but also includes issues regarding systems capacity.

As noted earlier, a closely related issue is whether organizational resilience should be focused on response to crisis, or instead, emphasize adaptive capacity over time. Some are concerned with survival rather than innovation, such as to Lisack and Letiche (2002), who state that the aim of resilience is "the preservation of qualities, functions, or identity" (p. 83). Others suggest that the focus should be on building capacity, not just surviving a single, massive challenge. As Hamel and Valikangas (2003) view it, "Resilience is not about responding to a one-time crisis. … It's about continuously anticipating and adjusting to deep, secular trends that can permanently impair … earning(s). … It is about having the capacity for change before change becomes desperately obvious" (pp. 53–54). Organizational resilience "requires innovation with respect to those organizational values, processes, and behaviors that systematically favor perpetuation over innovation. … The goal is an organization that is constantly making its future rather than defending it past" (p. 55).

It should be recognized that responding to challenges, dire or not, enables organizations to develop adaptive capacity. Similar to the adage "that which does not kill us makes us stronger," building the capacity for resilience requires an organization to confront challenges. As Lengnick-Hall and Beck (2005) express it, organizations become more resilient by overcoming "just manageable" threats over time. The key is whether the organization responds to these challenges in a way the leaves it brittle and inflexible, or more flexible and adaptive.

This is the point made by Sutcliffe and Vogus (2003) when they observe that, under threat, organizations can respond rigidly, and decision makers can reduce the variety and complexity of information, thereby narrowing the available behavioral responses. A resilient response, on the other hand, emerges from "reactively ordinary adaptive processes that promote competence, restore efficacy, and encourage growth, as well as the structures and practices that bring about these processes" (p. 94). Another dimension of building resilience is *development*, or the "capacity for adaptability, positive functioning, or competence following chronic stress or prolonged trauma" (p. 95). Most importantly, "an entity not only survives/thrives by positively adjusting to current adversity, but also, in the process of responding, strengthens its compatibilities to make future adjustments" (p. 97).

Although in some ways it can be argued that resilience may only be assessed retrospectively in evaluating whether an organization survived and prospered in the face of a significant challenge or disaster, such a perspective is not very useful to organizations and the people who lead them. The focus here is on building the capacity for resilience in anticipation of challenges. Lengnick-Hall and Beck define *resilience capacity* as a "unique blend of cognitive, behavioral, and contextual properties that increase a firm's ability to understand its current situation and to develop customized response that reflect that understanding." This perspective,

they state, "encourages a firm to develop a grand and varied repertoire of routines for responding to uncertainty" (2005, p. 12).

According to Hamel and Valikangas (2003), organizations that want to become more resilient face four key challenges. The first is a *cognitive* challenge. Organizations seeking to become more resilient must be free of denial. They must have a realistic view of their capacities and the challenges they face, or could face in the future. This means that organizations recognize that sometimes the problems they face in the present are different that those faced in the past, and therefore require a new and unique responses. The second major challenge is *strategic*: How can organizations develop new alternatives and options in responding to challenges? How can they plan for an uncertain future? The third challenge is *political*. Responding adaptively requires organizations to be able to divert resources and support "experiments" seeking new and novel approaches to problems. The final challenge is *ideological*: Organizations must become opportunity-driven rather than focusing on the optimization of existing models and systems.

Taken together, then, the literature suggests that resilient organizations have a number of important characteristics. First, they are redundant. Redundancy or excess capacity allows an organization to survive even if one component of the organization fails. Second, resilient organizations are robust. They are vigorous, active organizations that promote the mental and psychological health of their employees. Third, resilient organizations are flexible. They are willing and ready to try new approaches rather than relying only on standard operating procedures. Reliability is also a characteristic of resilient organization. To build and maintain resilience, the organizational "infrastructure" must be sound, providing reliable and accurate data, working communication channels, and management of resources. Finally, resilient organizations foster a culture of respect and trust. Organizational members will not be willing to take necessary risks and experiment if the organizational culture and management punish mistakes and failures.

Horne and Orr (1998) suggest that seven "streams" of practical behavior contribute to resilience:

1. Community: A shared sense of purpose and identity.
2. Competence: The capacity and skills to meet demands.
3. Connections: Relationships and linkages that expand capacity and flexibility.
4. Commitment: Trust and goodwill.
5. Communication: Strong communication to make sense and derive order.
6. Coordination: Good timing to ensure alignment.
7. Consideration: Attention to the human factor.

These characteristics of resilient organizations and the elements that must be in place to foster resilience can now be considered in relationship to traditional and contemporary organizational and management theory.

Traditional Organization and Management: Constraints on Resilience

Questions about the most useful way to understand organizational resilience are closely related to how we conceive of organizations themselves. Traditional conceptions of organizations and management are largely hostile to the notion of resilience and counter to the goal of building adaptive capacity. Much of traditional organizational theory can be traced to the work of a Max Weber, a German sociologist who wrote about the emergence of large-scale organizations in the late 19th and early 20th centuries. He defined *bureaucracy*, as any large organization, public or private, with a fixed and stable hierarchical authority structure, with a clear division of labor, recruitment based on qualifications, formal rules and regulations, and written records (Weber, cited in

Gerth & Mills, 1946). According to Weber, the primary advantage of this organizational form was efficiency: "Experience tends to universally show that the purely bureaucratic type of administration [is] capable of attaining the highest degree of efficiency and is in this sense formally the most rational known means of carrying out imperative control over human beings" (p. 337). In fact, bureaucracies were likened to impersonal machines, structured to achieve consistency and control, and people in the organization were seen as interchangeable "cogs" in that machine.

Although Weber lauded the efficiency of bureaucracy, he, and many scholars who followed, has critiqued the bureaucratic organizational form on at least two counts: (1) that once fully developed, it is difficult to control through democratic governance; and (2) that it has a deleterious effect on individuals who work in such organizations, retarding normal adult psychological development. Nonetheless, the bureaucratic ideal is deeply engrained in how we think about organizations and informs many of the management practices used in organizations today. Specifically, the bureaucratic values of rationality, efficiency, and control are very much a part of how contemporary organizations are designed and managed.

Consistent with the bureaucratic view of organizations, traditional views of management are based on the idea that, like machines, organizations should be precisely controlled, mechanical, and efficient. Within this perspective, it is management's job to control the organization by ensuring that rules are followed; that authority is limited; that variation, and therefore discretion, is avoided; and that careful records are kept. Again, the purpose is efficiency and consistency. For example, the famous French management theorist and practitioner Henri Fayol (1949) identified five general functions that managers should perform: planning, organizing, commanding, coordinating, and controlling. This perspective was also reflected in the work of Frederick W. Taylor, who developed what he termed *scientific management*, an approach based on carefully defined "laws, rules, and principles" (1923, p. 7). Taylor focused on studying work scientifically to obtain detailed measurements of time and motion to optimize efficiency. Once the "best way" is discovered, the manager's job is to enforce it strictly and control people to avoid variation.

What becomes immediately clear is that this approach to organizational design and management is at odds with what is needed to foster organizational resilience. Traditional organizational theory and management do not allow for practicing the needed improvisation, adaptation, and experimentation characteristic of resilient organizations. For example, key to traditional views of organizations and management are the ideas of the division of labor and unity of command. The logic behind the division of labor is that because people differ in knowledge and skills and have limited time, dividing the work of the organization into identifiable areas allows people to gain expertise, thereby increasing efficiency and avoiding duplication. Once the division of labor is established, the organization has a structure of authority to coordinate and control its various parts. Unity of command requires that there be a single authority at the top of the organization to which all subordinates ultimately report through a "chain of command." Finally, "under hierarchy, knowledge is treated as a scarce resource and is therefore concentrated, along with the corresponding decision rights, in specialized functional units and at higher levels in the organization" (Adler, 2001, cited in Wise, 2006, p. 310).

Again, these organizational precepts conflict with the imperatives of resilience. If the sole value is efficiency, then the redundancies needed for building resilience will be avoided. Strict division of labor and unity of command produce workers who may know their own specific jobs very well but are ill-equipped and unable to step into new roles when circumstances change. In some cases,

they will simply lack the needed information to identify a problem correctly and respond appropriately. Hierarchical controls and strict supervisory relationships limit information and access, and quash attempts to deviate from the rules. As Yukl points out,

> Efficiency can be increased by refining work processes, establishing norms and standard procedures, investing in specialized personnel, facilities, or equipment, and organizing around strategy. However, these practices tend to reduce flexibility and make it more difficult to change strategies and work processes at a future time in response to environmental threats and opportunities. (2004, p. 81)

Nonetheless, these ideas are deeply embedded in our thinking about organizations; it may be the natural tendency of organizational leaders, when under threat, to respond by becoming more rather than less bureaucratic. In doing so, they impose greater rigidity, leading to less rather than more resilient behavior. In a moment when everything seems to be flying "out of control," it may seem rational to put in place more controls and strict hierarchical management practices, excessive dependence on standard rules of procedure, and limitations on the variability of communications.

Unfortunately, this may be exactly the wrong set of activities to get the organization through the situation. Rational planning assumes at least some measure of predictability, some understanding of what the future is likely to bring. But when everything is unfolding in completely unpredictable ways, rationality is actually counterproductive. What is needed instead is a capacity for "acting in the moment," something that is better attained through quick adaptability, imagination, ingenuity, spontaneity, creativity, rapidly shifting networks and patterns, and highly improvised behavior.

There are interesting parallels here in terms of the management of natural resources and ecosystem resilience. As noted earlier, traditional natural resource management focuses on reducing natural variation in an effort to make an ecosystem more predictable, economically viable, and controllable. But this reduction in natural variation actually can lead to a loss of resilience in a system, leaving it more vulnerable to environmental crisis. In much the same way, a resilient organization is not continually subject to rational controls or standard operating procedures. Rather, such an organization is more likely to have lost the capacity for resilience.

Contemporary Expressions of Organization and Management: Opening the Door to Resilience

While traditional organizational theory focuses on structure and controls, organizations are also made up of individuals who, rather than being like "cogs in a machine," are complex human beings with needs and capacities that go far beyond what earlier organizational and management theories allowed. In other words, these newer conceptions of organizations also consider the human element, a key factor in organizational resilience.

This shift in perspective can be largely traced back to the mid-1920s, when a group of Harvard researchers conducted a study at the Hawthorne Works of the Western Electric Company. The study was originally designed within the scientific management tradition and focused on the relationship between working conditions (e.g., lighting and the arrangement of work) and worker productivity. After multiple failed experiments, however, the researchers found that the human aspects of organizational life were more important than the structure or conditions of the work in determining efficiency and effectiveness. This opened the door to the study of how management can influence the behavior of individuals through the social aspects of work and the role managers play in fostering worker satisfaction.

This human relations perspective was exemplified in Douglas MacGregor's (1960) Theory X and Theory Y. MacGregor critiqued the assumptions about human behavior that formed the basis for traditional management techniques (Theory X). Theory X, according to MacGregor, assumes that human beings are lazy and dislike work, that they must be forced to do so, they do not want responsibility, and that they want and need supervision. MacGregor argued that Theory Y assumptions would lead to better outcomes: that work is as natural as play, that people do not need to be forced or coerced, that they want responsibility, and that they will make commitments and devote energy to meet objectives.

Also within the human relations tradition, writers such as Herbert Simon questioned traditional notions of authority. He suggested that authority flows from the bottom-up rather the top-down. He argued that each individual "establishes an area of acceptance within which the subordinate is willing to accept the decisions made for him by his superior" (Simon, 1957, pp. 74–75). Others, such as Chris Argyris (1970), argued that formal organizations and traditional management practices were inconsistent with the growth and development of healthy adult personalities. Argyris suggested that in order for children to move into adulthood, they must move from passivity to activity, from dependence to independence, from a limited to a greater range of behaviors, from shallow to deeper interests, from a shorter to a longer time perspective, from a position of subordination to a position of equality, and from lack of awareness to greater awareness. Yet, argued Argyris, these developmental paths are thwarted by traditional management practices that give individuals little or no control over their work, control how they can respond, and encourage passivity through close controls.

These perspectives caused a shift in focus away from the strict control of organizations and people to consider questions of human behavior and human needs. In large measure, however, theses approaches were and continue to be superimposed on systems of bureaucratic authority. From a cynical perspective, it can be argued that the purpose of these approaches was merely to make workers feel more satisfied, so that they would produce more in a bureaucratic setting. But later theoretical developments built on human relations, especially contemporary ideas about organizational culture, organizational learning, and the importance of emotional intelligence, have led to the creation of management principles that can support and foster organizational resilience, particularly as it relates to individuals. Before considering these developments, however, it is necessary to look at how the dominant conception of organizations themselves has shifted away from a machine metaphor toward a biological systems metaphor.

In the systems view of organizations and management, the focus shifts away from structure and human behavior to concentrate on the organization's adaptation to its environment. According to the systems approach, organizations are not like machines but are best viewed as organisms pursuing particular goals within a complex environment. Systems theory clearly relies on a biological/ecological metaphor. In this view, the organizational system takes in human, financial, and material resources it requires from the environment and responds to environmental demands, much like a living organisms takes in nourishment and responds to demands or challenges from its environment. The organization as "organism" then processes these resources and inputs, and produces outputs (products, services, etc.) that are placed back into the environment. The environmental responses to these outputs become new inputs. These environmental interactions and feedback loops are what allow the organization to adapt and survive (see, e.g., Katz & Kahn, 1996).

From a systems perspective, the primary imperative is organizational survival. It urges managers to focus on the organizational environment to ensure that the needed inputs are reliably available, that the environmental factors that may impinge on the organization are identified and addressed, and that

the environment values (and will thus pay for) the outputs being produced. Particularly important from the standpoint of resilience, a systems view of organizations suggests the need for variability. As noted by Weick and Sutcliffe, "The lesson from complex systems thinking is that management processes can be improved by making them adaptable and flexible, able to deal with uncertainty and surprise, and by building capacity to adapt to change" (2007, p. 79).

Unlike traditional organizational theory, the systems view recognizes that to gain stability in the entire system, one has to allow instability in the component parts (Wildavsky, 2003), in order for them to respond to environment factors. Again, however, the question arises as to meaning of "stability." As already noted, the systems view of the organizational system relies specifically on a biological/ecological metaphor. In biological/ecological systems, stability is achieved when the system returns to its previous state after it has been subjected to a challenge. In organizations, to use challenges and problems to build adaptive capacity, "stability" might involve finding a new, stronger, and more flexible state rather than returning to the previous state. It is perhaps a subtle distinction, but an important one. If the goal is simply to return to a previous state, then, almost by definition, the organization cannot become "better" and more responsive to future challenges.

A second way that the systems view of organizations departs from traditional organizational theory is in the area of redundancy and failure. As already noted, the primary imperative of traditional organizational theory is efficiency; therefore, redundancy is to be avoided. In systems theory, however, redundancy is a necessary part of system survival. Wildavsky (2003) quotes Martin Landau in this regard: "The theory of redundancy is a theory of system reliability" (p. 115). Redundancy is necessary to systems because overlap permits both adaptability and failure, and "failure is the seamy side of success, without which there could be no survival" (p. 115). This calls into question, for example, bureaucratic assumptions about a strict division of labor based on specialization. Although such structural arrangements are efficient, they are brittle to the extent that failure in one part of the organization cannot be easily accommodated by other parts of the organization because specialization limits the range of knowledge and skills to a particular area. As a result, Wildavsky notes that this "overspecialization" may actually make a system unstable in times of change.

As such, the systems view of organization is more consistent with the imperatives of organizational resilience. By recognizing the need for variability, this perspective provides for experimentation, change, and flexibility. By embracing the need for redundancy, systems theory recognizes that component parts of the organization must, on some level, be at least partially interchangeable—that units and the individuals in them do not become so highly specialized that only one person or one group "owns" critical information or skills sets.

Although the systems view of organizations gets us closer the capacity to build resilient organizations, it is limited in two important areas. The first relates to the use of strategic planning processes to deal with environmental challenges. As opposed to the rational planning model suggested by bureaucracy and the machine metaphor, the systems perspective calls for a shift away from "rational" planning to find the "correct" solutions, and toward strategic planning. Strategic planning involves an analysis of an organization and its environment in terms of strengths, weaknesses, opportunities, and threats (or SWOT analysis) to help align organizational resources with organizational realities to reach strategic objectives. The problem as it relates to resilience is that this approach to planning presupposes that future challenges can be anticipated. The whole point of resilience, on the other hand, is to enable the organization to deal

with unanticipated problems. As Weick and Sutcliffe observe,

> Organizations create plans to prepare for the inevitable, preempt the undesirable, and control the controllable. Rational as all this may sound, planning has its shortcomings. Because planners plan in stable, predictable contexts, they are lulled into thinking that the world will unfold in a predetermined manner, a lapse that Mintzberg calls "the fallacy of predetermination." When people are in the thrall of predetermination, there is simply no place for unexpected events that fall outside the realm of planning. (2007, p. 79)

The second major weakness of systems theory in relation to resilience is that it largely neglects questions of internal organizational management. The organization is, in effect, treated like a "black box" into which inputs go and from which outputs emerge. By looking to the literature on organizational culture, learning, and emotional intelligence, we can fill in these last missing pieces of the organizational resilience puzzle.

Over the past several decades, organizational theorists have begun to conceptualize organizations not as machines or as natural systems, but as social constructs. Within this general framework, some theorists have emphasized the importance of understanding the "culture" of the organization. *Organizational culture* is the basic pattern of attitudes, beliefs, and values held by members of the organization. Edgar H. Schein (1997, pp. 8–10) notes that culture can be manifested in many ways, including the following:

1. *Observed behavioral regularities in human interaction.* These include language, customs, traditions, and rituals employed in a particular organization.
2. *Group norms.* These are the implicit standards and values that evolve in working groups, including, for example, the approach to problems or what constitutes a "good day's work."
3. *Espoused values.* These are the articu-

lated, publicly known principles and values that the organization wants to achieve.

4. *Formal philosophy.* These are the official policies and ideological principles that guide the organization's actions toward those inside and outside the organization.

5. *Rules of the game.* These are the informal, implicit rules for getting along in the organization, and "the ropes" that a new employee must learn and practice to be accepted. It is "the way we do things around here."

6. *Climate.* This is the general feeling conveyed by the physical layout of the organization, and the way its members interact with each other and those outside the organization.

7. *Embedded skills.* These are the special skills and competencies that group members use in accomplishing tasks. These skills may be passed on informally.

8. *Habits of thinking, mental models, and/ or linguistic paradigms.* These are the shared cognitive frameworks or ways of thinking that guide the perceptions, thought processes and approaches to problem solving taught to new members in the early socialization process.

9. *Shared meanings.* These are the understandings and implicit agreements that emerge when organizational members interact with each other.

10. *"Root metaphors" or integrating symbols.* These include ideas, feelings, and images that organizations use to define and characterize themselves, which may or may not be consciously known, but which become embedded in the physical layout and other material artifacts of the group.

Understanding organizational culture is a key element in understanding how to foster resilience. Because culture has a profound effect on how organizational members perceive and address problems, interact with each other, and define their roles and values in relation to the organization, it can in many ways determine whether an organization and its members demonstrate resilient behaviors. If the organizational culture is one that encourages innovation, learning from failures rather than punishing them, and cooperation and collaboration, thus engendering trust and a psychologically safe environment to take risks, then resilient behavior would be expected to increase (Denhardt & Denhardt, 2002). If, on the other hand, the culture is one of competition and fear, the avoidance of failure, conformity and submission to authority, then it is it is much less likely that individuals will demonstrate resilient behavior.

Culture is a relatively stable element in organizations and changes only very slowly. Leadership plays a particularly important role in shaping how and whether organizational culture evolves over time. Particularly important in an organization's cultural history are moments of crisis. Because of the heightened emotions and attention during a crisis, a leader's reactions and behavior can have particular importance in highlighting the organization's culture values. These often are the stories told to newcomers during the socialization process to acquaint them with key norms and expectations. Unfortunately, as already noted, these are the moments when leaders sometimes revert to control and command strategies, much to the detriment of resilient behaviors, both at the time and into the future. If a challenge or crisis is responded to with flexibility, trust, confidence, it can leave the organization better off over time because it reinforces a culture that encourages resilience. This is so *despite the outcome* of the problem at hand.

Closely related to organizational culture is the concept of organizational learning. Learning organizations recognize that much of human behavior in organizations (Argyris, 1993) can be understood as grounded in the organization's collective consciousness. Therefore, to change and improve, management must address both surface behavior and the underlying levels of collective values and culture in the organization.

Peter Senge, writing in *The Fifth Discipline*, suggested five elements that contribute to building a learning organization. *Personal mastery* is a discipline that connects individual learning, personal skills, and spiritual growth with organizational learning. It involves our capacity to focus continuously on what is most important, while ensuring that the view of reality remains clear and truthful (Senge, 1990, p. 141). *Mental models* link the ways we view the world and our assumptions about "how things work" with innovation and learning. Our mental models may create substantial barriers to new ideas (particularly if they conflict with our understanding of reality), or they may become a source of new knowledge and creativity learning (Senge, 1990, pp. 174–178). *Shared vision* occurs when an image or idea becomes transformed into a powerful force that is shared throughout the organization or group. The organization that has a shared vision is "connected, bound together by a common aspiration" (p. 206). *Team learning* is the capacity of a group of individuals to coalesce, to engage their collective energies into an integrated team. The team remains connected through its shared vision, and individual learning becomes translated into a group or shared experience. Finally, *systems thinking* shows how human action represents a systemic, interrelated set of events. So, to understand and effect change, we must recognize the interconnectedness of our actions and their consequences in the broader system. Those who are able to achieve this type of systems thinking—what Senge calls "the fifth discipline"—have embodied the concept of individual and organizational learning (p. 7).

This "learning" organization model, then, combines systems thinking, organizational culture, shared vision, and individual development as hallmarks of an adaptive organization. As such, this model has a number of elements and characteristics that can support

the development of organizational resilience in relatively obvious ways. The literature on organizational resilience, as already noted, has close parallels with Senge's focus on individual learning and growth, an undistorted view of reality, common aspirations, recognition of the interconnectedness of individuals, and the structural and functional interdependencies within organizations.

Emerging Frameworks for Developing Resilient Organizations

Recently several organizational scholars have begun more explicitly to employ the resilience perspective in understanding organizational behavior, especially under conditions of risk. Aaron Wildavsky, in his classic *Searching for Safety* (2003), first published in 1988, sought to demonstrate that as a matter of public policy, safety cannot be achieved by avoiding risk but only by taking active, even risky steps toward safe conditions. These steps might include entrepreneurial strategies such as trial-and-error risk taking, which, Wildavsky argues, promotes resilience—"learning from adversity how to do better" (p. 2) Risk taking can produce gains, including gains in safety. Thus, the trick is not to avoid risk but to employ risk in the pursuit of gains, not losses. The jogger, for example, places the most stress on the heart while he or she is running. That's a risk. But by taking that risk, the jogger's heart is ultimately in better condition for the rest of the time.

The alternative strategy would require trial without error; that is, no change would be allowed without evidence that the proposed action would do no harm. Under this approach, the testing of a vaccine that might help millions but harm dozens would not be allowed, even though the overall health of the society might be improved. Wildavsky (2003) argues that such an approach, if followed closely, would likely prevent almost any large-scale social or technological improvement. A policy of trial without error would likely strangle growth and change because any new development almost surely will harm someone, though many others may benefit. But trial without error is the strategy of choice among the risk averse. Consequently, "if you can do nothing without knowing first how it will turn out, you cannot do anything at all. An indirect implication ... is that if trying new things is made more costly, there will be fewer departures from past practice; this very lack of change may itself be dangerous in foregoing chances to reduce existing hazards" (p. 38).

Of particular interest to students of organizational life is Wildavsky's (2003) discussion of anticipation versus resilience. In cases of anticipation, an effort is made to predict and prevent dangers before they occur. In cases of resilience, we seek to cope with unanticipated dangers after they occur, to bounce back, and even to become better than before. If we could absolutely predict future outcomes and effectively avoid the dangers they might hold, anticipation would be the preferred alternative. But uncertainty is so great with respect to either natural or man-made occurrences that it is extremely hard to predict what is likely to happen. And even if we can make an effective prediction, we may be limited in our capacity to act in a way that avoids the negative consequences.

The alternative is to build a capacity for resilience. Indeed, a failure to do so may limit the capacity of an organization or society to maintain itself under conditions of change and uncertainty. "The experience of being able to overcome unexpected danger may increase long-term safety; but maintaining a state of continuous safety may be extremely dangerous in the long run to the survival of the living species since it reduces the capacity to cope with unexpected hazards" (Wildavsky, 2003, p. 79). Under conditions of certainty, a strategy of anticipation may be most effective. But under conditions of uncertainty and change, a strategy of building the capacity of an organization to be resilient is the preferable strategy. "Where risks are highly predictable and verifiable, and rem-

edies are relatively safe, anticipation makes sense. Where risks are highly uncertain and speculative, and remedies do harm, resilience makes more sense because we cannot know which possible risks will actually become manifest" (p. 221). In a world of change and uncertainty, that is, in the "real" world, increasing the capacity of organizations and societies to understand evolving complexity and to adapt effectively is increasingly the correct strategy; indeed, it is often the only strategy.

The same reliance on resilience rather than anticipation is found in Karl Weick and Kathleen Sutcliffe's 2007 book *Managing the Unexpected*, which is interestingly subtitled *Resilient Performance in an Age of Uncertainty*. Weick and Sutcliffe focus more directly on resilient *organizations*, and begin by exploring factors that allow organizations, such as nuclear aircraft carriers or emergency medical treatment teams, to maintain their reliability even under changing and even surprising circumstances, including those in which the potential for error and disaster is overwhelming. Weick and Sutcliffe call these high-reliability organizations, or HROs. Although they operate under difficult conditions, HROs have less than their share of accidents. These organizations, they argue, are most successful when they are mindful about what is happening around and to them. This in turn allows them to update their ideas about themselves and their environment so as to adapt more quickly to unpredictable dilemmas.

HROs are successful because they engage in certain practices that allow them to be aware of emerging problems, and to adapt and recover quickly when things do go wrong. Among the practices that Weick and Sutcliffe highlight as typical to HROs and recommend to other organizations are building a capacity for resilience and taking advantage of expertise, wherever it might reside in the organization. Following Wildavsky (2003), Weick and Sutcliffe (2007) distinguish between anticipation and resilience, arguing that organizations may try to deal with surprises through anticipation, but their capacity to anticipate is limited. Instead, they must rely on their capacity for resilience, responding to surprises as they occur and bouncing back from errors quickly. The capacity for resilience means that these organizations "work to develop knowledge, capability for swift feedback, faster learning, speed and accuracy of communication, experiential variety, skill at recombination of existing response repertoires, and comfort with improvisation" (p. 73). A special component of resilience is *mindfulness*, a more nuanced appreciation of context and the willingness to restructure categories of thinking, so that they better correspond to emerging situations.

Another interesting recommendation for increasing the organization's capacity for resilience is to take advantage of expertise, wherever it exists. Many organizations, Weick and Sutcliffe (2007) note, operate on the assumption that expertise accumulates at the top of the organization, that those at top of the hierarchy are always the ones best positioned to come up with the right answers. But, of course, this typically is not the case. Expertise for dealing with particular problems is distributed throughout the organization, and one characteristic of a resilient organization is that the search for expertise moves down and through the organization rather than relying on those at the top. Not only does such a strategy ensure the most appropriate responses, but it also minimizes the potentially damaging effect of errors at the top. Again, it is important to note that Weick and Sutcliffe study HROs to learn lessons that can and should be applied in all organizations to deal more effectively with change and uncertainly.

Complementing the work of Wildavsky and that of Weick and Sutcliffe, both of which emphasize the importance of resilience in organizations, is the concept of adaptive management. *Adaptive management* is in many ways the antithesis of traditional command and control management strategies. It is based on the idea that change and vari-

ability are like experiments that allow organizations to learn and adapt continuously.

The concept of adaptive management emerged from industrial operation theory in the 1950s and was later adapted as a natural resource management approach in the 1970s (Johnson, 1999). Ecologists during this time period were voicing dissatisfaction with traditional approaches and moving toward the idea that natural resource management approaches must recognize that ecosystems always involve great uncertainty about the future. This uncertainty demanded that "control" strategies give way to approaches that treat natural resource management policies as "experiments" from which information could be gained and policies reformulated. As Habron defined it, the *adaptive management of natural resources* is "a series of linked iterative steps involving problem identification, collaborative brainstorming, model development, hypothesis testing, planning, experimentation, monitoring, evaluation and behavioral change" (2003, p. 29). Or, as Walters puts it more succinctly, "We generally use the term to refer to a structured process of 'learning by doing' that involves much more than simply better ecological monitoring and response to unexpected management impacts" (1997, p. 1).

The concept of adaptive management has since been applied to organizational management, and provides key insights into how leaders and managers can foster resilience in their organizations. Perhaps most importantly, the adaptive management approach distinguishes between what Glover, Friedman, and Jones (2002) call *adaptive* and *maladaptive change*. These authors point out that organizations change all the time, but that it is possible, even common, to create change that is not adaptive for the organization:

Change involves any new allocation of time, resources, or priorities by people within an organization. But change is no guarantee of successful adaptation. ... Adaptation always involves creative problem solving in which the change leaders bring about a successful and sustainable alternation in the nature of the relationship between the organization and its environment. When change does not involve adaptation, the result may be only additional activity layered on top of an organizations culture, often creating a situation worse than the starting place. (p. 19)

This speaks directly to the issue of building the capacity for resilience, suggesting that organizations can change in a manner that either fosters or detracts from the capacity for future adaptation. Building resilience requires attention to not only the substance but also the process of change. When changes are implemented as rational "solutions" to "problems," it is assumed that that the full nature of the problem is known, that behavioral responses are predictable, and that management decrees can override organizational culture. Using this set of assumptions, when change does not go as planned, managers frequently try to apply additional force to secure implementation and place the blame for failures on uncooperative employees and intractable systems. In fact, "in many cases, organizations are far worse off after a failed change attempt than they were in the first place. In this regard, suffering with an inadequate status quo may often be better than introducing further problems with a maladaptive change effort" (Glover et al., 2002, p. 17).

If, however, we accept that information can be incomplete, that situations are changeable, that systems are complex, and that there are multiple influences on behavior, then a "learn as you go" strategy allows us to modify our approach in response to new information. This increases the likelihood that the change will be sustainable and help to maintain rather than constrict innovation and flexibility. To manage adaptively requires strong values, as opposed to rational analysis. It requires leaders to manage their emotions, and to have little fear of conflict and great humility (Westley, 2002).

In fact, Vera and Rodriguez-Lopez (2004) argue that humility is a particularly important resource in building resilience. Humility ensures that people have a realistic view of themselves and their organization. Humility is associated with organizational learning, service, and resilience, as demonstrated by "acceptance of success with simplicity, pragmatic acceptance of failure, avoidance of narcissism and resilience against adulation, avoidance of self-complacency, and frugality" (Vera & Rodriguez-Lopez, 2004).

Finally, adaptive management is related to the key role that leaders and managers play in creating shared values and shaping culture. The leader's behavior, values, and emotional authenticity create a platform or culture from which individuals can respond to change with flexibility, confidence, and improvisation. What is needed is not just an environment in which people are free from reprisal and punishment, but one in which they feel that in trusting others and being open to creative solutions, they are just behaving in a manner that is consistent with "way things are done around here." This requires a strong and positive organizational culture of innovation, along with the psychological safety that comes from an emotionally intelligent leader.

Conclusion

Management today requires a new way of thinking about how to organize for and build organizational resilience and adaptive management. In contrast to the rationalist language of bureaucracy, we need to focus on a systems perspective, human needs and motivations, and organizational culture. Although these approaches do not always achieve the most efficient results, they do build an organization's capacity to adapt to the unexpected. A resilient organization requires an adaptive manager to use challenges as an opportunity to build capacity. When the worst occurs, rational dynamics no longer apply, and the manager who seeks technically rational answers will often end up doing more organizational harm than good. On the other hand, the manager who can quickly discern emerging patterns, imaginatively create new ways of capturing and shaping human energy, and capture the flow of the moment will most likely build an adaptable and resilient organization that can not only survive challenges but also prosper when the unexpected happens.

References

Argyris, C. (1970). *Intervention theory and method*. Reading, MA: Addison-Wesley.

Argyris, C. (1993). *Knowledge for action*. San Francisco: Jossey-Bass.

Benard, B. (1995). *Fostering resilience in children*. Urbana, IL: ERIC Clearinghouse on Elementary and Early Childhood Education. (ERIC Reproduction Service No. ED386327)

Berkes, F. C., Colding, J., & Folke, C. (Eds.). (2003). *Navigating social-ecological systems*. Cambridge, UK: Cambridge University Press.

Coutu, D. (2002). How resilience works. *Harvard Business Review, 80*, 46–55.

Denhardt, J., & Denhardt, R. B. (2002). Creating a culture of innovation. In M. Abramson & I. Littman (Eds.), *What do we know about innovation?* (pp. 107–142). Lanham, MA: Rowman & Littlefield.

Fayol, H. (1949). *General and industrial management* (Trans. C. Storrs). London: Isaac Pitman & Sons.

Gerth, H. H., & Mills, C. W. (1946). *From Max Weber: Essays in sociology*. New York: Oxford University Press.

Glover, J., Friedman, H., & Jones, G. (2002). Adaptive leadership: When change is not enough. *Organizational Development Journal, 20*, 15–32.

Gunderson, L. (2000). Ecological resilience in theory and action. *Annual Review of Ecology and Systematics, 31*, 425–239.

Habron, G. (2003). The role of adaptive management for watershed councils. *Environmental Management, 31*, 29–41.

Hamel, G., & Valikangas, L. (2003). The quest for resilience. *Harvard Business Review, 81*, 52–63.

Horne, J. (1997). The coming of age of organizational resilience. *Business Forum, 22*, 24–28.

Horne, J., & Orr, J. (1998, Winter). Assessing behaviors that create resilient organizations. *Employment Relations Today*, pp. 29–39.

Johnson, B. L. (1999). Introduction to the special feature: Adaptive management—scientifically sound, socially challenged? *Ecology and Society, 3*, 10–13.

Katz, D., & Kahn, R. (1996). *The social psychology of organizations*. New York: Wiley.

Lengnick-Hall, C., & Beck, T. (2003, August). *Beyond bouncing back: The concept of organizational resilience*. Paper presented at the National Academy of Management Conference, Seattle, WA.

Lengnick-Hall, C., & Beck, T. (2005). Adaptive fit versus robust transformation. *Journal of Management, 31*, 1–20.

Lisack, M., & Letiche, H. (2002). Complexity, emergence, resilience, and coherence: Gaining perspective on organizations and their study. *Emergence, 4*, 72–94.

MacGregor, D. (1960). *The human side of the enterprise*. Columbus, OH: McGraw-Hill.

Mallack, L. (1998). Putting organizational resilience to work. *Industrial Management, 40*, 8–13.

Schein, E. H. (1997). *Organizational culture and leadership* (2nd ed.). San Francisco: Jossey-Bass.

Senge, P. M. (1990). *The fifth discipline: The art and practice of the learning organization*. New York: Currency/Doubleday.

Simon, H. A. (1957). *Models of man*. New York: Wiley.

Sutcliffe, K., & Vogus, T. J. (2003). Organizing for resilience. In K. Cameron, J. E., Dutton, & R. E. Quinn (Eds.), *Positive organizational scholarship* (pp. 94–110). San Francisco: Berrett-Koehler.

Taylor, F. W. (1923). *Scientific management*. New York: Harper & Row.

Vera, D., & Rodriguez-Lopez, A. (2004). Humility as a source of competitive advantage. *Organizational Dynamics, 33*, 393–408.

Walters, C. (1997). Challenges in adaptive management of riparian and coastal ecosystems. *Conservation Ecology, 1*(2). Available at *www.consecol.org/vol1/iss2/art1*

Weick, K., & Sutcliffe, K. (2007). *Managing the unexpected: Resilient performance in an age of uncertainty* (2nd ed.). San Francisco: Jossey-Bass.

Westley, F. (2002). The devil in the dynamics: Adaptive management on the front lines. In L. H. Gunderson & C. S. Holling (Eds.), *Panarchy* (pp. 333–360). Washington, DC: Island Press.

Westley, F., Carpenter, S. R., Brock, W. A., Holling, C. S., & Gunderson, L. H. (2002). Why systems of people and nature are not just social and ecological systems. In L. H. Gunderson & C. S. Holling, (Eds.), *Panarchy* (pp. 103–119). Washington, DC: Island Press.

Wildavsky, A. (2003). *Searching for safety.* New Brunswick, NJ: Transaction

Wise, C. (2006). Organizing for homeland security after Katrina: Is adaptive management what's missing? *Public Administration Review, 66,* 302–318.

Wolin, S., & Wolin, S. (1993). *The resilient self: How survivors of troubled families rise above adversity.* New York: Villard.

Yukl, G. (2004). Tridimensional leadership theory. In R. J. Burke & C. L. Cooper (Eds.), *Leading in turbulent times* (pp. 75–91). Malden, MA: Blackwell.

17

Indicators of Community Resilience

What Are They, Why Bother?

John Stuart Hall
Alex J. Zautra

"Growth" has been a buzzword in our society. More is better. But are more people, more highways, more factories, more consumption intrinsically better? Cancer, too, is growth—growth out of step with the body, the larger system it depends on. A co-intelligent community, conscious of its internal and external interconnectedness, would not seek endless growth of its material "standard of living." Rather, it would seek sustainable development of its "quality of life," as manifested in the welfare of its members, the vitality of its culture and the health of the natural environment in which it was embedded.
—*www.co-intelligence.org/S-sustainableSeattle.html*

Overview: Using Resilience Indicators to Chart Community Progress

Throughout history, communities and civilizations have sought to enhance the quality of community life and the well-being of their people. However, more recently we have seen greater interest in attending to the details of community development by capitalizing on the improved ability to define, measure, and extend community well-being and successes to all residents. With that interest has come attention to the development of indicators of progress in furthering well-being in the community.

Communities are vibrant, ever-changing, and challenging social worlds. A thoughtful-ly crafted comprehensive community index can inform us about the direction, negative or positive, of growth and change in those communities. A glance into the community indicator literature uncovers a formidable list of attempts by organizations and communities to tackle this daunting task. Each attempt aims to capture a picture of community functioning and status, reducing the complex phenomenon of community life into a few quantifiable mileposts for the purposes of evaluation and informing policy and programming. As with any measure, an indicator must outline the target phenomenon or condition, and the specific goals and desired outcomes for which it is being developed. The need to link community vision, goals, outcomes, and indicators within a community resilience framework requires attention to processes, as well as to outcomes.

A community that is building capacity is one that plans for positive growth as well as decline, integrates economic and social goals, and fosters connections across diverse groups within its borders. For these lofty ambitions to be more than pipe dreams, the community needs methods to chart its progress on social and economic goals using real data. The 21st-century metropolis that stays tuned in to a range of risk and resource factors rather than relying solely on a model of risk not only bucks the current and long-standing trends but also is moving toward a model of governance that provides a greater capacity to sustain and improve quality of life for its members.

What Is Community Resilience?

Healthy Communities

A take-off point for the development of community resilience indicators anywhere is an understanding of the operational meaning of community. *Community* has many definitions, and debate among social scientists and philosophers on the fine points of what a community is, and is not, will likely carry on indefinitely. Nevertheless, there are many useful common threads with which a working definition can be woven together for the purpose of informing the development of a functional Community Resilience Index (CRI). In essence a community is defined by the presence of sustained and substantial positive social interaction among people who share common ground. Past definitions focused on the patterns of social engagement bounded by geographic areas such a neighborhoods, towns, and school districts—what Black and Hughes (2001) refer to as *communities of location*. In addition, social networks of people with shared identities and purposes define what Black and Hughes refer to as *communities of interest*. These clusters of people, bounded by common val-

ues rather than by geography, are no less important in our understanding of community. A focus on community, then, embraces both the shared geographic and the conceptual spaces that constitute what social scientists have referred to as *weak ties* (Granovetter, 1973). These webs of social interconnection determine the extent of civic engagement and social capital. From the perspective of resilience, a key domain of interest is how communities further the capacities of their constituents to develop and sustain well-being, and partner with neighboring communities of location and interest to further the aims of the whole region.

The definition of *health* as the absence of disease has held sway in public policy debates for the greater part of the 20th century. This narrow view has been gradually overtaken by a broader and more comprehensive approach that includes the capacity for quality of life, as well as the absence of pathology.[1] In terms of physical health, this transition has led to greater attention to functional capacity and less on prevalence estimates of "caseness." In mental health, a similar transformation has taken place in referring to disablement as the criterion for poor mental health rather than a diagnosis of mental disorder (American Psychiatric Association, 1994).

Inquiries into the processes that allow for resilience in physical and mental health led us to a deeper appreciation of human capacities than are found in the standard paradigms that underlie clinical research and practice. Paradigms within the clinical sciences have focused so much on revealing hidden pathologies within us that we have ignored the natural capacities of people, even those who are ill, to resolve problems, to bounce back from adversity, and to find and sustain energy in the pursuit of life's goals. Instead of focusing on attributes of people and their social worlds that confer risk, ideas such as recovery and sustainability invite us to examine qualities of the person and his or her social and community environments that confer optimism, hope, purpose, positive and lasting social ties, and self- and collective efficacy. These are qualities that permit flourishing within dynamic, challenging, even threatening environments that characterize rapidly changing metropolitan areas.

In parallel fashion, we often define the quality of life within a community by the absence of crime, safe streets, convenience to stores selling everyday commodities, and a relatively unfettered path from home to work and back again. People need the structure of a coherently organized physical environment that affords them basic goods. They want to live within communities that support their needs for social connection and psychological growth. Resilient community structures build on peoples' hopes, as well as provide a means of circling the wagons to provide a "defensible space." We need definitions that go beyond the absence of problems: not just risk but also capacity, thoughtfulness, planning, and a forward-leaning orientation, including attainable goals and a realistic vision for the community as a whole.

Boothroyd and Eberle (1990) defined a *healthy community* as one in which all organizations, large and small, formal and informal, work together successfully to enhance the quality of life of all its members. We agree. From our resilience perspective, *health* refers not simply to attending to levels of illness, pain, and psychological disturbance but also to taking a social account of balance of opportunities for enrichment in work, family and civic life, the qualities that sustain well-being for individuals and build vibrant communities that can sustain healthy lifestyles for generations.

Needed: A CRI

By taking the broad view of human and community health, and focusing on qualities that promote resilience, we make the task of identifying yardsticks for community resilience a challenging one. However daunting the complexities that underlie that effort, to attempt anything less would be to shortchange the communities we study,

and diminish our chances of preserving the local resources that provide for sustainable growth and development.

One temptation is to embrace the conceptual foundations outlined thus far but stop short of completing the difficult work of operationalization. In so doing we only "talk the talk," leaving behind the legacy of an academic exercise or, worse yet, a framework so open to interpretation that all efforts, or the lack thereof, are justifiable. Community indicators integrated into an index of resilience provide a means of making tangible progress toward our goals, yielding critical feedback on the success of our efforts. Our efforts at strengthening community can then be evaluated in terms of resilient processes and outcomes informing us of what works and what programs need to be reexamined in light of the data.

Advancing Beyond Existing Methodologies

Indicator development to date has laid substantial groundwork from which we begin to build a CRI. However, there are several opportunities to improve on existing indicators and to further our thinking, measurement, and analysis of community resilience. Thus far, indicators have largely relied on descriptive statistics, without a guiding theory. Also, the social issues that the indicators aim to address remain vague and ambiguous. For example, the health of constituents may be boiled down to number of hospital visits and infant mortality rates. These types of data serve as a crude estimates and tell us little about the physical functioning of individuals. In turn, this information has little impact on the community receiving such information and how it should inform their daily behaviors and understanding of community health.

Theoretical Advances

Resilience theory provides a framework to enhance existing indicators, which have tended to take a singular approach to measurement; that is, most have examined what constitutes a healthy or an unhealthy community, without attention to the underlying structure that defines the two constructs. A bidimensional or two-factor framework of resilience suggests that resilience factors are not simply qualities found at the positive end of a single continuum of risk. Models that contain at least two separate dimensions: One that estimates vulnerabilities, and another, strengths (Zautra, 2003) together confer unique advantages in the prediction of health not accounted for by one-dimensional assessments of relative risk.

This two-factor approach makes obvious the point that the absence of negative experiences does not *pari passu* imply the presence of positive ones. Conversely, the absence of positive experiences does not necessarily imply the presence of negative ones. Proceeding without an awareness of the distinct quality and meaning of positive versus negative aspects of mental health and social relations, however, leads to shortsightedness in the selection of measures and the construction of predictive indices of health, resulting in shortfalls in predicting differences between groups in health and well-being. Furthermore, the confusion that comes from mixing together disparate (and unrelated) indicators leads to lack of specificity in identifying active ingredients of the processes (social, cultural, interpersonal, and physiological) that could direct the design of preventive interventions and build theory (Castro, Cota, & Vega, 1999; Steptoe & Marmot, 2003). Communities are complex, and capturing their assets, as well as their liabilities, extends the two-dimensional approach of resilience properly to identification of indicators to chart progress toward greater health and well-being at the level of community.

Community Research

Another limitation to existing indicator selection has been the very practical constraints of data availability and cost of new data acquisition. At first glance, there seem to be fountains of information from various public, nonprofit, and private organizations at state, local, and national levels, so much information that many sound alarms about information overload. But not all information from the vast fields of websites and official reports is uniformly available for all communities. It is often possible to augment existing data with new research to provide the best set of indicators for a particular community. Indeed, when community members are brought together to talk about the best measures of progress for their neighborhood, town, or region, they are likely to suggest new measures that require individual data collection through surveys, focus groups, and other approaches, all of which is well and good as a community involvement and planning process, but also expensive.

There are many different types of communities, and the definitions used in indicators remain varied and vague. Communities have complex and dynamic features that our statistical measures and research questions are only beginning to appreciate. Sophistication in design and methods of inquiry, in addition to good theory, is essential for understanding them. Issues of how to define a community, measure its direct and indirect effects, and tease apart the relative importance of individual-, family-, and community-level factors are only beginning to be addressed. Advances in research over the last 10 years have begun to identify the impacts of neighborhood characteristics on individual health and well-being (Folland, 2007). These improvements in community research provide methodologies to move social indicators successfully beyond an era of descriptive statistics to making and testing predictions about what constitutes a resilient community.

Distinguishing Processes and Outcomes

The articulation of a conceptual framework for community resilience requires attention to processes, as well as to outcomes. The final test of resilient outcomes occurs when the community faces a formidable challenge. The assessment of progress toward resilience requires attention to those intermediary processes that increase the likelihood of resilience. Resources such as human and financial capital provide the raw materials for healthy communities. These and other factors influence the development of resilient processes, such as social capital and collective efficacy. Those processes lead to resilient communities. This model has feedback as well, and promotes the place of learning in governance. Communities that demonstrate resilience further develop their capacities for resilience.

Time Is of the Essence

Cities are vibrant and dynamic, and the measures used to capture them should be able to capture the breadth and movement of a city. Different histories, cultures, experiences, plans, and contexts are what differentiate communities. A resilient community is one that examines the long-term changes within the society, warding off ill outcomes before they arrive and enhancing quality of life over that of previous generations. Longitudinal research is an essential component of any community indicator product. The positive impact of programming and developments may not be seen in a matter of weeks, or certainly not in a one-time snapshot of life in a community.

Longitudinal analyses provide the opportunity to begin to understand causal processes, which cannot be assessed in cross-sectional data; that is, they can help to decipher programming that is facilitating positive change and that which is not. Statistical analyses are rapidly evolving, and opportunities to use longitudinal growth and dynamic systems modeling are improving by the day. Although many indicators have been collected consistently over time, there has been minimal examination of growth and trajectories within those datasets. In addition, we know little about models of change within communities.

Developing CRIs

An accurate depiction of community resilience requires a mix of strategies. First, a social accounting would rely on existing indicators with which to map and monitor trends in community resourcefulness and potential vulnerabilities. These indicators, if carefully chosen, may be used to capture resilient outcomes of communities following unplanned events that challenge its adaptive capacity. For example, the proportion of residents with 4 or more years of higher education provides one indicator of workforce flexibility in the event of an economic crisis. Second, a direct appraisal of key elements of resilience processes is needed to assess key dimensions of resourcefulness not detected with existing methods, and to capture emergent strengths that do not yet register on global outcome indices of social and economic progress. The extent of resident knowledge of and participation in community forums, and other means of active engagement in collective decisions that affect our lives, informs us of the degree of social connection and resident commitment to furthering the quality of life in our communities. Third, the social ecology of sustainability and recovery cannot be ignored. Along with measures of job growth and household income, for example, we need to assess budgets for family time and impacts of income disparity on community civility.

To illustrate, consider the following list of attributes of resilient processes for communities of location, reproduced in Table 17.1. These are key elements of community resilience theory that should be monitored for degrees of change in communities that aspire to develop greater resilience capacity.

Some indicators that are routinely collected may "stand in" as valid indicators for many of the qualities of community life depicted here, but not all of them. The measurement of "trust," for example, is a critical dimension that requires direct assessment. Household surveys have been used for this purpose and are the best methodology cur-

TABLE 17.1. Fundamentals of Neighborhood Resilience

Resilient communities ...

1. Have neighbors that trust one another (Kawachi, Kennedy, & Glass, 1999; Sampson, Raudenbush, & Earls, 1997; Subramanian, Kim, & Kawachi, 2002).

2. Have neighbors that interact on a regular basis (Berkman & Syme, 1979; Bolland & McCallum, 2002; Unger & Wandersman, 1985).

3. Have residents who own their houses and stay for awhile (Bures, 2003; Galster, 1998; Temkin & Rohe, 1998).

4. Have residents who have a sense of community and cohesion (Brodsky, O'Campo, & Aronson, 1999; Chavis & Wandersman, 1990; Cutrona, Russell, Hessling, Brown, & Murry, 2000; Farrell, Aubry, & Coulombe, 2004; Sarason, 1974).

5. Have residents who work together for the common good and are involved in community events and affairs (Duncan, Duncan, Okut, Strycker, & Hix-Small, 2003; Hyyppa & Maki, 2003; Perkins, Florin, Rich, Wandersman, & Chavis, 1990; Price & Behrens, 2003; Sampson et al., 1997).

6. Have formal and informal civic places for gathering (Oldenburg, 1991; Sharkova & Sanchez, 1999).

rently available. The cost of this method is often prohibitive, although the innovative use of Web-based technologies may make large samples for citizen interviews affordable in the near future.

We advocate a complementary, at times alternative, approach to acquiring information about community resilience. Citizen panels that comprise leaders and other concerned citizens who are members of the communities studied, could be developed to identify unique characteristics of their constituent areas that deserve close attention. These citizen panels can fill the gaps left by social accounting and address directly problems and prospects for community resilience. With care in selection of the citizen panel to ensure that it is representative of those most informed and concerned, the group mem-

bers may be enjoined to meet periodically to review the status of their communities; follow a well-facilitated, carefully designed, uniform framework for analysis; suggest new and better indicators of progress; and provide early warning of downturns in quality of life that are likely to leave their communities less resilient in the future.

If the goal is to uncover indicators of resilient communities, the challenges of measuring change are readily apparent. A city that plans and is future-oriented, connected, and not segmented, and that focuses on resources, as well as risk factors, bucks the current and long-standing trends. However, considerable effort is needed to generate such a dramatic shift in attention to community resourcefulness. Despite these challenges, there are reasons to believe that critical steps can be taken to move to more resilient governance, with substantial and sustainable gains in community well-being as a result. A "tipping point" in which the benefits outweigh the investment costs is required. To reach this critical point in community development requires resourceful people with keen insights and strong leadership skills, coupled with accurate data that can persuade the skeptics and reassure supporters that the path they have chosen is the correct one. An effective model depends on good data, high-quality feedback, leaders who are willing to listen and to act, and a citizenry that is informed and involved. Our resilience model is no different in this regard. Resilience fundamentals applied through civic engagements that further "learning governance" provide a path to community development that strengthens prospects for a sustainable future for all.

Resilience Indicators for Healthy Communities

The selection of meaningful community indicators is dependent on several factors, but the single, most important factor is the identification of an underlying model to guide the work. As Lewin (1951) once admonished, "Nothing is as practical as good theory." Indicators do not have meaning in themselves. In order for these measures to provide a coherent assessment of the community, we need to select an integrative approach to understanding what constitutes a healthy and strong community. Otherwise, data that arise from a set of indicators are more likely to be subject to interpretative whim and fancy. A strong model, important for building community, is essential to correctly focus and interpret the data, and to judge the extent and even the direction of positive change resulting from ambitious community programs.

We have chosen resilience as the key construct with which to build a model that informs our choices of community indicators. To inquire about resilience is to ask two fundamental questions about human adaptation. First is recovery: How well do people bounce back and recover fully from challenge (Masten, 2001; Rutter, 1987)? People who are resilient display a greater capacity quickly to regain equilibrium physiologically, psychologically, and socially following stressful events. Second and equally important is sustainability: the capacity to continue forward in the face of adversity (Bonanno, 2004). To address this aspect of resilience, we ask: How well do people sustain health and meaningful positive engagement within a dynamic and challenging environment? Healthy communities are those that confer these capacities for resilience to their constituents.

A community's resilience is best understood by applying ecological principles to the analysis of social systems in terms of these two defining features of resilience. With a focus on recovery, Black and Hughes (2001) defined *resilience* as "the ability of systems to cope with shocks and bounce back" (p. 16). Another definition offered in terms of *sustainability* is "the capacity of a system to tolerate disturbances while retaining its structure and function" (Fiksel, 2003, quoted in Fiksel, 2006, p. 16). Folke and colleagues (2002, p. 438) integrated these two proper-

ties when they identified three elements of resilience: "(1) the magnitude of shock that the system can absorb and remain within a given state; (2) the degree to which the system is capable of self-organization; and (3) the degree to which the system can build capacity for learning and adaptation."

The United Nations World Commission on Environment and Development (also known as the Brundtland Commission) in 1987 defined *sustainable development* as "development that meets the needs of the present without compromising the ability of future generations to meets their own needs" (Sustainable Pittsburgh, 2004, p. 82). As Folke and colleagues (2002, p. 439) point out, when resilience is synthesized in the context of sustainable development, at least three general policy recommendations can be drawn:

> The first level emphasizes the importance of policy that highlights interrelationships between the biosphere and the prosperous development of society; the second stresses the necessity of policy to create space for flexible and innovative collaboration towards sustainability; and the third suggests a few policy directions for how to operationalize sustainability in the context of social-ecological resilience.

We agree with Hancock (2000): A healthy community must also perforce be a resilient community, one that has the systems of governance and social capital needed to rebound from difficult times and sustain that which is most positive about its identity for its current and future inhabitants.

In summary, a resilience portfolio can help to inoculate communities against potential threats and crises, but it requires new perspectives, actions, and measures. Operationally this means a focus on identifying, conserving, and investing in human, social, intellectual, and physical capital, rather than expending large parts of that capital and the energy of its leadership in short-term, narrow programs, activities, and services (Churchill,

2003). Investment in valid indicators of social progress in keeping with a resilience perspective provides the kind of feedback needed to build more vibrant and sustainable communities. By taking the broad view of human and community health, and focusing on qualities that promote resilience, we make the task of identifying yardsticks for community resilience a challenging one. However daunting the complexities that underlie this approach, to attempt anything less would be to shortchange community potential and diminish chances of building on the positive forces of sustainable growth and development.

Finding and Applying the Right Indicators

According to the World Health Organization (WHO; 1986, as cited in Boothroyd & Eberle, 1990, p. 3), a *social indicator* is a "variable which helps to measure change." Innes (1990) defines an *indicator* as "simply a set of rules for gathering and organizing data so they can be assigned meaning." To enrich definition, analogies are often used to illustrate the concept. For example, a report from the Sustainable Seattle (1995, cited in Phillips, 2005) project likens indicators to "gauges and dials of an aircraft's instrument panel." This metaphor has meaning for the Seattle community, the home of Boeing and one of greatest concentrations of engineers in the United States. Review of the substantial community indicators literature shows that many analogies have been applied to clarify the meaning of indicators, and that indicators have been used to serve different overlapping primary functions. We have summarized these functions, which are shown in Table 17.2, and include description, simplification, measurement, trend identification, clarification, communication, and catalyst for action (Phillips, 2005).

Indicators also have great practical power. As noted in *Resilience: Health in a New Key*, "what gets measured gets done" (St. Luke's Health Initiatives [SLHI], 2003, p. 17). Since much of what has been measured to date focuses on risk rather than resilience, targets for action are often reactive and defensive, designed more to avoid deeper problems than to increase capacities.

Indicators of community life derive in part from the work of social scientists on the broader domain of social indicators. This work, begun in the latter half of the past century, focused on the development of measures of social progress that would parallel the gathering of data to provide "economic indicators" of the vitality of regions of the country. It was evident then, and subsequently reinforced by numerous observations of the uneven growth and decay of quality of life even in economically flourishing communities, that a balanced approach is needed to chart progress in regional community development (Swain, 2002). Indeed, founders of the United States acknowledged the importance of gathering data on the social condition of our nation by including in the U.S. Constitution the requirement that the government conduct a periodic census of its people. Although the original U.S. Census of 1790 comprised a mere six questions about the number, race, and age of people living in each household, the Census has evolved as the most comprehensive national dataset detailing the nation's demographic, social, and economic conditions and change. Social researchers have relied heavily on these data to interpret quality-of-life trends, progress, and challenges of the society.

Of interest as well has been the concern for inclusion of indicators of quality of life that include the perspectives of the community members themselves, as well as urban planners and social scientists. Following the lead of research pioneers in North America and Europe, social scientists in other regions of the world have adopted and refined social "barometers" to monitor progress in enhancing the welfare and well-being of citizens (Moller, Huschka, & Michalos, 2008). A distinctive feature is that these barometers

TABLE 17.2. Functions of Community Indicators

Function	Description	Answers the question ...
Description	Describe conditions or problems. Increase general understanding.	"What are things like?"
Simplification	Simplify complexity; provide a representative picture with significance extending to a larger phenomena of interest.	"What's the big picture?"
Measurement	Measure characteristics of quality of life; measure performance of activities or services.	"How much?"
Trend identification	Establish baseline data; identify trends or patterns; show direction, improvement, disintegration, and plateaus. Two types:	
	1. Past orientation. Indicators are chosen in light of their "historical trend–identification properties" (MacLaren, 1996, p. 9), showing how dimensions of an identified phenomenon have been changing;	"How did we do?"
	2. Future orientation. The indicator is a "forward-looking instrument" (MacLaren, 1996, p. 9), used as a predictive, forecasting device.	"Where are we headed?"
Clarification	Clarify analytical issues or long-term goals; highlight areas of concern or improvement.	"What's most important?"
Communication	Translate data into terms that are understandable by wide range of users.	"How do we explain ... ?"
Catalyst for action	Stimulate public, stakeholder, and political awareness, as well as interest and will to work toward change.	"What next?"

Note. Data from Phillips (2005).

measure both individual and societal quality of life. Designed to capture nuances in local definitions of progress, regional barometers are unique expressions of regional indicators of the good life.

Much of this work rests on inventories constructed by researchers to examine individuals' perceptions of their own health and well-being (Andrews & Withey, 1976; Campbell & Converse, 1972). In these efforts, individuals are asked to rate their well-being and satisfaction with their own lives. Interestingly, this work uncovered distinct differences between perceptions of quality of life, as defined by the subject, in contrast to those defined by social indicators. The disconnect between the two sets of findings suggests the need to incorporate ways of estimating both social and psychological well-being with community indicators.

One of the major advancements in field of social indicators has been the study of environmental issues. Cobb and Rixford (1998) highlight that this area of emphasis has made extraordinary advances in theory development. The ecological framework has advanced the indicator movement beyond solely descriptive statistics to an examination of theoretical frameworks of change and development of a future orientation. By looking to the future, environmental indicators can identify the impact of current systems and practices, and develop alternative means for enhancing future outcomes in the ecosystem.

Many Types of Indicators

The number of indigenous community indicator programs has grown in recent decades. Dluhy and Swartz (2006) identified over 200 community-based indicator projects in the United States alone. As a part of the international Social Indicators Research Series project, two volumes provide a compilation of cases of best work in community indicators research (Sirgy, Rahtz, & Lee, 2004; Sirgy, Rahtz, & Swain, 2008). These cases from around the globe, including several from the United States, use a uniform approach to describe and evaluate community indicator experiences:

- History of community indicators work within the region
- Planning of community indicators
- Actual indicators selected
- Data collection process
- Reporting of results
- Use of indicators to guide community development decisions and public policy

The recent community indicators movement has employed largely bottom-up planning, in which each community has set its own goals and monitored its own changes. This stands in contrast to previous efforts led primarily by governments to examine national trends. Indeed, democratic theory dictates that to some extent the desired outcomes and the important dimensions to evaluate vary across communities. However, one key limitation of a bottom-up, community-based approach is the lack of a unified conceptual framework in which communities of location and interest can work together for the benefit of the whole region. An effective response to this limitation would be a universal conceptual framework, with the flexibility to adapt, taking local characteristics and circumstances into account.

Ongoing Social and Community Indicator Programs

A number of U.S. communities are setting the pace for developing community indicators of resilient processes and incorporating those indicators into ongoing community building efforts. Table 17.3 describes some of the leaders in this emerging field.

Perhaps because of its relative longevity, the Jacksonville Community Council, Inc. ([JCCI], 2005) is repeatedly cited as one of the leading efforts and was highlighted in the well known book *Smart Communities: How Citizens and Local Leaders Can Use Strategic Thinking to Build a Brighter Future* by Morse (2004; see also Sirgy et al., 2008, pp. 1–22; see also Swain, 2002). JCCI was established in 1975 and has consistently worked to increase the dialogue of Jacksonville's current state and function, and the future it hopes to attain for itself. Their mission is to engage "diverse citizens in open dialogue, research, consensus building and leadership development to improve the quality of life and build a better community in Northeast Florida and beyond" (JCCI, n.d., paragraph 1). As is the case with many other indicator mission statements, the leaders of this nonpartisan civic organization proclaim the importance of indicators in opening a civic dialogue on the current status and functioning of their communities.

Although each of the cases mentioned in Table 17.3 has adopted different approaches, they share important common elements. To begin, each is a fully collaborative venture, incorporating ideas and resources from many sectors of the community, including governments, universities, nonprofits, private firms, and the general citizenry. They have all developed extensive processes to help derive and use key indicators. A major part of the process work focuses on stimulating and sustaining genuine grassroots participation, while including various community "experts" and policymakers in the processes. The result is that while chosen indicators and goals differ by community,

TABLE 17.3. Examples of Exemplary U.S. Community Indicator Projects

Sustainable Pittsburgh

Committed to affecting regional decision-making processes, so that regard for sustainability in economic, environmental, and social ventures alike is incorporated, the nonprofit organization Sustainable Pittsburgh developed and produced a set of performance indicators in 2002. This set of indicators proved to be only the beginning for Sustainable Pittsburgh, for they have led the organization to develop Affiliate Network Topic Teams, through which action items are developed by participating community members to move the region closer to its goals of creating a sustainable environment and economy, and sustainable system of social equity. For more information, log onto *www.sustainablepittsburgh.org.*

Community Indicators Initiative of Spokane

Harnessing the resources of partners such as Eastern Washington University, the City of Spokane, and the Spokane County United Way, the Community Indicators Initiative of Spokane, Washington, has been able to engage its community toward the lofty goal of democratizing data in the name of improving communities. From these indicators, which culminated in a comprehensive report in 2005, local organizations and community-based groups are able to glean data for making organizational and community decisions. For more information, log onto *www.communityindicators.ewu.edu.*

Jacksonville Community Council, Inc.

The Jacksonville Community Council, Inc. (JCCI) is a pioneer in the field of community indicators. For more than 20 years, the JCCI has collected and disseminated information on the quality of life in the Jacksonville area of Florida by utilizing a comprehensive list of more than 100 indicators in nine areas of interest, including arts and culture, education, public safety, and health. The JCCI—comprised of expert staff and citizen volunteers—is able to produce comprehensive reports for use by government, business leaders, and other citizens in making decisions and taking action to improve the community's state of being. For more information, log onto *www.jcci.org.*

Sustainable Seattle

For more than 15 years, the nonprofit organization Sustainable Seattle has sought to enhance quality of life in the Seattle area by providing communities with information to make choices that lead to a more sustainable future. As part of this effort, in the mid-1990s, the organization began developing a set of regional indicators through an inclusive process of community participation that drew on citizens' values and goals. While pleased with early efforts, which led to the publication of multiple reports of indicators for community use, Sustainable Seattle reassessed its indicator project in the early part of the 21st century, with an eye toward making the product more effective and beneficial to the community. This has led the organization to develop neighborhood-based indicators (to complement the ongoing system of regional indicators) and a comprehensive plan for moving the indicators from assessment to action to garner sustainability for the Seattle area in the long term. For more information, log onto *www. sustainableseattle.org.*

Truckee Meadows Tomorrow

Based in Reno, Nevada, the nonprofit organization Truckee Meadows Tomorrow is dedicated to providing information that will lead decision makers to create positive change within communities. Working with a set of 33 indicators of the quality of life in northern Nevada, Truckee Meadows Tomorrow publishes an annual Community Well-Being Report, which highlights not only the area's current state of being but also policies and programs that actively work toward counteracting negative trends in the community. But their work does not end there. They actively encourage community members to take a personal interest in changing their community's status by personally adopting an indicator as a tool to drive advocacy and service efforts, by participating in their online forum to discuss issues with like-minded community members, and by joining their organization. For more information, log onto *www. truckeemeadowstomorrow.org.*

(cont.)

TABLE 17.3. *(cont.)*

City of Santa Monica

In the mid-1990s, the City of Santa Monica heeded the community's concern that current progress might be coming at the price of future generations' well-being, by developing and adopting a plan to base citywide decisions on the premise of sustainability. In short, they keep an eye to the future when making decisions about the present. The City of Santa Monica does so through the assistance of its Sustainable City Plan (2006)—a set of goals and indicators for all segments of the community developed by city staffers and a group of community stakeholders that operated under an agreed-upon set of 10 guiding principles of sustainability. This plan for the City of Santa Monica has over time become embedded within the fabric of its decision-making processes, to the extent that the city finds itself not only meeting its targets but (in many instances) also exceeding them. For more information, log onto *www.smgov.net/epd/scp/index.htm.*

Boston Indicators

The Boston Foundation, Greater Boston's community foundation—grant maker, partner in philanthropy, key convener, and civic leader—coordinates the Boston Indicators Project in partnership with the City of Boston and the Metropolitan Area Planning Council. The Project relies on the expertise of hundreds of stakeholders gathered in multiple convenings to frame its conclusions, and draws data from the wealth of information and research generated by the region's excellent public agencies, civic institutions, think tanks, and community-based organizations. For more information, log onto *www.bostonindicators.com.*

there is substantial overlap of concepts and measures. In addition, these examples show significant signs of sustainability and impact on community dialogue, and in some cases policy actions.

Two potential flaws are also identifiable in these examples. First, they often identify many indicators that raise questions about community priorities and focus. Second, it is difficult to determine policy and theoretical accountability for some indicators. If the community group finds indicator(s) moving in an undesirable direction, they must determine the reason for change and who is likely to respond. Depending on the indicator, this can be a difficult assignment.

Community Resilience Indicators or Community Domains

At the heart of every community, system, or organization is a basic, underlying framework, or *infrastructure*. In communities of place, infrastructure is often used as a synonym for the *built environment*. Yet full community infrastructure means much more than the basic facilities, services, and

installations. Beyond physical and formal elements are other, evolving elements of community, including the social, civic, economic, environmental, and human connections that intersect in functioning communities. Building full community capacity is a long-term balancing act that requires reasoned investment in each of these community domains, and sustained evaluation of separate and combined effects on community infrastructure of such investments. Continuous appraisal that focuses on how these domains connect and reinforce each other is essential to building resilience processes and outcomes.

Important elements of resilience at individual and community levels dictate continuous learning and adapting to indicators of changing community infrastructure and capacity. For example, there is the central resilience concept of protective factors. Research reveals a list of protective factors that can reside within the individual, family, or community. These can be biological, psychological, social, or environmental, and they interplay with risk factors to set the threshold for likely susceptibility or resilience in the face of stress. Positive kith and kin relations are one example of protective factors. Extent of negative social ties is a risk factor. Members of a community may have varying levels of engagement in both beneficial and distressing social interactions (Finch, Okun, Barrera, Zautra, & Reich, 1989).

Resilience, which can help to inoculate communities against potential threats and crises, requires new perspectives, actions, and measures. Operationally this means a focus on identifying, conserving, and investing in the human, social, intellectual, and physical capital that make up its protective elements rather than expending large parts of that capital and energy of its leadership in short-term, narrow programs, activities, and services (Churchill, 2003, p. 357). Investments in these domains, linked to good indicators of impacts, help us to learn about, adapt, and harness the power of resilience to build more vibrant and sustainable communities.

Many items from the abundant list of actual and potential community indicators derived from examples described in this chapter can provide the kind of feedback and systems guidance that communities need for strategic choice and investment. In fact, when one begins to think seriously about operational community indicators, the first words that may come to mind are *information overload*. Data abound from the U.S. Census; local Councils of Government; a multitude of national, state, and local governments and agencies; educational institutions and think tanks; various public opinion polls; and many more sources. We are convinced that resilience and community health, broadly defined, require tracking a robust and relatively compact set of indicators as opposed to covering all likely measures. The key question is, how might such a powerful set of indicators be built? Can a resilience index be developed from these mountains of data: If so, how? Knowing that others have faced these challenges, and wanting to understand better community resilience indicators, processes, and outcomes,

we began by surveying the recent literature, websites, reports, and conferences that have piqued our curiosity about community indicators, and attempting to solve this particular Rubik's Cube. Here is what we found:

1. Great variation in communities represented. To begin with, the standard variation in definition of *community* mentioned early in this chapter is reflected by existing studies. More subtle but very important differences can be found in value preferences that are apparent when we compare these reports. Some communities emphasize environment, others economic development, still others education, and so forth. These differences are often the result of leadership and membership in groups sponsoring the various community indicators projects, or sometimes simply the result of researchers' interest in particular aspects of community. Whatever the roots of such differences, value preferences help to sort and select indicators. A pure focus on community resilience indicators needs to control for these biases and be fully transparent about values represented by indicators.

2. A tilt toward deficits, but assets are frequently represented. We expected to find many measures of community deficits in these studies and reports, and we were not disappointed. Crime rates, air quality violations, congestion measures, high school dropout rates, neighborhood violence indicators, and much more are used repeatedly to signal community decline and distress, whereas improvements on these dimensions are interpreted to mean improved community health. Yet among these studies we were also able to find many asset measures. A list of frequently retrieved traditional risk (deficit) and community resilience (asset) indicators is located in Table 17.4. A critical need in building resilient communities is realism. This means a balanced, as well as frequent, appraisal of assets and deficits. A robust system of community resilience indicators needs to promote feedback and balance.

3. Genuine, relatively widespread involvement of a diverse array of community stakeholders contributes to lasting and meaningful changes in community resilience processes and outcomes. Resilience thrives on conscious choice and is only enhanced by the thoughtfulness of a wide range of constituencies raising collective attention to shared frameworks that can advance and protect community well-being.

Communities differ greatly in history, past investments, leadership priorities, perceived and actual needs, and many other ways. For these reasons, development of various forms of capital investment and community capacity building need to involve community members who know the area well and use methods of engagement that fit the local culture. Yet, out of the mountains of available information, some frequently encountered indicators tie directly to central infrastructure investment choices despite great variation in community settings.

Almost any community would want to consider such "prime" indicators. A sample of indicators that can be tied directly to resilience propositions has been frequently advocated in several community building projects and studies, and has wide applicability for various types of communities. These indicators are described below by major categories or domains of community infrastructure. Importantly, some of these indicators cross the somewhat artificial boundaries of domain and type of community. We consider these boundary-crossing indicators to be particularly powerful "prime indicators" and potential candidates for a new CRI that can be used and adapted to many communities.

Physical Infrastructure

At the center of many communities is physical capacity—housing, transportation systems, energy resources, sustainable environment, land use, and so forth—that helps to define community and community readiness. Akin to individual "basic needs," some level of investment and planning in this realm is required for communities to exist and to aspire to greater resilience in other community realms. Vast data systems portray these dimensions of community change and development. In fast-growth areas such as the emerging Phoenix–Tucson Megapolitan region (Gammage, Hall, Lang, Melnick, & Welch, 2008; Lang & Dhavale, 2005), there is much focus on indicators of congestion, response time for emergencies, high environmental and capital costs of rapid growth, and the enormously important major issues of sustainability, carrying capacity, prosperity, and well-being that result from growth for all residents.

A deficit perspective is often coupled with a perceived need to "catch up," resulting in substantial investments in the basic needs of growing urban places. There is plenty of information about miles of roadways under construction, cost of housing units being built, various forms of air pollution, and so forth. But what do these measures mean? What are the full implications of increase miles of new freeways, thousands of new homes per month, hundreds of millions of dollars invested in new office buildings, and so forth? And what about asset measures such as:

- Per capita new spending for alternative forms of transportation
- Affordable housing index
- Parks and open space, actual and planned
- Rates and types of human adaptation to dramatic changes in the physical environment
- Annual loss of open desert acreage to new development

Healthy communities need to dig deeper to look for measures sensitive to capital investment and development that promote greater connectivity, less isolation, and effective communication channels. Communities should be able to track physical infrastructure responses to rapidly changing, diversifying forces and technologies to answer the question: Within this context of fast change and enormous growth, what are the impacts of physical infrastructure on human connectivity?

Social Infrastructure

Social capital has been much more widely discussed in recent years due in large part to Robert Putnam's comprehensive and well-articulated argument in the book *Bowling Alone* (2001). Social capital, the derivative of networks of people who trust and assist each other, is an extremely important community asset. By tracking indicators of social capital, such as membership in organizations that traditionally have provided forums for developing community networks, Putnam argues that this valuable community commodity is in decline. But the social capital discussion, which has been going on for some time in scholarly articles, lacks unanimity for very good reasons that center on indicators.

First, there is the "strength of weak ties" argument (Granovetter, 1973); that is, in present and future community contexts of high rates of migration, population, and technological change, new opportunities and networks are being created and may to some extent be replacing older forums for social capital. Closely connected to this concern is the observation that organizations lamented as being in decline have often promoted a form of solidarity, resulting in high social capital for members and exclusion of nonmembers. The resulting impact can be less communitywide capacity to trust and assist in the face of threat. This is the "too much social capital" fear.

Communities need to pay careful attention to indicators of social capital development in both newer and older forms. Key indicators that help communities track and understand social capital formation might include the following:

- Places, public and private, for exchange, communication, and dialogue about community issues
- Sources of community news
- The full range and number of organizations that connect people at various levels of community (block watches, neighborhood associations, community centers, planning groups, etc.).
- "Trust index" rates that attempt to measure levels of trust within neighborhoods and communities (Putnam, 2001; Sampson, 1988)

Civic Infrastructure

Civic infrastructure is the formal and informal processes and networks through which communities make decisions, solve problems, and plot future courses. This governance process involves government actors as important players, but in most successful communities it is much more than government. Community governance follows formal and informal processes, and relies on interdependence of business, nonprofit organizations, government, and citizens. This is like the collaborative associational process described by Tocqueville early in the nation's history, avoided and at times abandoned by some political bosses over the evolution of community development and governance, that now increasingly is seen as the formula for communities that want to avoid political infighting and gridlock to make lasting decisions and seize opportunities. Like a community's physical infrastructure, a civic infrastructure that has deteriorated needs to be renovated and maintained on an ongoing basis. In newer communities, the civic infrastructure has to be built (National Civic League, 1999). The quality of the civic infrastructure is an important determinant of community health, broadly defined.

The *Civic Index*, which measures the skills and processes that a community must possess to deal with its unique concerns and aspirations, allows communities to inventory and unleash their powers and abilities by evaluating and improving their civic infrastructure (National Civic League, 1999). Key indicators drawn from that work include the following:

- Rates of participation in the political process (multilevel)
- Local indigenous leadership profiles, numbers, and quality measures. Who is making community decisions?
- Number of community committees, councils, and cross-sector groups focusing on community issues.
- Forms of governance, major changes in roles and rules of governance.

Economic Infrastructure

Many components connect to make up a community economy. Obvious strengths, such as vast supplies of valuable physical resources, have been considered as economic advantages for some places. Yet, as the global economy tips toward the primacy of knowledge-based products and services, a reevaluation of economic resources and capacities is needed. In addition to that determination of community economic assets, and ways to build on them, is the essential community health need to develop strategies that increase prosperity for all, while decreasing income inequalities between "haves" and "have nots."

From a resilience perspective, the challenge is to design ways to respond to community shocks by producing the goods and services needed, and by recovering economic capacity quickly. Economic resilience impacts various levels of the economic system, including the individual business and household, the market, and the regional economy as a whole. Economic resilience fosters ability to maintain normal economic function by actions such as conserving resources, importing needed goods, or reallocating resources according to price signals that indicate their relative scarcity. It also includes adaptive measures in the face of a crisis, such as conserving at greater than normal levels

or using various central planning interventions, such as information clearinghouses to match suppliers with customers. Indicators of a resilient economic infrastructure might include the following:

- Higher employment rates
- Creation of higher paying jobs
- Decrease in income inequality
- Rates of business and private sector representation in community planning

Human Development Infrastructure

This area includes investment in education and training, over the lifespan and broadly defined. As in the other areas of community infrastructure, resilience actions mean bringing all logical and available assets into the educational effort. A community's formal education system is like its formal government—heavily involved but not the only player. Communities that make the most of their educational resources promote mentoring, training, coaching, and so forth, in many different settings and among various volunteers and community leaders, as well as within the formal education system. Full development of human capital is central to community building and closely related to development of the community's economic infrastructure. Indicators of a more resilient human capital infrastructure might include the following:

- Lifelong learning opportunities
- Retraining, mentoring programs
- Measures of educational achievement and skills development
- Leisure activities
- Per capita education system–penal system spending ratios

Health and Well-Being Infrastructure

Investment in organizations, programs, and community collaborations that promote health and well-being, broadly defined, is obviously an important contribution to community resilience. It is also true that invest-ment in particular public health prevention and education efforts may reap large and long-term public benefits for the commu-nity. The outcomes of these efforts may be revealed in health and well-being improve-ments across a wide spectrum of conditions. Here, attention may be focused on those ill-nesses most affected by psychological, social, and environmental conditions. For example, cardiovascular risk reduction involves more attention to healthy lifestyle and stress man-agement than to cancer prevention. More-over, concern for health resilience needs to extend beyond the prevention of ill health to include attention to restoration of well-being and the sustainability of functioning among those with chronic illness. How much capac-ity for independent functioning is sustained among persons with potentially disabling conditions, such as osteoarthritis, is the kind of resilience-based approach to the selection of indicators of favorable health outcomes that we advocate.

It is also quite important to realize that in-dicators are imperfect in many ways. Chang-ing conditions, new data sources, degree of confidence in inference, and theoretical advance frequently call for refinement and change in indicators, which, after all, merely "indicate" phenomena. For example, an im-portant indicator of obesity, the *body mass index* (BMI), divides weight by the square of a person's height. Yet recent research points to the danger of "internal fat" surrounding vital organs, and invisible to the naked eye, which is not well represented by this stan-dard indicator.

It is essential in this, as in all other areas of community infrastructure, that profession-als interact closely with nonprofessionals in planning and implementing health and well-being efforts. Indicators that may be useful in this domain include the following:

- Marriage/divorce ratios
- Physical, social, and emotional health
- Life expectancy

- Infant health measures
- Vitality (energy vs. fatigue)

Toward a CRI: Community Dialogue and Prime Indicators of Resilience

As reviewed earlier, our process of close examination of indicators used to measure community change and progress was fruit-ful. Many good measures of key community dimensions are available and being used. Yet selection of "prime indicators" required ad-ditional analysis and consideration. To start that process, we reviewed this domain clas-sification and resulting indicators with a diverse group of Phoenix area community leaders and stakeholders with substantial experience in the language and practice of community health and resilience. In focus group sessions we probed for depth of mean-ing and refinements, and had rich and robust discussions of potential resilience indicators for the Phoenix region.[2]

Following these meetings, we then looked very closely at the pool of good indicators to find the best ones—those that appeared frequently in the literature and generated the most enthusiasm among experienced community reviewers. Finally, building on our appraisal of indicator literature and dialogues with community stakeholders and leaders, we selected as prime indicators mea-sures that seemed to be central to community resilience. Importantly, we searched for and found indicators that crossed the boundaries of community domains and types of com-munities and in themselves were unifying connecting rods of community resilience.

Before reviewing the actual prime indica-tors selected, we should alert the reader to important considerations in the selection of prime indicators.

Wide Variation in Type of Community

As described earlier in this chapter, there is great variation in type of community represented in the literature and participants around the table at such community meetings. Despite the virtually universal importance of certain concepts, such as social cohesion, to resilience in virtually any community, differences in data availability, community vision and purpose, and much more, make development of indicators equally applicable to all communities problematic. The central message here is twofold. First, prime indicators should apply to and be measurable for many communities. Yet community variability requires that prime indicators be carefully reviewed and often supplemented in inclusive community processes.

As noted in the *Health in a New Key* pocket guide, this means that different communities need to remain open to multiple resilience indices. "Individual and community development proceeds across and among the buckets and silos of specific index factors. Everything singular becomes plural. Don't rush to develop one 'bottom line' index" (SLHI, 2005, p. 14).

Account for Qualitative Dimensions

Several indicators of important resilience concepts rest on basic, generally available descriptive data. Number of acres of parks, number of public employees (e.g., police and teachers), miles of highways, and much more, are examples of the one-dimensional, descriptive nature of many indicators. In our community focus group discussions, the need to understand quality, what lies beneath the numbers, was emphasized. For example, in addition to the number of neighborhood organizations, the importance of measuring the vitality, quality, and productivity of these organizations, as well as the quality of the changing social network that links them together, was repeatedly emphasized. This concern also compels communities to look carefully at ways to augment and better understand prime indicators, and to understand the limits inferred by these indicators. Our earlier recommendation concerning the

development of citizen panels provides one methodology for dealing with this concern.

Understand the Complex Connections between Community Indicators and Actions

Some indicators are more likely than others to change, based on direct community action. Exogenous forces beyond the control of many communities may result in greater or lesser resources and capacities. Closely related, the causal distinction between process and outcome indicators is easily made in some cases, more blurry in others. Understanding this, some communities may want to focus on indicators of resilience that are clearly and directly impacted by community action. Yet a long-term, comprehensive view suggests tracking and accounting for important baseline measures that are not easily changeable.

The Prime Indicators

With these considerations in mind, we developed a list of those indicators that seem most valuable and valid across domains and types of communities (Table 17.4). These appear frequently in other community indicator projects and studies, were reflected in our discussion sessions with community stakeholders, and represent key elements of resilience theory. The "prime indicators" selected for reasons noted earlier are not presented as an inclusive and complete list. Nevertheless, they are measurable, overlapping concepts that provide a useful baseline for many communities. A community that improves over time on several of these indicator dimensions is likely to build resilience capacity. One that shows improvement on all dimensions would almost certainly be on the path to greater resilience. And, perhaps most importantly, a community that uses these indicators as a launching pad to develop a forward-looking resilience program for its constituency will have made great progress in moving toward a more resilient future.

TABLE 17.4. Twelve Prime Indicators of Community Resilience Capacity

Traditional risk indicators →	Community resilience indicators
1. Homeless rates	1. Affordable housing
2. Families below poverty line	2. Income equality
3. Illiteracy rates	3. Home Internet access
4. High school dropout rates	4. Educational attainment
5. Low voter turn out/registration	5. Elected leadership diversity
6. Prevalence rates for chronic illness	6. Rates of recovery of healthy functioning following illness
7. Rank on City Stress Index	7. Rank on United Way "State of Caring Index"
8. Emergency room utilization	8. Access to health care
9. Traffic congestion	9. Public space, including public park acreage, bike and walking paths, open space, etc.
10. Air pollution	10. Air quality
11. Crime rates	11. Recidivism rates
12. Discrimination	12. Perceptions of social trust and cohesion

Notes

1. In 1984, the World Health Organization (WHO) first extended the concept of health from the individual level to both individual and group levels. It says, "Heath is defined as the extent to which an individual or group is able, on one hand, to realize aspirations and satisfy needs; and, on the other hand, to change or cope with the environment. Health is, therefore, seen as a resource for everyday life, a dimension of our 'quality of life,' and not the object of living; it is a positive concept emphasizing social and personal resources, as well as physical capabilities" (WHO, 1986, quoted in Boothroyd & Eberle, 2000, p. 3).
2. For more detail on our Phoenix area community development work, see Hall and Zautra, (2008), and Zautra, Hall, and Murray (2008).

Acknowledgments

We wish to acknowledge the dedication and diligence of Billie Sandberg and Kate Murray in preparation of this chapter. Order of authorship for this chapter was determined by the toss of a coin.

References

American Psychiatric Association. (1994) *Diagnostic and statistical manual of mental disorders* (4th ed.). Washington, DC: Author.

Andrews, F. M., & Withey, S. B. (1976). *Social indicators of well-being: Americans' perceptions of life quality.* New York: Plenum Press.

Berkman, L. F., & Syme, S. L. (1979). Social networks, host resistance, and mortality: A nine-year follow-up study of Alameda County residents. *American Journal of Epidemiology, 109,* 186–204.

Black, A., & Hughes, P. (2001). *The identification and analysis of indicators of community strength and outcomes.* Canberra, Australia: Department of Family and Community Services.

Bolland, J. M., & McCallum, D. M. (2002). Neighboring and community mobilization in high-poverty inner-city neighborhoods. *Urban Affairs Review, 38,* 42–69.

Bonanno, G. A. (2004). Loss, trauma, and human resilience: Have we underestimated the human capacity to thrive after extremely aversive events? *American Psychologist, 59,* 20–28.

Boothroyd, P., & Eberle, M. (1990). *Healthy communities: What they are, how they're made.* Vancouver, BC, Canada: UBC Centre for Human Settlements.

Brodsky, A. E., O'Campo, P. J., & Aronson, R. E. (1999). PSOC in community context: Multi-level correlates of a measure of psychological sense of community in low-income, urban neighborhoods. *Journal of Community Psychology, 27,* 659–679.

Bures, R. M. (2003). Childhood residential stability and health at midlife. *American Journal of Public Health, 93,* 1144–1148.

Campbell, A., & Converse, P. E. (1972). *The human meaning of social change.* New York: Russell Sage Foundation.

Castro, F. G., Cota, M. K., & Vega, S. C. (1999). Health promotion in Latino populations: A sociocultural model for program planning, development, and evaluation. In R. M. Huff & M. V. Kline (Eds.), *Promoting health in multicultural populations: A handbook for practitioners* (pp. 137–168). Thousand Oaks, CA: Sage.

Chavis, D. M., & Wandersman, A. (1990). Sense of community in the urban environment: A catalyst for participation and community development. *American Journal of Community Psychology, 18,* 55–81.

Churchill, S. (2003). Resilience, not resistance. *City, 7*(3), 349–360.

Cobb, C. W., & Rixford, C. (1998). *Lessons learned from the history of social indicators.* San Francisco: Redefining Progress.

Cutrona, C. E., Russell, D. W., Hessling, R. M., Brown, P. A., & Murry, V. (2000). Direct and moderating effects of community context on the psychological well-being of African American women. *Journal of Personality and Social Psychology, 79,* 1088–1101.

Dluhy, M., & Swartz, N. (2006). Connecting knowledge and policy: The promise of community indicators in the United States. *Social Indicators Research, 79,* 1–23.

Duncan, T. E., Duncan, S. C., Okut, H., Strycker, L. A., & Hix-Small, H. (2003). A multilevel contextual model of neighborhood collective efficacy. *American Journal of Community Psychology, 32,* 245–252.

Farrell, S. J., Aubry, T., & Coulombe, D. (2004). Neighborhoods and neighbors: Do they contribute to personal well-being? *Journal of Community Psychology, 32,* 9–25.

Fiksel, J. (2003). Designing resilient, sustainable systems. *Environmental Science and Technology, 37,* 5330–5339.

Fiksel, J. (2006). Sustainability and resilience: Toward a systems approach. *Sustainability: Science, Practice, and Policy, 2,* 14–21. Retrieved June 26, 2007, from *ejournal.nbii.org/archives/vol2iss2/0608-028.fiksel.html.*

Finch, J. F., Okun, M. A., Barrera, M., Jr., Zautra, A. J., & Reich, J. W. (1989). Positive and negative social ties among older adults: Measurement models and the prediction of psychological distress and well-being. *American Journal of Community Psychology, 17,* 585–605.

Folke, C., Carpenter, S., Elmqvist, T., Gunderson, L., Holling, C. S., & Walker, B. (2002). Resilience and sustainable development: Building adaptive capacity in a world of transformations. *AMBIO: A Journal of the Human Environment, 31,* 437–440.

Folland, S. (2007). Does "community social capital" contribute to population health? *Social Science and Medicine, 64,* 2342–2354.

Galster, G. (1998). *An econometric model of the urban opportunity structure: Cumulative causation among city markets, social problems, and underserved areas.* Washington, DC: Fannie Mae Foundation.

Gammage, G., Hall, J. S., Lang, R. E., Melnick, R., & Welch, N. (2008). *The Sun Corridor: Arizona's megapolitan.* Phoenix: Morrison Institute for Public Policy, Arizona State University.

Granovetter, M. (1973). The strength of weak ties. *American Journal of Sociology, 78,* 1360–1380.

Hall, J. S., Jones, P. M., Snook, M., & Springer, C. G. (1998). *The Information Partnership: Planning a community information-sharing network for metropolitan Phoenix.* Phoenix: Arizona State University.

Hall, J. S., & Zautra, A. J. (2008). *Working toward the good life: Creating indicators of community resilience.* Unpublished workbook. Phoenix, AZ: Resilience Solutions Group and St. Luke's Health Initiatives.

Hancock, T. (2000). Healthy communities must also be sustainable communities. *Public Health Reports, 115,* 151–156.

Hyyppa, M. T., & Maki, J. (2003). Social participation and health in a community rich in stock of social capital. *Health Education Research, 18,* 770–779.

Innes, J. E. (1990). *Knowledge and public policy.* New Brunswick, NJ: Transaction.

Jacksonville Community Council, Inc. (2005). *Quality of life progress report: A guide for building a better community.* Jacksonville, FL: Author.

Jacksonville Community Council, Inc. (2006). *2006 Quality of Life Progress Report.* Jacksonville, FL: Author.

Jacksonville Community Council. (n.d.). Mission statement. Retrieved September 4, 2008, from *www.jcci.org/about/missionstatement.aspx.*

Kawachi, I., Kennedy, B. P., & Glass, R. (1999). Social capital and self-rated health: A contextual analysis. *American Journal of Public Health, 89,* 1187–1193.

Lang, R., & Dhavale, D. (2005). *Beyond megalopolis: Exploring America's new Megapolitan geography* (Census Report Series 05:01). Alexandria: Metropolitan Institute at Virginia Tech.

Lewin, K. (1951). *Field theory in social science: Selected theoretical papers.* New York: Harper & Row.

MacLaren, V. M. (1996). *Developing indicators of urban sustainability: A focus on the Canadian experience.* Toronto: ICURR Press.

Masten, A. S. (2001). Ordinary magic: Resilience processes in development. *American Psychologist, 56*(3), 227–238.

Moller, V., Huschka, D., & Michalos, A. C. (2008). *Barometers of quality of life around the globe: How are we doing?* Dordrecht: Springer.

Morse, S. W. (2004). *Smart communities: How citizens and local leaders can use strategic thinking to build a brighter future.* San Francisco: Jossey-Bass.

National Civic League. (1999). *The Civic Index: Measuring your community's civic health* (2nd ed.). Denver, CO: National Civic League.

Oldenburg, R. (1991). *The great good place.* New York: Marlowe.

Perkins, D., Florin, P., Rich, R., Wandersman, A., & Chavis, D. M. (1990). Participation and the social and physical environment of residential blocks: Crime and community context. *American Journal of Community Psychology, 18,* 83–115.

Phillips, R. (2005). *Community indicators measuring systems.* Aldershot, UK: Ashgate.

Price, R. H., & Behrens, T. (2003). Working Pasteur's quadrant: Harnessing science and action for community change. *American Journal of Community Psychology, 31,* 219–223.

Putnam, R. D. (2001). *Bowling alone: The collapse and revival of American community.* New York: Simon & Schuster.

Rutter, M. (1987). Psychosocial resilience and protective mechanisms. *American Journal of Orthopsychiatry, 57*(3), 316–331.

Santa Monica Sustainable City Plan. (2006). Santa Monica, CA: City of Santa Monica.

Sampson, R. J. (1988). Local friendship ties and community attachment in mass society: A multilevel systemic model. *American Sociological Review, 53,* 766–779.

Sampson, R. J., Raudenbush, S. W., & Earls, F. (1997). Neighborhoods and violent crime: A multilevel study of collective efficacy. *Science, 277,* 918–924.

Sarason, S. B. (1974). *Psychological sense of community: Prospects for a community psychology.* San Francisco: Jossey-Bass.

Sharkova, I. V., & Sanchez, T. W. (1999). *An analysis of neighborhood vitality: The role of local civic organizations.* Portland, OR: Center for Urban Studies, Portland State University.

Sirgy, M. J., Rahtz, D., & Lee, D. J. (2004). *Community quality-of-life indicators: Best cases I.* Dordrecht: Springer.

Sirgy, M. J., Rahtz, D., & Swain, D. (2008). *Community quality-of-life indicators: Best cases II.* Dordrecht: Springer.

United Way of Missoula County. (2001). *Social Indicators 2001.* Missoula, MT: Author.

St. Luke's Health Initiatives (SLHI). (2003). *Resilience: Health in a new key.* Phoenix, AZ: Author.

St. Luke's Health Initiatives. (2005). *Health in a new key: A pocket guide to developing healthy, resilient communities.* Phoenix, AZ: Author.

St. Luke's Health Initiatives (2008). *Health in a new key.* Phoenix, AZ: Author. Retrieved September 4, 2008, from *www.slhi.org/new_key/index.shtml.*

Steptoe, A., & Marmot, M. (2003). Burden of psychosocial adversity and vulnerability in middle age: Associations with biobehavioral risk factors and quality of life. *Psychosomatic Medicine, 65,* 1029–1037.

Stone, A. A., & Neale, J. M. (1982). Development of a methodology for assessing daily experiences. In A. Baum & J. E. Singer (Eds.), *Advances in environmental psychology: Environment and health* (pp. 49–83). Hillsdale, NJ: Erlbaum.

Subramanian, S. V., Kim, D. J., & Kawachi, I. (2002). Social trust and self-rated health in U.S. communities: A multilevel analysis. *Journal of Urban Health*, 79, S21–S34.

Sustainable Pittsburgh. (2004). *Sustainable Pittsburgh: Southwestern Pennsylvania regional indicators report*. Pittsburgh, PA: Author.

Swain, D. (2002). *Measuring progress: Community indicators and the quality of life*. Jacksonville, FL: Jacksonville Community Council, Inc.

Temkin, K., & Rohe, W. M. (1998). Social capital and neighborhood stability: An empirical investigation. *Housing Policy Debate*, 9, 61–88.

Unger, D. G., & Wandersman, A. (1985). The importance of neighbors: The social, cognitive, and affective components of neighboring. *American Journal of Community Psychology*, 13, 139–169.

United Nations World Commission on Environment and Development. (1987). *Our common future*. Oxford, UK: Oxford University Press.

Watson, D., Wiese, D., Vaidya, J., & Tellegen, A. (1999). The two general activation systems of affect: Structural findings, evolutionary considerations, and psychobiological evidence. *Journal of Personality and Social Psychology*, 76, 820–838.

Zautra, A. J. (2003). *Emotions, stress and health*. New York: Oxford University Press.

Zautra, A. J., Hall, J. S., & Murray, K. (2008). Community development and community resilience: An integrative approach. *Community Development*, 39, 1–18.

III

ETHNIC AND CULTURAL DIMENSIONS OF RESILIENCE

18

Cultural Adaptation and Resilience

Controversies, Issues, and Emerging Models

Felipe González Castro
Kate E. Murray

In this chapter we examine multiple factors, both environmental and individual, that operate as determinants of resilience development among adult immigrant populations. Migration from one geographic region to another is a universal process that occurs worldwide and on a daily basis. Additionally, the process of migration offers a natural mechanism for the study of cultural adaptation and resilience development among immigrants, who must cope with the challenges and stressors they encounter within a new cultural environment. Depending on the circumstances of migration, a multitude of events can promote beneficial or detrimental outcomes, thus influencing the quality of life of immigrants and their families.

Cultural adaptation is a complex process of adjustment in which daily experiences and individual, familial, and community factors influence the quality of life of diverse immigrants. In particular, discrimination based on race, religion, physical appearance, or other factors constitutes a major stressor encountered by many immigrants, particularly within national environments in which economic downturns foment conditions of prejudice and discrimination against "foreigners," and "illegal aliens," who are perceived as "threats to the society."

This chapter examines various factors and processes that influence well-being and quality of life, and the development of resilience as a form of adaptive coping in response to the challenges of immigration. We examine this process of migration and adjustment through a resilience model that examines individual, familial, and community factors as they influence this dynamic process of adjustment to a new host environment. In line with other chapters in this resilience handbook, we also explore definitions and conceptions of resilience in terms of processes and outcomes, and within the context of migration and cultural adaptation.

The Extent of Immigration Worldwide

In the recent past, remarkable changes have occurred worldwide involving accelerated patterns of migration and sociocultural mobility, industrial globalization, and the emergence of "transnational communities and networks," to an extent never seen before (Friedman, 2005; Williams, 1998). According to the United Nations (UN; 2002), based on data for the period from 1975 to 2000, the number of individuals living in a country other than where they were born doubled to an estimated 175 million people. Moreover, for the first time in history, the majority of people in the world are living in an urban setting (UN, 2008), an environment that invites greater levels of intercultural contact and exchange. These changing worldwide trends demand a greater understanding of human mobility as a consequence of greater cross-cultural contact, along with thoughtful planning to develop culturally responsive policies and programs to these complex changes.

The consequences of global migration are pervasive and significant. An abiding controversy involves whether to restrict border crossings given concerns over terrorism (LeGrain, 2006), and how to respond to globalization and the interdependency of individuals and nations (Friedman, 2005). The emergence of restrictive immigration policies can profoundly affect immigrants' life experiences, both for those who migrate before such policies are enacted, and for those hoping to migrate after these changes are in effect.

In recent years, research on migration and, in particular, acculturation research, have been roundly criticized (e.g., Hunt, Schneider, & Comer, 2004; Rudmin, 2006). Although acculturation has been a major focus of research with migrants and minority populations, such research has been compromised by weak definitions and the lack of methodological rigor. Accordingly, these studies have often yielded contradictory results and conclusions (Hunt et al., 2004). Based on these perspectives, within this chapter we (1) discuss a history of the migration and the acculturation literature; (2) examine the links between migration and resilience theory; and (3) explore racial/ethnic identity within the context of the experience of migration. Migration, either voluntary or forced, provides a unique opportunity to examine cultural adaptation and resilience outcomes that may occur as consequences of this dynamic process.

Overview of Stress and Resilience among Immigrant Populations

Resilience theory provides a useful framework for understanding the experience of migration. Resilience has been widely and variably used throughout the literature to describe various life experiences within diverse populations (Rutter, 1999). Nonetheless, the debate persists over how best to define and measure resilience, whether it is best conceptualized as an outcome, a dynamic process, a trait, or a state. In a comprehensive review of the resilience literature, Luthar (2006) defines *resilience* as "a phenomenon or process reflecting relatively *positive adaptation despite experiences of significant adversity or trauma*" (p. 742, original emphasis). Within this chapter, we also define *resilience* as positive adaptation to the stressors and challenges of migration, that is, an outcome that develops from persistent efforts at coping with the multiple and often chronic stressors encountered within the new environment. A major question here is, "Among immigrants, what constitutes positive adaptation, and what are the major determinants of this positive adaptation?"

Persons who migrate from one community to a new and distinctly different community face multiple stressors and related challenges that prompt the need for adaptation to these stressors. Among immigrants, a pervasive motivational factor that initially prompts migration is the quest for a better life (Portes & Rumbaut, 1996). However, several "setting" contexts influence the experience of migration and the severity of the stressors encountered. Such basic setting contexts include the conditions that precede the act of migration. These distinct setting contexts in turn have produced certain distinct immigrant groups, including (1) manual laborers who migrate to attain better paying jobs; (2) professionals and entrepreneurs who migrate to conduct business and to enhance their standard of living; and (3) refugees and asylum seekers who flee from war and/or persecution (Portes & Rumbaut, 1996).

In relation to differences in motivations for migration, several individual and environmental factors introduce related challenges during migration and adaptation to a new environment. The various stressors that typically influence this adaptation include language barriers; navigation of new cultural landscapes; changes in social networks and supports; and the logistical details of securing lodging, food, and other basic necessities (Padilla, Cervantes, Maldonado, & Garcia, 1988). Thus, resilience research examines *how* people respond to and cope with such challenges. The likelihood of positive adaptation is influenced by factors that facilitate the immigrant's integration into a new society or environment, as well as other factors that aid in the acquisition of new *cultural competencies*, including (1) acquiring *new knowledge* about local and regional laws and social customs; (2) learning *new occupational skills* and *linguistic skills*; and (3) establishing *new networks* of neighbors, acquaintances, friends, and others who can offer social support. These resources and personal competencies aid in attaining positive outcomes as immigrants navigate throughout their new sociocultural environment.

Acculturation research has found that immigrants who participate in the larger community, while also maintaining their native heritage (i.e., bicultural integration), tend to exhibit lower levels of distress (Berry, 2005). However, this conclusion and line of research has been criticized recently. The first major limitation is that many acculturation studies have primarily examined the experiences of minority populations in three similar countries: Australia, Canada, and the United States (Hunt et al., 2004). Individuals and groups within these Western cultures may experience lower levels of reported stress when integrating into these mainstream societies. By contrast, experiences of minority groups in underdeveloped nations may be radically different than experiences within these three Western nations. More research is needed that examines the interaction of various types of immigrants and types of environments for a more detailed understanding of the processes involved in acculturation change as it occurs within various nations.

Second, the definition of a *resilient outcome* is likely biased by the selective use of measures of *positive adaptation*. This issue relates to the ways in which resilient outcomes are measured across cultures, and also to the definition of *successful migration*. Ungar (2003) argues that researchers should utilize culturally appropriate emic outcomes. *Emic*, "bottom-up" research studies that utilize qualitative and mixed-methods approaches (Hanson, Creswell, Clark, Petska, & Creswell, 2005) are essential for understanding cultural meanings, nuances, and interpretations of the migration experience. These approaches can move beyond the biases introduced by the *etic*, or "top-down" selection of outcome measures, that *a priori* impose constraints on the definition of *successful adaptation*. That which host society research investigators may regard as *successful adaptation* may not coincide with the migrant's own beliefs about successful adaptation. For example, a migrant may exhibit outward indicators of successful adaptation, such as developing a large network of supportive interpersonal connections, gainful employment, and the absence of diagnosable physical or mental disorders. However, that person may also long for lost cultural comforts from his or her homeland. He or she may also mourn the loss of the social status he or she enjoyed within his or her native country, as well as feel devalued within the new community. From this person's perspective, life has not necessarily "gotten better," despite his or her having "made it," as defined by Western standards.

Furthermore, resilience can be viewed as a cumulative product of several attained markers of successful adaptation, or it can be domain specific. From a multidomain perspective, successful adaptation, a resilient outcome in one domain, such as employment or language acquisition, does not necessarily establish resilience in another domain, such as within the domain of psychological or social well-being. For example, in a study of Soviet Jewish adolescent refugees who migrated to the United States, Birman, Trickett, and Vinokurov (2002) found that *acculturation*, that is, cultural orientation to either the American or to the Russian culture, was associated with different outcomes. Acculturation toward the American culture was related to getting better grades in school and attaining support from American peers, whereas acculturation toward the Russian culture was related to perceived support from Russian peers. Moreover, acculturation to both cultures predicted lower reported loneliness and greater parental support. These findings illustrate the need for conducting measurements within multiple life domains, and the advantage of utilizing diverse indices of adaptation rather than relying on a single measure.

Therefore, we advocate the use of an integrative mixed-methods approach that utilizes objective and subjective measures of adaptation (Castro & Coe, 2007), measures that are also culturally and contextually appropriate. To some extent, successful outcomes that emerge from the migration experience involve adaptations that are congruent with the host community's norms or cultural standards. However, as suggested earlier, such adaptation does not preclude preservation of the migrant's native culture, values, beliefs, and quality-of-life standards because these also influence the migrant's overall acculturative trajectory and subjective perceptions of "having made it" within the new environment. In summary, measures of resilient outcomes must aptly assess each of several domains to capture more fully the complexities of these migration and adaptation experiences.

Concepts of Culture

First we must define what we mean by *culture* (Hunt et al., 2004). Given the existence of over 100 varied definitions (Baldwin & Lindsley, 1994), *culture* can be conceptualized as a rich, complex, and multifaceted construct. It embodies diverse "worldviews" and "lifeways," as observed within and across populations, subpopulations, and ethnic groups. Many scholars have identified core features of the construct of *culture*, generally defining it as standards of behavior acquired from membership within a group (Harwood, 1981). Thus, culture comprises a group's collective system of beliefs, values, expectations, and norms that are transmitted from elders to children, and culture encodes forms of problem solving that are useful for coping, adaptation, and survival (Thompson, 1969, as cited by Baldwin & Lindsley, 1994). Moreover, a group's cultural heritage is the source of its collective stories about ancestors and their achievements, and this includes the group's sacred or revered customs and traditions. Psychologically, a group's cultural heritage and identity confer a sense of "peoplehood," unity, and belonging, and these operate as the foundation of the group's collective ethnicity (McGoldrick & Giordano, 1996). Culture also comprises a system of communication that includes shared symbols and meanings utilized by members of that ethnic group or community. Moreover, Triandis and Brislin (1984) have distinguished between *objective* and *subjective* elements of culture: Objective elements are cultural items, such as works of art and physical structures, whereas subjective elements include psychological factors, such as beliefs, attitudes, norms, roles, and values.

Significant issues have emerged within the migration literature regarding ways in which culture has been conceptualized. First, different ethnic groups have often been combined under a generic label, such as when the Hispanic population is examined in its totality. This approach can gloss over the considerable within-group heterogeneity that exists among peoples from distinct national heritages, such as Cuban versus Spanish versus Mexican, and so on (Rogler, Cortes, & Malgady, 1991). It is thus doubtful that a single racial or ethnic label, such as "Hispanic," can provide a definitive category that aptly captures the complexity of cultural influences that govern the migrant experience (Hunt et al., 2004), while also taking into account this within-group heterogeneity. This does not mean that the broad-based examination of culture is irrelevant. To the contrary, the complexity of culture implies just the opposite. It is, however, essential to examine the distinct cultural elements that influence individual and societal experiences. Also important is a transdisciplinary approach that integrates research from several fields, including anthropology, sociology, and psychology. This transdisciplinary approach can also benefit from the use of qualitative and mixed-methods approaches, which are essential for attaining a "deep structure" (Resnicow, Soler, Braithwait, Ahluwalia, & Butler, 2000) understanding of culture, the process of migration, and its complex effects on cultural adaptation and resilience outcomes. In this regard, the renowned anthropologist Clifford Geertz (1983) espouses a *semiotic* concept of culture, identifying the role of meaning and the interpretation of experiences as core features in studies of culture. We also believe that a semiotic concept of migration is very important.

In one effort to capture the complexity of culture, Chao and Moon (2005) have introduced a framework, called the *cultural mosaic*, that examines a collage of elements that comprise a person's sociocultural identity. Based on the composite set of cultural elements (cultural tiles), such as demographic (e.g., age, race, ethnicity, gender), geographic (e.g., urban–rural status, region, or country), and associative elements (e.g., family, religion, profession) for each individual, a unique combination of elements is used to describe that person's unique cultural identity. As an extension of this framework, individuals in a given ethnic collective share many common elements (e.g., ethnicity, region or origin, religion) that in combination comprise their common identity. This cultural mosaic framework thus recognizes the complexity of culture at the individual level by describing a complex and multielement system, albeit one that has a definite organizational structure. This mosaic may appear complex, yet upon closer inspection, it exhibits a coherent and clearly identifiable structure.

Acculturation and Assimilation

As noted previously, *acculturation* is a worldwide phenomenon that occurs when individuals and families migrate from one sociocultural environment to another, usually in a quest for better living conditions and opportunities. One of the earliest definitions of *acculturation* was provided by Redfield, Linton, and Herskovits (1936), who described it as "the phenomena which result when groups of individuals having different cultures come into continuous first-hand contact, with subsequent changes in the original culture patterns of either or both groups" (p. 149). Notwithstanding this definition, early conceptions of acculturation posited that it was a linear, unidirectional process. Under this "melting pot" notion, acculturation was seen as inevitably resulting in full assimilation, a group's or a person's loss of their "culture of origin," with the ultimate adoption of the prevailing cultural lifeways within a new environment.

As noted above, the term *assimilation*, as contrasted with acculturation, has been used to refer to this final outcome, which ostensibly involves this "loss of ethnic identity" upon "blending into" the new culture. From this "all or none" perspective, early acculturation research measured acculturation in terms of a unidimensional continuum (Cuellar, Arnold, & Maldonado, 1995). This conception suggested this unidimensional progression involving complete assimilation with greater time spent within the new culture. From this perspective, full assimilation would thus constitute the natural and perhaps most adaptive outcome, involving a complete "blending into" the "mainstream" culture.[1] More recently, an *orthogonal acculturation framework* has been introduced, describing variations in cultural identity that comprise not only acculturation toward the mainstream culture, but also acculturation (enculturation) toward the native culture as this occurs among young migrants, and/or the maintenance of native-culture lifeways among elder migrants. Under this *orthogonal model* (Oetting & Beauvais, 1990), certain variations in cultural identities can develop, including the development of a full and balanced *bicultural/bilingual identity* (Berry, 1994; Cuellar et al., 1995; Marin & Gamboa, 1996).

Among the most commonly cited models of acculturation, Berry's (1997) two-factor model defines four possible acculturation experiences or outcomes: (1) *marginalization* (low affiliation with the new culture/host and with the native cultures), (2) *separation* (high native-culture affiliation, low new-culture affiliation), (3) *assimilation* (high new-culture affiliation, low native-culture affiliation), and (4) *integration* (high affiliation with both cultures). Thus, acculturation represents not a single ideal outcome but a person's (or group's) particular pattern of orientations toward each of two distinct core cultures. Implicit in this framework is that acculturation is *not* a linear process, but a dual-culture process of adaptation that involves four distinct acculturation outcomes. And under this framework it is now argued that acculturation is *not* a "zero-sum" process given that the acquisition of elements of one new culture *do not*

automatically involve the loss of elements from the culture of origin (Rogler, 1994; Rogler et al., 1991).

In summary, acculturation is typically now broadly conceptualized as a two-factor, bidimensional, and orthogonal process: (1) acculturation toward a new culture, and (2) acculturation toward the original native culture or the retention of that culture (i.e., *enculturation*) (Cuellar et al., 1995; Marin & Gamboa, 1996), although this conceptualization is not without its critics (Rudmin, 2003, 2006). As one criticism, these cultural orientations are not "all or none" processes, as suggested by this model (complete acceptance of complete rejection of one or both orientations), but instead may involve the elective acquisition of some elements of one of these "cultures," and not others, and the same goes for the abandonment of certain cultural elements and not others.

Despite these advances in definitions and measurement, a question persists as to whether existing models and measures aptly capture the complexity of migrant experiences under such basic models of acculturation. In accord with the complexities involved in defining culture and acculturation, questions persist in favor of developing more accurate and testable models that better describe the complexity of various migration experiences, and the processes of acculturation and cultural adaptation. Given that the process of migration, sociocultural mobility, and acculturative change is ubiquitous, introducing novel stressors that demand adaptation and modifications in personal and ethnic identity, the need exists for theory-driven and in-depth analyses of various acculturative processes. Such analyses may benefit from innovative yet rigorous methodologies that would produce more generative and informative research knowledge about identity development and the process of cultural adaptation as this occurs among various migrant and other racial/ethnic minority populations (Castro, 2007). Resilience theory provides a useful framework for such investigations.

Context and Acculturation

From a systemic ecodevelopmental perspective, *context* is recognized as a condition that influences many outcomes and their meaning, including the role of context as a condition that influences the process of acculturation (Castro, Shaibi, & Boehm-Smith, 2009). Individual, familial, and/or community adaptations typically occur within specific contextual domains, including situations, environments, familial systems, personalities, and biological contexts. For example, the experience of a Sudanese family fleeing violent conflict in their home village (a forced and dangerous situational context) and resettling through a federal humanitarian program in Sweden (a new and unfamiliar environmental context) will be radically different from the migration experiences of a French businessman (a voluntary and planned entrepreneurial situational context) who relocates to England (a new but familiar environmental context) for the purpose of enhancing wealth. Similarly, the experience of ethnic minority groups in New York City today differ from the experiences of minority groups who dwell within small rural towns in the U..S. Midwest (ecologically different environmental contexts). Thus, situational, environmental, historical, sociopolitical, and other contexts cannot be

overlooked as "surrounding" contextual factors that influence significantly the migrant's life experiences (Castro et al., 2009).

To understand more fully these experiences we must also conduct multilevel analyses in our studies of migration (see Table 18.1). Moreover, mixed-methods quantitative and qualitative approaches that explore nuances occurring at these individual, familial, community, and sociopolitical levels can help to describe the multiple systemic influences on the "real-world" adaptations of immigrants and their families. For example, we can describe multilevel analyses that influence social support. At an individual level, we can examine an immigrant's perceived support and language barriers that may limit access to sources of support. At a family level, we can assess the influence of family members, based on their role and involvement within the family, as well as examine the levels of cohesion that exist within that family. At a community level, we can explore the activity and membership of many families within a local community organization and local cultural networks. At a sociopolitical level, the analysis of family reunification and migration policies can set the context for chronic environmental stressors that may adversely affect the life chances of immigrants and their families. Each level of analysis can thus provide unique and complementary data

TABLE 18.1. Risk and Resource Factors during Migration

Level of analysis	Risk factors	Resource factors
Individual	• Language barriers • Social isolation	• Opportunities for education • Social ties (bridging and bonding capital)
Family	• Family conflict • Parent–child acculturation gap	• Social support • Pooled resources
Community	• Collective trauma • Discrimination	• Community organizations and leadership • Availability of interpreters
Societal	• Sociopolitical history of marginalization and discriminatory policies	• Intercultural political dialogue • Culturally responsive social policies

based on a more integrative and contextual analysis of these effects examined at multiple systemic levels.

Within this systemic context, certain events may exert differential effects on the process of acculturative change (Berry, 1994). For example, a specific event, such as the police shooting of a young and unarmed male Haitian immigrant, may impose considerable stress among residents of this Haitian community. This violent episode may be perceived as discrimination, and may accentuate the need for adaptive coping and resilience as members of this community mourn the loss of one of their own. Such contexts may facilitate certain kinds of acculturation while discouraging others. In summary, among immigrants, these various systemic contexts may exert varied and even bidirectional influences during the ongoing process of acculturation.

Resilience Theory: Bidimensional Effects

Increasing evidence supports the presence of distinct resilience-related processes: one that protects against harm, and another that promotes growth and goal attainment (see Zautra, Hall, & Murray, 2008, for further review). Traditionally, psychology research has focused on risk factors that predict ill health, which can occur as a consequence of the cumulative effects of illness and pathology. However, risk factors account for only some of the explanatory variance; we must also examine resource factors that predict positive health and adaptive outcomes to understand more fully the life experiences of various migrants. Evidence from evolutionary processes also suggests the benefits of positive emotions as salubrious influences on health (Fredrickson, 1998). Just as bidimensional models of acculturation emphasize that identification with one culture does not preclude identification with another, examining both risk and resource factors permits the development of more complex models of adaptation and resilience. There

is growing evidence of the independence of these two dimensions, for example, in studies of physiological functioning (Canli et al., 2001; Watson, Wiese, Vaidya, & Tellegen, 1999), and in the experiences of positive and negative emotions (Zautra, 2003).

Although not necessarily identified within this framework, existing literature supports the influences of both risk and resource factors as determinants of life outcomes among migrant populations. In Table 18.1 we provide illustrative, although not exhaustive, examples of risk and resource factors that may influence migration outcomes. Here, the case of social relations provides a useful exemplar. For an individual who has migrated with his or her family, social relations may serve as a significant source of emotional support, likely elevating the levels of positive emotions and psychological "uplifts." Family conflict, which may result from an acculturation gap between parents and children, constitutes a separate risk factor that predicts higher levels of negative affect, and perhaps other indicators of poor individual and/or family outcomes (Farver, Narang, & Bhadha, 2002).

Acculturative Change and Resilience

Many investigators have written about the process of cultural adaptation as examined through the *process of acculturation*, although few studies have truly examined or modeled acculturation as a *process of acculturative change* across time. If we conceptualize acculturation as a dynamic temporal process, then in principle we must examine this process of cultural change as it unfolds over time. Large cross-sectional studies have contrasted differences between the experiences of newly arrived migrants and those who have lived in a new country for several generations. Accordingly, single assessments of acculturation in cross-sectional studies have provided a single glimpse in time, thus limiting a more complete understanding of the mechanisms or temporal processes that promote adaptation among various immigrants and migrating populations.

Furthermore, what may appear as resilience at one stage of migration could actually produce a pathological outcome at a latter stage of life. Similar to changes in resilience, as observed across developmental milestones (Luthar, 2006), there may exist differing markers of successful adaptation, depending on the stage of migration examined. For example, learning basic language skills during the initial weeks of migration may be remarkable, although this same level of language acquisition after decades in the new country may suggest limited success at cultural adaptation. On the other hand, early-stage emotional difficulties during a cross-cultural transition may reflect a mourning of losses relative to one's homeland (a short-term outcome) that could nonetheless constitute an adaptive response that may ultimately produce a healthy long-term adaptation into the new country (a long-term outcome). Process-related details and nuances can be glossed over by superficial and time-insensitive models and analyses. Such analyses do not consider the multiple trajectories of adaptive and maladaptive change that occur over time, and that differ for various immigrants. Often such superficial models are also limited by the use of singular or simplistic outcome measures, such as language facility or employment, or by the use of single-scale measures of acculturation status.

Migration, Sociocultural Challenges, and Resilience: Review of the Literature

Considerable research has been conducted on the experience of migration, particularly as related to acculturation. In this section, we review some of the literature on migration and sociocultural change, as examined through combined resilience and ecodevelopmental frameworks. To illustrate this approach, we review resilience issues from a systemic, multilevel perspective, that is, from the levels of the individual, family, community, and society (Castro et al., 2009).

Individual Factors

Migrant populations are extremely diverse, and exhibit varied experiences and likely diverse acculturation trajectories as these relate to the process of cultural adaptation. To enhance our understanding of how individuals cope with difficulties in this transition, much research has focused on how individual characteristics may facilitate or impede certain acculturation outcomes, including the development of resilience. Both risk and resource factors are implicated in the occurrence of these adaptive outcomes.

One initial factor that affects cultural adaptation is the immigrant's initial motivations for migration. Individuals can vary greatly in the time and preparation devoted to planning their migration, as well as in their intrinsic desire, voluntary or forced, to leave their homeland. *Refugees* are individuals who are forced to flee their native country for fear of persecution, and who frequently must abandon their homes in the midst of violent conflict, with little or no time to prepare (Stein, 1981). A meta-analysis by Porter and Haslam (2005) of 56 reports (which included people internally displaced as refugees) found that the mental health outcomes of refugees were significantly worse relative to a comparison group of nonrefugees, such as voluntary migrants (mean weighted effect size = .41). Clearly, individuals who are forcibly displaced from their homeland differ considerably from individuals who are able to plan their migration. Therefore, refugees are frequently considered as a population at great risk for mental and/or health problems given their forced migration, along with the added stressors of having a history of persecution, torture, and trauma. Thus, refugees can benefit greatly from programs and policies that provide protection, safety, and social supports when resettling into a new country (Davidson, Murray, & Schweitzer, 2008; Porter & Haslam, 2005).

Immigrants can also vary considerably in their levels of education, language facility, and the resources they bring into their new environment. Higher levels of education have typically been associated with positive outcomes after migration. Individuals who frequently engage in planned migrations also benefit from having higher levels of education (Berry, Poortinga, Segall, & Dasen, 2002). Generally, education serves as a powerful resource, and typically comprises marketable skills that enhance opportunities for employment and financial opportunities. Education also includes the knowledge and aptitudes that promote adaptive adjustment in diverse environments worldwide. However, among persons undergoing forced migration, higher education has also been associated with worse outcomes upon resettlement. Among such refugees who are forcibly displaced, it is hypothesized that for those with higher levels of education, the loss of the social status they enjoyed in their native country constitutes a significant loss that they mourn when dwelling within lower-income environments in the new society. In this regard, research has shown that refugees who report the loss of homeland social roles and life projects also report higher levels of psychological distress within their new host country (Colic-Peisker & Walker, 2003; Miller, 1999; Miller et al., 2002).

There also are differences between adults and children regarding the acquisition of key cultural competencies. As contrasted with migrating children, it appears more difficult for migrating adults to acquire new linguistic and other competencies. Especially among older adults, the acquisition of new skills may be impeded by conflicts with their established native-cultural values, norms, and behaviors (Coatsworth, Pantin, & Szapocznik, 2002). And, for youth as well as for older adults, the process of developing competencies in two cultural groups often introduces challenges greater than those experienced in the process of typical, single-culture development (Castro, Boyer, & Balcazar, 2000).

At the level of the family, a differential acculturation between children and older adults can impact family functioning, as we discuss later in this chapter. We also suggest that adults may typically need additional supports in the acquisition of a new language. In a study of adult Southeast Asian refugees in Canada, Beiser and Hou (2001) found that English ability was not a significant predictor of employment or of depression during the initial stages of resettlement. However, after 10 years in Canada, 8% of the sample did not speak English, and English ability was a significant predictor of better employment status and fewer depressive symptoms. Moreover, these authors suggest that early involvement in the labor market can also influence migrant trajectories.

Language is typically a critical marketable skill, and language mastery often influences people's capacity for acculturative change toward a new social culture. By contrast, language deficiencies can promote social isolation from this mainstream culture. Individuals who are unable to interact with the mainstream culture may also be more likely to feel separate and marginalized from the larger society. In fact, in several studies of refugee migrants, social isolation has been implicated in higher levels of psychopathology (Miller et al., 2002; Mollica et al., 2001). Individual differences exist in immigrants' social isolation and in the social networks from which they garner social support. Individual factors, such as age or level of education, can also operate as moderating influences on the social ties and connections a person may attain. An older adult struggling to develop competencies for survival within a new environment may nonetheless be surrounded by a secure network of family and friends who assist him or her in meeting basic daily needs. This however, can introduce a dependency on this network, which in turn can produce stress on occasions when network resources are not available. The influence of social networks can be examined at an individual level by assessing the size of the immigrant's social network and the extent of social support obtained, and based on the individual's self-reports, or through familial and community processes, as discussed in the following sections.

Family Factors

Differential Acculturation

Stress resulting from the acculturation process may compromise family values, attitudes, and familistic behaviors (Gil, Wagner, & Vega, 2000). Particularly among immigrants, acculturation-related conflicts between parents and children can weaken parent–child bonds. The resulting family dysfunction has been attributed to these faster rates of acculturation by children, compared with their parents, a process described as *differential acculturation* (Coatsworth et al., 2002). Parent–child communication and other conflicts resulting from these differential rates of acculturation have also been associated with higher rates of disease risk behaviors (Elder, Broyles, Brennan, Zuniga de Nuncio, & Nader, 2005) and adolescent substance use (Gil et al., 2000; Valez & Ungemack, 1995).

Among children and youth, *linguistic acculturation*, the acquisition of the language skills used in the new cultural environment, has been associated with an expansion of social networks. This network not only exposes immigrant youth to new lifeways and places them at greater risk for encountering drug-using peers and greater opportunities to use various substances (Escobar, 1998), but in some cases it also distances them from the protective effects of family and their culture of origin (Duncan, Duncan, Biglan, & Ary, 1998; Flannery, Williams, & Vazsonyi, 1999). In general, this parent–child "acculturation gap" is often characterized by conflict and disrupted parent–child communications.

In summary, impaired family function, identity conflicts, and the emergence of problem behaviors have been identified as core elements of disrupted family systems

that occur in immigrant families as a consequence of acculturation-related changes (Schwartz, Pantin, Prado, Sullivan, & Szapocznik, 2005). Many immigrant parents who settle within the United States complain that their acculturating adolescent children are becoming "too independent," irreverent, and lacking in respect for their parents. Moreover, among Asian Indian families, Farver and colleagues (2002) report that the *absence* of this acculturation gap has been associated with higher youth self-esteem and lower anxiety, and also suggests that *parental acculturation styles* directly influence children's ethnic identity development and psychological well-being. In that study, the parental acculturative styles that involved a *separatist orientation* (native culture–only orientation) and the *marginalized orientation* (an avoidance of both native and mainstream cultures) were associated with higher levels of family conflict when compared with the *integrated orientation* (a bicultural orientation) and the *assimilated orientation* (a mainstream culture–only orientation).

The Hispanic/Latino Health Paradox

The Hispanic/Latino paradox has emerged as the observation that despite exposure to low-income environments, certain Hispanics, primarily those of Mexican origin and/or immigrants, exhibit remarkably salubrious physical and mental health outcomes comparable to those attained by mainstream white Americans (non-Hispanic whites) (Abraido-Lanza, Dohrenwend, Ng-Mak, & Turner, 1999; Franzini, Ribble, & Keddie, 2001; Markides & Coreil, 1986). As a mechanism that may underlie this paradox, certain Hispanics may benefit from protective or resilience factors that maintain these healthy outcomes despite exposures to unfavorable environments (Alderete, Vega, Kolody, & Aguilar-Gaxiola, 2000; Palloni & Morenoff, 2001). In part, these protective factors may involve *familism* and/or *family traditionalism*, as well as the social and family supports that exist within many traditional rural and immigrant family systems. These supportive influences have been observed among more traditional Mexican and other Latino family systems (Mendoza & Fuentes-Afflick, 1999). However, such protective influences may erode with acculturation or assimilation (Castro & Coe, 2007), unless retained under bicultural development despite the occurrence of acculturative change into "the American mainstream culture" (Morales, Lara, Kington, Valdez, & Escarce, 2002). Regarding this process, one important question is whether these traditional familial factors confer resilience (Castro et al., 2007), and whether these protective effects appear only among certain Hispanics/Latinos (i.e., Mexicans) but not other Latinos (e.g., Puerto Ricans).

Community and Societal Factors

Social and Human Capital

Among immigrant populations, the concepts of social capital and human capital introduce the importance of resources necessary for successful adaptation. *Social capital* comprises the system of external resources, such as an extended family, community support networks, and mutual aid groups, that may offer support resources for immigrants and their families (Massey, Durand, & Malone, 2002), whereas *human capital* comprises "personal traits and characteristics that increase a worker's productivity" (p. 10). Generally, level of education may be regarded as a form of human capital given that education typically confers an immigrant marketable skills for productive functioning within a new environment.

From this perspective, *resilience*, when conceptualized as trait-like *personal competence* that may be regarded as another element of human capital, may contribute to the person's occupational productivity. Resilience as a form of human capital may include (1) *confident optimism*, (2) *productive activity*, (3) *insight* and *warmth*, and (4) *skilled expressiveness* (Klohnen, 1996), as

well as (5) the capacity for *self-regulation* of emotions and behavior (Buckner, Mezzacappa, & Beardslee, 2003; Tugade & Fredrickson, 2004) and (6) *goal-directed efforts* to attain important outcomes (Connor & Davidson, 2003). In combining the influences of social capital and human capital, the capacity for enacting resilient behaviors may be enhanced by these resources that facilitate the capacity to *navigate effectively* within the local environment. This capacity to "navigate" an environment in quest of a valued goal may constitute a critical skill for attaining adaptive short-term goals, while also avoiding maladaptive outcomes and rising above the adversities that occur along the way.

Community-Level Factors

Cultural factors at the community level may include (1) the normative environment, the racial/ethnic or immigrant mix of the local community (i.e., an ethnic enclave), and (2) local social policies and civic norms that support or oppose the arrival of new migrants. For these immigrants, the availability of a community that is accepting of outside customs and traditions offers a comfortable environment that promotes adjustment and integration into that new community. By contrast, whereas the structural characteristics of a community that exhibits *discrimination* and *racial segregation* may impose many stressors on immigrants and their families (Kulis, Marsiglia, Sicotte, & Nieri, 2007), community support groups may foster resilience in migrant individuals and their families by providing them with information, social supports, and beneficial resources, as offered by families and neighbors who share the immigrants' culture and are concerned about their welfare (Portes, 1997; Zhou, 1997). Conversely, some ethnic enclaves may contribute to risks by isolating individuals from a wider set of social and economic resources and opportunities within the mainstream society, thus setting the stage for potential *downward, segmented assimilation* (Portes & Zhou, 1993). A meta-analysis by Pettigrew and Tropp (2006) showed that across 516 studies, greater levels of intergroup contact were associated with lower levels of prejudice (mean effect size = −.21). This suggests that, at a community level, greater levels of interaction among diverse cultural groups would be associated with better intergroup relations.

As one sociopolitical context, expressions of hostility toward certain ethnic or cultural groups, such as immigrants or ethnic minorities, may ultimately foment a community-wide "oppositional culture" (Ogbu, 1995). In response, members of marginalized groups may reject mainstream society's values and goals, and identify with an alternative subculture that may include gang membership, drug trafficking, illegal drug use, and other antisocial behaviors. Stressors arising from social and economic deprivations, often resulting from acculturation conflicts, can also undermine traditional cultural values and family stability. The resulting parent–child conflicts may then manifest themselves as behavioral problems, such as substance use (Valez & Ungemack, 1995).

Furthermore, the lowered socioeconomic status (SES) and cultural losses that many migrants experience when transitioning into a new environment introduce several concerns. Many studies suggest that individuals exposed to low-SES community conditions experience the most negative health outcomes (Marmot & Wilkinson, 1999). Moreover, the combination of low individual and community SES predicts the poorest physical and mental health outcomes (Stafford & Marmot, 2003). Within the migration and acculturation literature there has been a varied and inconsistent examination of the impact of SES on health outcomes and how three major factors (acculturation, SES, and health) may interact (Salant & Lauderdale, 2003). The adverse effects of SES may be manifest through limited access to resources and/or the aversive characteristics of a low-SES community, including racial segregation and discrimination, high levels of crime, and exposure to toxins and other environmental stressors. For example, refugees to the United States are commonly resettled into neighborhoods in which they are at risk of violence and exposure to multiple traumatic events. A study by Fox, Cowell, and Montgomery (1999) showed that refugee children reported higher numbers of traumatic experiences in their host community compared with their community of origin (Wandersman & Nation, 1998). High levels of stress, coupled with low levels of personal control over adverse events, are two of many pathways by which SES can contribute to negative migration outcomes.

Person × Environment Interactive Effects: Social and Human Capital

As noted previously, *social capital* refers to social and interpersonal resources acquired from a social network of relationships. Social capital can thus grow upon the expansion of a social network that comprises kin, friends, and others from the same ethnic or religious background, which facilitates adaptive integration into the new environment. Accordingly, social capital constitutes a resource that can facilitate resilience. In this person × environment interaction, persons high in human capital and social capital are likely to adapt especially well during the process of migration, with existing human capital competencies enhanced by the availability of social capital, thereby facilitating cultural adaptation. In other words, the positive sociocultural conditions from the "sending community" and those of the "receiving community" can enhance the immigrant's initial life chances within the new environment. At the community level, as social capital grows, cultural integration can gain momentum and can become an ongoing and sustainable process (Massey et al., 2002). Of course, social capital also exists within the context of contemporary economic and political conditions that may encourage migration or discourage it. From an interactive perspective, the concept of social capital suggests that social resources facilitating adaptation within a new environment are not exclusively person variables, or environmental variables, but are instead *interactive effects* that are products of both the person and the environment. The concept of social capital thus offers implications for resilience development that may emerge as a product of these person × environmental interactive effects.

Segmented Assimilation

Social capital has also been identified as a resilience factor that may insulate or otherwise protect youth from antisocial conduct, including drug use (Nagasawa, Qian, & Wong, 2001). It has been noted that *human capital* refers to personal competencies, including education, work skills, and personal resources that facilitate social and economic mobility (Nagasawa et al., 2001). The joint influences of social and human capital can thus operate as key determinants of *segmented assimilation* (Portes & Zhou, 1993), which refers to the differing pathways to socioeconomic mobility that occur for differing groups of immigrants. According to Portes and Zhou (1993), these pathways are (1) assimilation into the white middle class and related upward mobility, (2) assimilation into an underclass, and (3) resistance to assimilation and the preservation of ethnic identity in the form of a *separatist identity*. Under this model, an abiding question is: "Which of these pathways may constitute the most adaptive form of cultural adaptation?" Will immigrants having high social and human capital, and by implication higher resilience, exhibit a greater likelihood of assimilation into the white middle class, coupled with upward socioeconomic mobility? Alternatively, will they develop a bilingual/bicultural identity and high personal agency? Whether growth in resilience occurs under an assimilation outcome or a bicultural outcome, or both, is a question for future research. By implication, immigrants with high social capital and, ostensibly, high resilience would

not be likely to exhibit segmented assimilation into the underclass (i.e., a "downward drift" into lower SES).

In the analysis of socioeconomic adaptation among immigrants, we concur with Churchill's (2003) call for "Resilience, Not Resistance"; that is, it is important that recovering communities work collaboratively with immigrants in a way that "respects difference but identifies common values and objectives and attempts to find legitimate means by which to moderate necessary conflict" (p. 353). Community norms, leadership, and societal policies play crucial roles in fostering accepting intercultural values. As Liu (2007) suggests, "Under some circumstances, psychological adjustment for mainstreamers (persons from the core "mainstream" sector of the society) might seem even more difficult … [as they] might not be equally well-prepared to accept or adjust to various changes in their lives brought about by the immigrant population" (p. 770). Therefore, ongoing dialogue that explores different and at times conflicting opinions and points of view is essential if we are to realize positive intercultural ideals (Churchill, 2003).

Resilience Development among Adult Immigrants and Their Children

Positive Ethnic Identity: Implications for Resilience among Adolescents and Adults

At the heart of the migrant experience lies the redefinition and development of individual and community identities. *Ethnic identity* refers to the extent to which a person identifies with his or her cultural, national, racial, or ethnic group. For some migrants raised in small towns or rural communities, preferred ethnic identity may involve identifying more with their local community or province (e.g., identifying as being a *Jarocho* or *Veracruzano* [a native of the state of Veracruz, Mexico], in preference to identifying as being a "Mexican").

Tajfel and Turner's (1986) social identity theory highlights the importance of a sense of belonging to a group, and the attitudes and feelings that emerge from that sense of group identification. Group identity, of which ethnic identity constitutes one subtype, can shape *self-concept* (how the person sees the self) and operate as a source of *self-esteem* (how the person like himself or herself) and group identity. This identity is likely also important in the development of resilience among immigrant children and youth, as well as adults.

Identity formation constitutes a fundamental life challenge for every human being, a developmental task that elicits fundamental questions about the self and shapes the person's unique individual identity. These fundamental questions include the following: Who are you? What do you believe in? Where you are going in life? Ostensibly, persons with low self-worth, confusing value orientations, and undefined or ambiguous life goals experience *identity confusion* and related feelings of emptiness, worthlessness, and/or aimlessness. Much of this literature has focused on identity development among ethnic/minority youth, although individuals of all ages across the lifecycle can face particular age-specific identity challenges that can comprise competing and often conflicting cultural value orientations that emerge when transitioning from one cultural environment to another.

Phinney (1990, 1993) proposed a three-stage model of ethnic identity development that has been accepted as a classic stage model. These three identity development stages are (1) *unexamined ethnic identity*, (2) *ethnic identity search*, and (3) *ethnic identity achievement*. During Stage 1: *Unexamined Ethnic Identity*, the youth exhibits an *unexplored identity* that consists of a lack of ethnic identity awareness or consciousness; accordingly, the youth accepts without question the values and attitudes communicated by the mainstream culture, including negative views of his or her ethnic group. At this stage, minority youth may regard themselves as being "white," or as belonging to the "mainstream culture," thus lacking aware-

ness and interest in exploring their ethnicity, and they may even avoid thinking about issues of ethnicity and race.

During Stage 2: *Ethnic Identity Search*, according to Phinney (1990, 1993), the ethnic youth develops an awareness of his or her own ethnic identity, often after experiencing a disturbing or consciousness-raising event. This event can prompt a sense of injustice, anger, outrage, and a growing awareness that certain attitudes or mainstream cultural values are detrimental or discriminatory, as expressed toward the youth's racial or ethnic group. This consciousness-raising stage is followed by Stage 3: *Ethnic Identity Achievement*, in which the youth ultimately develops a clear and more confident sense of self and attains comfort upon accepting his or her own racial/ethnic identity. Thus, this state involves a resolution of ethnic identity uncertainties, and acceptance and internalization of one's own ethnic identity. The youth thus develops a mature value and appreciation of his or her own ethnic self-concept, and can also express *ethnic pride* (Phinney, 1993). Within Phinney's three-stage model of ethnic identity development, the task of ethnic identity achievement would appear to be completed during late adolescence. From a different perspective, the development of ethnic and other forms of personal identity may constitute lifelong developmental tasks that extend into adulthood and are reactivated upon immigration, when the person faces the challenge of adopting new and more complex adult roles and responsibilities (becoming a parent, establishing a professional persona, etc.).

Thus, because this process of identity formation may be reactivated upon immigration to a new and different sociocultural environment, this new challenge may disrupt or destabilize a heretofore stable or "achieved" state of ethnic identity development. By extension, one form of ethnic identification can involve multiple identity dimensions, which have been conceptualized and described as involving (1) an identification with one's own ethnic group, (2) an identification with the mainstream group, and (3) in some instances, an identification with a generic "pan-ethnic" group (Chung, Kim, & Abreu, 2004). This *pan-ethnic identification* would involve referring to oneself as "Asian American," for Chinese, Japanese, Korean, and other related ethnic/national groups. Similarly, this would involve labeling oneself as "Latino" or "Hispanic" for Mexican American, Puerto Rican, Cuban, and other related groups. As suggested earlier, during adulthood, this complex task of multiple identity development may increase in complexity given that the adult persona typically comprises multiple adult life roles and their related dimensions of personal and ethnic identification.

In an analysis of the process of acculturation as it influences identity formation, Schwartz, Montgomery, and Briones (2006) conceptualized identity as a *complex construct* that comprises components including (1) *personal identity*—personal goals, values, and beliefs; (2) *social identity*—group identification and affiliation; and (3) *cultural identity*—a subset of social identity. From this perspective, cultural identity refers to solidarity and connectedness with one's cultural or ethnic group. According to Schwartz and colleagues, personal identity "anchors" the person. This anchoring is especially important for immigrants and ethnic minorities as they may struggle during the transition from their home cultural environment to a new, receiving cultural environment. The development of stable personal, social, and cultural identities (i.e., *identity integration*) would appear to be a potent resource that is instrumental for effective coping with cultural conflicts; it would afford migrants the competence to resolve cultural conflicts in a productive manner. Thus, a stable and integrated *bilingual/bicultural identity* may serve as a core competence that fosters resilience because it may aid in resolving dialectical cultural conflicts, such as those involving individualism versus collectivism, or traditionalism versus modernism, and so forth.

Toward an Achieved Ethnic Identity

Identity Development in the Presence of Discrimination

From a *cultural strengths* perspective, ethnic minorities who develop a well-defined *ethnic identity schema* (Alvarez & Helms, 2001), and who express *ethnic pride* in their identity, may benefit from the cultural strengths afforded by this identification: a sense of belonging to their ethnic group, coupled with a strong favorable attitude about their ethnicity (Castro, Stein, & Bentler, 2009). This personal competence may be enhanced by social supports provided by family and peers, which may impart confidence and a capacity for active decision making. This competence might also aid in resisting discriminatory assaults to one's racial or ethnic identity and character. Such assaults would be imposed by others in the form of prejudicial or discriminatory threats levied against the ethnic/minority person.

The processes of identity development or change, as prompted by acculturative change, has been regarded as stressful, especially for immigrants and ethnic minorities who face discrimination on the basis of their ethnicity, appearance, limited English proficiency, or immigrant status. For a sample of Latina/o adults, Moradi and Risco (2006) proposed a structural model that examines perceived discrimination, acculturation to the mainstream American culture and Latino acculturation orientation to own Latino ethnic culture as mediated by personal control because these factors may influence self-esteem and psychological distress. Not unexpectedly, Moradi and Risco found that perceived discrimination is positively associated with psychological distress and negatively associated with a sense of personal control. By contrast, a sense of personal control was associated positively with greater self-esteem and negatively with psychological distress. Also, acculturation toward the American mainstream culture correlated positively with enhanced self-esteem. Moreover, personal control/environmental mastery was observed as a mediator of the influence of perceived discrimination on the outcome variables of self-esteem and psychological distress. In other words, among these Latina/o adults, perceived discrimination prompted a lower sense of control, which in turn contributed to psychological distress. Ostensibly, as suggested by this model, social efforts to eliminate discrimination, along with empowering persons with greater control and mastery for enhanced resilience, may aid in reducing psychological distress and decrements to self-esteem resulting from exposure to discriminatory life stressors. This study also highlights the complex interrelationships among discrimination, self-esteem, and acculturation as precursors of psychological distress and well-being.

Bicultural and Multicultural Identity Development

Despite exposure to social and at times discriminatory experiences that can discourage identification as a "person of color," some scholars have described the positive effects of a dual-cultural identity that can build *bicultural competence* (LaFromboise, Coleman, & Gerton, 1993). Biculturally competent individuals have been described as having the capacity for *cultural flex*—the ability to "shuttle" or transition back and forth between majority and minority cultures (LaFromboise et al., 1993; Ramirez, 1999). As one example, some bicultural/bilingual Latino youth are capable of "language brokering"—that is, the capacity to translate for parents or others from English to Spanish and vice versa (Weisskirch, 2005). Children who act as language brokers appear to have a positive sense of self and a secure ethnic identity, and they may thrive under these conditions of dual-culture exposure. This bicultural orientation, which includes positive skills and attitudes toward both cultures, may foster positive emotions and a positive self-concept (Tugade & Fredrickson, 2004), which may in turn foster a growing sense of cultural competence (Izard, 2002) and resilience.

Parental Influences on Ethnic Pride and Resilience

Synergistic Effects of Ethnic Pride and Resilience

In general, greater ethnic "identity maturation" has been associated with better psychological adjustment (Alvarez & Helms, 2001). Here, the construct of *ethnic pride* appears similar or synonymous with the constructs "collective self-esteem" (Alvarez & Helms, 2001) and "group-esteem," in which group esteem reflects people's positive feelings about being a member of their own racial or ethnic group. Thus, Latinos who belong to a minority culture or ethnic group, and who proudly acknowledge their ethnic identity and express a positive self-appraisal despite their minority status, may be exhibiting *resilience* in the form of strong self-confidence and personal agency, resources that may aid in actively avoiding distress despite exposure to discrimination (Klohnen, 1996; Masten, 2001).

Wills and colleagues (2007) examined an ethnic pride variable, *positive ethnic esteem*, which was associated with low rates of substance use among African American adolescents. In a structural equations model analysis of 670 African American adolescents, parental endorsement of *racial socialization* (teaching racial consciousness) was also associated with greater positive ethnic esteem, which was in turn associated with greater substance resistance efficacy, and subsequently with lower youth substance use, as measured by lower rates of cigarette smoking and alcohol use. Thus, among these African American families, a youth's positive appraisal of his or her own racial/ethnic identity, coupled with parental endorsement and support of racial identity, operated jointly as a protective factor against substance use.

Reciprocal Parent–Child Influences on Resilience

The mother–daughter dyad can also serve as the locus for the development of resilience. As a focused strategic approach to resist discrimination, a qualitative study examined

Salvadorian mothers' consciousness-raising strategies to promote ethnic pride in their young daughters (Carranza, 2007). This strategic approach emphasized encouraging daughters to express pride in their indigenous heritage as a means of resisting discrimination and building capacity for resilience. This mother-initiated ethnic pride enhancement focused on several approaches: (1) fostering pride in one's own racial ancestry, (2) parental role modeling, (3) pride in and maintenance of one's own native language, and (4) fostering a sense of belonging to one's native ethnic group. This parental activity for enhancing ethnic pride appeared to promote self-esteem and to build resilience in the service of personal identity development, based on personal agency that would aid in resisting discriminatory assaults. This analysis by Carranza (2007) illustrates the process of promoting and maintaining resilience, which was beneficial for not only the young daughters but also the mothers. Studies of these potential reciprocal effects may aid understanding of the mutual benefits of cultural adaptation that occur within the context of parent–child relationships.

An Illustrative Case of Refugee Experiences

Peter[2] was a physician who fled his country about 15 years ago. He left his homeland for a neighboring country, where he could work each day without fearing that his four young children and wife would be missing when he returned home each night. He was lucky. He was able to get out before things got worse, whereas friends and neighbors who had stayed behind were forcibly expelled from their homes or killed. Furthermore, Peter was able to continue to work in his professional field, whereas many from his country were disparaged for their skin color each day as they struggled to make ends meet. However, as Peter's children got older, they too began to struggle in their schooling because his daughters were reaching the "glass ceiling" of secondary education, a place where they would not be welcome.

Peter decided it was time to move once again; this time for the sake of his children's future. After several years of sending off applications and completing interviews and tests, their refugee status was recognized and the family was moved to a third country through a humanitarian refugee resettlement program. Although several family members remained in their war-torn homeland, Peter's family was happy for another opportunity to gain freedom from discrimination and persecution. All members of the family could now access education, and they grasped at these opportunities in the spirit of reestablishing a sense of normality and renewed hope for the future.

However, things were not so easy for Peter. With considerable education and two decades of expertise as a physician within his new immigrant community he was forced to settle for manual labor positions, with few prospects for moving ahead. Despite his pleas to anyone who would listen, there seemed to be few options for Peter to move forward. While packing meat, he spent most days ruminating about leaving his family to move to a country in which he could practice medicine. Ultimately, he felt he could not leave his family to struggle alone without him. After 5 years of working and volunteering time in other positions to gain more professional experience, Peter's door finally opened. Although not in his area of professional specialty, he was offered a position in which his skills and abilities were valued and was able to provide for his family in a way that made him proud.

Peter's story highlights several important themes that depict the challenges and conflicts of many refugees. To succeed, Peter had to maintain perseverance, fortitude, and loyalty to family, as well as pride in his heritage. Peter and his family did not show a single upward trajectory during their migration pathway; rather, his pathway was marked by a series of improvements and setbacks. He recognized that although his identity as a professional was a central part of his identity as a health professional, his family was also central to his identity as a father and provider. If interviewed at the start of his tenure in resettlement, Peter would have met the diagnostic criteria for major depressive disorder. However, if we examine his family's overall immigration trajectory and their efforts at cultural adaptation, then we see his remarkable resilience, the importance of his family and of social supports, and his ability to adapt and persevere in the face of many difficult circumstances. Peter's story provides an example of the difficulties faced by the more than 60 million displaced persons around the globe (Office of the UN High Commissioner for Refugees, 2008).

A Developmental Model of Acculturation and Cultural Adaptation

Model Overview

For many immigrants, the process of cultural adaptation within a new environment can consist of several possible life pathways that proceed through a sequential series of mediating events, ultimately leading to healthy or to unhealthy short- and long-term outcomes. More specifically, for many immigrants, the process of cultural adaptation can be examined longitudinally in the form of several possible developmental pathways, or "life journeys," that comprise a progression across several stages or life milestones, as immigrants grapple with the challenges of adaptation to emergent challenging events and contexts experienced within the new host society. Figure 18.1 presents a sequential model of these migration pathways, a series of events that can lead to specific positive or negative long-term outcomes. This model is an expansion of a prior stress–mediation–coping model that describes the complex process of stress–appraisal–coping that leads to specific short- and long-term outcomes (Cervantes & Castro, 1985).

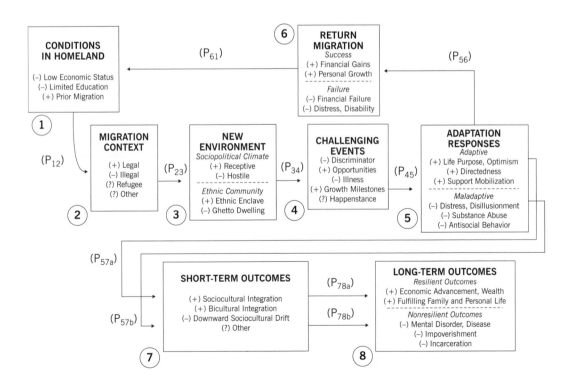

FIGURE 18.1. Sequential model of resilience-related pathways for immigrants.

Setting Conditions for Migration

For immigrants, this process of cultural adaptation begins with *predisposing conditions* within the homeland, *Conditions in the Homeland* (1), which comprise immigrants' personal resources, and their preparedness for migration and adaptation within a new environment (Portes & Rumbaut, 1996). "Human capital" and "social capital" factors, such as immigrants' socioeconomic position and social networks within their homeland, their level of education, preexperiences with migration as provided by prior migrating family members or others, and other sources of human and social capital, can influence their state of preparedness and set the personal context for their adaptation and life chances within a new environment (Portes & Rumbaut, 1996).

Migration then occurs within a specific *Migration Context* (2) and can involve migration under one of several immigrant identities: legal migration, illegal migration, migration as a refugee, or some other type of migration, such as migrating under a student visa or as a contract worker (Portes & Rumbaut, 1996). It can also involve situational, environmental, familial, and other contextual domains. Upon entering a new community, country, or society, the *New Environment* (3) and its specific environmental contexts, immigrants' life chances are greatly influenced by the abiding *Sociopolitical Climate* within that new environment. Although this climate can be receptive during times of economic prosperity, it can also be hostile during times of an economic downturn (Locke, 1998; Massey et al., 2002). Immigrants' life chances can also be influenced by migration into an *ethnic enclave* or community, an *Ethnic Community*, which provides venues to reconnect immigrants with experiences from the homeland. Ethnic enclaves can include other immigrants who speak an immigrant's language, and the availability of familiar foods and other commodities from the homeland (Schwartz et al., 2005). These enclaves make the process of adjustment more tolerable than other environments that lack these familiar life experiences and social resources. However, certain ethnic enclaves can also consist of lower-class ghetto neighborhoods, ravaged by the presence of illegal drugs, crime, and violence, may thus impede efforts at adaptive assimilation.

Early Stages of Cultural Adaptation

Within the new environment immigrants face a series of challenging experiences, *Challenging Events* (4), which they can frame either as threats or as opportunities. Immigrants' appraisal of these challenges as "threats to well-being" may frame these challenges as "stressors" that, if chronic, can produce ongoing distress and evolve into diagnosable mental disorders and/or a health-related problems. Conversely, appraisal of these challenges as "opportunities" may render them as obstacles to be surpassed and as achievable goals to be attained, thus motivating actions that may reap benefits from overcoming these challenges. These challenging events can include racial or other forms of *discrimination, novel opportunities, illnesses, growth milestones*, and even unexpected or uncontrollable events that involve *happenstance* or *luck*. For many immigrants, especially stressful and challenging events involve racial, ethnic, or job-related discrimination and racially motivated violence.

Recent studies have examined specific stressors and life difficulties that immigrants encounter as a result of active antiimmigrant attitudes (Carranza, 2007; Viruell-Fuentes, 2007; Walker, 2007). Another challenging life event includes the need to learn the local language in cases when the immigrant's native language differs from the predominant language of the new environment. Other challenges include learning the "local culture," that is, the major psychosocial norms and other subjective culture factors (Triandis & Brislin, 1984) that prevail and are rewarded within that new environment. These subjective factors include cultural values, social norms, cultural attitudes, cultural beliefs, and culturally sanctioned behaviors. Moreover, within any community there exists a diversity of subjective norms based on the diverse populations that inhabit that community. This diversity adds complexity to the tasks of cultural adaptation and its challenges as faced by various immigrants. In this regard, a culturally diverse enclave can comprise a multitude of subcultures that introduce diversity and at times conflict during the tasks of cultural adaptation. Within this context, another challenging task for the immigrant involves the establishment of new and supportive social networks of neighbors, friends, coworkers, and others.

Later Stages of Cultural Adaptation

Ostensibly, immigrants who are more likely to succeed within that new environment possess many personal resources (human capital), such as skills for attaining well-paying jobs that are compatible with and rewarded by the new social environment (Massey et al., 2002). Conversely, other immigrants who have low human capital reap limited rewards from the new environment because they lack the skills that are valued and rewarded by that new environment. Thus, at the core of resilience-related coping lies the immigrant's personal competence or skills, including the capacity for effective decision making, and for exercising self-control and self-regulation because these self-directive skills can be focused on attaining desirable, positive outcomes (Griffin, Scheier, Botvin, & Diaz, 2001).

As indicated previously, certain cognitive, affective, and behavioral responses, *Adaptation Responses* (5) have been associated with resilience in various populations. These adaptive responses include having a life purpose; exercising goal-directed cognitions and behaviors (Connor & Davidson, 2003); emotional self-regulation (Buckner, Mezzacappa, & Beardslee, 2003); developing a sense of mastery (Klohnen, 1996); and the capacity to mobilize social supports (Portes & Rumbaut, 1996). By contrast the absence

of low levels of these personal resources portends a low likelihood of successfully directing efforts toward attaining desirable and socially valued outcomes. Deficits in these personal competencies or the presence of negative social capital may constitute *maladaptive responses* and may include self-defeating cognitions that induce distress and disillusionment; substance abuse; and violence or other forms of antisocial behavior.

Cultural Adaptation Outcomes

Success or Failure in Short- and Long-Term Outcomes

After living for a period of time within a new environment, some immigrants may choose or alternatively be forced to return to their native community, *Return Migration* (6). Thus, immigrants can return after having succeeded in their sojourn, or after having failed (Massey et al., 2002). For some illegal (undocumented) immigrants, deportation constitutes involuntary return migration, an event that is typically ill-timed for the immigrants and their families, and this event is typically disruptive and stressful.

As noted previously, resilience-related pathways may be regarded as a product of a series of mediating events that ultimately produce various *Short-Term Outcomes* (7), including *sociocultural integration*—successful assimilation or integration into the new environment and upward socioeconomic mobility. The case of assimilation indicates that this mobility involves "effectively blending" into the new society, often coupled with a loss of one's own ethnic or native identity. However, as noted previously, sociocultural integration, which may also occur without necessarily involving full assimilation, involves *bicultural integration* (La Fromboise et al., 1993) and comprises successful integration into the new society, where immigrants also maintain most aspects of their native cultural identity, thus developing a bilingual/bicultural identity. In either case, both sociocultural integration and bicultural integration are often regarded as other forms of successful cultural adaptation. This suggests that in this temporal chain of events prior mediators operated favorably to facilitate adaptive coping, ostensibly resulting in improvements in the immigrant's quality of life and sense of well-being (Farver et al., 2002; Griffin et al., 2001). Such adaptation, which is likely successful, is to be contrasted with *downward sociocultural drift*, unsuccessful adaptation characterized by negative short-term outcomes in which an immigrant either fails to advance socioeconomically or even drifts further down in SES, and coupled with a deterioration in quality of life.

As time progresses, the noted short-term outcomes would set conditions for the occurrence of *Long-Term Outcomes* (8), which may serve as more stable standards for defining resilience. Major outcomes that suggest resilient coping and adaptation may include *economic advancement* or attaining *wealth* and/or *educational advancement*; and/or attaining a *fulfilling family and personal life* and a related sense of *well-being* (Massey et al., 2002). By contrast, *nonresilient outcomes* may include the occurrence of *mental disorder* or *somatic disease*; *impoverishment*; or *incarceration, illegal drug use*, or *other antisocial behaviors*. These contrasting favorable and unfavorable outcomes, respectively, generally may be regarded as instances of successful and unsuccessful cultural adaptation. However, as noted previously, the immigrant's own appraisal of the desirability and benefits of a particular outcome should be considered when concluding whether any outcome is truly successful or unsuccessful.

Changing Elements of Assimilation and of Resilience

In principle, cultural adaptation trajectories and outcomes among immigrants that involve increases in assimilation and resilience should involve changes in known core elements of both. Depending on the immigrant's initial state of human and social capital, increases or shifts toward full assimilation into the American "mainstream cul-

ture" would generally involve shifts toward certain core American ideals. Generally, these core ideals include (1) *linguistic acculturation*: the acquisition or enhancement of skills in speaking and reading in English; (2) *normative value changes*: changes in sociocultural norms in accord with prevailing white Anglo Saxon Protestant beliefs that involve the values of individualism, freedom, entrepreneurialism, Protestant ideals, a conversion from another religion to a Protestant denomination, and other related norms; (3) *belief and attitudinal changes*: beliefs in democracy, scientific rationality, and other American secular ideals; (4) *consumerism and related behavioral changes*: changes in behaviors involving consumerism, dietary and leisure-time behavior, work behaviors, and other behaviors associated with "the American way" (Locke, 1998). Clearly these changes are not independent of one another; for example, changes in beliefs and attitudes likely prompt changes in behaviors and even in value orientations. Moreover, this articulation of such acculturative changes becomes more complex and less clear in acculturative changes that involve a preference for and the development of a bilingual/bicultural identity.

Similarly, regarding increases in resilience (when conceptualized as personal competence), resilience enhancements depend on the initial level of resilience exhibited by the immigrant upon his or her migration to the United States. Here, also, based on core aspects identified as elements of resilience, shifts toward increased resilience in the context of cultural adaptation to the American society involve (1) having a *life purpose* that is consistent with normative American values and ideals; (2) exercising *goal-directed beliefs*, *attitudes*, and *behaviors* that include the pursuit of happiness and economic security or wealth; (3) increasing the capacity for *emotional self-regulation*; (4) developing a *sense of mastery* for success within America; and (5) having the capacity to *mobilize social supports* that include networks of white American neighbors and friends, as well as those from the immigrant's native culture. Of course, these criteria for resilience are based on studies with U.S. youth and adults, and one important cross-cultural issue involves how these criteria, as Westernized aspects of resilience, may or may not relate to resilience that is manifest in underdeveloped and/or non-Western countries. Furthermore, because in this instance resilience is conceptualized as an outcome rather than personal competence, increases in resilience involve the attainment of positive and adaptive short- and long-term outcomes. Such outcomes many include increases in SES and in personal well-being, aspects of quality of life that show improvements for immigrants and their families relative to their prior status within their native country.

Complexity in the Appraisal of Improved Quality of Life

Within the domain of adaptive outcomes, cultural issues and core values add complexity to the appraisal of outcomes that may be regarded as improvements in quality of life. In many instances, short- and long-term outcomes are mixed, and typically involve trade-offs (i.e., gains in one domain but losses in another). How may these be appraised as increments or decrements in an immigrant's overall quality of life? For example, if an immigrant from Italy becomes wealthy but experiences a loss of family unity and cohesion among his children and extended family, does that constitute an improvement in that immigrant's quality of life?

Similarly, an immigrant from Mexico may enjoy successful assimilation into the mainstream American culture by attaining wealth, marrying a young European American woman, and attaining a short-term outcome that involves full assimilation and the complete loss of all elements of his native Mexican culture. During these early years after entry into the United States, that Mexican immigrant may avoid introducing ethnic cultural experiences to his children, discourage the speaking of Spanish in his home, speak only English in order to "be American," and also encourage his children to associate only with European American children. Under these normative, household parental expectations, his children would be devoid of any aspects of a Mexican cultural identity; they become mainstream Americans. Despite becoming affluent and well positioned within American society, later in their adolescence the children of this Mexican immigrant may complain that their father deprived them of their Mexican cultural heritage because they cannot speak Spanish or relate culturally with their Latino friends. They feel that they "don't have a culture" because they cannot relate to their Latino friends with fond memories of early life experiences growing up within a Mexican community. How does this scenario relate to the quality of life of the immigrant and his children? In the converse scenario, a Latino mother from Guatemala inculcates her children with the value of learning the indigenous language and cultural norms from her native Guatemalan culture, only to find that her children show no interest in this native culture, and that in time they become mainstream young adult Americans, much to this mother's disappointment.

These complex intergenerational scenarios illustrate the diverse and intriguing patterns of cultural adaptation that should be examined in depth within future research. Future case study and group-level analyses can aid in clarifying the determinants and features of healthy and resilient cultural adaptation to a new and different sociocultural environment, as experienced by diverse groups of immigrants and their families.

Future Directions

With ever-increasing mobility and movement occurring around the world, a greater understanding is needed of immigration processes as they relate to the development of resilience among various immigrants. The implications for conflict, distress, and adjustment of cross-cultural contacts and migration are profound. Resilience theory provides a useful framework for the study of the dynamic process of adaptation as it occurs during various types of migration. Individual, familial, and community risks and resources can affect immigrant trajectories and the resulting forms of cultural adaptation (e.g., segmented assimilation). In this chapter, we have outlined a sequential model of adaptation that includes precipitating and environmental factors (within one's homeland and within the new host community) that present specific challenges in the process of migration, and adaptive coping. This model suggests the importance of studies on the determinants of resilient trajectories, studies that can influence culturally adaptive short- and long-term outcomes following migration, and also recognize the diverse contexts and circumstances in which these forms of cultural adaptation can occur.

Emerging Research Questions

Within the context of the cultural adaptation of immigrants, we may ask, "How do we best frame and define the construct of resilience?" From the perspective of the ecodevelopmental process described in the developmental model of acculturation and cultural adaptation we ask, "Is it best to regard resilience as a state, as a short-term situational outcome, or as stable and trait-like long-term competence?" Assuming that there is no single or absolute form of healthy cultural adaptation for immigrants that may be regarded as resilient, what set of life trajectories lies within the domain of *resilient adaptation*, as contrasted with other life trajectories that must be regarded as nonresilient or maladaptive forms of cultural adaptation? These pressing questions can be addressed with conceptual clarifications, and also with new, culturally sensitive empirical studies designed with sensitivity to the ethnic, cultural, and cross-cultural adaptation and resilience issues that we have examined within this chapter.

A Final Word

Although the experiences of migration can be as diverse as the peoples of the world, the study of migration is a valuable endeavor because new knowledge from these immigration studies can benefit hundreds of millions of migrants and refugees throughout the world. Despite ongoing efforts to build fences and close borders, an era of international movement and exchange appears inevitable. Therefore, it seems in our best interest to enhance our understanding of the processes of cross-cultural contact and migration, and to learn ways to foster resilient outcomes for individuals, families, and communities as they traverse the globe.

New ways of promoting harmony and minimizing conflict are also essential in an era in which diversity and global change seem to be snowballing at exponential rates. Rather than throwing our hands up in defeat, we advocate for the importance of acculturation and cultural adaptation studies from cross-disciplinary, ecodevelopmental, and resilience-based perspectives. From such multilevel, longitudinal, and culturally sensitive research, we can enhance our understanding the processes of healthy migration and acculturative change. In turn, policy, intervention programs, and health practices can be designed and developed to promote the well-being of diverse immigrant populations in these dynamic and challenging times.

Acknowledgments

This work was supported by Grant No. MGS0041, "Resilience in Arizona Hispanic Leader," from the Institute for Mental Health Research; from Grant No. R01 AG026006 from the National Institute on Aging; and from Grant No. P20MD002316 from the National Center on Minority Health and Health Disparities. The content of this chapter is solely the responsibility of the authors and does not necessarily represent the official views of the National Center on Minority Health and Health Disparities or the National Institutes of Health.

Notes

1. Despite frequent reference to "the mainstream culture" within the acculturation literature, there is considerable difficulty in operationally defining the "mainstream" culture into which a new migrant is assimilating. Any society consists of a "tapestry" of different cultures (e.g., rural vs. urban life, liberal vs. conservative values). Although we recognize the complexity involved in aptly of operationalizing "mainstream culture," within this chapter, we refer to the "mainstream" or the "new culture" for simplicity of expression in discussing various assimilation outcomes during the process of acculturation.
2. Key details of this person's narrative have been removed or altered. For example, his name and key demographic characteristics have been changed to protect his anonymity.

References

Abraido-Lanza, A. F., Dohrenwend, B. P., Ng-Mak, D. S., & Turner, J. B. (1999). The Latino mortality paradox: A test of the "salmon bias" and healthy migrant hypothesis. *American Journal of Public Health, 89,* 1543–1548.

Alderete, E., Vega, W. A., Kolody, B., & Aguilar-Gaxiola, S. (2000). Lifetime prevalence of and risk factors for psychiatric disorders among Mexican migrant farmworkers in California. *American Journal of Public Health, 90,* 608–614.

Alvarez, A. N., & Helms, J. E. (2001). Radical identity and reflected appraisals as influences on Asian Americans' racial adjustment. *Cultural Diversity and Ethnic Minority Psychology, 7,* 217–231.

Baldwin, J. R., & Lindsley, S. L. (1994). *Conceptualizations of culture.* Tempe: Urban Studies Center, Arizona State University.

Beiser, M., & Hou, F. (2001). Language acquisition, unemployment and depressive disorder among Southeast Asian refugees: A 10-year study. *Social Science and Medicine, 53,* 1321–1334.

Berry, J. W. (1994). Acculturative stress. In W. Lonner & R. Maplass (Eds.), *Psychology and culture* (pp. 211–215). Boston: Allyn & Bacon.

Berry, J. W. (1997). Immigration, acculturation, and adaptation. *Applied Psychology: An International Review, 46,* 5–68.

Berry, J. W. (2005). Acculturation: Living successfully in two cultures. *International Journal of Intercultural Relations, 29,* 697–712.

Berry, J. W., Poortinga, Y. H., Segall, M. H., & Dasen, P. R. (2002). *Cross-cultural psychology: Research and applications* (2nd ed.). New York: Cambridge University Press.

Birman, D., Trickett, E. J., & Vinokurov, A. (2002). Acculturation and adaptation of Soviet Jewish refugee adolescents: Predictors of adjustment across life domains. *American Journal of Community Psychology, 30,* 585–607.

Buckner, J. C., Mezzacappa, E., & Beardslee, W. R. (2003). Characteristics of resilient youths living in poverty: The role of self-regulation process. *Development and Psychopathology, 15,* 139–162.

Canli, T., Zhao, Z., Desmond, J. E., Kang, E., Gross, J., & Gabrieli, J. D. (2001). An fMRI study of personality influences on brain reactivity to emotional stimuli. *Behavioral Neuroscience, 115,* 33–42.

Carranza, M. E. (2007). Building resilience and resistance against racism and discrimination among Salvadoran female youth in Canada. *Child and Family Social Work, 12,* 390–398.

Castro, F. G. (2007). Is acculturation really detrimental to health? *American Journal of Public Health, 97,* 1162.

Castro, F. G., Boyer, G. R., & Balcazar, H. G. (2000). Healthy adjustment in Mexican American and other Latino adolescents. In R. Montemayor, G. R. Adams, & T. P. Gullotta (Eds.), *Adolescent diversity in ethnic, economic and cultural contexts* (pp. 141–178). Thousand Oaks, CA: Sage.

Castro, F. G., & Coe, K. (2007). Traditions and alcohol use: A mixed methods analysis. *Cultural Diversity and Ethnic Minority Psychology, 13,* 269–284.

Castro, F. G., Garfinkle, J., Naranjo, D., Rollins, M., Brook, J. S., & Brook, D. W. (2007). Cultural traditions as "protective factors," among Latino children of illicit drug users. *Substance Use and Misuse, 42,* 621–642.

Castro, F. G., Shaibi, G. Q., & Boehm-Smith, E. (2009). Ecodevelopmental contexts for preventing type 2 diabetes in Latino and other racial/ethnic minority populations. *Journal of Behavioral Medicine, 32,* 89–105.

Castro, F. G., Stein, J. A., & Bentler, P. M. (2009). Ethnic pride, traditional family values, and acculturation in early cigarette and alcohol use among Latino adolescents. *Journal of Primary Prevention, 30,* 265–292.

Cervantes, R. C., & Castro, F. G. (1985). Stress, doping and Mexican American mental health: A systematic review. *Hispanic Journal of Behavioral Sciences, 7,* 1–73.

Chao, G. T., & Moon, H. (2005). The cultural mosaic: A metatheory for understanding the complexity of culture. *Journal of Applied Psychology, 90,* 1128–1140.

Chung, R. H., Kim, B. S., & Abreu, J. M. (2004). Asian American Multidimensional Acculturation Scale: Development, factor analysis, reliability, and validity. *Cultural Diversity and Ethnic Minority Psychology, 10,* 66–80.

Churchill, S. (2003). Resilience, not resistance. *City, 7,* 349–360.

Coatsworth, J. D., Pantin, H., & Szapocznik, J. (2002). Familias Unidas: A family-centered ecodevelopmental intervention to reduce risk for problem behavior among Hispanic adolescents. *Clinical Child and Family Psychology Review, 5,* 113–132.

Colic-Peisker, V., & Walker, I. (2003). Human capital, acculturation and social identity: Bosnian refugees in Australia. *Journal of Community and Applied Social Psychology, 13,* 337–360.

Connor, K. M., & Davidson, J. R. T. (2003). Development of a new resilience scale: The Connor–Davidson Resilience Scale (CD-RISC). *Depression and Anxiety, 18,* 76–82.

Cuellar, I., Arnold, B., & Maldonado, R. (1995). Acculturation rating scale for Mexican-Americans II: A revision of the original ARMSA scale. *Hispanic Journal of Behavioral Sciences, 17,* 275–304.

Davidson, G. R., Murray, K. E., & Schweitzer, R. (2008). Review of refugee mental health and wellbeing: Australian perspectives. *Australian Psychologist, 43,* 160–174.

Duncan, S. C., Duncan, T. E., Biglan, A., & Ary, D. (1998). Contributions of the social context to the development of adolescent substance use: A multivariate latent growth modeling approach. *Drug and Alcohol Dependence, 50,* 57–71.

Elder, J. P., Broyles, S. L., Brennan, J. J., Zuniga de Nuncio, M. L., & Nader, P. R. (2005). Acculturation, parent–child acculturation differential, and chronic disease risk factors in a Mexican-American population. *Journal of Immigrant Health, 7,* 1–9.

Escobar, J. I. (1998). Immigration and mental health: Why are immigrants better off? *Archives of General Psychiatry, 55,* 781–782.

Farver, J. A., Narang, S. K., & Bhadha, B. R. (2002). East meets West: Ethnic identity, acculturation, and conflict in Asian Indian families. *Journal of Family Psychology, 16,* 338–350.

Flannery, D. J., Williams, L. L., & Vazsonyi, A. T. (1999). Who are they with and what are they doing?: Delinquent behavior, substance use, and early adolescents' after-school time. *American Journal of Orthopsychiatry, 69,* 247–253.

Fox, P. G., Cowell, J. M., & Montgomery, A. C. (1999). Southeast Asian refugee children: Violence experience and depression. *International Journal of Psychiatric Nursing Research, 5,* 589–600.

Franzini, L., Ribble, J. C., & Keddie, A. M. (2001). Understanding the Hispanic paradox. *Ethnicity and Disease, 11,* 496–518.

Fredrickson, B. L. (1998). What good are positive emotions? *Review of General Psychology, 2,* 300–319.

Friedman, T. L. (2005). *The world is flat.* New York: Farrar, Straus & Giroux.

Geertz, C. (1983). Thick description: Toward an interpretive theory of culture. In C. Geertz, *Local knowledge: Further essays in interpretative anthropology* (pp. 3–30). New York: Basic Books.

Gil, A. G., Wagner, E. F., & Vega, W. A. (2000). Acculturation, familism, and alcohol use among Latino adolescent males: Longitudinal relations. *Journal of Community Psychology, 28,* 443–458.

Griffin, K. W., Scheier, L. M., Botvin, G. J., & Diaz, T. (2001). Protective role of personal competence skills in adolescent substance use: Psychological well-being as a mediating factor. *Psychology of Addictive Behaviors, 15,* 194–203.

Hanson, W. E., Creswell, J. W., Clark, V. L. P., Petska, K. S., & Creswell, J. D. (2005). Mixed methods research designs in counseling psychology. *Journal of Counseling Psychology,* 52, 224–235.

Harwood, A. (1981). *Ethnicity and medical care.* Cambridge, MA: Harvard University Press.

Hunt, L. M., Schneider, S., & Comer, B. (2004). Should "acculturation" be a variable in health research?: A critical review of research on US Hispanics. *Social Science and Medicine, 59,* 973–986.

Izard, C. E. (2002). Translating emotion theory and research into preventive interventions. *Psychological Bulletin, 128,* 796–824.

Klohnen, E. C. (1996). Conceptual analysis and measurement of the construct of ego-resiliency. *Journal of Personality and Social Psychology,* 70, 1067–1079.

Kulis, S., Marsiglia, F. F., Sicotte, D. M., & Nieri, T. (2007). Neighborhood effects on youth substance use in a southwestern city. *Sociological Perspectives,* 50, 273–301.

LaFromboise, T., Coleman, H. L. K., & Gerton, J. (1993). Psychological impact of biculturalism: Evidence and theory. *Psychological Bulletin,* 114, 395–412.

LeGrain, P. (2006). *Immigrants: Your country needs them.* London: Little, Brown.

Liu, S. (2007). Living with others: Mapping the routes to acculturation in a multicultural society. *International Journal of Intercultural Relations,* 31, 761–778.

Locke, D. C. (1998). *Increasing multicultural understanding: A comprehensive model* (2nd ed.). Thousand Oaks, CA: Sage.

Luthar, S. (2006). Resilience in development: A synthesis of research across five decades. In D. Cicchetti & D. J. Cohen (Eds.), *Developmental psychopathology: Risk, disorder, and adaptation* (2nd ed., pp. 739–795). New York: Wiley.

Marin, G., & Gamboa, R. J. (1996). A new measurement of acculturation for Latinos: The Bidimensional Acculturation Scale for Latinos (BAS). *Hispanic Journal of Behavioral Sciences,* 18, 297–316.

Markides, K. S., & Coreil, J. (1986). The health of Hispanics in the southwestern United States: An epidemiologic paradox. *Public Health Reports,* 101, 253–265.

Marmot, M., & Wilkinson, R. G. (Eds.). (1999). *Social determinants of health.* New York: Oxford University Press.

Massey, D. S., Durand, J., & Malone, N. J. (2002). *Beyond smoke and mirrors: Mexican immigration in an era of economic integration.* New York: Russell Sage Foundation.

Masten, A. S. (2001). Ordinary magic: Resilience processes in development. *American Psychologist,* 56, 227–238.

McGoldrick, M., & Giordano, J. (1996). Overview: Ethnicity and family therapy. In M. McGoldrick, J. Giordano, & J. K. Pearce (Eds.), *Ethnicity and family therapy* (2nd ed., pp. 1–27). New York: Guilford Press.

Mendoza, F. S., & Fuentes-Afflick, E. (1999). Latino children's health and the family-community health promotion model. *Western Journal of Medicine,* 170, 85–92.

Miller, K. E. (1999). Rethinking a familiar model: Psychotherapy and the mental health of refugees. *Journal of Contemporary Psychotherapy,* 29, 283–304.

Miller, K. E., Weine, S. M., Ramic, A., Brkic, N., Bjedic, Z. D., Smajkic, A., et al. (2002). The relative contribution of war experiences and exile-related stressors to levels of psychological distress among Bosnian refugees. *Journal of Traumatic Stress,* 15, 377–387.

Mollica, R. F., Sarajlic, N., Chernoff, M., Lavelle, J., Vukovic, I. S., & Massagli, M. P. (2001). Longitudinal study of psychiatric symptoms, disability, mortality, and emigration among Bosnian refugees. *Journal of the American Medical Association,* 286, 546–554.

Moradi, B., & Risco, C. (2006). Perceived discrimination experiences and mental health of Latino/a American persons. *Journal of Counseling Psychology,* 53, 411–421.

Morales, L. S., Lara, M., Kington, R. S., Valdez, R. O., & Escarce, J. J. (2002). Socioeconomic, cultural, and behavioral factors affecting Hispanic health outcomes. *Journal of Health Care for the Poor and Underserved,* 13, 477–503.

Nagasawa, R., Qian, Z., & Wong, P. (2001). Theory of segmented assimilation and the adoption of marijuana use and delinquency by Asian Pacific youth. *Sociological Quarterly,* 42, 351–372.

Oetting, E. R., & Beauvais, F. (1990). Orthogonal cultural identification theory: The cultural identification of minority adolescents. *International Journal of Addictions,* 25(5A–6A), 655–685.

Office of the UN High Commissioner for Refugees. (2008). *2007 global trends: Refugees, asylum-seekers, returnees, internally displaced and stateless persons.* Geneva: Author.

Ogbu, J. U. (1995). Cultural problems in minority education: Their interpretations and consequences—Part One: Theoretical background. *Urban Review, 27,* 189–205.

Padilla, A. M., Cervantes, R. C., Maldonado, M., & Garcia, R. E. (1988). Coping responses to psychosocial stressors among Mexican and Central American immigrants. *Journal of Community Psychology, 16,* 418–427.

Palloni, A., & Morenoff, J. D. (2001). Interpreting the paradoxical in the Latino paradox: Demographic and epidemiological approaches. *Annals of the New York Academy of Sciences, 954,* 140–174.

Pettigrew, T. F., & Tropp, L. R. (2006). A meta-analytic test of intergroup contact theory. *Journal of Personality and Social Psychology, 90,* 751–783.

Phinney, J. S. (1990). Ethnic identity in adolescents and adults: Review of research. *Psychological Bulletin, 108,* 499–514.

Phinney, J. S. (1993). A three-stage model of ethnic identity development in adolescence. In M. E. Bernal & G. P. Knight (Eds.), *Ethnic identity: Formation and transmission among Hispanics and other minorities* (pp. 61–79). Albany: State University of New York Press.

Porter, M., & Haslam, N. (2005). Predisplacement and postdisplacement factors associated with mental health of refugees and internally displaced persons: A meta-analysis. *Journal of the American Medical Association, 294,* 602–612.

Portes, A. (1997). Immigration theory for a new century: Some problems and opportunities. *International Migration Review, 31,* 799–825.

Portes, A., & Rumbaut, R. G. (1996). *Immigrant America: A portrait.* Berkeley: University of California Press.

Portes, A., & Zhou, M. (1993). The new second generation: Segmented assimilation and its variants. *Annals of the American Academy of Political and Social Science, 530,* 74–96.

Ramirez, M. (1999). *Multicultural psychotherapy: An approach to individual and cultural differences* (2nd ed.). Boston: Allyn & Bacon.

Redfield, R., Linton, R., & Herskovits, M. J. (1936). Memorandum for the study of acculturation. *American Anthropologist, 38,* 149–152.

Resnicow, K., Soler, R., Braithwait, R. L., Ahlu-walia, J. S., & Butler, J. (2000). Cultural sensitivity in substance abuse prevention. *Journal of Community Psychology, 28,* 271–290.

Rogler, L. H. (1994). International migrations: A framework for directing research. *American Psychologist, 49,* 701–708.

Rogler, L. H., Cortes, D. E., & Malgady, R. G. (1991). Acculturation and mental health status among Hispanics. *American Psychologist, 46,* 585–597.

Rudmin, F. W. (2003). Critical history of the acculturation psychology of assimilation, separation, integration, and marginalization. *Review of General Psychology, 7,* 3–37.

Rudmin, F. W. (2006). Debate in science: The case of acculturation [Electronic version]. *AnthroGlobe Journal.* Retrieved July 6, 2008, from *malinowski.kent.ac.uk/docs/rudminf_acculturation_061204.pdf.*

Rutter, M. (1999). Resilience as the millennium Rorschach: Response to Smith and Gorrell Barnes. *Journal of Family Therapy, 21,* 159–160.

Salant, T., & Lauderdale, D. S. (2003). Measuring culture: A critical review of acculturation and health in Asian immigrant populations. *Social Science and Medicine, 57,* 71–90.

Schwartz, S. J., Montgomery, M. J., & Briones, E. (2006). The role of identity in acculturation among immigrant people: Theoretical propositions, empirical questions, and applied recommendations. *Human Development, 49,* 1–30.

Schwartz, S. J., Pantin, H., Prado, G., Sullivan, S., & Szapocznik, J. (2005). Family functioning, identity, and problem behavior in Hispanic immigrant early adolescents. *Journal of Early Adolescence, 25,* 392–420.

Stafford, M., & Marmot, M. (2003). Neighborhood deprivation and health: Does it affect us all equally? *International Journal of Epidemiology, 32,* 357–366.

Stein, B. N. (1981). The refugee experience: Defining the parameters of a field of study. *International Migration Review, 15,* 320–330.

Tajfel, H., & Turner, J. (1986). The social identity theory of intergroup behavior. In S. Worchel & W. Austin (Eds.), *Psychology of intergroup relations* (pp. 7–24). Chicago: Nelson-Hall.

Thompson, L. (1969). *The secret of culture: Nine community studies.* New York: Random House.

Triandis, H. C., & Brislin, R. W. (1984). Cross-cultural psychology. *American Psychologist*, *39*, 1006–1016.

Tugade, M. M., & Fredrickson, B. L. (2004). Resilient individuals use positive emotions to bounce back from negative emotional experiences. *Journal of Personality and Social Psychology*, *86*, 320–333.

Ungar, M. (2003). Qualitative contributions to resilience research. *Qualitative Social Work*, *2*, 85–102.

United Nations. (2002). *Number of world's migrants reaches 175 million mark* (No. Press Release POP/844). New York: Author.

United Nations. (2008). *World urbanization to hit historic high by year's end*. New York: Author.

Valez, C. N., & Ungemack, J. A. (1995). Psychosocial correlates of drug use among Puerto Rican youth: Generational status differences. *Social Science and Medicine*, *40*, 91–103.

Viruell-Fuentes, E. A. (2007). Beyond acculturation: Immigration, discrimination, and health research among Mexicans in the United States. *Social Science and Medicine*, *65*, 1524–1535.

Walker, R. L. (2007). Acculturation and acculturative stress as indicators for suicide risk among African Americans. *American Journal of Orthopsychiatry*, *77*, 386–391.

Wandersman, A., & Nation, M. (1998). Urban neighborhoods and mental health: Psychological contributions to understanding toxicity, resilience, and interventions. *American Psychologist*, *53*, 647–656.

Watson, D., Wiese, D., Vaidya, J., & Tellegen, A. (1999). The two general activation systems of affect: Structural findings, evolutionary considerations, and psychobiological evidence. *Journal of Personality and Social Psychology*, *76*, 820–838.

Weisskirch, R. S. (2005). The relationship of language brokering to ethnic identity for Latino early adolescents. *Hispanic Journal of Behavioral Sciences*, *27*, 286–299.

Williams, R. B. (1998). Asian Indian and Pakistani religions in the United States. *Annals of the American Academy of Political Science*, *558*, 178–195.

Wills, T. A., Murry, V. M., Brody, G. H., Gibbons, F. X., Gerrard, M., Walker, C., et al. (2007). Ethnic pride and self-control related to protective and risk factors: Test of the theoretical model for the strong African American families program. *Health Psychology*, *26*, 50–59.

Zautra, A. J. (2003). *Stress, emotions and health*. New York: Oxford University Press.

Zautra, A. J., Hall, J. S., & Murray, K. E. (2008). Resilience: A new integrative approach to health and mental health research. *Health Psychology Review*, *2*, 41–64.

Zhou, M. (1997). Growing up American: The challenge confronting immigrant children and children of immigrants. *Annual Review of Sociology*, *23*, 63–95.

19

Cultural Dimensions of Resilience among Adults

Michael Ungar

The construct of resilience remains largely unknown outside a few Western, English-speaking nations. Conceptually, however, there is evidence from studies of children, youth, and adults of coping patterns within stressful environments, illustrating mechanisms that mitigate the impact of risk and promote well-being (Ungar, 2005; Wong & Wong, 2006). In this chapter, I review the conceptual and empirical challenges that we encounter when trying to understand (and nurture) resilience across different cultures and contexts. Definitional ambiguity and contextual influences muddy the conceptual waters; research design and measurement similarly confound efforts to investigate resilience empirically. This is especially true when resilience as a culture-bound construct is studied beyond what Kagitçibasi (2006) characterizes as the *minority world* (the small percentage of people living in Western nations with a Eurocentric perspective and attachment to an objectivist scientific discourse). To address both the conceptual and

empirical problems culture introduces to the study of resilience, I offer a definition that accounts for both processes and outcomes associated with adaptation in culturally meaningful ways. I also review the literature that does exist for a construct that still finds its empirical footing mostly in the minority world. Based on what is available, I argue that there is both homogeneity and heterogeneity in outcomes and processes associated with resilience when cultural pluralism and contextual variation are introduced into how we both conceptualize and investigate stress and coping in resource-poor ecologies.

Conceptual Issues

Resilience is a conceptual nameplate for a body of research and interventions focused on positive developmental outcomes among populations that face substantial amounts of risk. Typically the term is used in two ways. First, as an outcome, *resilience* is associated with the acquisition of both internal and external assets that work together to potentiate a state of mental and physical well-being when individuals are exposed to non-normative levels of psychosocial stress. The term may also be used to indicate engagement in protective processes associated with the development of preferred outcomes. In other words, we may say that an individual *is resilient* (when referring to positive outcomes despite exposure to risk) or *shows resilience* (when referring to the individual's participation in processes that lead to well-being under stress). These positive developmental outcomes have been shown to result from processes as diverse as changing growth trajectories; buffering the impact of exposure to risk; promoting self-esteem through relationships; and augmenting access to health-enhancing resources, such as mentors, social supports, meaningful employment, political efficacy, and a positive cultural identity (Garmezy, 1983; Luthar, Cicchetti, & Becker, 2000; Rutter, 1987; Ungar, 2004b).

In an effort to reconcile these disparate definitions and to introduce into the definition the fluidity necessary to account for contextual and cultural variability, I have suggested that *resilience* be defined as follows:

> In the context of exposure to significant adversity, whether psychological, environmental, or both, resilience is both the capacity of individuals to navigate their way to health-sustaining resources, including opportunities to experience feelings of well-being, and a condition of the individual's family, community and culture to provide these health resources and experiences in culturally meaningful ways. (Ungar, 2008, p. 225)

To illustrate why a more ecological definition of resilience is necessary, we might consider the experience of an adult immigrant who has witnessed the genocide perpetrated against his or her people because of their ethnicity. There are many examples of such experiences, including victims of the Holocaust, the Rawandan genocide, the Lost Boys who fled Sudan in the late 1980s, and the ethnic cleansings that took place in the former Yugoslavia. As immigrants and refugees, people's capacity to heal is only partly the consequence of their ability to create psychological well-being (in the form of personal efficacy or a positive identity as a survivor). The term *resilience* also reflects their capacity to navigate to a safer physical ecology (e.g., a humanitarian refugee camp) and a facilitative social ecology (e.g., relationships with others who share similar experiences). Both ecological dimensions must be provided by those on whom the refugees depend. Underlying a culturally and contextually relevant definition of resilience (for any population under stress) is, therefore, aspects of *navigation*, the agentic exercise of personal power directed toward the acquisition of resources. Arguably, these resources may only be selected from those that are both available and accessible within the individual's physical and social ecologies, or latent within his or her psychological and genetic predisposition. This first principle of navigation, therefore, is multidimensional. Navigation cannot only be the individual's capacity to "beat the odds": It must also be a measure of the capacity of service providers, governments, churches, families, and communities to help individuals facing significant adversity "change the odds" stacked against them (see Seccombe, 2002). In this sense, resilience is a process that is reliant upon the physical and social ecologies in which it unfolds and, therefore, is necessarily culture bound by the everyday practices and sociopolitical decisions of one's society. Conceptually, it is a misnomer to talk of the resilient individual without also talking about the resilient environment that facilitates survival.

To the process of navigation must be added cultural sensitivity. By *culture*, I am referring to everyday practices that are ritualized into a set of values and systems of codified beliefs that reflexively perpetuate orderly social relations. Cultural norms and expectations are transmitted vertically between generations and horizontally between individuals who are of the culture and those who are compelled or choose to acculturate. The relevance of culture to resilience is that it shapes the availability and accessibility of facilitative resources (both internal and external) necessary for positive development under stress. For example, a community may decide to limit the availability of postsecondary education to women or, even when that education is available, make school attendance prohibitively expensive and therefore inaccessible. These political decisions regarding resources shape the majority of people's capacity to navigate to what they need, even if they are endowed with psychological and genetic qualities that predispose them toward success. Even internal qualities such as temperament and intelligence differ in their availability because different cultural contexts may value or diminish in importance specific characteristics, encouraging the individual to deny him- or herself free self-expression (Chen, DeSouza, Chen, & Wang, 2006).

The second principle of resilience must therefore be *negotiation*. Individuals and communities may overcome stress and engage in processes that sustain well-being when they are able to *negotiate* for health-sustaining resources to be provided in culturally meaningful ways. In many instances, this produces cultural disharmony as one group (in the previous example, refugees) may make demands for resources, such as social services and religious tolerance, that challenges the biases of those in the dominant culture. Negotiation means successfully securing not only physical resources, such as housing, food, education and safety, in the quality and quantity required but also the discursive power to define one's self and one's coping strategies as successful.

Returning to the example of the refugee, personal motivations and talents help individuals to cope with trauma, but a safe community, adequate financial assistance, and access to retraining opportunities ensure that one's personal talents can be used. The nature of the services provided to facilitate integration, however, must be culturally relevant. Resettlement that results in social isolation from one's cultural peers, education that does not match the identity formation needs of the individual, and employment opportunities that fail to provide status (as defined by the individual's culture) do not provide for the psychological well-being of those relocated, even if materially their safety is assured. Furthermore, individual-level variables also vary in their contribution to well-being, with aspects of personality being devalued (therefore diminishing one's coping capacity) when one is out of step with the norms of the dominant culture.

Homogeneity versus Heterogeneity

Paradoxically, defining *resilience* as dual processes of navigation and negotiation provides a universal way to conceptualize the processes associated with adaptation to stress, while tolerating heterogeneity in the outcomes associated with the construct. Research by Ungar and his colleagues in 14 communities globally has documented both processes at work in the lives of older youth facing significant risk as they transition to adulthood (Ungar et al., 2007, 2008). Whereas some processes were found to be common across cultures, the specificity of their expression and the outcomes that are negotiated as valuable (and therefore culturally determined) permit a more fluid postmodern treatment of stress and coping. In this culturally relative understanding of stress, normative and non-normative life events cause individuals anxiety only to the extent that events are perceived as challenging (see Johnson & McCutcheon, 1980). Within any single cultural context, the nature of negotiations to define events as positive or negative (stressful) may be difficult to deconstruct when cultural insiders' assumptions of normality discourage critical reflection. Outcomes associated with positive development become tautologies: The successful adult is the one everyone agrees is performing in culturally approved ways. Alternative expressions of coping that fall outside the norm may be seen as a sign of vulnerability instead of resilience. For example, the need to acculturate may be more burdensome in the United States, where cultural norms encourage a "melting pot," whereas resistance to acculturation (isolationism) in Canada may be encouraged because of federal policies that promote "multiculturalism." Neither national process is necessarily good or bad. Both are simply cultural norms that seek to order relationships between social groups to everyone's benefit.

It has long been understood that stress and coping interact both empirically and conceptually (Reich & Zautra, 1988). Across varying social ecologies, these interactions become even more complex. Two aspects of this relationship may be better accounted for when we overlay this model of navigation and negotiation onto processes related to stress and coping. First, coping is always a judgment made within discursive spaces that involve people with varying degrees of power engaging in definitional practices to honor how they understand success. By way of illustration, in her doctoral research, Singh (2007) documents the complexity in how South Asian women navigate the terrain of sexual abuse. As a cultural value "emotional restraint" is highly prized, but "this valuation of silence and restraint serves as a double-bind for South Asian women who are survivors of sexual trauma, as the cultural command of silence about their experiences of abuse manifests in long-term psychologically damaging effects" (p. 3). Herein lies the paradox. Enduring violence without complaint brings these women a sense of coherence (Antonovsky, 1987), the orderly positioning of themselves within a matrix of relationships upon which they depend: "that silence then becomes a method of empowerment, negotiation, and resilience for South Asian women in their families" (p. 4). Singh is not naive to the consequences of this cop-

ing strategy, noting that it reflects the privilege and oppression of those who employ it. However, her qualitative work with women ages 22–48 suggests that the use of silence (a strategy that they say promotes their resilience) helps to preserve their families' standing in the community and their own well-being. Such collectivist ideas are difficult for Westerners to appreciate, but within the South Asian community a child's rape can compromise her ability to marry and the respect her family receives in their community. Silence was described by the women Singh interviewed as a way they maintain a sense of hope. The silence imposed on them, and that which is self-imposed, becomes a mode of coping:

> Informants described how they used the cultural command of silence about child sexual abuse as a way to introvert and separate from others so they could heal. None of the informants described feeling positively about being silenced about their abuse. However, they described transforming the South Asian demand of women's silence about abuse into a positive coping strategy. (p. 36)

This example is one of many in the literature, mostly documented through qualitative research with narrowly defined populations (Ungar, 2003). Often the culturally based coping strategy employed is one that the dominant culture defines as pathological (in the previous example, the women might be said to show "learned helplessness"; Abramson, Seligman, & Teasdale, 1978) or oppressive. Discursive dissonance results when majority world cultures challenge Eurocentric bias and the supposition of universality in outcomes. Arguably, there is a need to appreciate that universal processes may proceed with multifinality. A few good processes may produce many different outcomes.

This terrain where resilience is defined becomes even more contestable when stress and coping are understood as variable in their relationship even within one set of cultural boundaries. Among individuals who share a similar culture, contextual differences, such as degree of poverty, or rurality, may influence the degree to which particular stressors confound developmental outcomes. There is an interaction between the context and stress exposure. Resilience researchers are very clear on this point. A promotive factor acts differently for individuals under stress than for those whose level of stress exposure is more normative (Luthar et al., 2000). To illustrate, an individual from a privileged background may improve his or her life chances by attaining higher education, but the amount of variance accounted for in a model of successful development may be very low when there is little exposure to prior risk. Alternatively, for a student from a racial minority with very low levels of postsecondary school attendance, the effect of a university degree on life course development would account for a large proportion of variance in explanatory models of resilience (Hannon, 2003). Without contextualization and appreciation of the relevant experience of the individuals involved, the impact of stressors and coping strategies are difficult to predict. Phenomenologically, stress and coping depend on context. Studies of resilience therefore provide a useful way to understand these associations. Context, of which culture is one dimension, creates variability in how the processes of navigation and negotiation unfold.

What this means is that resilience (like coping) must be distinct from simple expressions of strengths. Those from low-stress, privileged backgrounds also navigate and negotiate. *Resilience*, though, refers to navigations and negotiations in exceptional physical and social ecologies that burden individuals. The processes may be similar, but the qualitative nature of one's navigations and negotiations, and the influence of particular outcomes, will vary. Returning to Singh's example (2007) of South Asian women and their coping strategies following sexual abuse, normal social processes, such as acculturation, take on a very different

meaning. Studies of acculturation among both adult women (Grant et al., 2004) and youth (Berry, Phinney, Sam, & Vedder, 2006) have shown that immigrants who do not acculturate may actually do better psychologically than those who adopt new cultural identities, when doing so threatens their adherence to their own cultural norms. Not acculturating to the dominant values of those around them may actually provide a culturally relevant set of strategies to survive the psychological pain of the abuse. In these women's case, relationships are very important to this strategy, both constraining self-expression and co-constructing the individual as powerful within this uniquely feminized definition of control. Relationships may be universally helpful, but their function, form, and impact in this context are immensely important to sustaining well-being. Understood this way, culture (and its everyday practices) both shapes the nature of one's navigations and negotiations for health-enhancing resources and is itself an outcome. Holding on to one's culture well (*cultural adherence*) may help to buffer stress in abnormally difficult situations.

A Developmental Perspective

The principles of navigation and negotiation that undergird a culturally variant definition of resilience can help to scaffold an inquiry into the substantive building blocks of positive development across populations. Understanding navigations that influence resilience requires sensitivity to several dimensions, among which are developmental age or stage (including the life phase of the adult); personal barriers to community and institutional participation (in schools, recreation, social networks) that change with age-related status; individual and collective strengths (locus of control, temperament, intelligence, ethnoracial identity, cultural rituals and rites of passage); the toxicity or sustainability of the physical ecology (the quality of water and air in natural and manufactured environments); and the economic and political dimensions of interaction that decide which resources are provided and to whom. The more each of these dimensions facilitates adaptation under stress, the more likely there is to be navigation to health-sustaining resources that people say are meaningful to them.

The processes are necessarily developmental, with individuals and their environment demonstrating plasticity in interactions that change over time (Lerner, Dowling, & Anderson, 2003). For example, as Yates, Egeland, and Sroufe (2003) have shown through their 25-year longitudinal study, the processes that potentiate resilience begin early, both shaping the opportunity structures that surround the child and later the adult, and influencing individuals' capacities to make the most of opportunities. Referring specifically to the focal population of their work, Yates and colleagues write:

> The successful negotiation of early developmental issues provides a foundation for the process of resilience among disadvantaged youth. This process originates in early transactional exchanges between the child and her or his caregiver that scaffold the child's developing capacities for adaptive emotion regulation, social engagement, and positive expectations of the social world and of the self. (pp. 257–258)

Evidence from equally mature longitudinal studies, such as those by Werner and Smith (2001) begun in the 1950s with a birth cohort of 697 children, has shown that early developmental gains and social advantages are associated with later resilience. However, these pathways are neither linear nor without setbacks. Although most individuals who show good coping early continue to do well, a portion of individuals who overcome early disadvantage succumb to the challenges of adult developmental tasks. In Werner and Smith's study, 16% of the total sample of men and women were not doing well at midlife. Of these individuals, two-thirds of the males and four-fifths of the women had

been troubled teens. Phrased this way, the focus is on the persistence of maladaptive coping strategies. However, although this would seem to argue for the inevitability of maladaptation, a prospective look at the findings shows that "by age forty, only one out of four of the individuals who had been troubled teens were still doing poorly. Three out of four were coping with the demands of midlife without any major problems" (p. 54). The significance of such longitudinal work is the optimism that disadvantaged populations can navigate their way through developmental tasks even during their adult years. Far more succeed than fail. Werner and Smith explain these positive trajectories as being potentiated by both early access to resources and the availability of the resources that facilitate recovery later in life.

Findings such as these point to the need for a process of constant inquiry to understand the adult's navigations and negotiations for resources. Resources that are more or less valued as developmental goals will fluctuate. In this sense, identity formation as one who is healthy is best seen as "liquid" (Bauman, 2000). There are a great many choices available to individuals in a globalized pastiche of colliding culturally determined definitions of what it means to be *doing well*.

Empirical Issues

As already shown, understanding resilience means not only conceptualizing the threats facing individuals but also deconstructing the culturally normative meaning of successful development amid exposure to risk. Generic factors across populations, such as a meaningful role in one's community, self-efficacy, self-esteem, secure attachments, safety, and optimism (see Kirby & Fraser, 1997), may contribute to resilience but culturally embedded expressions of each factor (e.g., patterns of interaction with parents, feelings of responsibility for others, rites of passage, religious affiliations, a sense of humor, and gender-based expectations) combine to shape how a sense of well-being is achieved when risk is present (McCubbin et al., 1998; Ungar, 2005).

Empirically, resilience is difficult to account for across cultures because navigations and negotiations are variable in their expression. There are several ways, however, that cultural sensitivity to variation and research methodologies can find epistemological convergence. First, research is made easier when resilience and vulnerability are maintained as two factors rather than opposite ends of a unidimensional variable. Like understandings of mental health and mental illness, the measure of an individual's vulnerability (risk) may be high or low, with only minimal covariance demonstrated with his or her resilience. *Resilience* refers only to the positive aspects of development under stress. The absence of strengths does not necessarily mean that one's vulnerability increases. This is particularly important when understanding resilience across cultures. For example, shyness was previously valued as a positive quality among urban Chinese when Chen and colleagues (2006) evaluated young people in the early 1990s. More shyness was associated with more successful academic achievement and desirability among peers, but less shyness did not necessarily mean that one was at risk of being ignored or failing school. It was a unidimensional construct. Being outgoing, however, is a separate dimension of personality and can be associated with vulnerability because outgoing individuals may have more delinquent peers, which increases their exposure to risk and detracts them from their studies. All this is entirely variable within the cultural collisions now taking place in modern China. In Chen and colleagues' follow-up research a decade later, urban Chinese youth showed that they no longer valued shyness, instead demonstrating patterns of desirability typical of Western youth. Being shy switched to a vulnerability factor, putting one's social relationships in peril. Likewise, outgoingness became a resilience factor, predicting better coping in the competitive

environment of Shanghai's schools. Keeping these two factors, resilience and vulnerability, separate simplifies empirical investigations of resilience when researchers account for cultural variation.

The second thing we can do to facilitate the study of resilience is to work with multiple methods. Empirically, the problem with studying resilience is who decides what are positive indicators of resilience across cultures and contexts. Research can resolve this by working with both quantitative and qualitative investigations to inquire into the phenomological expressions of resilience. Working across cultures, it is difficult to imagine a study whose construct validity (in the qualitative paradigm, authenticity) is not challenged by those from the culture studied if multiple methods are not employed.

Empirically, then, there must remain tension between the *emic*, or idiosyncratic, understanding by a homogeneous population regarding the antecedents of well-being under stress, and the *etic*, or transcultural and generalizable, aspects of resilience common to heterogeneous populations. The problem with much of the resilience research is lack of transparency with regard to which perspective is being used. The standpoint bias of those who do the research is seldom made clear. Whereas the Western scientific tradition has helped to generate a list of supposed universals with regard to stress and coping, a Eurocentric, social democratic tradition of psychological science has yet to prove its generalizability to the majority world, to those people living outside Western democracies, and to those marginalized by race and ethnicity (including Aboriginal peoples) who reside therein (Smith, 1999). Reasonably, one's ethnoracial background would be expected to shape most aspects of what we mean by *resilience*. After all, as Sisneros, Stakeman, Joyner, and Schmitz (2007) explain,

> Ethnicity is fluid, flexible, layered, and dependent on circumstances and context; ethnic identity is affected by cultural elements, af-

filiative dimensions (selection of friends and acquaintances from one's own ethnic group, as well as behavior and dress), and subjective dimensions (perceptions of those within and outside the ethnic group of which one is a member). (p. 42)

Investigating resilience outside Western contexts (where authenticity of the concept has not yet been shown) requires accounting for variations in people's physical and social ecologies, and the negotiated meaning systems they use every day.

Even if we want to account for differences, the task can become terribly cumbersome. When culture is accounted for, there can be a naive assumption of differences when in fact homogenization of culture has already muted variation between groups that are only superficially categorized as separate. This can be seen when studies of well-being account for ethnicity or race within environments in which one culture dominates (see, e.g., Alegria, Takeuchi, et al., 2004). One's expressed ethnicity reflects one's sense of attachment to a group identity, which in turn shapes values and behavior. Race, too, is just as much a social construction as ethnicity, with a set of beliefs that are as permeable and temporal. Superficial qualities, such as skin color and shape of facial features, may cue us to an individual's racial category, but the designation overlooks the much more important similarities we share in the human genome, or phenomenologically because of our social class. Not surprisingly, then, one's immersion in any one particular group brings with it historical antecedents that facilitate or prevent access to social and economic opportunities, identity conclusions, and experiences associated with psychological well-being under stress.

The problem, however, is not so simple as to suppose a crisp division between ethnoracial groups and their experiences regarding developmental processes. Even when we naively assume differences and design qualitative studies with unique and bounded populations, there remains much that is shared between groups when development takes place within shared spaces that constrain navigations and negotiations. The process by which ethnoracial identity informs people's lives is a two-way street, with an individual's culture colliding with that of the dominant culture that surrounds him or her. According to McGoldrick (2003), "Ethnicity refers to a group's common ancestry through which individuals have evolved shared values and customs. It is deeply tied to the family, through which it is transmitted over generations, and it is reinforced—and at times invalidated—by the surrounding community" (p. 236). Processes of globalization, the discursive power of Western scientific method, and the dynamics of acculturation and cultural imperialism all make study data practically indecipherable unless multiple methods are employed. After all, just because an individual is perceived to be representative of ethnoracial diversity, it does not necessarily follow that he or she is influenced by the culture in which he or she is thought to be a member. While such a powerful aspect of ourselves may be transmitted transgenerationally, McGoldrick is conscious in her clinical work that people also exercise their right to ignore or reject aspects of their heritage. Importantly, when understanding resilience across cultures, both cultural adherence and cleaving one's self from ethnoracial and cultural traditions are more or less adaptive coping strategies, depending on the individual's context (Ungar et al., 2007). Affiliation may bring access to a network of supports, whereas assimilation with the dominant culture may be an attempt to "pass" among cultural elites who control access to education, employment, and other structural opportunities. Given this dynamic interchange and people's personal agency in ethnocultural self-definition, the benchmarks of resilience are bound to be ambiguous when viewed both within and across populations.

Empirically, this problem of culture as it relates to positive coping also affects those from the dominant (typically white) cultural group. In the cultural mosaic of the West, being white with European ancestry may be overlooked as one's cultural identity. This white privilege is made invisible when the dominant group talks of diversity as a quality of other groups but not itself. Supported by a transnational privileging of one set of cultural norms, whiteness can make white culture imperceptible. Interestingly, the concept of whiteness was originally developed to classify men who would enjoy the rights of citizenship in early American society. As Sisneros and colleagues (2007) remind us: "One of the hidden phenomena of membership in a privileged group is the assumption of normality, according to which others are not normal" (p. 25). As a culturally relative judgment of normative positive functioning under stress, definitions of resilience that are operationalized in studies across cultures are at risk of reifying value systems that are always changing. A survey of the literature concerned with resilience and coping among adults across cultures suggests there is *more a need to ask than to tell*. Both clinical interventions and research that use the construct of resilience are biased when they do not include a process of inquiry into the localized meaning of positive development under stress.

The third empirical issue that needs attention in culturally sensitive investigations of resilience, then, is the investigation of what is universal and what is unique to different populations. Many studies overlook the difficult terrain of culture and context in which resilience is realized, assuming construct homogeneity. For example, in a study of 450 Russian immigrants to northern Israel (Aroian & Norris, 2000), resilience was found to be related to depression but not to the overall level of distress experienced by immigrants whose average time of resettlement was 3 years. The study quantified resilience as nine items on a reduced version of Wagnild and Young's (1993) Resilience Scale. The items measured included constructs such as self-reliance, independence, determination, and perseverance. No effort was made to under-stand whether such characteristics were most relevant to the population of Soviet Jews who came from a more collectivist society than Israel. Though other studies have demonstrated the validity of the Resilience Scale across cultures (see Pesce et al., 2005), there are often assumptions of generalizability of the underlying constructs. Researchers commonly overlook more indigenous factors relevant to survival. Equally troubling, studies such as this make little or no effort to understand the conditions in which personal traits are activated or suppressed when individuals are in transition between contexts, with variable access to health-enhancing resources. How common the population's experience really is may go unstudied.

Caution is needed, therefore, when interpreting culture and its influence on people's adaptations. Totalizing a group's experience as culture bound can falsely imply impermeable boundaries between individuals and the values held by others who control the social discourse found in the media, in educational systems, and in the economy that surrounds them. In an example of Israeli and Arab parenting practices, the findings suggest a separation between the two groups, when in fact all that is observed is a continuum of experience on a single factor (e.g., social support). Thus, despite my previous argument regarding cultural specificity, in fact there may also be cause to believe that universal processes are at play. Herein lies the problem for empirical investigations of resilience: There always remains the challenge to account for the intersection of culture and context. Factors accepted as indicators of positive development change depending on people's adherence to their culture across contexts (at one's place of employment, cultural differences may be more muted as people try to fit in) and time (developmentally, older adults are more likely to adhere more strongly to their culture; Knyazev, Supancic, & Slobodskaya, 2008). The Israeli–Arab study would be more compelling with evidence as to the degree of differentiation along lines of both collectivism and individualism, and if bias toward a certain type of child play and responsiveness were not implied by the analysis. In a more collectivist Arab culture (an assumption for which no test is provided), the question is whether the type of parenting practices used and the more compliant child that results is seen as advantageous.

How, then, are we to know which culturally determined factors are likely predictive of a population's success? And how small a unit of analysis should we examine in our research if we are to understand what resilience means for different cultural groups? The best we can do is demonstrate sensitivity to the pluralism that comes with multicultural perspectives on healthy development and ask people to define for themselves the boundaries to their sociocultural affiliations. If, for example, we look at why young adults go to college, sensitivity is needed to account for differences across populations. In a study of 713 freshmen, Phinney, Dennis, and Osorio (2006) found that for ethnic/minority and lower-income students, helping family and proving worth through postsecondary education were important factors that had not previously appeared in the research using common measures to account for student motivation. Coté and Levine (1997) found in their studies (which were not explicitly investigating cultural variability) only general support for both these concepts: family and self-worth. However, when only ethnically diverse and lower-income students were studied, both themes were distinct and overlapping. Therefore, although there is a trend here toward homogeneity across cultural minorities and majorities with regard to why adults go to college, there is also heterogeneity in the influence of different motivations. The possible contagion effect is a dominant culture that values education for particular reasons and influences the values of minorities. Whenever we study the values of groups (especially a younger, more culturally mobile group, such as well-educated young adults), we need to pay attention to culture as a negotiated space, with the definition of positive behavior contingent on aspects of culture to

which the individual adheres most. None of this need necessarily tumble us into the abyss of endless differentiation. Some aspects of culture, such as education, appropriate use of violence, social support, and contribution to one's community, can be assumed to be nearly universal across cultures (see Georgas, Berry, van de Vijver, Kagitçibasi, & Poortinga, 2006; Ungar, 2008).

Researching Resilience across Cultures

Nuanced understandings such as these are likely to require a research paradigm that is more tolerant of the emic perspectives of participants (subjects). Sanchez, Spector, and Cooper (2006) note that a serious limitation in cross-cultural/cross-national (CC/CN) stress research is the "reliance on measures that are developed in a single country and exported for use elsewhere. Even if the items are successfully translated linguistically, there exists the possibility that the individual items do not do a good job of reflecting the construct universally. In other words the scale suffers from ethnocentricity in its development" (p. 197). Similarly, Tweed and Conway (2006) explain in regard to coping: "The very idea of what makes a good 'outcome' is itself subject to cultural variability, and researchers should be wary of over-applying particular measures of psychological coping success (e.g., increases in self-esteem) in cultures where these measures have less meaning for that purpose" (p. 148). Both cautions warn resilience researchers seeking to understand the concept to view it as a social construction. Culture is more than a confounding variable when we appreciate that for individual populations and subpopulations, the specificity of coping requires us to look for uniquely local characteristics that may not be reflected in the literature. Even among marginalized groups within a single country, such as minority populations of Hispanic peoples in the United States, there may be great variability within groups when individuals claim different geographic and historical traditions (i.e.,

Cuban Americans and Mexican Americans). Without establishing the degree of construct invariance across groups, structural pathways from predictor variables to outcomes are not interpretable (Tragesser, Beauvais, Swaim, Edwards, & Oetting, 2007). As van de Vijver and Leung (1997) explain, deconstructing culture means that we make careful choices regarding the context variables to be measured and how findings are understood.

When Alegria, Woo, and her colleagues (2004) sought standardized measures applicable to ethnic/minority populations, they realized that the heterogeneity of the populations they were studying for the National Latino and Asian American Study would confound the use of most measures:

> Although a thorough understanding of concepts relevant to one culture is obtained using the emic approach, these concepts are not necessarily comparable to those of other cultures. On the other hand, the etic approach emphasizes reliability by standardizing the measures at the expense of validity (measuring what is supposed to be measured). Validity may be compromised by imposing artifactual cross-cultural homogeneity due to a constricted conceptualization (omitting differences across groups) embedded in the instrumentation. (p. 272)

Getting around these shortcomings inevitably leads to unsatisfactory compromises if generalizability is the goal. Mixed-method approaches, and more focused quantitative research, may provide results with greater construct validity (Luthar & Brown, 2007; Ungar & Liebenberg, 2005).

There are few good examples of culturally sensitive resilience research involving adults; the majority of the work in this field has been with children. However, what does exist often involves adults following disasters and war. An American example is Weiss and Berger's (2006) study following the World Trade Center attacks in New York in 2001. The highest rates of posttraumatic stress disorder (PTSD) among people living in New York were found among Hispanic women, even though they were the least likely as a group to have had firsthand experience with the disaster (the direct loss of a relative, or having worked near the Towers). Weiss and Berger speculated that these women's social isolation, lack of education, and poor income made them more vulnerable to the effects of social turmoil. Although these factors may be relevant for many different cultures, they were particularly influential in the lives of these women given their social location within a society in which most of them were only marginally involved. Nurturing resilience among these women would necessarily involve addressing each aspect of their vulnerability (e.g., building their social capital), while also identifying localized constructions of strengths most relevant to them.

Widening Our Perspective of Resilience

Globally, efforts are being made to broaden how we conceptualize and measure resilience. The ethnocentrism of psychological theory is being challenged by many multicultural research teams. For example, Georgas and colleagues (2006), using Berry's (1969) ecocultural framework, are investigating family behavior across global contexts with sensitivity to ecological and sociopolitical factors. As Berry and Poortinga (2006) write: "As a discipline, psychology tends to be both culture-bound and culture-blind" (p. 52). Although their work focuses on identifying "pan-human validity" (p. 52), the goal is unlikely to be realized except for the broadest of generalities. Valid models to explain human interaction are likely to be negotiated when the perspectives of majority world cultures are privileged. Those with less representation in the Western psychological discourse (notably, in the journals that publish funded research) are sorely disadvantaged in arguing for their perspective of healthy developmental trajectories. The relative power of the Western researcher or clinician trumps the social location of people whose cultural experience is not well represented. One might see this more clearly if the situation were reversed. One can imagine the controversy if Western families were judged by the standards of more collectivist societies, as found in Islamic, Asian, and Aboriginal communities (see Kagitçibasi, 2006). By such standards, many suburban middle-class adults would be shown to be highly disordered if the benchmarks of successful functioning were fully inverted to privilege less economically developed but socially cohesive populations globally. The social capital that Putnam (2000) warns is endangered in North America still exists in less economically developed nations. One might imagine an entire nosology of psychological symptoms associated with Western lifestyles: alienation, materialism, declining focus on the family, institutionalization of older adults, lack of shared public spaces, and paucity of physical contact. All these factors would be evidence of severe dysfunction among Westerners.

As cultural myopia is challenged through the empowerment of marginalized voices, broader understandings of positive development under stress are found. For example, the phylogenetically blind view of the Western family as the ideal structure is being questioned by the positive reframing of more diverse adult and child social relations. The matriarchal family of the Caribbean, in which fathers are transient and children are raised by their extended family in kinship adoption systems during crises (as in some Aboriginal communities; Blackstock & Trocmé, 2005) are examples of variability in how successful attachment, a frequent benchmark of resilience, is achieved.

Methodologically, we can find new (and often muted) understandings of resilience when we engage those who are invisible in the literature in participatory processes that provide a forum in which to be heard. In Brown's (2004) look at blackness among young, urban black men, he found that what helps these men survive systemic racism may

not always be seen as prosocial when judged by the standards of the dominant culture. There is a need to see resilience-related processes and outcomes within their social and historical context. As Brown explains: "Determing resilience should not be judged by the outcomes and values that others deem relevant" (p. 14). Working with a small group of black men, Brown showed that blackness is not associated with health outcomes directly. Instead, blackness as a construct is a way the men measure connections:

> The respondents did not describe Blackness in terms of healthy or unhealthy. Instead, they posited that Blackness was organized and differentiated along a continuum of connectedness. People were described as having either higher or lesser levels of Blackness. These levels were based on an individual's sense of commitment and relatedness to the struggles, ills, and plight of Black people and their promotion and preservation of Black culture. Individuals with higher levels of Blackness were described as people who stayed connected, gave back to the Black community, and promoted Black culture according to their resources. (p. 179)

It would seem that blackness is not a risk factor but a resource that brings about the social cohesion that buffers risk.

On a much larger scale, an ongoing program of resilience-related research across more than a dozen countries, the International Resilience Project (IRP; Ungar et al., 2007, 2008; Ungar, Lee, Callaghan, & Boothroyd, 2005) employs multiple research methods to capture both the homogeneity of resilience as a process across cultures and the heterogeneity in psychosocial outcomes. The research uses concurrent quantitative and qualitative methods. Through team meetings of more than 35 researchers, and consultations with their communities, the IRP developed a single measure of resilience as it is understood across all of the original 14 research sites spanning five continents. The Child and Youth Resilience Measure (CYRM) was designed to capture individual, relational, community, and cultural aspects of resilience. Results from initial testing with 1,451 youth showed good construct validity and, as hypothesized, low factorial invariance. Participants in majority and minority world contexts recorded varying response patterns on the original 58-item instrument (the CYRM was subsequently shortened to 28 items). While boys and girls from North American non-Aboriginal communities responded as predicted, boys and girls, and boys from high- and low-cohesion communities, formed distinct subgroups of respondents. Qualitative interviews, analyzed with grounded theory methods with at-risk young people thought to be thriving in those same 14 communities, helped to explain variability in the results. Interestingly, there was no direct correspondence between the models developed to account for the findings from both the quantitative and qualitative investigations. Specifically, the quantitative data could not be sorted under the seven tensions (themes) that emerged in the qualitative study: access to material resources, relationships, identity, cohesion, power and control, social justice, and cultural adherence. Results showed that no single pattern to the resolution of these "tensions" predicted resilience better than any other pattern when researchers accounted for culture and context. The lack of predetermination in the relationship between the seven tensions means that each maintained its fluid and multidimensional contribution to resilience. For example, cultural adherence was shown to be more or less valued by participants depending on how well it helped to secure safe and meaningful relationships, material resources, and a powerful identity. Youth juggle their cultural adherences between their local culture and globalized (homogenized) culture based on how well their affiliation helped to guarantee their survival. When expedient, they fit in with broad community norms or family norms, depending on what makes most sense at the time in a particular context. Empirically, such contextually relative definitions of constructs make it difficult to standard-

ize measures or determine outcomes, even though there is homogeneity in the themes that emerge across cultures.

Nine catalyst questions used to elicit localized discourses of resilience are presented in Appendix 19.1. Adaptations of the questionnaire and its probing questions have been used in a number of studies around the world (Colombia, Thailand, China, Canada, and India, to name a few). These questions, addressed to individuals and groups of stakeholders (either professionals or laypeople), help to synthesize a picture of what resilience as an outcome and process looks like on the ground in culturally variant contexts. The process works best when it is dialogical, allowing participants to comment on findings as they develop from one interview to the next (Rodwell, 1998). Results may be used to inform the development of quantitative measures, though concurrence of results following administration is unlikely. Still, the questions have been useful in deconstructing the culturally embedded aspects of resilience that relate to people's navigations and negotiations for resources under stress. Paradigmatically, it seems that the empirical assumptions of quantitative research reify processes associated with resilience that phenomological investigations (including postpositivist approaches such as grounded theory) may fail to validate.

The problem, then, with writing about culturally variant perspectives of resilience is that there can be no final conclusions, only the generation of principles by which to continue inquiry. A kaleidoscope of possible factors interact in patterns that reflect the cultural confluence and subsequent disentanglement of a global community of migrants. For both clinicians and researchers, understanding resilience as a cultural construction, an artifact of patterned interactions and beliefs that are fluid, requires a postmodern perspective that tolerates ambiguity in assessment of the relative influence that factors exert on one another. There is a need for constant inquiry. It is not that we cannot generalize or transfer substantive theory generated in one cultural zone to another. It is that the act of generalizing is always less than satisfying without a contextualized perspective that lets others speak from their locality. If we talk less and listen more, then we may be able to make cultural variance knowable to those trained to intervene and observe. However, there continues to be a dearth of studies outside Western countries that can demonstrate whether there is convergence between factors associated with resilience across different cultures. Where such work has occurred (Hjemdal, 2007; Ungar, 2008) results remain tentative.

Hidden Resilience

When individual negotiations for culturally variable definitions of success are appreciated, a challenge is posed to the teleological nature of the resilience discourse. There is multifinality in adult developmental pathways, with many good ends resulting from many different protective processes. At the intersection of individual definitions of success and the appraisal of what resources an environment realistically has to offer lies *hidden resilience* (Ungar, 2004b), which is patterns of coping that allow individuals to experience their lives subjectively as successful whether or not others outside their culture and context see them that way. In a similar vein, Luthar (1999) explains that there are "innumerable ways in which potentially powerful risk and protective factors do not operate in directions that may be intuitively anticipated, but often can reflect complicated, conditional and even counterintuitive trends" (p. 3). Both conceptually and empirically, hidden resilience can be shown to exist when epistemological assumptions are challenged through indigenizing processes of knowledge production (participatory methods to include localized constructions of hypothesized processes in empirical studies) and phenomenology is given status equal to that of empiricism.

This was done successfully in a cross-sectional study of individuals from one village in Sri Lanka that was particularly hard hit by the tsunami in 2005. Hollifield and colleagues (2008) examined the impact of the devastation on the mental health of 89 adults 20–21 months afterward. Using standardized measures (originating in economically developed countries) they assessed for signs of PTSD, depression, and related somatic symptoms and impairment. Though theirs was not explicitly a study of resilience, they also examined people's coping practices, as identified during focus groups with residents prior to the study's implementation. The strategies suggested by townspeople included relying on one's own strengths; family/friends; general religious practices; *Ayurveda* (a traditional system of health care); Western-model medical doctor and health system; *Thovil, Bodhi-puja*, and other cultural and religious rituals of local significance; and horoscope. While women more than men relied on many of these coping strategies, more than half of respondents said they use at least one of these strategies regularly. Of course, not all of these strategies are unique to this village in Sri Lanka. A survey of the literature on PTSD reveals that other studies have found social support from family and friends to be equally predictive of positive outcomes for Western populations. Charuvastra and Cloitre (2008), in their survey of studies that investigated social bonds and PTSD, found that lack of social support was among the strongest predictors of the disorder. The studies they reviewed, such as that with American Legionnaires who returned home from Vietnam, show clearly an interactional effect between the environment in which individuals interact and the impact of trauma on functioning. It should be no surprise, then, that some protective factors were just as relevant to the Sri Lankan townspeople as to populations of Western veterans. Religious practices, for example, a generic factor in many studies of PTSD, were associated with individuals in Sri Lanka being above the clinical cutoff for anxiety and PTSD. Other strategies (*Ayurveda*, religious rituals, and horoscope) that were indigenous to the Sri Lankans have not been studied for their relevance in Western contexts.

The empirical problem is that the observer and the observed are likely to disagree in their phenomological account of what they consider to be a factual representation of their experience. There is unlikely to be concurrence between self-reports and reports by others in situations where there is the potential for discursive variation resulting from cultural and contextual difference. In such cases, as in all cross-cultural research, there is the need for confirmatory factor analysis to test the degree of factorial invariance (van de Vijver & Leung, 1997).

One does not have to make research exotic to see the applicability of the hidden resilience concept. Among all marginalized populations, discursive resistance can, when heard, call forth new understandings of the everyday expressions of resilience. To illustrate, there is a bias in the literature toward formal education as the only learning that has value, despite evidence that even if education is valued by a particular ethnoracial group, it may not appear accessible or useful for populations that are marginalized and expect to encounter barriers to employment and advancement no matter what their educational attainment (Dei, Massuca, McIsaac, & Zine, 1997). A more emic perspective would appreciate learning as it is understood by heterogeneous groups. As Dei and colleagues (1997) remind us in their study of African Canadians who drop out of school, "Dropping out was recognized as a process which had much broader social and cultural implications. ... These behaviours may be symptoms of a larger problem and can often tell us something about the process of schooling rather than simply about the individual" (p. 62). The resistance to formal education shown by minorities may be interpreted as a way to preserve dignity and personal efficacy, and to cope with racism by asserting

independence from normative expectations. Even here, though, an emic perspective reminds us to avoid generalization. Although some minority groups struggle with making education meaningful (and thus a pathway to positive outcomes), many others do not. Furthermore, within any single group, individuals and individual families may differ widely depending on their values or context. Members of an ethnic minority might hold one set of values regarding education in their country of origin and another when immersed inside a culture to which they have emigrated that is different from their own. It has been suggested, for example, that racial differences are relatively inconsequential to development outcomes among Aboriginal people if community resources are plentiful and a group's cultural identity is promoted (Lalonde, 2006). The poverty associated with immigration, colonization, marginalization, and racism is the mechanism that skews adaptation. While this makes intuitive sense, and has been demonstrated empirically, different cultural and racial groups may perceive different potential futures, and therefore different pathways to resilience because of their varying abilities and desires to acculturate (Yeh, Kim, Pituc, & Atkins, 2008).

Teasing out this dynamic interplay between resources and meaning that gives rise to hidden resilience for different ethnoracial groups requires research that accounts for people's unique experiences. Studies and interventions based on an assumption of sameness are likely to miss their mark. Returning to the theme of immigration, we find in Weiss and Berger's (2006) work with Latinas in the United States a consideration for the positive aspects of the immigrant experience and its impact on stress. Adapting the Posttraumatic Growth Inventory (PTGI) to this population, they investigated five dimensions of change: new possibilities; relating to others; personal strength; appreciation of life; and spiritual change. When previously translated, the PTGI has shown good psychometric properties but low factorial invariance with two- and four-factor models accounting for the responses of different populations for which a five-factor model was expected. Using data from 100 Latinas in the New York metropolitan area with 1–10 years of U.S. residency (ages 23–79, from 16 different countries of origin), a highly contextualized understanding of the immigrant experience emerged. Noteworthy is that items related to spirituality were not found to correlate significantly with positive growth despite expectations that they would do so.

The Indigenization of Resilience

Once we shift our focus from the individual to the interaction among the individual, the individual's culture (and that of the individual's family and community), and the individual's broader physical and social ecologies, much changes in how we understand resilience. There is little likelihood of standardized pan-human validity when models of resilience as innate are challenged. Evolution in the way we understand resilience since Anthony's (1987) chapter in *The Invulnerable Child* and Higgins's (1994) *Resilient Adults Overcoming a Cruel Past* has opened doors to both conceptual clarity and better research. We are coming to understand that culture matters as the study of resilience become increasingly indigenized. Whether one lives in an affluent family in the United States, a South African township, an Aboriginal community in northern Canada, or on a Brazilian street, the factors associated with survival under stress are going to vary by both context and culture. The values and beliefs of the society surrounding the individual decide what resources are provided and valued (education for women; mental health counseling for the mentally ill; subsidized housing for poor people; community cultural centers for ethnoracial minorities; etc.).

Understanding resilience (and health-related phenomena in general) as embedded in culture and discursive practices opens up opportunities to discover new concepts that may contribute to coping well under stress. An optimistic survey of the field as new voices emerge reveals the possibility of importing into the dominant Western literature on resilience the research findings and intervention approaches of less well-known researchers (Liebenberg & Ungar, 2008). Luthar and colleagues (2000) suggest that resilience researchers need to find ways to create "high fidelity between the theoretical underpinnings of their work and the specific criteria they select to operationalize 'successful adaptation' within particular at-risk samples" (p. 549). The advice, if taken to heart, encourages dialogue across borders and languages. Rather than exporting concepts, a constructionist understanding of resilience suggests the possibility of seeking indigenous understandings of positive development (Ungar, 2004a). It also invites the import of new ways of conceptualizing resilience from those outside the dominant scientific discourse. Cultural pluralism is not only good for investigations with the minorities who are a growing part of communities in Western countries where immigration policies have liberalized, but it is also a necessity if we are to expand our thinking and reflect carefully on what may be absent from Western developmental theories (Robinson, 2007). By expanding our repertoire of interventions, our results are likely to benefit adults who encounter turmoil. Cultural sensitivity to what resilience means can inform better intervention for both minority and majority groups.

Though the resilience construct remains controversial, and the indicators uncertain, there is growing evidence that many adults who encounter challenges still thrive. Arguably, their success is an interactive, complex process that requires sensitivity to the risks they face, their internal and external assets, and the culture and context in which coping occurs.

APPENDIX 19.1. The International Resilience Project Adult Interview Guide

- "What would I need to know to grow up well where you live?"
  Probing Questions:
  1. What roles do religious organizations play in your life? Has this changed over time?
  2. What do other members of your family think about the way you live your life, your beliefs (those regarding gender roles, etc.)?
  3. How do you handle change at an individual level, and the changes taking place for everyone in your community? Are things now better or worse than when you were a child? Why?
  4. How do you contribute to your community?
  5. What is it like for you when people around you succeed?
  6. Do you have a life philosophy? What is it?
  7. Do you identify in any way(s) with your culture? Can you describe your culture? Can you describe (or show me) day-to-day activities that are part of your culture and the way things are done in your community?
- "How do you describe people who grow up well here despite the many problems they face? What word(s) do you use?"
- "What does it mean to you, to your family, and to your community, when bad things happen?"
  Probing Questions:
  1. Can you tell me what some of these bad things are?
  2. What do people do to cope?
  3. What do they say about these things when they happen?
  4. Who talks about them most? Least? And who is most likely to come up with the solutions to problems when they occur?
  5. What do other people think of these solutions? Can you give me examples?
- "What kinds of things are most challenging for you growing up here?"
  Probing Questions:
  1. Have you or people you know been exposed to violence? How do you avoid this in your family, community, and when with peers?
  2. How does the government play a role in providing for your safety, recreation needs, housing, and jobs? Has this role changed over time?
  3. Do you feel equal to others? Are there others you do not feel equal to? How do these others make you feel? What do they do that makes you feel this way?
  4. Do you have access to work and education opportunities? How do you get this access? Who provides it to you?
- "What do you do when you face difficulties in your life? Has this changed as you got older?"
- "What does being healthy mean to you and others in your family and community?"
  Probing Questions:
  1. Could you describe the way your parents or caregivers looked after you?
  2. How do your family members express themselves and how do you know what they think of you?
  3. Do you have someone you consider a mentor or role model? Can you describe him or her?
  4. Do you have other meaningful relationships with people at school, home, work, or in your community?
- "What do you do, and others you know, do to keep healthy mentally, physically, emotionally, and spiritually?"
  Probing Questions:
  1. Do you have a sense of control over your world? How does this affect your life?
  2. How much uncertainty are you able to live with? Has this changed over time?
  3. Do you value self-awareness, insight? How does this affect your life and what you do day to day?
  4. Would you describe yourself as optimistic or pessimistic about life? Why?
  5. Do you have personal goals and aspirations? What are these?
  6. How much can you be independent, and how much do you have to rely on others in your life for your survival?
  7. How much do you use substances like alcohol and drugs? What do others around you think about this?
- "Can you share with me a story about someone who has coped well in your community despite facing many challenges?"
- "Can you share a story about how you have managed to overcome challenges you face personally, in your family, or outside your home in your community?"

Acknowledgments

Preparation of this chapter is supported in part by grants from the Social Sciences and Humanities Research Council of Canada. I wish to thank the many members of the International Resilience Project (*www.resilienceproject.org*) for their collaboration in the development of the theory presented in this chapter.

References

Abramson, L. Y., Seligman, M. E., & Teasdale, J. D. (1978). Learned helplessness in humans: Critique and reformulation. *Journal of Abnormal Psychology, 87*(1), 49–74.

Alegria, M., Takeuchi, D., Canino, G., Duan, N., Shrout, P., Meng, X.-L., et al. (2004). Considering context, place and culture: the National Latino and Asian American Study. *International Journal of Methods in Psychiatric Research, 13*(4), 208–220.

Alegria, M., Vila, D., Woo, M., Canino, G., Takeuchi, D., Vera, M., et al. (2004). Cultural relevance and equivalence in the NLAAS instrument: Integrating etic and emic in the development of cross-cultural measures for a psychiatric epidemiology and services study of Latinos. *International Journal of Methods in Psychiatric Research, 13*(4), 270–288.

Anthony, E. J. (1987). Children at high risk for psychosis growing up successfully. In E. J. Anthony & B. J. Cohler (Eds.), *The invulnerable child* (pp. 147–184). New York: Guilford Press.

Antonovsky, A. (1987). The salutogenic perspective: Toward a new view of health and illness. *Advances, Journal of the Institute for Advancement of Health, 4*(1), 47–55.

Aroian, K. J., & Norris, A. E. (2000). Resilience, stress, and depression among Russian immigrants to Israel. *Western Journal of Nursing Research, 22*(1), 54–67.

Bauman, Z. (2000). *Liquid modernity.* Cambridge, UK: Polity.

Berry, J. W. (1969). On cross-cultural comparability. *International Journal of Psychology, 4,* 119–128.

Berry, J. W., Phinney, J. S., Sam, D. L., & Vedder, P. (2006). Immigrant youth: Acculturation, identity, and adaption. *Applied Psychology: An International Review, 55*(3), 303–332.

Berry, J. W., & Poortinga, Y. H. (2006). Cross-cultural theory and methodology. In J. Georgas, J. W. Berry, F. J. R. van de Vijver, C. Kagitçibasi, & Y. H. Poortinga (Eds.), *Families across cultures: A 30-nation psychological study* (pp. 51–71). New York: Cambridge University Press.

Blackstock, C., & Trocmé, N. (2005). Community-based child welfare for Aboriginal children: Supporting resilience through structural change. In M. Ungar (Ed.), *Handbook for working with children and youth: Pathways to resilience across cultures and contexts* (pp. 105–120). Thousand Oaks, CA: Sage.

Brown, A. L. (2004). *Exploring blackness as a site of resilience in street life oriented young Black men living in the inner-city.* Doctoral dissertation, Seton Hall University, South Orange, NJ.

Charuvastra, A., & Cloitre, M. (2008). Social bonds and posttraumatic stress disorder. *Annual Review of Psychology, 59,* 301–328.

Chen, X., DeSouza, A., Chen, H., & Wang, L. (2006). Reticent behavior and experiences in peer interactions in Canadian and Chinese children. *Developmental Psychology, 42,* 656–665.

Coté, J. E., & Levine, C. (1997). Student motivations, learning environments, and human capital acquisition: Toward an integrated paradigm of student development. *Journal of College Student Development, 38*(3), 229–243.

Dei, G. J. S., Massuca, J., McIsaac, E., & Zine, J. (1997). *Reconstructing "drop-out": A critical ethnography of the dynamics of Black students' desengagement from school.* Toronto: University of Toronto Press.

Garmezy, N. (1983). Stressors of childhood. In N. Garmezy & M. Rutter (Eds.), *Stress, coping, and development in children* (pp. 43–84). New York: McGraw-Hill.

Georgas, J., Berry, J. W., van de Vijver, F. J. R., Kagitçibasi, C., & Poortinga, Y. H. (Eds.). (2006). *Families across cultures: A 30-nation psychological study.* New York: Cambridge University Press.

Grant, B. F., Stinson, F. S., Hasin, D. S., Dawson, D. A., Chou, S. P., & Anderson, K. (2004). Immigration and lifetime prevalence of DSM-IV psychiatric disorders among Mexican Americans and non-Hispanic whites in the United States: Results from the National Epidemiologic Survey on Alcohol and Related Conditions. *Archives of General Psychiatry, 61*(12), 1226–1233.

Hannon, L. (2003). Poverty, delinquency, and educational attainment: Cumulative disadvantage or disadvantage saturation? *Sociological Inquiry, 73*(4), 575–594.

Higgins, G. O. (1994). *Resilient adults overcoming a cruel past*. San Francisco: Jossey-Bass.

Hollifield, M., Hewage, C., Gunawardena, C. N., Kodituwakku, P., Bopagoda, K., & Weerarathnege, K. (2008). Symptoms and coping in Sri Lanka 20–21 months after the 2004 tsunami. *British Journal of Psychiatry, 192*, 39–44.

Hjemdal, O. (2007). Measuring protective factors: The development of two resilience scales in Norway. *Child and Adolescent Psychiatric Clinics of North America, 16*(2), 303–322.

Johnson, J. H., & McCutcheon, S. (1980). Assessing life stress in older children and adolescents: Preliminary findings with the Life Events Checklist. In I. G. Sarason & C. D. Spielberger (Eds.), *Stress and anxiety* (Vol. 7, pp. 111–125). Washington, DC: Hemisphere.

Kagitçibasi, C. (2006). Theoretical perspectives on family change. In J. Georgas, J. W. Berry, F. J. R. van de Vijver, C. Kagitçibasi, & Y. H. Poortinga (Eds.), *Families across cultures: A 30-nation psychological study* (pp. 72–89). New York: Cambridge University Press.

Kirby, L. D., & Fraser, M. W. (1997). Risk and resilience in childhood. In M. Fraser (Ed.), *Risk and resilience in childhood: An ecological perspective* (pp. 10–33). Washington, DC: NASW Press.

Knyazev, G. G., Supancic, M., & Slobodskaya, H. R. (2008). Child personality in Slovenia and Russia: Structure and mean level of traits in parent and self-ratings. *Journal of Cross-Cultural Psychology, 39*(3), 317–334.

Lalonde, C. E. (2006). Identity formation and cultural resilience in Aboriginal communities. In R. J. Flynn, P. M. Dudding, & J. G. Barber (Eds.), *Promoting resilience in child welfare* (pp. 52–71). Ottawa, ON, Canada: University of Ottawa Press.

Lerner, R. M., Dowling, E. M., & Anderson, P. M. (2003). Positive youth development: Thriving as the basis of personhood and civil society. *Applied Developmental Science, 7*(3), 172–180.

Liebenberg, L., & Ungar, M. (2008). *Resilience in action*. Toronto: University of Toronto Press.

Luthar, S. S. (1999). *Poverty and children's adjustment*. Thousand Oaks, CA: Sage.

Luthar, S. S., & Brown, P. J. (2007). Maximizing resilience through diverse levels of inquiry: Prevailing paradigms, possibilities, and priorities for the future. *Development and Psychopathology, 19*, 931–955.

Luthar, S. S., Cicchetti, D., & Becker, B. (2000). The construct of resilience: A critical evaluation and guidelines for future work. *Child Development, 71*(3), 543–562.

McCubbin, H. I., Fleming, W. M., Thompson, A. I., Neitman, P., Elver, K. M., & Savas, S. A. (1998). Resiliency and coping in "at risk" African-American youth and their families. In H. I. McCubbin, E. A. Thompson, A. I. Thompson, & J. A. Futrell (Eds.), *Resiliency in African-American families* (pp.287–328). Thousand Oaks, CA: Sage.

McGoldrick, M. (2003). Culture: A challenge to concepts of normality. In F. Walsh (Ed.), *Normal family processes* (3rd ed., pp. 61–95). New York: Guilford Press.

Pesce, R. P., Assis, S. G., Avanci, J. Q., Santos, N. C., Malaquias, J. V., & Carvalhaes, R. (2005). Cross-cultural adaptation, reliability and validity of the Resilience Scale. *Cadernos de Saude Publica, 21*(2), 436–448.

Phinney, J. S., Dennis, J., & Osorio, S. (2006). Reasons to attend college among ethnically diverse college students. *Cultural Diversity and Ethnic Minority Psychology, 12*(2), 347–366.

Putnam, R. D. (2000). *Bowling alone: The collapse and revival of American community*. New York: Simon & Schuster.

Reich, J. W., & Zautra, A. J. (1988). Direct and stress-moderating effects of positive life experiences. In L. H. Cohen (Ed.), *Life events and psychological functioning: Theoretical and methodological issues* (pp. 149–180). Newbury Park, CA: Sage.

Robinson, L. (2007). *Cross-cultural child development for social workers*. London: Palgrave.

Rodwell, M. K. (1998). *Social work constructivist research*. New York: Garland.

Rutter, M. (1987). Psychosocial resilience and protective mechanisms. *American Journal of Orthopsychiatry, 57*, 316–331.

Sanchez, J. I., Spector, P. E., & Cooper, C. L. (2006). Frequently ignored methodological issues in cross-cultural stress research. In P. T. P. Wong & L. C. J. Wong (Eds.), *Handbook of multicultural perspectives on stress and coping* (pp. 187–201). New York: Springer.

Seccombe, K. (2002). "Beating the odds" versus "changing the odds": Poverty, resilience, and family policy. *Journal of Marriage and Family, 64*(2), 384–394.

Singh, A. A. (2007). *Resilience strategies of South Asian women who have survived child sexual abuse*. Doctoral dissertation, Georgia State University, Atlanta.

Sisneros, J., Stakeman, C., Joyner, M. C., & Schmitz, C. L. (2007). *Critical multicultural social work*. Chicago: Lyceum.

Smith, L. T. (1999). *Decolonizing methodologies: Research and indigenous peoples*. New York: Zed Books.

Tragesser, S. L., Beauvais, F., Swaim, R. C., Edwards, R. W., & Oetting, E. R. (2007). Parental monitoring, peer drug involvement, and marijuana use across three ethnicities. *Journal of Cross-Cultural Psychology, 38*, 670–694.

Tweed, R. G., & Conway, L. G. (2006). Coping strategies and culturally influenced beliefs about the world. In P. T. P. Wong & L. C. J. Wong (Eds.), *Handbook of multicultural perspectives on stress and coping* (pp. 133–154). New York: Springer.

Ungar, M. (2003). Qualitative contributions to resilience research. *Qualitative Social Work, 2*(1), 85–102.

Ungar, M. (2004a). A constructionist discourse on resilience: Multiple contexts, multiple realities among at-risk children and youth. *Youth and Society, 35*(3), 341–365.

Ungar, M. (2004b). *Nurturing hidden resilience in troubled youth*. Toronto: University of Toronto Press.

Ungar, M. (2005). Introduction: Resilience across cultures and contexts. In M. Ungar (Ed.), *Handbook for working with children and youth: Pathways to resilience across cultures and contexts* (pp. xv–xxxix). Thousand Oaks, CA: Sage.

Ungar, M. (2008). Resilience across cultures. *British Journal of Social Work, 38*, 218–235.

Ungar, M., Brown, M., Liebenberg, L., Othman, R., Kwong, W. M., Armstrong, M., et al. (2007). Unique pathways to resilience across cultures. *Adolescence, 42*, 287–310.

Ungar, M., Lee, A. W., Callaghan, T., & Boothroyd, R. (2005). An international collaboration to study resilience in adolescents across cultures. *Journal of Social Work Research and Evaluation, 6*(1), 5–24.

Ungar, M., & Liebenberg, L. (2005). The International Resilience Project: A mixed methods approach to the study of resilience across cultures. In M. Ungar (Ed.), *Handbook for working with children and youth: Pathways to resilience across cultures and contexts* (pp. 211–226). Thousand Oaks, CA: Sage.

Ungar, M., Liebenberg, L., Boothroyd, R., Kwong, W. M., Lee, T. Y., Leblanc, J., et al. (2008). The study of youth resilience across cultures: Lessons from a pilot study of measurement development. *Research on Human Development, 5*(3), 166–180.

van de Vijver, F. J. R., & Leung, K. (1997). Methods and data analysis of comparative research. In J. W. Berry, Y. H. Poortinga, & J. Pandey (Eds.), *Handbook of cross-cultural psychology: Vol. 1. Theory and method* (2nd ed., pp. 257–300). Needham Heights, MA: Allyn & Bacon.

Wagnild, G. M., & Young, H. M. (1993). Development and psychometric evaluation of the resilience scale. *Journal of Nursing Management, 1*(2), 165–178.

Weiss, T., & Berger, R. (2006). Reliability and validity of a Spanish version of the Posttraumatic Growth Inventory. *Research on Social Work Practice, 16*(2), 191–199.

Werner, E. E., & Smith, R. S. (2001). *Journeys from childhood to midlife: Risk, resilience, and recovery*. Ithaca, NY: Cornell University Press.

Wong, P. T. P., & Wong, L. C. J. (Eds.). (2006). *Handbook of multicultural perspectives on stress and coping*. New York: Springer.

Yates, T. M., Egeland, B., & Sroufe, L. A. (2003). Rethinking resilience: A developmental process perspective. In S. S. Luthar (Ed.), *Resilience and vulnerability: Adaptation in the context of childhood adversities* (pp. 243–266). Cambridge, UK: Cambridge University Press.

Yeh, C. J., Kim, A. B., Pituc, S. T., & Atkins, M. (2008). Poverty, loss, and resilience: The story of Chinese immigrant youth. *Journal of Counseling Psychology, 55*(1), 34–48.

IV

INTERVENTIONS FOR ENHANCING RESILIENCE

20

The Emergence of Capacity-Building Programs and Models of Resilience

Martha Kent
Mary C. Davis

The study of adult resilience is emerging as a vibrant area of research. The course of its development shares the formative qualities of most pioneering activities: a concern with definition, territorial boundaries, stakeholder interests, orthodoxies of approach and method. In their conceptual definition of resilience, Lepore and Revenson (2006) base their understanding of resilience on answers to three questions: What is resilience? Who has it? How do we get it? This chapter follows the course of these three questions as we review the emerging adult resilience literature. We find resilience treated as traits, as process, and emerging in interventions. Our goals are (1) to convey the context that has given rise to the study of adult resilience, (2) to review the main strength-based, treatment approaches relevant to the development of resilience interventions, and (3) to introduce intervention programs and new resilience models developing locally in Phoenix, Arizona. In reviewing this emerging field we have an opportunity to consider

anew the nature of resilience and how we can best promote it.

Studies of adult resilience and resilience intervention programs are rooted in two separate strands of research: One is the older coping and stress tradition of the 1970s, the other covers the recent therapeutic treatment programs of the past decade. The strands converge in the studies and writings about recent extreme events, such as the 9/11 World Trade Center attacks or current combat in Iraq and Afghanistan, and in studies on trauma and resilience associated with these events. Whereas the study of resilience in children growing up in adversity (Garmezy, 1971; Rutter, 1979) represented a paradigm shift in developmental psychopathology from deficits to the inclusion of strengths, the present emergence of adult resilience studies has continued that shift, in a similar recognition that the experience of challenge does not necessarily result in deficient adaptation and psychopathology but may more often express adaptive resilience.

427

What Is Resilience?

Definitions of resilience are addressed in one form or another in various chapters of this volume, offering an opportunity for much more textured and richer understanding of the construct. Our own understanding is meant to be a contribution to this evolving process and to leave the quest for a definition with an open-ended appreciation of resilience as an adaptive process and a positive outcome in the face of major adversity. Resilience is likely to be a slow process (Masten & Reed, 2002) that may become apparent only with time. It may be cultivated over the lifespan. In the constant interplay of person and environment over the course of a life, resilience may emerge and reveal both process and outcome. Our own focus on developing resilience interventions aims to bring about process changes that may result in improved adaptive outcomes.

Who Is Resilient?

Concerns over protective factors and resilience as soldiers are being deployed to Iraq and Afghanistan have brought to the fore the study of trait attributes that buffered and preserved the well-being of soldiers during World War II, the Vietnam War, the Persian Gulf War, and service in Iraq and Afghanistan. In an early study to address strength in adversity, Hunter (1993) collected data between 1971 and 1978 on American prisoners of war (POW), who had been held in North Vietnam from 1964 through 1973. In a dose-dependent manner, harshness of treatment and length and location of detention were related to effects on health and adjustment to normal life, family, work roles, and emotional functions. Despite large variability, most people were stronger than they thought they were, Hunter observed. Among the strengths were preserving contact with other POWs during captivity, such as communicating by tap code; using the mind; gaining clarity; and finding strengths in recalling family

ties and maintaining ties to fellow prisoners. After their release, key variables were taking direct action, self-confidence, ability to communicate, a will to live, service to others, a future orientation, a personal cause, and finding benefits from captivity.

In more recent studies of former POWs in Vietnam's infamous Hanoi Hilton, Charney and Southwick (in Rosenbaum & Covino, 2005) identified 10 characteristics of resilience exemplified by them: optimism; altruism; having a moral compass or beliefs that cannot be shattered, faith and spirituality, a sense of humor, role models, and a mission or meaning in life; facing fear; and training to become resilient. These qualities overlap with Hunter's findings in the 1970s. Haglund, Nestadt, Cooper, Southwick, and Charney (2007) extracted a similar typology from a variety of studies with combat and civilian populations: a positive attitude of optimism and humor; active rather than passive coping; cognitive flexibility; finding meaning; growth; having core beliefs, faith, and spirituality; and use of physical exercise, social support, and role models. These qualities are also described by Hoge, Austin, and Pollack (2007) in their review of resilience factors that buffer or decrease vulnerability to posttraumatic stress disorder (PTSD) in combat and civilian experiences, by Southwick, Vythilingam, and Charney (2005) in their review of the psychobiology of depression and resilience, and by Agaibi and Wilson (2005) in their review of trauma, PTSD, and resilience. A condensed summary is provided in Table 20.1.

In this list of resilience traits it is easy to recognize the influences of the large body of earlier research on coping and stress, and antecedent work on positive emotions, hardiness, and posttraumatic growth. Table 20.1 also provides a brief description of concepts and of findings cited in support of the main traits. The list of trait attributes claimed for resilience are among the most enduring adaptations identified in the extensive literature on coping and stress, optimism, and positive emotions.

TABLE 20.1. Resilience as Qualities of the Person

Ten qualities	Descriptions, findings	Authors
1. Positive emotions		
Optimism, hope, humor, see options, positive outcomes, ability to laugh at oneself, humor, positive emotions	Decrease stress-related illness, mood and arousal, are restorative, increase well-being and health, broaden-and-build theory, hope theory	Carver et al. (1993); Scheier et al. (1989); Folkman & Moskowitz (2000); Affleck & Tennen (1996); Fredrickson (2001); Snyder et al. (2002)
2. Control		
Locus of control, self-esteem and pride, control, challenge, commitment, control over stressors	Lower levels of PTSD, components of hardiness, predict mental health in soldiers	King et al. (1998); Soet et al. (2003); Kobasa (1979); Florian et al. (1995)
3. Active coping, engagement, facing fear		
Task-focused versus emotion-focused versus avoidant coping, passive coping, avoidance versus engagement, facing fear, leaving comfort zone, adaptive coping	Making plans versus venting versus denial, how you engage with risk, exposure increases self-efficacy, courage, stress inoculation, coping through emotional approach	Johnsen et al. (2002); Beaton et al. (1999); Maddi (1999a, 1999b); Rutter (1987); Regehr et al. (2000); Meichenbaum (1985); Stanton et al. (2002)
4. Cognitive flexibility		
Alternative explanations, positive reframing, acceptance, problems are temporary and limited	Tolerate highly stressful events, redefining as challenge, rebuilding assumptive world, acceptance in extreme hardship and in illness, explanatory style	Southwick et al. (2005); Schaefer & Moos (1992, 1998); Janoff-Buhlman (1992); Manne et al. (2003); Wade et al. (2001); Seligman et al. (1988); Seligman (2002)
5. Meaning and value in adversity		
Posttraumatic growth, learning from crises, benefits from adversity	Value life, relationships	Tedeschi et al. (1998); Park et al. (1996)
6. Altruism		
Altruism, required helpfulness, survivor mission, empathy and compassion	Successful adaptation; fewer traumatic symptoms; helping as coping; turn tragedy into activism; PTG is training in empathy	Bleuler (1984); Rachman (1979); Midlarsky (1991); Anderson & Anderson (2003); Tedeschi et al. (1998)
7. Spirituality		
Framework for understanding, making sense of tragedy, moral compass	Physical and emotional protective survival, health, less depression, core beliefs, and guiding principles	McCullough et al. (2000); Koenig et al. (1998, 2004); Janoff-Bulman (1992)
8. Training		
Previous experience of trauma, stress inoculation	Training in stoicism, prior training on stressors—torture, emergency work; prior experience with stress can foster adaptation	Alvarez & Hunt (2005); Hagh-Shenas et al. (2005); Meichenbaum (1985)

How Do We Become Resilient?

Resilience as Process: Resources and Capacities of Resilience

Component Trait Models

Resilience researchers are increasingly aware of the complexity of the concept of resilience and the need for complexity in studies of resilience that extends beyond protective factors of traits and risk factors of context or environment (Curtis & Cicchetti, 2003). The next level of complexity evident in the research literature on adult resilience is represented by the component attribute approach to resilience (see Table 20.2). Hardiness is such an attribute, and it comprises of sense of control, commitment, and challenge (Maddi, 1999b). In a study of hardiness and postcombat social support as well as postcombat stressful life events, hardiness was negatively associated with PTSD or fewer PTSD symptoms in a sample of Vietnam War veterans (King, King, Fairbank, Keane, & Adams, 1998). Hardiness emerged as showing a strong negative association with PTSD. Moderating variables affecting this relation were found in the quality of postcombat social support and postcombat additional stressful life events.

In their study of Persian Gulf War troops, Sutker, Davis, Uddo, and Ditta (1995) estimated that the prevalence of PTSD in that conflict reached 16–19%. These investigators noted that subgroups of survivors of extreme events, such as POW survivors, were free of psychiatric symptoms. They studied the association between personal and environmental resources, and psychological outcomes subsequent to combat experience in the Persian Gulf War. Results showed that commitment items of *hardiness* (a sense of meaning, purpose, perseverance), avoidance coping, and less perceived family cohesion (less helpful and supportive responses of family members) were consistent predictors of PTSD diagnoses. Thus, personal characteristics and environmental factors moderated vulnerability to war stress. In a study of a National Guard unit deployed to the Persian Gulf (Bartone, 1999), hardiness emerged as a significant predictor of health across a variety of health indicators. In interaction with combat stress, hardiness predicted fewer symptoms under stress.

Thus, qualities of person alone were not sufficient to predict resilience, but required social support to make resilience effects happen. In an elegant study, Benotsch and colleagues (2000) addressed directly the question of person and environment resources, and their relation to combat stress and PTSD symptoms. They added a longitudinal dimension (Time 1) prior to deployment to the Gulf War region and 2 years later (Time 2). From Time 1 to Time 2, the resources of hardiness and problem-solving coping decreased significantly, while avoidance coping increased significantly. During this time interval, PTSD symptoms increased significantly. Thus, troops returning from combat had both increased symptoms and decreasing personal resources. However, avoidance and low family cohesion at Time 1 predicted PTSD symptoms at Time 2. Moreover, initial high PTSD at Time 1 was associated with more avoidance coping and less family cohesion at Time 2. A cyclical pathological process between increasing PTSD and diminishing resources was set in motion, resulting in a loss spiral first described by Hobfoll (1989).

Studies of resilience resources and capabilities, associated with earlier wars prior to the Vietnam conflict or earlier POW experiences, are actually quite recent and were and continue to be conducted decades after the actual events themselves. Zeiss and Dickman (1989) identified correlates of PTSD in World War II POWs 40 years after the war. Only rank was a powerful predictor of current symptoms, with higher rank predicting less severe symptoms. Gold and colleagues (2000) corroborated severe psychological sequelae for POWs in World War II and the Korean Conflict 40–50 years after captivity, namely, that trauma severity, and age and education at time of captivity were the best predictors of current PTSD symptoms, with age and education acting as resilience factors.

The relation between hardiness and the POW experience was investigated in two Israeli studies. Waysman, Schwarzwald, and Solomon (2001) studied hardiness as protective against negative outcomes and promotive of positive outcomes in ex-POWs of the 1973 Yom Kippur War and a matched group of combat controls. In rating ex-POWs on how they were at present and how they were before the war, the investigators found a main association between hardiness and positive change. The more hardy the POWs, the more positive the change they reported in a process termed *transformational coping* that transformed meaning of events in a positive manner. Zakin, Solomon, and Neria (2003) replicated these findings.

Posttraumatic growth (PTG), another multicomponent construct, was found to be unrelated to PTSD (Powell, Rosner, Butollo, Tedeschi, & Calhoun, 2003), to be related to self-deception (Maerker & Zoellner, 2004), and likely to have a complex relationship to PTSD, reflecting the multifactorial structure of the Posttraumatic Growth Inventory (Morris, Shakespeare-Finch, Rieck, & Newbery, 2005).

Integrative Models of Traits and of Emotions

Integrative models of traits, of emotions, or of both comprise the next level of complexity beyond component models. These are best represented by the extensive research programs of Hobfoll and associates and of Zautra and associates. An integrative model is proposed by Hobfoll (2002) in his conservation of resources (COR) model, in which positive traits and coping constructs are viewed as adaptive "resources" that interact in ways that conserve a person's resources when under stress. This model treats resources (or traits and coping) as part of a larger dynamic process of well-being. Resources of traits and coping change under stressful challenge. Possession of a reliable resource reservoir is critical for well-being and health. Thus, the emphasis is not on the workings of a single trait, such as optimism, or even on component constellations of resources, but on the larger dynamic picture of what supports or hinders adaptation.

Hobfoll and associates have explored the main three factors comprising COR: social support resources (social support, social networks), personal resources (self-esteem, mastery, social competency), and environmental factors (Hobfoll, 1989; Hobfoll, Freedy, Lane, & Geller, 1990). It is a dynamic model in which conservation of resources is mobilized in the face of resource loss and concomitant stress. When faced with adversity, people mobilize resources. The negative outcome depends on the extent to which they can limit resource loss. Resource gain has less of an impact than resource loss. A sampling of studies show that economic stress altered personal (mastery) and social resources (social support), thus affecting anger and depression in inner-city women (Hobfoll, Johnson, Ennis, & Jackson, 2003); childhood abuse was associated with interpersonal resource loss, PTSD, and depression (Schumm, Hobfoll, & Keogh, 2004; Schumm, Stines, Hobfoll, & Jackson, 2005); and resource loss predicted PTSD and depression following the World Trade Center attacks (Hobfoll, Tracy, & Galea, 2006).

In a series of studies, the team of Zautra, Reich, and Davis address the question of whether positive and negative affects function independently of each other, or whether they form a single bipolar dimension in which they are inversely related, and a rise in positive affect brings with it a decline in negative affect. Both models, bivariate and bipolar, have extensive empirical support (Reich, Zautra, & Davis, 2003). The unique contribution of this team is that they tested the two models against each other and were able to affirm the validity of both, and to demonstrate the conditions under which one model prevailed and the other receded. They proposed the dynamic model of af-

TABLE 20.2. Resilience as Resources and Capacities to Challenge

Capacities	Descriptions, findings	Authors
Hardiness		
Hardiness and social support	Stressful life events, Vietnam veterans	King et al. (1998)
Hardiness and PTSD	Commitment, control, and challenge and PTSD in Persian Gulf veterans	Sutker et al. (1995)
Hardiness and symptoms	Psychological and health related symptoms in Persian Gulf veterans	Bartone (1999)
Social support, coping style	Severity of PTSD symptoms in Persian Gulf veterans	Benotsch et al. (2000)
Approach coping	PTSD in Persian Gulf veterans	Sharkansky et al. (2000)
Hardiness, attachment style	Lower level of symptoms and PTSD in Israeli ex-POWs	Zakin et al. (2003)
Hardiness	Stress symptoms, negative life change in Israeli ex-POWs	Waysman et al. (2001)
Posttraumatic growth (PTG)		
PTG	No relationship with symptoms of PTSD in refugees of Bosnia and Herzegovena	Powell et al. (2003)
PTG	Janus-faced model of PTG or self-perception of PTG is self-deception in survivors of Dresden bombing	Maercker & Zoellner (2004)
Strengths, assessment, PTG	Assessing PTG to guide interventions	Tedeschi & Kilmer (2005)
Education		
Education and age	Inverse relation with distress in POWs World War II and Korean Conflict ex-POWs	Gold et al. (2000)
Education and rank	Better outcome with PTSD in POWs and World War II ex-POWs	Zeiss & Dickman (1989); Speed et al. (1989)
Conservation of resources (COR)		
Resource loss, resource gain	Economic stress alters personal and social resources and impacts anger and depression, inner-city women	Hobfoll et al. (2003)
Mastery and social support	Resources in reported child physical and sexual abuse, Native American women	Hobfoll (2002)

(cont.)

TABLE 20.2. *(cont.)*

Capacities	Descriptions, findings	Authors
Dynamic model of activation (DMA)		
Stressful events and affect	Positive and negative affect and stressful events	Zautra et al. (2000)
DMA and chronic pain	Application of DMA to chronic pain	Zautra et al. (2001)
Emotion and stress in everyday life	Dynamic approaches to emotions and stress	Zautra, Affleck, et al. (2005)
Emotions, stress, and health	Dimensions of emotions and health adaptation	Zautra (2003)
Resilience, emotions, and adaptation	Role of trait resilience and positive emotions in stress process	Ong et al. (2006)
Complexity of emotions	Complexity of emotions and resilience in later life	Ong & Bergeman (2004)

fect (DMA), which subsumed the bivariate and univariate models by joining them in a dynamic relationship. In comprehensive reviews (Zautra, 2003; Reich et al., 2003) they extract a number of basic principles. The context of affective experiences modifies the dynamic relationship. When the context is safe and predictable, information from multiple sources is processed, including both negative and positive information of the context. Positive and negative affective information does not overlap during low stress. A context of increased stress contains greater uncertainty, as well as narrowly focused attention, and simplified rapid judgment in responding to threat. During increased stress, the independent positive and negative affects collapse to form a simple bipolar dimension and an inverse relationship. The bivariate and bimodal dimensions were studied as they diverged or coalesced under conditions of acute and/or chronic stress in populations that ranged from college students (Reich & Zautra, 1981) to subjects with chronic pain (Zautra, Smith, Affleck, & Tennen, 2001), fibromyalgia (Davis, Zautra, & Smith, 2004), dimensions of simplicity–complexity (Reich, Zautra, & Potter, 2001), and others. Additional discussions of this DMA model and its applications are found in other chapters in this volume. Ong (Ong, & Bergeman, 2004; Ong, Bergeman, Bisconti, & Wallace, 2006) continues the study of DMA by exploring the dynamic relationship between emotions and trait resilience and how these modulate and mediate the adaptive process of stress.

Capacity-Building Interventions

September 11, 2001, is a watershed date for the mental health community. Agencies and institutions across the United States prepared for a torrent of psychological trauma and depression in the wake of the World Trade Center attacks. Emergency mental health hot lines, and programs for free screening and brief counseling sprang up across the country. Mental health workers, indeed, the entire country, became one coherent community, galvanized to take care of the aftereffects of the attacks. There was not an epidemic of trauma, but there was a lot of resilience. Five years later, Aaron Levin (2006) wrote in *Psychiatric News* (p. 20), "Resilience rather than pathology should become the standard expectation in the aftermath of trauma." The experts he cited are well known in the trauma research community: Arieh Shalev stated, "We need to define and study the non-PTSD outcome" (p. 20), which means exploring resilience, and Matthew Friedman (p. 20) acknowledged, "We've gone from nonrecognition to over recognition of PTSD." Rather than expect trauma, we should expect good adaptation. The emphasis on the study of resilience in the context of trauma is reinforced by the International Society for Traumatic Stress Studies. The Society dedicated its 22nd Annual Meeting in 2006 to the theme "The Psychobiology of Trauma and Resilience Across the Lifespan."

Changes in therapeutic approaches that emphasize capacities slightly antedate or overlap with the 9/11 World Trade Center attacks. The correspondence and overlap with that seminal event contributed to the growing examination of best practices guidelines published by the International Society for Traumatic Stress Studies in 2009 (Foa, Keane, Friedman, & Cohen, 2009) and the American Psychiatric Association in 2004. At the same time, new therapeutic directions developed as a response to the recognition that traditional therapies were not meeting major gaps in patients' needs and adjustment. The new wave of therapeutic approaches made the absence of capacities the center of treatment intervention, while including elements of traditional therapies and developing more holistic approaches to emotional treatment.

In developing dialectical behavior therapy (DBT), Linehan (1993a, 1993b) recognized that a treatment focused on change would not work with the chronically suicidal patients, who were exceedingly sensitive to criticism that easily resulted in emotion dysregulation. Therapy was not possible without addressing emotion dysregulation. Cloitre (Cloitre, Koenen, Cohen, & Han, 2002) addressed two symptoms found in adult survivors of child abuse (CA)—affect dysregulation and interpersonal difficulties—that were not treated effectively by existing therapies. Najavits and colleagues (1998) filled another gap in treatment approaches. In her manual *Seeking Safety* (2002), she explains, "Although this treatment draws on the traditions of many existing treatments … , it was developed to meet needs that did not appear to be addressed thus far" (p.

19). Najavits saw that treatment outcomes for patients with PTSD and substance abuse were much worse than those for any other dual-diagnosis group. Moreover, PTSD was frequently left undiagnosed and untreated in many substance abuse treatment programs, in the context of a culture of treatment that emphasized ameliorating substance abuse. She introduced Seeking Safety and adapted cognitive-behavioral therapy (CBT) to her dual-diagnoses population. We briefly review four representative capacity-building interventions and conclude with a fifth group of approaches that have mindfulness as a core element.

The two-phased *skills training* approach developed by Cloitre and associates (2002) consists of Phase 1, eight weekly sessions of skills training in affect and interpersonal regulation; Phase 2, eight weeks of modified prolonged exposure. Each session focuses on a particular skills deficit associated with CA trauma: (1) labeling and identifying feelings; (2) emotion management; (3) tolerating distress; (4) acceptance of feelings and enhancing positive emotions; (5) identification of trauma-based interpersonal schemas; (6) identification of trauma-generated feelings and conflict with current goals; (7) role plays of power and control; and (8) role plays of flexibility and power difficulties. The role plays emphasize emotions, problematic interpersonal behaviors, and new alternative behaviors. Homework consists of the application of skills.

Phase 2 covers prolonged imaginal exposure modeled on Foa and Rothbaum (1998). Patients repeatedly describe their traumatic events in a detailed, emotional fashion. Three additional components cover postexposure stabilization through coping skills to modulate feelings, postexposure identification of feelings during exposure, and identification of negative interpersonal schemas that are then contrasted with more adaptive schemas to highlight personal resources. Finally, individuals review coping skills and new schemas, and apply them to their current lives.

The two-phase treatment of skills training in affect and interpersonal regulation was tested in a controlled clinical trial. It proved effective in reducing PTSD symptoms and improving affective functions, reflected in standardized measures of depression, anxiety, dissociation, and alexithymia.

The *Seeking Safety* intervention by Najavits (2002), also a manualized program, comprises a modified CBT approach that covers cognitive, behavioral, and interpersonal domains. Each domain addresses a safe coping skill relevant to both PTSD and substance abuse. Safety is the dominant philosophy that is raised with each issue that impacts the individual's life: stopping use, reducing suicidality, reducing exposure to HIV risk, letting go of dangerous relationships, and stopping self-harm. Many self-destructive behaviors repeat the trauma that was inflicted on the individual. Seeking Safety helps patients to avoid repeating the cycle of violence. The violations of safety are replaced by establishing safety as a main life goal and teaching safety skills that preserve individuals' lives. The program integrates treatment of both PTSD and substance abuse. There is a focus on the reestablishment of ideals because both disorders exemplify major loss of ideals and meaning, a shattered world, and living "at the bottom." The program covers four content areas: cognitive, behavioral, interpersonal functions, and case management. CBT is present- and problem-oriented. There is an emphasis on the rehearsal of new skills, commitment to action, and practical solutions. Language focuses on potential rather than on pathology, terms of strengths, and is humanistic. Exploration of past trauma is not part of the Seeking Safety treatment approach.

Several studies have evaluated the effectiveness of this treatment program. In an early study Najavits and colleagues (1998) found significant reductions in substance use, trauma-related symptoms, suicide risk and thoughts, and improvement in social and family functioning, cognition, and knowledge about substance use and treatment. In a second study, Najavits and colleagues (2001, cited in Najavits, 2002) found improvement in participants' drug use, trauma symptoms, family and social functioning, and sense of meaning.

Behavioral activation, although first developed by Lewinsohn (1975), has reappeared in the work of Jacobson, Martell, and Dimidjian (2001) and Martell, Addis, and Dimidjian (2004).The approach is in the tradition of behavioral analysis and contextualism. *Depression* is defined as avoidance behavior in which individuals responds to avoidance contingencies with inactivity and rumination. Individuals respond primarily to deprivation, such as feeling lonely and calling a friend to complain. Individuals avoid negative feelings and disrupt routines rather than attain goals or engage in proactive approaches. The targets of treatment are inertia, avoidance behaviors, routine disruption, and passive rumination. This avoidance pattern is the "TRAP" from which the person can escape through "ACTION." With ACTION, the person assesses the function of the behavior, chooses to continue avoidance or chooses to change, tries the chosen behavior, integrates the new behavior into a routine, observes results of the new behavior, and never gives up. Individuals are also asked to set goals, and act toward their goals and not according to their mood.

Well-being therapy by Fava (1999) and associates (Fava, Rafanelli, Cazzaro, Conti, & Grandi, 1998) has as its goal the treatment of residual symptoms of mood and anxiety disorders following successful treatment of these conditions. Ryff and Singer (1996) held that the absence of illness is not equivalent to health and well-being. Recovery should not only alleviate negative symptoms but also foster positive wellness, and therapy should not necessarily just reduce symptoms but also increase personal effectiveness. Fava's therapeutic approach is based on Ryff's conceptual model of well-being (Ryff, 1989; Ryff & Singer, 1996). Treatment comprises eight sessions. Patients are asked to keep a diary of well-being episodes. In the first two sessions patients identify well-being episodes and their context. In the next three sessions, they identify automatic thoughts that interrupt well-being. In the final three sessions, Ryff's well-being dimensions are applied, and specific impairments are identified. The goal of therapy is to guide patients through the transition from impairment to well-being. Mastery and pleasure tasks, as well as exposure to feared situations, are encouraged. Ryff's well-being dimensions are summarized in her Scale of Psychosocial Well-Being as Autonomy, Environmental Mastery, Personal Growth, Positive Relations with Others, Purpose in Life, and Self-Acceptance. An early study (Fava et al., 1998) comparing well-being therapy and CBT found that well-being therapy was associated with a significant increase in perceive well-being and a significant decrease in symptomatic distress, beyond the positive effects of CBT.

Perhaps the boldest innovations belong to those therapies exploring the inclusion of *mindfulness meditation in established therapies*, such as the CBTs that comprise what Hayes (2004) termed the *third wave*, or generation, that is moving therapy into a different direction. In the first wave of behavior therapy and the second wave of cognitive therapy, a reduction of symptoms was clearly the central goal of treatment. The therapeutic focus was on changing maladaptive ways of thinking and feeling to promote improvement in functioning. In contrast, a mindfulness-based approach encourages acceptance of current experiences. There is no "problem" to be solved. Rather, thoughts and feelings are acknowledged without judgment and are accepted in the reality of the moment by an observing self that stands apart from the thoughts that enter consciousness (e.g., Kabat-Zinn, 1994; Segal, Williams, & Teasdale, 2002). Similar to traditional CBT, dysfunctional thought patterns are identified, but rather than promoting attempts to neutralize or control such thoughts through the processes of reframing and reappraisal, a mindful approach promotes detached observation. The effect of detached observation

is seen in the increased individual's capacity to tolerate difficult emotions. The accompanying exposure transforms such emotions into innocuous states. Anxiety symptoms and panic sensations, for example, typically amplify emotional reactivity. This cycle may be interrupted by halting the automatic tendency to avoid the sensations, and instead intentionally observe the sensations without judgment (Kabat-Zinn, 1990). By fostering objective awareness of feelings, thoughts, behaviors, and choices, mindfulness increases awareness of the whole range of choices available to individuals at any given moment.

Mindfulness is one aspect shared by several prominent third-wave behavior therapies, represented here by DBT, *acceptance and commitment therapy* (ACT), and *mindfulness-based cognitive therapy* (MBCT). Linehan (1993) makes mindfulness the center of DBT. It is the core skill taught to clients with borderline personality disorder, to "allow" difficult experiences rather than to suppress or avoid them. DBT draws mainly from the practice of Zen, with the focus on acceptance, validation, and tolerance instead of change. Thus, acceptance is opening oneself to the context, waiting for understanding, and acknowledging distress as an understandable outcome of the self rather than a problem to be solved. Thus, acceptance is very important in working with very sensitive, impulsive, and reactive clients. Validation defuses the emotional arousal of failure, shame, and fear. Acceptance focuses on the current moment, sees reality as it is, without delusions, and accepts reality without judgment. It encourages letting go of attachments, using skillful means, and finding a middle way. Linehan in DBT and Hays in ACT offer complex theoretical approaches, and detailed treatment procedures and manuals. A comprehensive review of either therapy is beyond the scope of this chapter. They are mentioned briefly, as an indication of where the burgeoning innovations in psychotherapies and interventions are heading. Only a brief outline is summarized in Table 20.3.

TABLE 20.3. Capacity-Building Therapeutic Interventions

Interventions	Descriptions	Authors
1. Life skills training for PTSD related to childhood abuse		
Training in life skills	Manualized program: 8 weeks in affect and interpersonal regulation; 8 weeks of modified exposure	Cloitre et al. (2002)
2. Safety skills for PTSD and substance abuse		
Establishing safety as life skill	Manualized program: 25 sessions; focus is on four content areas (cognitive, behavioral, interpersonal, case management); focus is on potential not pathology; attention to language as humanistic; promotes strengths, creates meaning; avoids exploration of past trauma and interpretive psychodynamic approach	Najavits (2002)
3. Behavioral activation		
Increase action despite nonmotivation	Depression is avoidance, inactivity, rumination; engage in behaviors that will be positively reinforced: meaningful activity, personal goals, be proactive, commit to action, have routines. Four targets: inertia, avoidance, routine disruption, rumination Therapy strategies: keep activity log, Three strategies to combat avoidance: avoid TRAP, get back on TRACK, and take ACTION, set goals and carry out behaviors to meet goals	Jacobson et al. (2001)
4. Well-being therapy		
Enhance psychological well-being	Psychotherapeutic approach based on Ryff's multidimensional model: environmental mastery, personal growth, purpose in life, autonomy, self-acceptance, positive relations with others	Fava (1999)
5. Mindfulness and change therapies		
A. Dialectical behavior therapy		
DBT core elements	Manualized program: achieve acceptance and change in therapy; tolerate pain, behavioral inhibitions, and simultaneously change Five elements: biosocial theory of the disorder; stages of treatment as a developmental process; each stage consists of a hierarchy of treatment targets; treatment must serve functions; identify sets of acceptance strategies, change strategies, and dialectical strategies	Linehan (1989); Linehan et al. (1991); Linehan & Schmidt (1995)
B. Mindfulness-based cognitive therapy		
Prevention of relapse in depression	Eight weeks, influenced by use of mindfulness by Hayes, Linehan; changing patient's relationship to depressive thoughts and feelings through "decentering," not *what* but *how* of processing moment-to-moment experience and openness and acceptance of the unpleasant; become aware of and relate differently to thoughts, feelings, and bodily sensations	Teasdale et al. (2000); Ma & Teasdale (2000)
C. Acceptance and commitment therapy		
ACT approach	To change one's relationship to one's thought rather than alter content of one's thoughts; based on analysis of language and cognition; relational frame theory (RFT) explains cognitive fusion and avoidance; change principles include contextualism, live according to chosen values and goals, change the context that supports a thought, alter context through cognitive diffusion and mindfulness: acceptance—experience events as they are; commitment—build larger patterns of flexible responding	Hayes (2004, 2007)

Resilience Approaches in Phoenix, Arizona

Psychological science has pointed to a host of attributes and skills linked to the capacity of individuals to sustain well-being in the face of more common life difficulties, as well as extremely traumatic experiences. A growing body of work suggests that we can foster those capacities to promote well-being and functional health. In our work with colleagues in the Resilience Solutions Group at Arizona State University, we are engaged in testing theory-driven interventions that focus on three particular dimensions of resilience capacities: personal mastery, mindfulness, and agency. Much of our effort has been directed toward addressing disruptions in emotion regulation that can occur in the face of chronic disabling conditions, including depression, chronic pain, and PTSD.

After decades of research, there is widespread agreement that a sense of personal mastery is fundamental to mental health and well-being. Perceiving that one's decisions and actions have an effect on one's outcomes is related to better adjustment across a host of challenges, ranging from physical illness (Affleck, Tennen, Croog, & Levine, 1987) to depression (Lewinsohn & Gotlib, 1995), to stressful life events (Thompson, 1981), and even to chronic difficulties (Perlmuter & Langer, 1982; Reich & Zautra, 1988). To what extent can we intervene to increase individuals' sense of mastery? A body of research has developed to investigate that possibility. It has demonstrated that mastery can be enhanced (Langer & Rodin, 1976; Rodin & Langer, 1977; Schulz, 1976), that mastery interventions can yield positive benefits, such as improved adjustment and mental health, and can enhance cellular immunocompetence (Blazer, 2002; Laudenslager, Ryan, Drugan, Hyson, & Maier, 1983). Our colleagues Reich and Zautra (1990) tested the benefits of a 10-week mastery intervention compared to a no-treatment control condition in a group of over 200 aging adults. The mastery intervention was designed to increase participants' active engagement in self-chosen positive activities and boost the development of coping skills to manage uncontrollable circumstances. The intervention had its intended effects: The mastery-enhancing group reported increased engagement in desirable activities, and significantly decreased psychological distress and negative affect.

As are mastery and control, positive affective resources are key to long-term adaptation. Lazarus, Kanner, and Folkman (1980) were among the first to recognize the potential utility of positive affect, suggesting that such affective experiences serve as useful restorative mechanisms, replenishing needed energy to cope with adverse events. Similarly, Lewinsohn and colleagues (e.g., Lewinsohn & Gotlib, 1995) have studied the beneficial effects of positive events on depression and mental health. The salience of positive affective engagement in adaptation is most pronounced during times of high stress (Fredrickson & Levenson, 1998; Zautra, Affleck, Tennen, Reich, & Davis, 2005). Positive emotions influence physiological responses to stress, for example (Fredrickson, 2001), by dampening arousal and speeding recovery from a stressful event, thereby allowing a more rapid return to a resting state. Being able to engage positive emotions during stressful times, when one's resources are taxed, may not only alleviate acute responses to stress but may also provide long-term benefits. Fredrickson posits that positive emotions are worth cultivating as a means to achieve psychological growth and improved well-being over the long term. Positive emotions may propel an "upward spiraling" toward emotional well-being, where the more positive emotions a person has, the more likely he or she is to cope effectively and create more positive emotions in the future (Fredrickson & Joiner, 2002). This kind of capacity building may be responsible for the kinds of effects recently observed in a longitudinal study of the onset of frailty with 1,558 Hispanic older adults (Ostir, Ottenbacher, & Markides, 2004). Healthy older adults who reported greater happiness, enjoyment of life, and hopefulness at the initial interviews were significantly less likely to be classified as frail during the 7-year follow-up assessment.

Many investigators who have focused on negative affect regulation have not realized that factors influencing positive affective states are often independent of negative affective states (Bradburn, 1969; Gable, Reis, & Elliot, 2000; Watson, Clark, & Tellegen, 1988). Traditional approaches that focus on regulation of negative affect may have little influence on positive affective regulation. Can we cultivate positive affective experiences that promote resilience in the face of stress? The answer seems to be "yes." For example, Reich and Zautra (1981) conducted a targeted, 2-week intervention that randomly assigned individuals to (1) engage in 12 positive events from a longer list of pleasurable activities that individuals indicated they had not experienced but would like to do so, (2) engage in two activities from the list, and (3) return for retesting only, with no intervening activity experience. In follow-up assessment, the two activity groups reported more pleasantness in their daily event and a better quality of life than did controls. Thus, simply engaging in pleasant activities increased individuals' sense of well-being. But more important from a resilience perspective, the 12-event, high-positive activity group showed significantly less psychological distress in response to stressful life events than the two-event and no-event control groups. Thus, being encouraged to engage in many positive activities was a source of resilience for people experiencing high levels of life stress.

Clearly, mastery and positive affective engagement are important keys to resilience. A third avenue to sustaining well-being during times of difficulty focuses on individuals' capacity to regulate emotions through awareness and acceptance of their emotional experiences, and to find meaning and purpose in these experiences. As we noted earlier, in the psychotherapy literature over the past decade, acceptance-based approaches have figured more and more prominently in cognitive-behavioral interventions for a variety of conditions, and have garnered substantial empirical support (e.g., Jacobson & Christensen, 1996; Linehan, 1993; Segal et al., 2002). According to Segal and colleagues (2002), heightened awareness coupled with acceptance of existing experience acts to interrupt the maladaptive automatic responding that commonly occurs during negative emotional states. Greater attention to the whole range of experiences also facilitates awareness of positive affective states, even when one is coping with stress (Shapiro et al., 2006). Positive affect, in turn, facilitates more adaptive, flexible responses to current circumstances, with the potential to enhance well-being and functional health (Fredrickson & Levenson, 2000; Zautra, Johnson, & Davis, 2005), and reduce helplessness in the management of everyday life problems.

We have been incorporating mindfulness meditation (MM) into our treatment approaches as a useful method to enhance the ability to regulate emotion through awareness and acceptance (Baer, 2003; Kabat-Zinn, 1990; Segal et al., 2002). Training in MM includes regular practice of exercises to increase self-regulation of attention from moment to moment, which helps to promote more intentional, considered responses to everyday events. Recently, we have examined the benefits of resilience-oriented interventions promoting mastery, positive affective engagement, and emotion regulation among individuals managing the demands of a chronic pain condition. In randomized clinical trial with rheumatoid arthritis (RA) patients, we contrasted a mastery-oriented approach based on established CBT to target pain (CBT-P), with an emotion regulation approach based on MM and positive social engagement (Zautra et al., 2008). The CBT-P intervention drew on strategies that emphasized active coping and behavioral pain management, whereas the MM intervention emphasized emotional awareness and acceptance. We contrasted both active treatments with an established arthritis education curriculum to determine whether CBT-P and MM produced greater benefits than education. Our findings suggest that both CBT-P and MM promote better adaptation in RA, albeit for different outcomes. Consistent with the emphasis on mastery-based strategies in CBT-P, patients receiving CBT-P showed the greatest improvement in pain control and disease activity, as measured by the proinflammatory marker interleukin-6. In line with the promotion of emotional awareness and acceptance in MM, patients receiving MM showed greater improvements in vitality than did the other two groups. Both active treatment groups showed more improvement in mental health and coping efficacy than did the education group. The relative value of the treatments varied as a function of depression history, however. Patients with RA and a history of recurrent depressive disorder benefited most from MM, suggesting that a focus on building emotion regulation skills was most beneficial to those with the most difficulty with emotion regulation. We are now testing whether CBT-P and MM offer similar benefits to individuals with *fibromyalgia*, a condition characterized by widespread chronic pain and fatigue, and frequently comorbid affective disturbance.

How can a resilience perspective be harnessed to promote well-being among those devastated by traumatic experiences? Kent (2008; Kent et al., 2007) has designed an experience- and theory-based intervention to restore resilience in conditions where it is lost or compromised, such as for individuals with PTSD, depression, or chronic illness. The intervention grew out of the understanding of good survival in extreme situations. These situations informed the overarching goal of Kent's model, which is to reestablish resilience and to reengage individuals' capacities for resilient actions that include qualities of approach/engagement and social relatedness. Once established, these qualities are then used by individuals to return to their own traumatic experiences or other difficulties in a resilient way. In

short, the intervention encourages individuals to develop and deploy the same resilient approach that is found among those who are naturally able to sustain well-being in extreme situations.

First tested with PTSD, this model stands in marked contrast to the widely used psychosocial interventions for PTSD (exposure, eye movement desensitization and reprocessing [EMDR], CBT), where individuals are directed toward reexperiencing traumatic events (and not their strengths), with a primary emphasis on alleviating distress. Kent's manualized treatment first restores approach/engagement and social relatedness strengths, then uses the restored strengths to return to traumatic and distressing experiences in a way that disarms the stress, takes the suffering out of trauma, and turns trauma into an ordinary memory. At the outset of treatment, individuals are asked to take their traumatic experiences "offline," temporarily setting aside those experiences from their thoughts and emotions. Instead, individuals are asked to bring "online" an experience from the past in which they felt cherished. This is to serve as an anchoring experience individuals can turn to when distressed instead of reestablishing their distress. In subsequent phases of treatment, individuals are asked to reexperience instances of approach/engagement from childhood and early adulthood, that is, occasions that were marked by feelings of interest and curiosity, awareness of beauty, and similar approach experiences. To heighten the vividness of these recalled experiences, individuals are encouraged to develop elaborated verbal descriptions and visual illustrations that describe their memory of approach/engagement events. They are also to locate these experiences in their bodies. In another phase of the intervention, individuals are asked to reexperience instances of social relatedness, reflected in occasions marked by such feelings as empathy, compassion, friendship, and love. In essence, individuals reestablish the strengths that constitute resilience in challenging situations. These renewed strengths are available as individuals are directed to reenter into traumatic experiences, starting with less distressing experiences and progressively moving toward more distressing ones. As individuals revisit difficult episodes, they are able to adopt the role or perspective of approach/engagement or social relatedness based on instances they have practiced. In doing so, they return to the traumatic as an agent rather than as a victim. The intervention is one of learning to practice resilience in response to past traumatic experiences. The therapist concludes the intervention by asking individuals to consider the question "What is a good life?" as a means of helping them reweave their life narrative into one that brings their strengths forward. The emphasis throughout the program is on rebuilding engagement and agency. These experiences are deeply integrated with the neuroendocrine/neurophysiological, psychological, and cognitive functions of the individual.

Evidence from a recently completed pilot study points to the remarkable promise of this resilience approach. Thirty-six patients with a long-standing history of PTSD were randomized to either the building resilience for change (BRC) treatment or to a waiting-list control group in a 12-week manualized treatment program. Individuals were assessed pre- and posttreatment on measures of PTSD and depression symptoms, well-being, and cognitive functioning. The groups were comparable on all dimensions at pretesting. At posttesting, those in the BRC group not only reported substantial improvement in PTSD and depression symptoms but also showed significant increases in well-being, memory, attention, and mental flexibility. The control group, in contrast, remained virtually unchanged across all measures. These are the first data we are aware of that assess such diverse outcomes that have both theoretical and practical implications for our understanding of the qualities of resilience and PTSD, and the potential for resilience approaches in the development of treatments.

Simulation and practice of resilience and agency in response to old trauma are at the core of our BRC intervention. To be sure, resilience and trauma are complex, multidimensional processes. In our work, and in this review, we have attempted to identify some of the basic building blocks in which multiple elements are concentrated, giving rise to the complexity we see in resilience and challenge. In the process, we have altered the focus from an emphasis on challenge, stress, and trauma toward a strengths-based orientation of agency. The resulting integration is pervasive in connecting disparate areas of experience, brain structures, neural networks, endocrine systems, and in expanding potentials for a self that can more easily leave old moorings.

Conclusion

Resilience interventions are firmly rooted in traditions that began decades ago and are now experiencing a new wave of growth. The science of resilience continues to advance by integrating theory-driven approaches with state-of-the-art technologies to develop and test new resilience treatments. What lies ahead? Our hope is that investigators will make interventions more readily accessible to those most in need of them (e.g., Mahoney, Tarlow, & Jones, 2003). In our own work, we are moving into the community to test whether brief, daily resilience interventions via cell phone and the Internet help individuals who face challenges such as chronic pain and depression. Our goal, one that we share with other resilience interventionists, is to encourage individuals to "practice" resilience in their daily lives.

Postscript

In considering resilience in its most fundamental and broadly human aspects, the need to consider a firm definition of resilience and its cross-cultural applicability are indeed important. We consider our own firm definition of resilience at the end rather than at the outset of this chapter, simply to give voice and acknowledgment to the various directions and efforts that have preceded us, and to leave open the possibilities of what an evolving process may contribute to our understanding. Since the goal in the building our resilience (BRC) intervention was to restore resilience in PTSD, we had to be clear about what both resilience and PTSD are. Given the literature we have reviewed and the developmental literature on resilience, we conclude that resilience is a response to challenge, just like stress and trauma are responses to challenge. Both occur in similar contexts that are characterized by noncontingency, or contexts in which individuals have little effect on that context or environment. Faced with an arbitrary, life-threatening event, the resilient response is characterized by (1) an efficient stress response, (2) an approach/engagement orientation, and (3) social relatedness. This contrasts with traumatic stress as exemplified in PTSD, which is characterized by a dysregulated stress response and the symptom triad of hyperreactivity, reexperiencing of trauma, and avoidance (American Psychiatric Association, 2000). These symptoms demonstrate loss or distortion of resilience. A broad behavioral dimension emerges, one of approach/engagement and withdrawal/defense that is biologically supported by major physiological, endocrine, and brain mechanisms, including the autonomic nervous system, ventral vagus, hypothalamic–pituitary–adrenal (HPA) axis, oxytocin/vasopression, cortisol, and left- and right-hemisphere functions, just to name a few.

The goal of traditional therapies is to ameliorate symptoms. New wave therapies incorporate the development of capacities within the context of established therapies and emphasize acceptance rather than change of symptoms. Our goal is to restore and build resilience at the outset, use resilient strengths to transform trauma, and reconsider life themes in ways that brings strengths forward.

To what extent is our understanding of stress and resilience applicable to all cultures? We believe that the biological mechanisms hold for all of humankind. We also believe that the dimension of approach/engagement and withdrawal/defense also holds for all humanity. Indeed, it could be said that the dimension characterizes all of life, extending from lowly one-celled organisms to *Homo sapiens*; all organisms approach what sustains them and avoid or defend against what harms. How the dimensions of approach/engagement and withdrawal/defense are expressed in a culture will vary widely and have different consequences for the adaptation to challenge and for the quality of life of its people.

In our review focused on resilience and capacity-building interventions, we have encountered only few instances of cross-cultural comparisons. These are limited mainly to comparisons of mindfulness practice in experienced meditators of the Buddhist tradition and naive Western individuals in the recent work on mindfulness and brain mechanisms launched by Davidson and colleagues (Davidson et al., 2003; Lutz, Greischar, Rawlings, Ricard, & Davidson, 2004). The result is the present flurry of seminars, retreats, research programs, and publications (e.g., Begley, 2007; Siegel, 2007). Broader cross-cultural questions of these two traditions are not addressed. The study of mindfulness is nevertheless a very important opening to the broader question of how cultures adapt to challenge, be they acute or chronic. What cultural traditions foster resilience? Which customs magnify threat and thereby foster stress resistance or weaken resilience? What buffering social relationships and social institutions enhance resilient adaptations? Has Western emphasis on individualism weakened social networks, thereby weakening individual resilience? In the dichotomy of individualism versus community, what are the gains and costs to each in resilience adaptations to challenge? These are most interesting questions awaiting investigation.

We believe that resilience and cross-cultural studies of resilience comprise the new frontier of social, biological, and cultural science, a direction that holds much promise in the development of well-being and harmonious relations.

Acknowledgments

This work is partly supported by the Phoenix VA Health Care System and the Institute for Mental Health Research for contributions by Martha Kent and by the National Institute of Musculoskeletal, Immune, and Skin Disease (Grant No. R01 AR41687, Alex J. Zautra, Principal Investigator). The contents of this chapter do not represent the views of the Department of Veterans Affairs or of the U.S. Government. The contents represent the positions of the authors Martha Kent and Mary C. Davis.

References

Affleck, G., & Tennen, H. (1996). Construing benefits from adversity: Adaptational significance and dispositional underpinnings. *Journal of Personality, 64*, 899–922.

Affleck, G., Tennen, H., Croog, S., & Levine, S. (1987). Causal attribution, perceived benefits, and morbidity following a heart attack: An eight-year study. *Journal of Consulting and Clinical Psychology, 55*, 29–35.

Agaibi, C. E., & Wilson, J. P. (2005). Trauma, PTSD, and resilience: A review of the literature. *Trauma, Violence, and Abuse, 6*, 195–216.

Alvarez, J., & Hunt, M. (2005). Risk and resilience in canine search and rescue handlers after 9/11. *Journal of Traumatic Stress, 18*, 497–505.

American Psychiatric Association. (2000). *Diagnostic and statistical manual of mental disorders* (4th ed.). Washington, DC: Author.

American Psychiatric Association. (2004). Practice guidelines for the treatment of acute stress and posttraumatic stress disorder. *American Journal of Psychiatry, 161*, 1–31.

Anderson, N. B., & Anderson. P. E. (2003). *Emotional longevity: What really determines how long you live?* New York: Viking.

Baer, R. A. (2003). Mindfulness training as a clinical intervention: A conceptual and empirical review. *Clinical Psychology: Science and Practice, 10*, 125–143.

Bartone, P. T. (1999). Hardiness protects against war-related stress in army reserve forces. *Consulting Psychology Journal: Practice and Research, 51*, 72–82.

Beaton, R., Murphy, S., Johnson, C., Pike, K., & Corneil, W. (1999). Coping responses and posttraumatic stress symptomatology in urban fire service personnel. *Journal of Traumatic Stress, 12*, 293–308.

Begley, S. (2007). *Train your mind, change your brain: How a new science reveals our extraordinary potential to transform ourselves.* New York: Ballantine Books.

Benotsch, E. G., Brailey, K., Vasterling, J. J., Uddo, M., Constans, J. I., & Sutker, P. B. (2000). War zone stress, personal and environmental resources, and PTSD symptoms in Gulf War veterans: A longitudinal perspective. *Journal of Abnormal Psychology, 109*, 205–213.

Blazer, D. G. (2002). Self-efficacy and depression in late life: A primary prevention proposal. *Aging and Mental Health, 6*, 315–324.

Bleuler, M. (1984). Different forms of childhood stress and patterns of adult psychiatric outcome. In N. F. Watt, A. L. Wynne, & J. E. Rolf (Eds.), *Children at risk for schizophrenia: A longitudinal perspective* (pp. 537–542). Cambridge, UK: Cambridge University Press.

Bradburn, N. (1969). *The structure of psychological well-being.* Chicago: Aldine.

Carver, C. S., Pozo, C., Harris, S. D., Noriega, V., Scheier, M. F., Robinson, D. S., et al. (1993). How coping mediates the effect of optimism on distress: A study of women with early stage breast cancer. *Journal of Personality and Social Psychology, 65*, 375–390.

Cloitre, M., Cohen, L. R., & Koenen, K. C. (2006). *Treating survivors of childhood abuse: Psychotherapy for the interrupted life.* New York: Guilford Press.

Cloitre, M., Koenen, M. C., Cohen, L. R., & Han, H. (2002). Skills training in affective and interpersonal regulation followed by exposure: A phase-based treatment for PTSD related to childhood abuse. *Journal of Consulting and Clinical Psychology, 70*, 1967–1074.

Curtis, W., & Cicchetti, D. (2003). Moving research on resilience into the 21st century: Theoretical and methodological considerations in examining the biological contributions to re-silience. *Development and Psychopathology, 15*, 773–810.

Davidson, R. J., Kabat-Zinn, J., Schumacher, J., Rosenkranz, M., Muller, D., Santorelli, S. F., et al. (2003). Alterations in brain and immune function produced by mindfulness meditation. *Psychosomatic Medicine, 65*, 564–570.

Davis, M. C., Zautra, A. J., & Smith, B. W. (2004). Chronic pain, stress, and the dynam-ics of affective differentiation. *Journal of Per-sonality, 72*, 1133–1159.

Fava, G. A. (1999). Well-being therapy: Concep-tual and technical issues. *Psychotherapy and Psychosomatics, 68*, 171–179.

Fava, G. A., Rafanelli, C., Cazzaro, M., Conti, S., & Grandi, S. (1998). Well-being therapy. A novel psychotherapeutic approach for residual symptoms of affective disorders. *Psychologi-cal Medicine, 28*, 475–480.

Florian, V., Mikulincer, M., & Taubman, O. (1995). Does hardiness contribute to mental health during a stressful real-life situation?: The roles of appraisal and coping. *Journal of Personality and Social Psychology, 68*, 687–695.

Foa, E. B., Keane, T. M., Friedman, M. J., & Cohen, J. A. (Eds.). (2009). *Effective treat-ments for PTSD: Practice guidelines for the International Society for Traumatic Stress Studies* (2nd ed.). New York: Guilford Press.

Foa, E. B., & Rothbaum, B. O. (1998). *Treating the trauma of rape: Cognitive-behavioral ther-apy for PTSD*. New York: Guilford Press.

Folkman, S., & Moskowitz, J. T. (2000). Positive affect and the other side of coping. *American Psychologist, 55*, 647–654.

Fredrickson, B. L. (2001). The role of positive emotions in positive psychology: The broaden-and-build theory of positive emotions. *Ameri-can Psychologist, 56*, 218–226.

Fredrickson, B. L., & Joiner, T. (2002). Positive emotions trigger upward spirals toward emo-tional well-being. *Psychological Science, 13*, 171–175.

Fredrickson, B. L., & Levenson, R. W. (1998). Positive emotions speed recovery from the cardiovascular sequelae of negative emotions. *Cognition and Emotion, 12*(2), 191–220.

Gable, S. L., Reis, H. T., & Elliot, A. J. (2000). Behavioral activation and inhibition in every-day life. *Journal of Personality and Social Psy-chology, 6*, 1135–1149.

Garmezy, N. (1971). Vulnerability research and the issue of primary prevention. *American Journal of Orthopsychiatry, 41*, 101–116.

Gold, P. B., Engdahl, B. E., Eberly, R. E., Blake, R. J., Page, W. F., & Frueh, B. C. (2000). Trau-ma exposure, resilience, social support, and PTSD construct validity among former prison-ers of war. *Social Psychiatry and Psychiatric Epidemiology, 35*, 36–42.

Hagh-Shenas, H., Goodarzi, M. A., Dehbozorgi, G., & Farashbandi, H. (2005). Psychological consequences of the Bam earthquake on pro-fessional and nonprofessional helpers. *Journal of Traumatic Stress, 18*, 477–483.

Haglund, M. E., Nestadt, P. S., Cooper, N. S., Southwick, S. M., & Charney, D. S. (2007). Psychobiological mechanisms of resilience: Relevance to prevention and treatment of stress-related psychopathology. *Development and Psychopathology, 19*, 889–920.

Hayes, S. C. (2004). Acceptance and commit-ment therapy and the new behavior therapies: Mindfulness, acceptance, and relationship. In S. C. Hayes, V. M. Follette, & M. M. Linehan (Eds.), *Mindfulness and acceptance: Expand-ing the cognitive-behavioral tradition* (pp. 1–29). New York: Guilford Press.

Hayes, S. C. (2007). Acceptance and commit-ment therapy, relational frame theory, and the third wave of behavioral and cognitive thera-pies. *Behavior Therapy, 35*, 639–665.

Hobfoll, S. E. (1989). Conservation of resourc-es: A new attempt at conceptualizing stress. *American Psychologist, 44*, 513–524.

Hobfoll, S. E. (2002). Social and psychological resources and adaptation. *Review of General Psychology, 6*, 307–324.

Hobfoll, S. E., Freedy, J. R., Lane, C., & Geller, P. (1990). Conservation of social resources: Social support resource theory. *Journal of So-cial and Personal Relationships, 7*, 465–478.

Hobfoll, S. W., Johnson, R. J., Ennis, N., & Jackson, A. P. (2003). Resource loss, resource gain, and emotional outcomes among inner city women. *Journal of Personality and Social Psychology, 84*, 632–643.

Hobfoll, S. E., Tracy, M., & Galea, S. (2006). The impact of resource loss and traumatic growth on probable PTSD and depression fol-lowing terrorist attacks. *Journal of Traumatic Stress, 19*, 867–878.

Hoge, E. A., Austin, E. D., & Pollack, M. H. (2007). Resilience: Research evidence and conceptual considerations for posttraumatic stress disorder. *Depression and Anxiety, 24,* 139–152.

Hunter, E. J. (1993). The Vietnam prisoner of war experience. In J. P. Wilson & B. Raphael (Eds.), *International handbook of traumatic stress syndromes* (pp. 297–303). New York: Plenum Press.

Jacobson, N. S., & Christensen, A. (1996). *Acceptance and change in couple therapy.* New York: Norton.

Jacobson, N. S., Martell, C. R., & Dimidjian, S. (2001). Behavioral activation for depression: Returning to contextual roots. *Clinical Psychology: Science and Practice, 8,* 255–270.

Janoff-Bulman, R. (1992). *Shattered assumptions.* New York: Free Press.

Johnsen, B. H., Eid, J., Laberg, J. C., & Thayer, J. E. (2002). The effect of sensitization and coping style on post-traumatic stress symptoms and quality of life: Two longitudinal studies. *Scandinavian Journal of Psychology, 43,* 181–188.

Kabat-Zinn, J. (1990). *Full catastrophe living: Using the wisdom of your body and mind to face stress, pain, and illness.* New York: Delacorte.

Kabat-Zinn, J. (1994). *Wherever you go, there you are: Mindfulness meditation in everyday life.* New York: Hyperion.

Kabat-Zinn, J. (2003). Mindfulness-based interventions in context: Past, present, and future: Commentaries. *Clinical Psychology: Science and Practice, 10,* 144–160.

Kent, M., Matt, K., Seidel, A., Carpenter, J., Highberger, L., & Davis, M. (2007). *Dissociation and the experience of trauma as subject and object.* Paper presented at the annual meeting of the International Society for the Study of Trauma and Dissociation, Philadelphia.

King, L. A., King, D. W., Fairbank, J. A., Keane, T. M., & Adams, G. A. (1998). Resilience-recovery factors in post-traumatic stress disorder among female and male Vietnam veterans: Hardiness, postwar social support, and additional stressful life events. *Journal of Personality and Social Psychology, 74,* 420–434.

Kobasa, S. C. (1979). Stressful life events, personality, and health: An inquiry into hardiness. *Journal of Personality and Social Psychology, 37,* 1–11.

Koenig, H. G., George, L. K., & Titus, P. (2004).

Religion, spirituality, and health in medically ill hospitalized older patients. *Journal of the American Geriatric Society, 52,* 554–562.

Koenig, H. G., George, L. M., & Peterson, B. L. (1998). Religious importance and remission of depression in medically ill older patients. *American Journal of Psychiatry, 155,* 536–542.

Langer, E. J., & Rodin, J. (1976). The effects of choice and enhanced personal responsibility for the aged: A field experiment in an institutional setting. *Journal of Personality and Social Psychology, 34,* 191–198.

Laudenslager, M. I., Ryan, S. M., Drugan, R. C., Hyson, R. I., & Maier, S. F. (1983). Coping and immunosuppression: Inescapable but not escapable shock suppresses lymphocyte proliferation. *Science, 221,* 568–570.

Lazarus, R. S., Kanner, A. D., & Folkman, S. (1980). Emotions: A cognitive–phenomenological analysis. In R. Plutchik & H. Kellerman (Eds.), *Theories of emotion* (Vol. 1, pp. 189–217). New York: Academic Press.

Lepore, S., & Revenson, T. (2006). Relationships between posttraumatic growth and resilience: Recovery, resistance, and reconfiguration. In L. G. Calhoun & R. G. Tedeschi (Eds.), *Handbook of posttraumatic growth* (pp. 24–46). Mahwah, NJ: Erlbaum.

Levin, A. (2006). PTSD not sufficient to explain responses to trauma. *Psychiatric News, 41,* 20.

Lewinsohn, P. M. (1975). The behavioral study and treatment of depression. In M. Hersen, R. M. Eisler, & P. M. Miller (Eds.), *Progress in behavior modification* (Vol. 1, pp. 19–65). New York: Academic Press.

Lewinsohn, P. M., & Gotlib, I. H. (1995). Behavior theory and treatment of depression. In E. E. Beckham & W. R. Leber (Eds.), *Handbook of depression* (2nd ed., pp. 352–375). New York: Guilford Press.

Linehan, M. M. (1989). Cognitive and behavior therapy for borderline personality disorder. In A. Tasman, R. E. Hale, & A. J. Frances (Eds.), *Review of psychiatry* (Vol. 8, pp. 84–102). Washington, DC: American Psychiatric Press.

Linehan, M. M. (1993a). *Cognitive behavioral treatment for borderline personality disorder.* New York: Guilford Press.

Linehan, M. M. (1993b). *Skills training manual for treating borderline personality disorder.* New York: Guilford Press.

Linehan, M. M., Armstrong, H. E., Suarez, A., Allmon, D., & Heard, H. L. (1991). Cognitive-behavioral treatment of chronically parasuicidal borderline patients. *Archives of General Psychiatry, 48*, 1060–1064.

Linehan, M. M., & Schmidt, H. (1995). The dialectics of effective treatment of borderline personality disorder. In W. O. O'Donohue & L. Krasner (Eds.), *Theories in behavior therapy: Exploring behavior change* (pp. 553–584). Washington, DC: American Psychological Association.

Lutz, A., Greischar, L. L., Rawlings, N. B., Ricard, M., & Davidson, R. J. (2004). Long-term meditators self-induce high-amplitude gamma synchrony during mental practice. *Proceedings of the National Academy of Sciences USA, 101*, 16369–16373.

Ma, S. H., & Teasdale, J. D. (2004). Mindfulness-based cognitive therapy for depression: Replications and exploration of differential relapse prevention effects. *Journal of Consulting and Clinical Psychology, 72*, 31–40.

Maddi, S. R. (1999a). Hardiness and optimism as expressed in coping patterns. *Consulting Psychology Journal: Practice and Research, 51*, 95–105.

Maddi, S. R. (1999b). The personality construct of hardiness: Effects on experiences, coping and strain. *Consulting Psychology Journal: Practice and Research, 51*, 83–94.

Maercker, A., & Zoellner, T. (2004). The Janus face of self-perceived growth: Toward a two-component model of posttraumatic growth. *Psychological Inquiry, 15*, 41–48.

Mahoney, D. F., Tarlow, B. J., & Jones, R. N. (2003). Effects of an automated telephone support system on caregiver burden and anxiety: Findings from the REACH for TLC intervention study. *Gerontologist, 43*, 556–567.

Manne, S., Duhamel, K., Ostrofr, J., Parsons, S., Martini, R., Williams, S. E., et al. (2003). Coping and the course of mother's depressive symptoms during and after pediatric bone marrow transplantation. *Journal of the American Academy of Child Adolescent Psychiatry, 42*, 1055–1068.

Martell, C., Addis, M., & Dimidjian, S. (2004). Finding the action in behavioral activation. In S. C. Hayes, V. M. Follette, & M. M. Linehan (Eds.), *Mindfulness and acceptance: Expanding the cognitive-behavioral tradition* (pp. 152–167). New York: Guilford Press.

Masten, A. S., & Reed, M. G. (2002). Resilience in development. In C. S. Snyder & S. J. Lopez (Eds.), *The handbook of positive psychology* (pp. 74–88). New York: Oxford University Press.

McCullough, M. E., Hoyt, W. T., Larson, D. B., & Koenig, H. G. (2000). Religious involvement and mortality: A meta-analytic review. *Health Psychology, 19*, 211–222.

Meichenbaum, D. (1985). *Stress inoculation training.* New York: Pergamon Press.

Midlarsky, E. (1991). Helping as coping. *Review of Personality and Social Psychology, 12*, 238–264.

Morris, B. A., Shakespeare-Finch, J., Rieck, M., & Newbery, J. (2005). Multidimensional nature of posttraumatic growth in an Australian population. *Journal of Traumatic Stress, 18*, 575–585.

Najavits, L. M. (2002). *Seeking Safety: A treatment manual for PTSD and substance abuse.* New York: Guilford Press.

Najavits, L. M., Gastfriend, D. R., Barber, J. P., Reif, S., Muenz, L. R., Blaine, J., et al. (1998). Cocaine dependence with and without posttraumatic stress disorder among subjects in the NIDA Collaborative Cocaine Treatment Study. *American Journal of Psychiatry, 155*, 214–219.

Ong, A. D., & Bergeman, C. S. (2004). The complexity of emotions in later life. *Journal of Gerontology B: Psychological Sciences and Social Sciences, 59*, P117–P122.

Ong, A. D., Bergeman, C. S., Bisconti, T. L., & Wallace, K. A. (2006). Psychological resilience, positive emotions, and successful adaptation to stress in later life. *Journal of Personality and Social Psychology, 91*, 730–749.

Ostir, G. V., Ottenbacher, K. J., & Markides, K. S. (2004). Onset of frailty in older adults and the protective role of positive affect. *Psychology and Aging, 19*, 402–408.

Park, C. L., Cohen, L., & Murch, R. (1996). Assessment and prediction of stress-related growth. *Journal of Personality, 64*, 71–105.

Perlmuter, L. C., & Langer, E. J. (1982). The effects of behavioral monitoring on the perception of control. *Clinical Gerontology, 1*, 37–43.

Powell, S., Rosner, R., Butollo, W., Tedeschi, R. G., & Calhoun, L. G. (2003). Posttraumatic growth after war: A study with former refugees and displaced people in Sarajevo. *Journal of Clinical Psychology, 59*, 71–83.

Rachman, S. (1979). The concept of required helpfulness. *Behavioural Research and Therapy, 17,* 1–6.

Regehr, C., Hill, J., & Glancy, G. D. (2000). Individual predictors of traumatic reactions in firefighters. *Journal of Nervous and Mental Disease, 188,* 333–339

Reich, J. W., & Zautra, A. (1981). Life events and personal causation: Some relationship with satisfaction and distress. *Journal of Personality and Social Psychology, 41,* 1002–1012.

Reich, J. W., & Zautra, A. J. (1988). Direct and stress-moderating effects of positive life experiences. In L. Cohen (Ed.), *Life events and psychological functioning: Theoretical and methodological issues* (pp. 149–180). Newbury Park, CA: Sage.

Reich, J. W., & Zautra, A. J. (1990). Dispositional control beliefs and the consequences of a control-enhancing intervention. *Journals of Gerontology B: Psychological Sciences and Social Sciences, 45,* P46–P51.

Reich, J. W., & Zautra, A. J. (1991). Experimental and measurement approaches to internal control in at risk older adults. *Journal of Social Issues, 46,* 143–158.

Reich, J. W., Zautra, A. J., & Davis, M. (2003). Dimensions of affect relationships: Models and their integrative implications. *Review of General Psychology, 7,* 66–83.

Reich, J. W., Zautra, A. J., & Potter, P. T. (2001). Cognitive structure and the independence of positive and negative affect. *Journal of Social and Clinical Psychology, 20,* 99–115.

Rodin, J., & Langer, E. J. (1977). Long-term effects of a control-relevant intervention with the institutionalized aged. *Journal of Personality and Social Psychology, 35,* 897–902.

Rosenbaum, J. J., & Covino, J. M. (2005). Stress and resilience: Implications for depression and anxiety. *Medscape Psychiatry and Mental Health, 10.* Retrieved September 30, 2006, from *www.medscape.com/viewarticle/518761.*

Rutter, M. (1987). Psychosocial resilience and protective mechanisms. *American Journal of Orthopsychiatry, 57,* 316–331.

Rutter, M. (1979). Protective factors in children's responses to stress and disadvantage. In M. W. Kent & J. E. Rolf (Eds.), *Primary prevention of psychopathology: Social competence in children* (Vol. 3, pp. 49–74). Hanover, NH: University Press of New England.

Ryff, C. D. (1989). Happiness is everything, or is it?: Explorations on the meaning of psychological well-being. *Journal of Personality and Social Psychology, 57,* 1069–1081.

Ryff, C. D., & Singer, B. (1996). Psychological well-being: Meaning, measurement, and implications for psychotherapy research. *Psychotherapy and Psychosomatics, 65,* 14–23.

Schaefer, J. A., & Moos, R. H. (1992). Life crisis and personal growth. In B. N. Carpenter (Ed.), *Personal coping: Theory, research and application* (pp. 149–170). Westport, CT: Praeger.

Schaefer, J. A., & Moos, R. H. (1998). The context for posttraumatic growth: Life crises, individual and social resources, and coping. In I. B. Weinger (Ed.), *Posttraumatic growth: Positive changes in the aftermath of crisis* (pp. 99–125). Mahwah, NJ: Erlbaum.

Scheier, M. F., Matthews, K. A., Owens, J. F., Magovern, G. J., Sr., Lefbvre, R. C., Abbott, R. A., et al. (1989). Dispositional optimism and recovery from coronary artery bypass surgery: The beneficial effects of physical and psychological well-being. *Journal of Personality and Social Psychology, 57,* 1024–1040.

Schulz, R. (1976). Effects of control and predictability on the physical and psychological well-being of the institutionalized aged. *Journal of Personality and Social Psychology, 33,* 563–573.

Schumm, J. A., Hobfoll, S. E., & Keogh, N. J. (2004). Revictimization and interpersonal resource loss predicts PTSD among women in substance-use treatment. *Journal of Traumatic Stress, 17,* 173–181.

Schumm, J. A., Stines, L. R., Hobfoll, S. E., & Jackson, A. P. (2005). The double-barreled burden of child abuse and current stressful circumstances on adult women: The kindling effect of early traumatic experience. *Journal of Traumatic Stress, 18,* 467–476.

Segal, Z. V., Williams, J. M. G., & Teasdale, J. D. (2002). *Mindfulness-based cognitive therapy for depression.* New York: Guilford Press.

Seligman, M. E. P. (2002). *Authentic happiness.* New York: Free Press.

Seligman, M. E. P., Castellon, C., Cacciola, J., Schulman, P., Luborsky, L., Ollove, M., et al. (1988). Explanatory style change during cognitive therapy for unipolar depression. *Journal of Abnormal Psychology, 97,* 13–18.

Shapiro, S. L., Carlson, L. E., Astin, J. A., & Freedman, B. (2006). Mechanisms of mindfulness: Review article. *Journal of Clinical Psychology, 62,* 373–386.

Sharkansky, E. J., King, D. W., King, L. A., Wolfe, J., Erickson, D. J., & Stokes, L. R. (2000). Coping with Gulf War combat stress: Mediating and moderating effects. *Journal of Abnormal Psychology, 109,* 188–197.

Siegel, D. J. (2007). *The mindful brain: Reflection and attunement in the cultivation of well-being.* New York: Norton.

Snyder, C. R., Rand, K. L., & Sigman, D. R. (2002). Hope theory: A member of the positive psychology family. In C. R. Snyder & S. J. Lopez (Eds.), *Handbook of positive psychology* (pp. 257–276). New York: Oxford University Press.

Soet, J. E., Brack, G. A., & DiIorio, C. (2003). Prevalence and predictors of women's experience of psychological trauma during childbirth. *Birth, 30,* 36–46.

Southwick, S. M., Vythilingam, M., & Charney, D. S. (2005). The psychobiology of depression and resilience to stress: Implications for prevention and treatment. *Annual Review of Clinical Psychology, 1,* 255–291.

Speed, J., Engdahl, B. E., Schwartz, J., & Eberly, R. E. (1989). Posttraumatic stress disorder as a consequence of the prisoner of war experience. *Journal of Nervous and Mental Disease, 177,* 147–153.

Stanton, A. L., Parsa, A., & Austenfeld, J. L. (2002). The adaptive potential of coping through emotional approach. In C. R. Snyder & S. J. Lopez (Eds.), *Handbook of positive psychology* (pp. 148–158). New York: Oxford University Press.

Sutker, P. B., Davis, J. M., Uddo, M., & Ditta, S. R. (1995). War zone stress, personal resources, and PTSD in Persian Gulf War returnees. *Journal of Abnormal Psychology, 104,* 444–453.

Teasdale, J. D., Segal, Z. V., Williams, J. M. G., Ridgeway, V. A., Soulsby, J. M., & Lau, M. A. (2000). Prevention of relapse/recurrence in major depression by mindfulness-based cognitive therapy. *Journal of Consulting and Clinical Psychology, 68,* 615–623.

Tedeschi, R. G., & Kilmer, R. P. (2005). Assessing strengths, resilience, and growth to guide clinical interventions. *Professional Psychology: Research and Practice, 36,* 230–237.

Tedeschi, R. G., Park, C. L., & Calhoun, L. G.

(Eds.). (1998). *Posttraumatic growth: Positive changes in the aftermath of crisis.* Mahwah, NJ: Erlbaum.

Thompson, S. C. (1981). A complex answer to a simple question: Will it hurt less if I can control it? *Psychological Bulletin, 90,* 89–101.

Wade, S. L., Borawski, E. A., Taylor, H. G., Drotar, D., Yeates, K. O., & Stancin, T. (2001). The relationship of caregiver coping to family outcomes during the initial year following pediatric traumatic injury. *Journal of Consulting and Clinical Psychology, 69,* 406–415.

Watson, D., Clark, L. A., & Tellegen, A. (1988). Development and validation of brief measures of positive and negative affect. *Journal of Personality and Social Psychology, 54,* 1063–1070.

Waysman, M., Schwarzwald, J., & Solomon, Z. (2001). Hardiness: An examination of its relationship with positive and negative long term changes following trauma. *Journal of Traumatic Stress, 14,* 531–548.

Zakin, G., Solomon, Z., & Neria, Y. (2003). Hardiness, attachment style, and long-term psychological distress among Israeli POWs and combat veterans. *Personality and Individual Differences, 34,* 819–829.

Zautra, A. J. (2003). *Emotions, stress, and health.* New York: Oxford University Press.

Zautra, A. J., Affleck, G. G., Tennen, H., Reich, J. W., & Davis, M. C. (2005). Dynamic approaches to emotions and stress in everyday life: Bolger and Zuckerman reloaded with positive as well as negative affects. *Journal of Personality, 76,* 1511–1538.

Zautra, A. J., Davis, M. C., Reich, J. W., Nicassio, P., Tennen, H., Finan, P., et al. (2008). Comparison of cognitive behavioral and mindfulness meditation interventions on adaptation to rheumatoid arthritis for patients with and without history of recurrent depression. *Journal of Consulting and Clinical Psychology, 76,* 408–421.

Zautra, A. J., Johnson, L., & Davis, M. C. (2005). Positive affect as a source of resilience to pain and stress for women in chronic pain. *Journal of Consulting and Clinical Psychology, 73,* 212–220.

Zautra, A. J., Potter, P. T., & Reich, J. W. (1997). The independence of affects is context-dependent: An integrative model of the relationship between positive and negative affect.

Annual Review of Gerontology and Geriatrics, 17, 75–103.

Zautra, A. J., Reich, J. W., Davis, M. C., Potter, P. T., & Nicolson, N. A. (2000). The role of stressful events in the relationship between positive and negative affects: Evidence from field and experimental studies. *Journal of Personality, 68,* 927–951.

Zautra, A. J., Reich, J. W., & Guarnaccia, C. A. (1990). Some everyday life consequences of disability and bereavement for older adults.

Journal of Personality and Social Psychology, 59, 550–561.

Zautra, A. J., Smith, B., Affleck, G., & Tennen, H. (2001). Examinations of chronic pain and affect relationships: Applications of a dynamic model of affect. *Journal of Consulting and Clinical Psychology, 69,* 786–795.

Zeiss, R. A., & Dickman, H. R. (1989). PTSD 40 years later: Incidence and person–situation correlates in former POWs. *Journal of Clinical Psychology, 45,* 80–87.

21

Boosting Happiness, Buttressing Resilience
Results from Cognitive and Behavioral Interventions

Sonja Lyubomirsky
Matthew D. Della Porta

The experience of frequent positive emotions—such feelings as joy, contentment, serenity, interest, vitality, and pride—is the hallmark of happiness (Diener, Sandvik, & Pavot, 1991; Urry et al., 2004). Positive emotions are also advantageous during the process of recovery from negative experiences (Fredrickson, 2001; Fredrickson & Cohn, 2007). This chapter examines research on boosting happiness and its implications for resilience. We first describe obstacles to increasing long-term well-being and present a sustainable model of happiness (Lyubomirsky, Sheldon, & Schkade, 2005) that attempts to circumvent those obstacles. Next, we describe several randomized controlled interventions that have tested predictions from this model. Finally, we examine the relation between happiness, positive emotions, and resilience, and consider what can be learned from happiness interventions to inform efforts to increase resilience.

Before continuing, the issue of terminology must be addressed. Frequent positive affect, high life satisfaction, and infrequent negative affect all comprise *subjective well-being* (Diener, Suh, Lucas, & Smith, 1999), the more formal label for the colloquial term *happiness* (Sheldon & Lyubomirsky, 2004). Thus, the terms *well-being* and *happiness* are used interchangeably throughout this chapter.

Can Happiness Be Lastingly Increased?

The pursuit and attainment of happiness is of great interest to millions of people. One need only browse the "self-help" shelves at the nearest bookstore to behold dozens of books advising the best way to obtain a happier life. However, the vast majority of these books are based on little or no scientific theory and rarely offer empirical evidence to support their claims (Bergsma, 2008; Norcross et al., 2000). Despite the lack of scientific data to validate the contentions of much of the trade literature, happiness is pursued vigorously in not only the United States and Western nations but also across the globe (Diener, Suh, Smith, & Shao, 1995; Freedman, 1978; Triandis, Bontempo, Leung, & Hui, 1990).

If most people desire to be happier, it is instructive to ask whether being happy is truly beneficial. Researchers have determined that the answer is "yes." For example, a meta-analysis examined 225 cross-sectional, longitudinal, and experimental studies that relate happiness to success in multiple life domains (Lyubomirsky, King, & Diener, 2005). This review found happiness to be associated with relatively stronger social relationships (e.g., Berry & Hansen, 1996; Harker & Keltner, 2001; Marks & Fleming, 1999; Okun, Stock, Haring, & Witter, 1984); superior work outcomes (e.g., Estrada, Isen, & Young, 1994; George, 1995; Staw, Sutton, & Pelled, 1994); and more activity, energy, and flow (e.g., Csikszentmihalyi & Wong, 1991; Mishra, 1992; Watson, Clark, McIntyre, & Hamaker, 1992). In addition, relative to their less happy peers, happy people have been found to be less likely to display symptoms of psychopathology (e.g., Diener & Seligman, 2002; Koivumaa-Honkanen et al., 2001) and more likely to show good coping abilities (e.g., Aspinwall, 1998; Bonanno & Keltner, 1997; Carver et al., 1993; Chen et al., 1996; Fredrickson & Joiner, 2002), to act cooperatively and prosocially (e.g., Cunningham, Shaffer, Barbee, Wolff, & Kelley, 1990; Isen, 1970; Williams & Shiaw, 1999), to have bolstered immune systems (e.g., Dillon, Minchoff, & Baker, 1985; Stone et al., 1994), and even to live longer (e.g., Danner, Snowdon, & Friesen, 2001; Maruta, Colligan, Malinchoc, & Offord, 2000; Ostir, Markides, Black, & Goodwin, 2000).

These results persuasively suggest that increasing happiness is a worthwhile scientific goal—because being happy not only feels good but it is also associated with (and often precedes) successful outcomes in life. However, until recently, the feasibility of sustained shifts in individuals' happiness had not been tested empirically. The neglect of this research question is likely due to three historical sources of pessimism regarding sustainable changes in happiness: the existence of a genetically determined happiness "set point," the long-term stability of personality, and the construct of hedonic adaptation (Lyubomirsky, Sheldon, & Schkade, 2005).

The notion of a genetically determined set point for happiness has been supported by a number of twin and adoption studies (e.g., Lykken & Tellegen, 1996; Tellegen et al., 1988). This research indicates that the heritability of well-being is approximately 50% (Braungart, Plomin, DeFries, & Fulker, 1992; see also Hamer, 1996; Williams & Thompson, 1993). Consistent with this finding, Suh, Diener, and Fujita (1996) found that following increases (or even decreases) in their well-being, people tend to return to their baseline levels of happiness over time. This research literature suggests that although well-being can change temporarily, people eventually return to their genetically determined happiness baseline.

The long-term stability of personality traits also presumably highlights the futility in pursuing sustainable increases in well-being. In a longitudinal study, stable individual differences were found to be more accurate predictors of well-being than life circumstances (Costa, McCrae, & Zonderman, 1987). Also, McCrae and Costa (1990) and others have shown that extraversion and neuroticism are strongly correlated with well-being. Thus, levels of well-being should remain relatively constant throughout life because of this strong link to stable personality traits (Diener & Lucas, 1999).

Finally, perhaps the biggest obstacle to increasing chronic happiness is *hedonic adaptation* (Lyubomirsky, 2009)—that is, the gradual process of diminishing emotional responses to positive or negative stimuli over time (Frederick & Loewenstein, 1999; see also Wilson & Gilbert, 2008). Although hedonic adaptation to negative events is welcome and adaptive, studies show that such adaptation is often slow or incomplete. For example, longitudinal studies demonstrate that people typically do *not* return to their baseline levels of well-being after negative life events, such as a disability (Lucas, 2007), unemployment (Lucas, Clark, Georgellis, & Diener, 2004), divorce (Lucas, 2005), and widowhood (Lucas, Clark, Georgellis, & Diener, 2003). By contrast, people adapt relatively quickly and completely to *positive* experiences (Lyubomirsky, 2009). For example, hedonic adaptation appears to be complete to positive life events, such as marriage (Lucas et al., 2003; see also Lucas & Clark, 2006) or a voluntary job change (Boswell, Boudreau, & Tichy, 2005). These findings suggest that people cannot become lastingly happier because they may not fully adapt to negative life events and will adapt all too fully to *positive* life events. However, as we see later in the chapter, it is important to note that the rate with which a person adapts to a positive or negative experience can be at least partially controlled through conscious intentional activity (Lyubomirsky, 2009).

In summary, several lines of theory and research serve to underscore the difficulty—if not impossibility—of lastingly enhancing well-being. Despite these formidable causes for concern, Lyubomirsky and her colleagues proposed a model specifying how sustainable change in happiness can be achieved (Lyubomirsky, 2008; Lyubomirsky, Sheldon, & Schkade, 2005).

A Model of Sustainable Happiness Change

Given the aforementioned sources of pessimism, how can an individual increase his or her baseline level of happiness for a sustained period of time? To begin, Lyubomirsky, Sheldon, and Schkade (2005) concede the conclusions of previous studies and integrate research on well-being into a single conceptual model. Specifically, they propose that a person's chronic happiness level is determined by three factors: a genetically based happiness set point (accounting for approximately 50% of the individual differences in

chronic happiness), life circumstances that affect happiness (10%), and intentional activities and practices (the remaining 40%). To be sure, the percentages of variance are averages of estimates from previous studies, and these three factors undoubtedly interact with one another.

The genetically determined set point for happiness (Lykken & Tellegen, 1996; Tellegen et al., 1988) is perhaps best indicated by an average of several self-reported well-being scores assessed over time (Lykken, 1999) and can be thought of as a point that can move within a "set range" for happiness (Sheldon & Lyubomirsky, 2004). For example, individuals may get promoted (or demoted) at work and experience a boost (or decline) in happiness. However, they eventually revert to their set point (Headey & Wearing, 1989). Due to its fixed nature, the set point is likely to be immune to influence or control. This lack of long-term malleability makes the happiness set point an unlikely and unproductive avenue by which to increase chronic happiness (Lyubomirsky, Sheldon, & Schkade, 2005).

In addition to the set point, a person's life circumstances also impact chronic happiness. Life circumstances are the stable "facts" of a person's life. These include life status conditions (e.g., health, location of residence, material possessions) and various demographic details, such as income, ethnicity, and religious affiliation. What is wrong with trying to attain ideal life circumstances as a prime strategy for increasing happiness? First, life circumstances are typically stable and are therefore vulnerable to the emotionally desensitizing effects of hedonic adaptation (Lyubomirsky, 2009; Sheldon & Lyubomirsky, 2004, 2006a). For example, Sheldon and Lyubomirsky (2006a) found that positive circumstantial changes (e.g., receiving an unexpected scholarship or initiation into a fraternity) were associated with only a temporary boost in well-being. Second, attempting to produce changes in life circumstances can consume time, energy, or resources that a person may not have and, in some cases (e.g., a real estate down-turn when one desires to move) is practically impossible. In sum, changing one's circumstances to increase happiness is not likely to be fruitful.

In contrast to the inadequacy of seeking happiness by changing one's set point or life situation, *intentional activities* appear to offer the best potential for lastingly increasing well-being. As described above, intentional activities and practices can account for as much as 40% of the individual differences in happiness. The scope of these activities and practices is very broad (Sheldon & Lyubomirsky, 2004) and can be cognitive (e.g., having an optimistic attitude; King, 2001; Lyubomirsky, Dickerhoof, Boehm, & Sheldon, 2008; Sheldon & Lyubomirsky, 2006b), behavioral (e.g., writing or sharing a letter of gratitude once a week; e.g., Lyubomirsky, Sheldon, & Schkade, 2005), or motivational (e.g., developing and pursuing life goals; Sheldon & Houser-Marko, 2001). These intentional activities allow people to *act* on their circumstances—through their thoughts, plans, and behaviors—rather than simply reacting to circumstances that are often uncontrollable. Engaging in particular intentional activities is the most effective method of boosting chronic happiness because such activities impede the process of hedonic adaptation (Lyubomirsky, 2009; Lyubomirsky, Sheldon, & Schkade, 2005). Intentional practices are relatively dynamic and episodic, which means that the nature of the activity or the process through which they are completed is varied. By definition, it is difficult to adapt to a context or stimulus that is continually changing. Hence, one is less likely to adapt to and eventually take for granted one's intentional activities than one's static circumstances.

Variation in how intentional activities are implemented can unfold in several ways. For example, activities can be kept fresh and interesting through optimal frequency or timing, such as counting one's blessings once a week as opposed to three times a week (Lyubomirsky, Sheldon, & Schkade, 2005). *Changing*

the activities—such as practicing different acts of kindness rather than the same acts week after week (Boehm, Lyubomirsky, & Sheldon, 2009)—can also prevent tedium and produce long-term increases in well-being (Sheldon & Lyubomirsky, 2006a). Furthermore, novel and unexpected activities can yield new experiences that are relatively more salient to an individual and that create lasting recollections (Wilson & Gilbert, 2008). Finally, all of these factors—timing, variety, and surprise—serve to entice attention to the activity, and, as Lyubomirsky (2009) argues, adaptation is less likely when an individual is able to maintain sustained awareness of the activity.

As mentioned earlier, our model of sustainable happiness has been tested in a number of randomized controlled interventions. The results of these interventions provide insight into the causal mechanisms through which intentional practices produce increases in sustainable happiness and forestall hedonic adaptation, and can serve as models for developing ways to enhance resilience in the face of stress or trauma.

Randomized Controlled Interventions

Committing Acts of Kindness

To test the efficacy of implementing a happiness-enhancing strategy, as well as the importance of timing (or frequency), our laboratory conducted a randomized controlled intervention in which participants were instructed to practice random acts of kindness for a period of 6 weeks (Lyubomirsky, Sheldon, & Schkade, 2005). Each week, students performed five acts of kindness, either all in one day or spread over the week. Short-term increases in happiness were found, but only for participants who practiced all five acts of kindness in a single day. This finding supports the idea that timing is critical. In this instance, committing kind acts throughout the week (as opposed to all in one day) may have diminished the salience of each act, perhaps making it less distinguishable from other kind acts the student typically performed. In another kindness study, participants who simply counted their acts of kindness over the course of a week reported relatively higher levels of subjective happiness compared to a control group (Otake, Shimai, Tanaka-Matsumi, Otsui, & Fredrickson, 2006).

Another intervention conducted by our laboratory required students to practice acts of kindness for 10 weeks (Boehm et al., 2009). Participants performed kind acts either three times or nine times each week, and either repeated essentially the same act weekly or varied it. By contrast, a control group simply listed events of the past week. Surprisingly, the results indicated that the frequency of performing kind acts did not affect well-being. However, students who varied their kind acts showed an increase in happiness immediately after the intervention and up to 1 month later. Participants who were not given the opportunity to change their kind acts actually reported lower happiness midway through the intervention but eventually returned to their baseline level at the follow-up assessment. In summary, the kindness interventions conducted to date illustrate that happiness can be amplified by intentional activity, and that both timing and variety moderate the effectiveness of practicing a happiness-enhancing strategy.

Expressing Gratitude and Optimism

In another randomized controlled intervention from our laboratory we instructed participants to express gratitude regularly (Lyubomirsky, Sheldon, & Schkade, 2005). We adapted the methodology of Emmons and McCullough (2003), who found promising evidence for the efficacy of this intervention, suggesting that grateful thinking promotes the savoring of positive events; however, they did not measure pre- and postintervention levels of well-being. In another relevant study, Seligman, Steen, Park, and Peterson (2005) found that writing and sharing a gratitude letter produced an increase in hap-

piness up to 1 month after the intervention. In our 6-week intervention, experimental participants listed in a "gratitude journal" up to five things for which they were grateful, either once a week or three times a week, whereas control participants simply completed the happiness assessments. Participants reported an increase in well-being only if they "counted their blessings" once a week. Once again, this finding supports the notion that the frequency of a happiness-increasing activity is crucial. In this instance, students who were instructed to write in their gratitude journal three times a week may have found the activity to be less fresh and meaningful (and more chore-like) over time than did those who only expressed gratitude once a week (Lyubomirsky, Sheldon, & Schkade, 2005).

In another intervention from our laboratory we tested the moderating effect of *motivation* by allowing participants to choose between one of two experiments. Those who opted to enroll in an experiment described as being designed to boost happiness comprised the "motivated" group, and those who opted into an experiment described as involving "cognitive exercises" served as the "nonmotivated group" (Lyubomirsky, Dickerhoof, Boehm, & Sheldon, 2008; Study 1). All students were then asked to express gratitude (by writing gratitude letters), to express optimism (by writing in a journal about the future accomplishment of their life goals and dreams; Markus & Nurius, 1986), or to complete a comparison control activity once a week over 8 weeks.

Participants who were apparently motivated to become happier, regardless of the intervention activity, had higher levels of well-being at the end of the study compared with participants who were not so motivated. In addition, the highest well-being benefits of our intervention accrued to those students who had a high degree of "fit" with their assigned activity (i.e., those who found the activity enjoyable and natural to perform), who exerted more effort in the activity during the 8-week intervention period, and who continued to practice the activity after the intervention period was finished. Finally, the gratitude and optimism interventions led people to have more positive thoughts and experiences, which in turn increased happiness (Lyubomirsky et al., 2008). These findings demonstrate the importance of four variables that moderate the effectiveness of practicing particular activities—namely, motivation to become happier, fit with the happiness-enhancing activity, effort in completing the activity, and continued practice of the activity, as well as the significance of one mediator (positive thoughts and events).

A follow-up study sought to test whether the effects of happiness-increasing practices, and the mechanisms that underlie them, generalize across cultures. Using an experimental design nearly identical to that used in the study described above, we found that, relative to a control group, both Anglo Americans and Asian Americans who practiced gratitude or optimism for 6 weeks reported significant increases in well-being immediately after the intervention had ended and up to 1 month later, but Anglo Americans put more effort into the intervention and benefited from it more (Lyubomirsky et al., 2008; Study 2). However, during the actual intervention, Asian Americans showed larger increases in sense of connectedness and feelings of gratitude than did Anglo Americans, and were later more likely to continue to engage in the exercises. These findings highlight intriguing cultural differences in the effectiveness of happiness-enhancing activities, which may be accounted for by differences in "independent" versus "interdependent selves" found in Anglo versus certain Asian cultures (Markus & Kitayama, 1991). However, some processes appear to be shared across cultures. For example, we found that increases in happiness in *all* our participants were mediated by increases in gratitude, optimism, relatedness, autonomy, and the experience of positive events.

Finally, Sheldon and Lyubomirsky (2006b) conducted a 4-week intervention that included an optimism condition (e.g., visualizing and writing about one's best possible selves), a gratitude condition (e.g., counting one's blessings), and a control condition (outlining the typical events of one's day). Corroborating previous findings that visualizing one's best possible selves is associated with increased optimism and higher levels of well-being (King, 2001), significant increases in positive affect were found for participants who practiced optimism (but, interestingly, not for those who practiced gratitude). Notably, however, *self-concordant motivation* (i.e., identification with the activity and interest in continued practice; Sheldon & Elliot, 1999) had a moderating effect on the effectiveness of this intervention. This study provides further support for the efficacy of practicing optimism and reveals the moderating effect of self-concordant motivation.

Taken together, these four gratitude and optimism interventions highlight the importance of moderating and mediating variables that underlie the efficacy of intentional activities to improve happiness.

Processing Unhappy and Happy Life Experiences

A series of studies from our lab tested which ways of processing unhappy and happy life experiences serve to enhance well-being (Lyubomirsky, Sousa, & Dickerhoof, 2006). In Study 1, students were instructed to write, talk, or think privately about their worst life experience for 15 minutes on 3 consecutive days. Students who wrote or talked about a negative past experience reported higher levels of well-being and physical health compared to students who thought privately about the experience. This pattern was also found 4 weeks later.

These results have interesting implications for the best way to cope with a negative event. The process of writing or talking about a traumatic event requires that words be organized into a coherent story. This inherent structure-making function of writing or talking about a trauma may have allowed students to make sense of the experience and "let go" of the negativity surrounding it (Pennebaker, 1993; Pennebaker & Francis, 1996). In contrast, thinking about a traumatic event tends to be relatively more image-based and chaotic, and does not lend itself as easily to organization and structure. Indeed, focusing repetitively on negative cognitions can lead individuals to reexperience and ruminate about negative experiences (for reviews, see Nolen-Hoeksema, 1991; Nolen-Hoeksema, Wisco, & Lyubomirsky, 2008).

In Study 2, students were instructed to write, talk, or think privately about their *happiest* life event. In a result that was essentially the converse of that in Study 1, participants who thought privately about their happiest experience reported a greater increase in life satisfaction than did those who wrote or talked about such an experience. Finally, to examine the mechanisms underlying these differing patterns of results, in Study 3 we instructed students to analyze (i.e., make sense of and try to understand) or replay (i.e., reexperience) their happiest life event while writing or thinking about it. Results indicated that participants who thought about and replayed their happiest life experience—without systematically trying to figure out why it happened—reported the highest well-being over time compared with participants who wrote about and analyzed such an event (who reported the lowest well-being). In summary, this research suggests that seeking systematically to understand one's negative life events is beneficial to happiness. In contrast, when it comes to positive life events, savoring and reexperiencing them (*without* analysis) is more adaptive (cf. Wilson & Gilbert, 2003).

Enhancing Psychological Resilience

The studies we have described thus far all tested the efficacy of the practice of happiness-enhancing strategies by individuals who, on average, were psychologically healthy and not facing severe stressors. How-

ever, the use of happiness-enhancing strategies is potentially valuable not just for normal, well-adjusted individuals but also for those suffering from both subclinical symptoms and clinical disorders, including both reactive and chronic depression and anxiety (Lyubomirsky & Dickerhoof, in press).

An important framework related to positive behavioral activities involves the enhancement of psychological resilience. Defined as the ability to recover from negative emotional experiences (J. H. Block & Block, 1980; Block & Kremen, 1996; Lazarus, 1993), *resilience* involves a process by which a person experiences positive emotion in the face of adverse circumstances (Carver, 1998; Tugade & Fredrickson, 2004).

The process of resilience generally unfolds in response to the experience of *stress*, which occurs when a circumstance or event is "appraised by the person as relevant to his or her well-being and in which the person's resources are taxed or exceeded" (Folkman & Lazarus, 1985, p. 152). In the event of a stressful experience, resilience is the mechanism that allows a person to cope with and recover from the harmful effects of negative emotional appraisals that often accompany stress. This is accomplished primarily by managing negative emotion and by mustering behavioral reactions to improve the stressful circumstance (Folkman & Lazarus, 1980). Thus, resilience helps people to cope with stressful life events and to take proactive behavioral actions to ensure more positive emotional appraisals of the events (Folkman & Lazarus, 1985).

Resilient individuals have also been found to build supportive social networks that facilitate coping (Demos, 1989; Kumpfer, 1999) and to show faster cardiovascular recovery after negative events (Tugade, Fredrickson, & Barrett, 2004). In summary, research indicates that resilience is a desirable psychological characteristic. Thus, an important question concerns whether an individual can purposefully enhance his or her level of resilience through the use of happiness-enhancing strategies. Prior work has suggested that increases in well-being can facilitate coping with future negative experiences (Reich & Zautra, 1981). This, and evidence from several other empirical studies, suggests that the answer to whether resilience can be bolstered is "yes."

Previous research using happiness-enhancing strategies with a clinical population has shown that the use of several mood-boosting "exercises" helped to alleviate symptoms of depression (Seligman et al., 2005; Seligman, Rashid, & Parks, 2006), and the expression of gratitude and optimism among healthy students led to a reduction of depressive symptomatology for up to 6 months after the intervention ended (Lyubomirsky et al., 2008). Indeed, in comparison to the maladaptive strategies (e.g., rumination) typically used by depressed and dysphoric people to cope with negative events, these positive activities can serve as relatively more effective alternative coping strategies (Lyubomirsky & Dickerhoof, in press).

Why do we expect that happiness interventions can be successfully applied to individuals facing severe stressors, traumas, or clinical disorders? The critical mechanism involves *positive emotions*—that is, feelings of joy, pride, curiosity, peacefulness, vigor, or affection—that are generated from continued practice of intentional happiness-boosting strategies. Notably, although the studies described above offer persuasive evidence that particular activities increase happiness, their results also reveal *how* and *why* such increases arise. For example, in one study, we found that one reason committing acts of kindness for others led to increases in happiness is that the actors perceived gratitude in the recipients of their kind act (Boehm et al., 2009). In two other studies, described above, individuals who practiced either gratitude or optimism reported more positive daily experiences (Lyubomirsky et al., 2008; Studies 1 and 2), and increased feelings of connectedness, gratitude, autono-

my, and optimism (Study 2), leading them to become happier. In all cases, a positive shift in how people perceived themselves and the world around them mediated the relationship between the practice of happiness-increasing intentional activities and reported increases in well-being (Lyubomirsky & Dickerhoof, in press).

These mediating factors—more positive construals, more positive experiences, and more positive emotions—are critical to understanding how and why happiness interventions can be effective in the wake of negative events and in clinical contexts. The key mechanism, as Fredrickson and Levenson (1998) have argued, is that positive emotions can "undo" the harmful effects of negative emotions. For example, participants induced to experience positive emotions—namely, joy and contentment—show increased cardiovascular recovery after an anxiety-inducing stimulus (Fredrickson, Mancuso, Branigan, & Tugade, 2000). In addition, positive emotions have been found to aid in coping with stress (Ong, Bergeman, Bisconti, & Wallace, 2006; for a review, see Folkman & Moskowitz, 2000) and bereavement (Bonanno & Keltner, 1997). Recent data from our laboratory extended this finding to depression (Dickerhoof, 2006). Those who were instructed to practice gratitude or optimism reported experiencing more frequent positive emotions, such as contentment and pleasure, for as long as 3 months after our intervention had ended. Notably, those very positive emotions in turn led the same individuals to show reduced depressive symptoms as long as 6 months after the study.

These studies highlight ways that happiness interventions—mostly through their impact on positive emotions, positive thoughts, and positive events—can help people build resilience in the face of adversity and bounce back from negative experiences. This process can occur via three mechanisms. First, emotions such as joy, satisfaction, and interest, marshaled by positive interventions provide individuals with a sort of "psychological time-out" in the face of stress and help them perceive the "big picture" of their situations. Hence, a negative or even traumatic circumstance can become less overwhelming and less impactful on all life domains.

Second, happiness activities can counteract negative, dysfunctional thoughts and, instead, bolster positive thinking. For example, hopeful expectations produced by the optimism strategy can replace thoughts of hopelessness and powerlessness. As mentioned above, two studies from our laboratory showed that those who actively and regularly practiced either gratitude or optimism over a 6- to 8-week period came to regard their routine experiences in more positive ways (e.g., finding everyday events—meeting a friend, commuting to work, cooking dinner—more satisfying; Lyubomirsky et al., 2008; Study 1) and to report more grateful, optimistic, autonomous, and relationship-enhancing thoughts (Study 2). These more positive thoughts and interpretations in turn triggered improvements in well-being.

Finally, happiness activities often bring about positive experiences. For example, practicing acts of kindness produces moments in which people feel efficacious and appreciated, and can even generate new friendships. Consistent with this notion, we found that people who expressed optimism or gratitude reported experiencing more positive events that linger with them, and that these experiences mediated increases in their happiness (Lyubomirsky et al., 2008; Study 2). Nonetheless, it is important to note that people who face stressors would do well not only to increase positive emotions but also to decrease negative emotions through a variety of empirically verified techniques, including cognitive-behavioral therapy (Beck, Rush, Shaw, & Emery, 1987; Hollon, Haman, & Brown, 2002), mindfulness-based stress reduction (Kabat-Zinn, 1990), and, when appropriate, psychopharmacological treatment (Klein, Gittelman-Klein, Quitkin, & Rifkin, 1980). In summary, happiness-enhancing intentional activities produce positive emotions that can counteract the effects of negative emotions, as well as generate positive thoughts and positive experiences. Through these processes, we argue that such activities are likely to be effective in enhancing psychological resilience.

Future Directions and Conclusions

Much remains to be learned about the efficacy, implementation, and mechanisms underlying happiness-enhancing strategies. First, long-term follow-up is required to determine whether the effects of activities such as expressing gratitude or optimism remain beyond 6 to 9 months after the intervention (Lyubomirsky et al., 2008; Seligman et al., 2005). Because our laboratory is interested specifically in how and why people can enhance and maintain happiness (and, hence, resilience) for the *long term*, we need to test the effects of various happiness-enhancing strategies over extended periods of time. Second, further research is needed on the effects of happiness interventions on not only long-term negative states and syndromes (e.g., depression) but also daily stressful experiences related to short-term psychological hardship. Third, the consequences of practicing happiness-boosting activities are yet to be associated with all of the benefits related to happiness itself (Lyubomirsky, Sheldon, & Schkade, 2005). Although we have already begun to address this issue in our laboratory (e.g., Boehm et al., 2009), more investigation is required to identify the spillover advantages of practicing happiness interventions (e.g., with respect to improved relationships, enhanced optimism and self-esteem, increased income and work productivity, or bolstered immune function) beyond a boost in well-being. Of course, many of these "fringe benefits" of increased happiness can also serve as bona fide mechanisms that underlie and impact resilience.

Finally, it will be crucial to advance our knowledge of *how* and *why* positive interventions are effective. As one example, the benefits of such interventions may be moderated by a person's actual or perceived effort toward them (Zautra & Reich, 1980), as well as by a person's motivation to improve and by degree of "fit" with the type of intervention (Sheldon & Elliot, 1999); indeed, preliminary evidence from our laboratory supports these suggestions (Lyubomirsky et al., 2008). Interventions that enhance efficacy (Blazer, 2002) are also likely to be associated with increased well-being and resilience. Our laboratory is currently conducting a set of studies that is testing a number of moderators underlying strategy effectiveness. This research aims to answer several questions: Does belief in the importance of being happy, and the degree to which one desires to pursue happiness, matter when one practices a happiness activity (Lyubomirsky, 2000)? Does social support (e.g., having a reassuring and helpful friend or family member) bolster the benefit of a happiness activity? Does one's unique personality trait profile moderate the effectiveness of practicing a happiness activity? Does the ability to slowly and reflectively solve problems or make decisions impact the practice of a happiness activity (Frederick, 2005)? Can placebo effects explain the activity's benefits? And, finally, does one's initial level of depression matter when one practices a happiness activity?

In addition to the strategies mentioned above, numerous alternative happiness-boosting techniques can be further tested and implemented independently or in conjunction with traditional happiness interventions. As a case in point, environmental interventions—for example, those involving using pleasant artificial scents, cheerful music, or warm white lighting—have been shown to increase positive affect and efficiency in task performance (Baron, 1990), creativity (Adaman & Blaney, 1995), and collaborative conflict resolution (Baron, Rea, & Daniels, 1992; Study 2), respectively. Indeed, combining environmental manipulations or other techniques that boost well-being with cognitive and behavioral interventions might produce synergistic or multiplicative effects on happiness and other positive outcomes.

Positive emotions are essential not only for producing durable happiness, but also for bolstering coping and resilience in the face of adversity. However, little current empirical research bears directly on this notion. As highlighted above, future studies should explore the extent to which happiness interventions can increase resilience by producing positive emotions, positive construals, and positive experiences. It is our hope that the results of future studies will further elucidate the complexity of positive intentional activities and provide insight into how these interventions can help to enhance happiness and psychological resilience in healthy, stressed, and clinical populations.

References

Adaman, J. E., & Blaney, P. H. (1995). The effects of musical mood induction on creativity. *Journal of Creative Behavior, 29*, 95–108.

Aspinwall, L. G. (1998). Rethinking the role of positive affect in self-regulation. *Motivation and Emotion, 22*, 1–32.

Baron, R. A. (1990). Environmentally induced positive affect: Its impact on self-efficacy, task performance, negotiation, and conflict. *Journal of Applied Social Psychology, 20*, 368–384.

Baron, R. A., Rea, M. S., & Daniels, S. G. (1992). Effects of indoor lighting (illuminance and spectral distribution) on the performance of cognitive tasks and interpersonal behaviors: The potential mediating role of positive affect. *Motivation and Emotion, 16*, 1–33.

Beck, A. T., Rush, A. J., Shaw, B. F., & Emery, G. (1987). *Cognitive therapy of depression*. New York: Guilford Press.

Bergsma, A. (2008). Do self-help books help? *Journal of Happiness Studies, 9*, 341–360.

Berry, D. S., & Hansen, J. S. (1996). Positive affect, negative affect, and social interaction. *Journal of Personality and Social Psychology, 71*, 796–809.

Blazer, D. G. (2002). Self-efficacy and depression in late life: A primary prevention proposal. *Aging and Mental Health, 6,* 315–324.

Block, J., & Kremen, A. M. (1996). IQ and ego-resiliency: Conceptual and empirical connections and separateness. *Journal of Personality and Social Psychology, 70,* 349–361.

Block, J. H., & Block, J. (1980). The role of ego-control and ego-resiliency in the origination of behavior. In W. A. Collings (Ed.), *The Minnesota Symposia on Child Psychology* (Vol. 13, pp. 39–101). Hillsdale, NJ: Erlbaum.

Boehm, J. K., Lyubomirsky, S., & Sheldon, K. M. (2009). *Spicing up kindness: The role of variety in the effects of practicing kindness on improvements in mood, happiness, and self-evaluations.* Manuscript in preparation.

Bonanno, G. A., & Keltner, D. (1997). Facial expressions of emotion and the course of conjugal bereavement. *Journal of Abnormal Psychology, 106,* 126–137.

Boswell, W. R., Boudreau, J. W., & Tichy, J. (2005). The relationship between employee job change and job satisfaction: The honeymoon-hangover effect. *Journal of Applied Psychology, 90,* 882–892.

Braungart, J. M., Plomin, R., DeFries, J. C., & Fulker, D. W. (1992). Genetic influence on tester rated infant temperament as assessed by Bayley's Infant Behavior Record: Nonadoptive and adoptive siblings and twins. *Developmental Psychology, 28,* 40–47.

Carver, C. S. (1998). Resilience and thriving: Issues, models and linkages. *Journal of Social Issues, 54,* 245–266.

Carver, C. S., Pozo, C., Harris, S. D., Noriega, V., Scheier, M., Robinson, D., et al. (1993). How coping mediates the effect of optimism on distress: A study of women with early stage breast cancer. *Journal of Personality and Social Psychology, 65,* 375–390.

Chen, C. C., David, A., Thompson, K., Smith, C., Lea, S., & Fahy, T. (1996). Coping strategies and psychiatric morbidity in women attending breast assessment clinics. *Journal of Psychosomatic Research, 40,* 265–270.

Costa, P. T., McCrae, R. R., & Zonderman, A. B. (1987). Environmental and dispositional influences on well-being: Longitudinal follow-up of an American national sample. *British Journal of Psychology, 78,* 299–306.

Csikszentmihalyi, M., & Wong, M. M. (1991). The situational and personal correlates of happiness: A cross-national comparison. In F. Strack, M. Argyle, & N. Schwarz (Eds.), *Subjective well-being: An interdisciplinary perspective* (pp. 193–212). Elmsford, NY: Pergamon Press.

Cunningham, M. R., Shaffer, D. R., Barbee, A. P., Wolff, P. L., & Kelley, D. J. (1990). Separate processes in the relation of elation and depression to helping: Social versus personal concerns. *Journal of Experimental Social Psychology, 26,* 13–33.

Danner, D. D., Snowdon, D. A., & Friesen, W. V. (2001). Positive emotions in early life and longevity: Findings from the nun study. *Journal of Personality and Social Psychology, 80,* 804–813.

Demos, E. V. (1989). Resiliency in infancy. In T. F. Dugan & R. Cole (Eds.), *The child of our times: Studies in the development of resiliency* (pp. 3–22). Philadelphia: Brunner/Mazel.

Dickerhoof, R. (2007). Expressing optimism and gratitude: A longitudinal investigation of cognitive strategies to increase well-being (Doctoral dissertation, University of California, Riverside). *Dissertation Abstracts International, 68,* 4174.

Diener, E., & Lucas, R. E. (1999). Personality and subjective well-being. In D. Kahneman, E. Diener, & N. Schwartz (Eds.), *Well-being: The foundations of hedonic psychology* (pp. 213–229). New York: Russell Sage Foundation.

Diener, E., Sandvik, E., & Pavot, W. (1991). Happiness is the frequency, not the intensity, of positive versus negative affect. In F. Strack, M. Argyle, & N. Schwarz (Eds.), *Subjective well-being: An interdisciplinary perspective* (pp. 119–139). Elmsford, NY: Pergamon Press.

Diener, E., & Seligman, M. E. P. (2002). Very happy people. *Psychological Science, 13,* 81–84.

Diener, E., Suh, E. M., Lucas, R. E., & Smith, H. L. (1999). Subjective well-being: Three decades of progress. *Psychological Bulletin, 125,* 276–302.

Diener, E., Suh, E. M., Smith, H., & Shao, L. (1995). National differences in reported subjective well-being: Why do they occur? *Social Indicators Research, 34,* 7–32.

Dillon, K. M., Minchoff, B., & Baker, K. H. (1985). Positive emotional states and enhancement of the immune system. *International Journal of Psychiatry in Medicine, 15*, 13–18.

Emmons, R. A., & McCullough, M. E. (2003). Counting blessings versus burdens: An experimental investigation of gratitude and subjective well-being in daily life. *Journal of Personality and Social Psychology, 84*, 377–389.

Estrada, C., Isen, A. M., & Young, M. J. (1994). Positive affect influences creative problem solving and reported source of practice satisfaction in physicians. *Motivation and Emotion, 18*, 285–299.

Folkman, S., & Lazarus, R. S. (1980). An analysis of coping in a middle-aged community sample. *Journal of Health and Social Behavior, 21*, 219–239.

Folkman, S., & Lazarus, R. S. (1985). If it changes it must be a process: Study of emotion and coping during three stages of a college examination. *Journal of Personality and Social Psychology, 48*, 150–170.

Folkman, S., & Moskowitz, J. T. (2000). Positive affect and the other side of coping. *American Psychologist, 55*, 647–654.

Frederick, S. (2005). Cognitive reflection and decision making. *Journal of Economics Perspectives, 19*, 25–42.

Frederick, S., & Loewenstein, G. (1999). Hedonic adaptation. In D. Kahneman, E. Diener, & N. Schwarz (Eds.), *Well-being: The foundations of hedonic psychology* (pp. 302–329). New York: Russell Sage Foundation.

Fredrickson, B. L. (2001). The role of positive emotions in positive psychology: The broaden-and-build theory of positive emotions. *American Psychologist, 56*, 218–226.

Fredrickson, B. L., & Cohn, M. A. (2007). Positive emotions. In M. Lewis, J. M. Haviland-Jones, & L. F. Barrett (Eds.), *Handbook of emotions* (3rd ed.). New York: Guilford Press.

Fredrickson, B. L., & Joiner, T. (2002). Positive emotions trigger upward spirals toward emotional well-being. *Psychological Science, 13*, 172– 175.

Fredrickson, B. L., & Levenson, R. W. (1998). Positive emotions speed recovery from the cardiovascular sequelae of negative emotions. *Cognition and Emotion, 12*, 191–220.

Fredrickson, B. L., Mancuso, R. A., Branigan, C., & Tugade, M. M. (2000). The undoing effect of positive emotions. *Motivation and Emotion, 24*, 237–258.

Freedman, J. (1978). *Happy people: What happiness is, who has it, and why.* New York: Harcourt Brace Jovanovich.

George, J. M. (1995). Leader positive mood and group performance: The case of customer service. *Journal of Applied Social Psychology, 25*, 778–795.

Hamer, D. H. (1996). The heritability of happiness. *Nature Genetics, 14*, 125–126.

Harker, L., & Keltner, D. (2001). Expressions of positive emotions in women's college yearbook pictures and their relationship to personality and life outcomes across adulthood. *Journal of Personality and Social Psychology, 80*, 112–124.

Headey, B., & Wearing, A. (1989). Personality, life events, and subjective well-being: Toward a dynamic equilibrium model. *Journal of Personality and Social Psychology, 57*, 731– 739.

Hollon, S. D., Haman, K. L., & Brown, L. L. (2002). Cognitive-behavioral treatment of depression. In I. H. Gotlib & C. L. Hammen (Eds.), *Handbook of depression* (pp. 383–403). New York: Guilford Press.

Isen, A. M. (1970). Success, failure, attention, and reaction to others: The warm glow of success. *Journal of Personality and Social Psychology, 15*, 294–301.

Kabat-Zinn, J. (1990). *Full catastrophe living: The program of the Stress Reduction Clinic at the University of Massachusetts Medical Center.* New York: Delta.

King, L. A. (2001). The health benefits of writing about life goals. *Personality and Social Psychology Bulletin, 27*, 798–807.

Klein, D. F., Gittelman-Klein, R., Quitkin, F. M., & Rifkin, A. (1980). *Diagnosis and drug treatment of psychiatric disorders.* Baltimore: Williams & Wilkins.

Koivumaa-Honkanen, H., Honkanen, R., Viinamaeki, H., Heikkilae, K., Kaprio, J., & Koskenvuo, M. (2001). Life satisfaction and suicide: A 20-year follow-up study. *American Journal of Psychiatry, 158*, 433–439.

Kumpfer, K. L. (1999). Factors and processes contributing to resilience: The resilience framework. In M. D. Glantz & J. L. Johnson (Eds.), *Resilience and development: Positive life adaptations* (pp. 179–222). New York: Kluwer Academic/Plenum Press.

Lazarus, R. S. (1993). From psychological stress

to the emotions: A history of changing out-looks. *Annual Review of Psychology*, *44*, 1–21.

Lucas, R. E. (2005). Time does not heal all wounds: A longitudinal study of reaction and adaptation to divorce. *Psychological Science*, *16*, 945–950.

Lucas, R. E. (2007). Long-term disability has lasting effects on subjective well-being: Evidence from two nationally representative longitudinal studies. *Journal of Personality and Social Psychology*, *92*, 717–730.

Lucas, R. E., & Clark, A. E. (2006). Do people really adapt to marriage? *Journal of Happiness Studies*, *7*, 405–426.

Lucas, R. E., Clark, A. E., Georgellis, Y., & Diener, E. (2003). Reexamining adaptation and the set point model of happiness: Reactions to changes in marital status. *Journal of Personality and Social Psychology*, *84*, 527–539.

Lucas, R. E., Clark, A. E., Georgellis, Y., & Diener, E. (2004). Unemployment alters the set point for life satisfaction. *Psychological Science*, *15*, 8–13.

Lykken, D. (1999). *Happiness: What studies on twins show us about nature, nurture, and the happiness set-point.* New York: Golden Books.

Lykken, D., & Tellegen, A. (1996). Happiness is a stochastic phenomenon. *Psychological Science*, *7*, 186–189.

Lyubomirsky, S. (2000, October). *In the pursuit of happiness: Comparing the United States and Russia.* Paper presented at the annual meeting of the Society for Experimental Psychology, Atlanta, Georgia.

Lyubomirsky, S. (2008). *The how of happiness: A scientific approach to getting the life you want.* New York: Penguin Press.

Lyubomirsky, S. (2009). Hedonic adaptation to positive and negative experiences. In S. Folkman (Ed.), *Oxford handbook of stress, health, and coping.* New York: Oxford University Press.

Lyubomirsky, S., & Dickerhoof, R. (in press). A construal approach to increasing happiness. In J. P. Tangney & J. E. Maddux (Eds.), *Social psychological foundations of clinical psychology.* New York: Guilford Press.

Lyubomirsky, S., Dickerhoof, R., Boehm, J. K., & Sheldon, K. M. (2008). *Becoming happier takes both a will and a way: Two experimen-tal longitudinal interventions to boost well-being.* Manuscript under review.

Lyubomirsky, S., King, L. A., & Diener, E. (2005). The benefits of frequent positive affect: Does happiness lead to success? *Psychological Bulletin*, *131*, 803–855.

Lyubomirsky, S., Sheldon, K. M., & Schkade, D. (2005). Pursuing happiness: The architecture of sustainable change. *Review of General Psychology*, *9*, 111–131.

Lyubomirsky, S., Sousa, L., & Dickerhoof, R. (2006). The costs and benefits of writing, talking, and thinking about life's triumphs and defeats. *Journal of Personality and Social Psychology*, *90*, 692–708.

Marks, G. N., & Fleming, N. (1999). Influences and consequences of well-being among Australian young people: 1980–1995. *Social Indicators Research*, *46*, 301–323.

Markus, H. R., & Kitayama, S. (1991). Culture and the self: Implications for cognition, emotion, and motivation. *Psychological Review*, *98*, 224–253.

Markus, H. R., & Nurius, P. (1986). Possible selves. *American Psychologist*, *41*, 954–969.

Maruta, T., Colligan, R. C., Malinchoc, M., & Offord, K. P. (2000). Optimists vs. pessimists: Survival rate among medical patients over a 30-year period. *Mayo Clinic Proceedings*, *75*, 140–143.

McCrae, R. R., & Costa, P. T. (1990). *Personality in adulthood.* New York: Guilford Press.

Mishra, S. (1992). Leisure activities and life satisfaction in old age: A case study of retired government employees living in urban areas. *Activities, Adaptation and Aging*, *16*, 7–26.

Nolen-Hoeksema, S. (1991). Responses to depression and their effects on the duration of depressive episodes. *Journal of Abnormal Psychology*, *100*, 569–582.

Nolen-Hoeksema, S., Wisco, B. E., & Lyubomirsky, S. (2008). Rethinking rumination. *Perspectives on Psychological Science*, *3*, 400–424.

Norcross, J. C., Santrock, J. W., Campbell, L. F., Smith, T. P., Sommer, R., & Zuckerman, E. L. (2000). *Authoritative guide to self-help resources in mental health.* New York: Guilford Press.

Okun, M. A., Stock, W. A., Haring, M. J., & Witter, R. A. (1984). The social activity/subjective well-being relation: A quantitative synthesis. *Research on Aging, 6,* 45–65.

Ong, A. D., Bergeman, C. S., Bisconti, T. L., & Wallace, K. A. (2006). Psychological resilience, positive emotions, and successful adaptation to stress in later life. *Journal of Personality and Social Psychology, 91,* 730–749.

Ostir, G. V., Markides, K. S., Black, S. A., & Goodwin, J. S. (2000). Emotional well-being predicts subsequent functional independence and survival. *Journal of the American Geriatrics Society, 48,* 473–478.

Otake, K., Shimai, S., Tanaka-Matsumi, J., Otsui, K., & Fredrickson, B. L. (2006). Happy people become happier through kindness: A counting kindnesses intervention. *Journal of Happiness Studies, 7,* 361–375.

Pennebaker, J. W. (1993). Social mechanisms of constraint. In D. M. Wegner & J. W. Pennebaker (Eds.), *Handbook of mental control* (pp. 200–219). Englewood Cliffs, NJ: Prentice-Hall.

Pennebaker, J. W., & Francis, M. E. (1996). Cognitive, emotional, and language processes in disclosure. *Cognition and Emotion, 10,* 601–626.

Reich, J. W., & Zautra, A. (1981). Life events and personal causation: Some relationships with satisfaction and distress. *Journal of Personality and Social Psychology, 41,* 1002–1012.

Seligman, M. E. P., Rashid, T. E., & Parks, A. (2006). Positive psychotherapy. *American Psychologist, 61,* 774–788.

Seligman, M. E. P., Steen, T. A., Park, N., & Peterson, C. (2005). Positive psychology progress: Empirical validation of interventions. *American Psychologist, 60,* 410–421.

Sheldon, K. M., & Elliot, A. J. (1999). Goal striving, need satisfaction, and longitudinal well-being: The self-concordance model. *Journal of Personality and Social Psychology, 76,* 482–497.

Sheldon, K. M., & Houser-Marko, L. (2001). Self-concordance, goal-attainment, and the pursuit of happiness: Can there be an upward spiral? *Journal of Personality and Social Psychology, 80,* 152–165.

Sheldon, K. M., & Lyubomirsky, S. (2004). Achieving sustainable new happiness: Prospects, practices, and prescriptions. In A. Linley & S. Joseph (Eds.), *Positive psychology in practice* (pp. 127–145). Hoboken, NJ: Wiley.

Sheldon, K. M., & Lyubomirsky, S. (2006a). Achieving sustainable gains in happiness: Change your actions, not your circumstances. *Journal of Happiness Studies, 7,* 55–86.

Sheldon, K. M., & Lyubomirsky, S. (2006b). How to increase and sustain positive emotion: The effects of expressing gratitude and visualizing best possible selves. *Journal of Positive Psychology, 1,* 73–82.

Staw, B. M., Sutton, R. I., & Pelled, L. H. (1994). Employee positive emotion and favorable outcomes at the workplace. *Organization Science, 5,* 51–71.

Stone, A. A., Neale, J. M., Cox, D. S., Napoli, A., Valdimarsdottir, V., & Kennedy-Moore, E. (1994). Daily events are associated with a secretory immune response to an oral antigen in men. *Health Psychology, 13,* 440–446.

Suh, E. M., Diener, E., & Fujita, F. (1996). Events and subjective well-being: Only recent events matter. *Journal of Personality and Social Psychology, 70,* 1091–1102.

Tellegen, A., Lykken, D. T., Bouchard, T. J., Wilcox, K. J., Segal, N. L., & Rich, S. (1988). Personality similarity in twins reared apart and together. *Journal of Personality and Social Psychology, 54,* 1031–1039.

Triandis, H. C., Bontempo, R., Leung, K., & Hui, C. H. (1990). A method for determining cultural, demographic, and personal constructs. *Journal of Cross-Cultural Psychology, 21,* 302–318.

Tugade, M. M., & Fredrickson, B. L. (2004). Resilient individuals use positive emotions to bounce back from negative emotional experiences. *Journal of Personality and Social Psychology, 86,* 320–333.

Tugade, M. M., Fredrickson, B. L., & Barrett, L. F. (2004). Psychological resilience and positive emotional granularity: Examining the benefits of positive emotions on coping and health. *Journal of Personality, 72,* 1161–1190.

Urry, H. L., Nitschke, J. B., Dolski, I., Jackson, D. C., Dalton, K. M., Mueller, C. J., et al. (2004). Making a life worth living: Neural correlates of well-being. *Psychological Science, 15,* 367–372.

Watson, D., Clark, L. A., McIntyre, C. W., & Hamaker, S. (1992). Affect, personality, and social activity. *Journal of Personality and Social Psychology, 63,* 1011–1025.

Williams, S., & Shiaw, W. T. (1999). Mood and organizational citizenship behavior: The effects of positive affect on employee organizational citizenship behavior intentions. *Journal of Psychology, 133,* 656–668.

Williams, D. E., & Thompson, J. K. (1993). Biology and behavior: A set-point hypothesis of psychological functioning. *Behavior Modification, 17,* 43–57.

Wilson, T. D., & Gilbert, D. T. (2003). Affective forecasting. *Advances in Experimental Social Psychology, 35,* 345–411.

Wilson, T. D., & Gilbert, D. T. (2008). Explaining away: A model of affective adaptation. *Perspectives on Psychological Science, 3,* 370–386.

Zautra, A., & Reich, J. (1980). Positive life events and reports of well-being: Some useful distinctions. *American Journal of Community Psychology, 8,* 657–670.

22

Positive Affect at the Onset of Chronic Illness
Planting the Seeds of Resilience

Judith Tedlie Moskowitz

Living with a serious chronic illness such as HIV, diabetes, or cancer means coping with an accumulation of stressors that can ultimately give rise to depression, anxiety, and even symptoms of posttraumatic stress disorder (PTSD) (Alonzo, 2000; Chalfant, Bryant, & Fulcher, 2004; Stevens & Doerr, 1997). In fact, the *Diagnostic and Statistical Manual of Mental Disorders* lists chronic illness as a stressor that can lead to PTSD (DSM-IV; American Psychiatric Association, 1994). Diagnosis is generally the point at which the cascade of stressors associated with chronic illness begins to build. Although receiving a diagnosis of a serious illness is likely to be one of the most stressful life events an individual experiences, it does not inevitably lead to adverse mental health outcomes. In fact, there is a great deal of variability in response to a diagnosis, with some individuals experiencing extreme distress, others demonstrating a more resilient

pattern with little perturbation in levels of psychological well-being, and still others reporting positive psychological and physical consequences in the wake of the diagnosis (Adriaanse et al., 2004; Fife, 2005; Groake, Curtis, Coughlin, & Gsel, 2005; Jadresic et al., 1994; Park, Lechner, Antoni, & Stanton, 2009; Valle & Levy, 2008; Van't Spijker, Trijsburg, & Duivenvoorden, 1997).

What predicts resilience in the face of a diagnosis of a serious chronic illness? A growing body of theory and empirical evidence suggests that positive affect at this critical point is of fundamental importance and contributes to more resilient psychological and physical health trajectories in people coping with diagnosis of a serious illness. This evidence is presented below, followed by a description of a newly developed intervention designed to increase positive affect in people recently diagnosed with a serious medical illness.

Resilience

In the context of a challenging medical diagnosis, *resilience* is defined as the ability to maintain normative levels of psychological well-being, or to return rapidly to prediagnosis levels. "Normative levels of psychological well-being" includes not only the avoidance of clinical levels of depression, anxiety, or PTSD, but also the capacity to experience positive affective states. Almost everyone experiences at least one stressful life event that poses a challenge to well-being. Individuals who have a resilient response to a stressful event may well experience some negative psychological effects of a stressful event but tend to return to their preevent levels of well-being more rapidly than do individuals who do not have a resilient response.

The majority of studies that look at predictors of resilience in response to a medical diagnosis have employed samples of people with cancer and, taken together, these studies suggest that factors predicting resilience tend to have positive affective characteristics. For example, certain types of coping (e.g., positive reappraisal—Hack & Degner, 2004; Stanton & Snider, 1993), dispositional variables (e.g., optimism—Carver et al., 1993, 2005; Stanton & Snider, 1993), positive appraisals of the illness (labeling oneself as a "survivor" or "cancer conqueror" vs. "victim"—Bellizzi & Blank, 2007), and finding benefit in the experience (Carver & Antoni, 2004; Urcuyo, Boyers, Carver, & Antoni, 2005) at the time of diagnosis or initial treatment are prospectively associated with more resilient patterns of adjustment. These findings are generally consistent with the broader literature on resilience in adults and children, which indicates that positive dispositional variables such as an easy temperament, sense of meaning in life, a positive outlook, and sense of humor (Masten & Reed, 2002), and resources such as social support (Bonanno, Galea, Bucciarelli, & Vlahov, 2007; Ozer, Best, Lipsey, & Weiss, 2003) are associated with a higher likelihood of resilient responses to a variety of life stressors.

Additional support for the role of positive affect in resilience comes from studies of how individuals high in *trait* resilience cope with stress. *Trait resilience*, also known as *ego resilience*, is the dispositional ability to "bounce back" from stressful experiences (Block & Kremen, 1996; Tugade & Fredrickson, 2004). It is usually assessed with a self-report measure of how one generally responds to new or unexpected situations. For example, the most commonly used measure of dispositional or trait resilience, the Ego Resiliency Scale (Block & Kremen, 1996) asks participants to rate themselves on items such as "I quickly get over and recover from being startled," and "I enjoy dealing with new and unusual situations." In laboratory studies in which participants were told to prepare to present a speech, those who were high on trait ego resilience were more likely to experience positive affect, both in general and in response to the speech preparation stressor. In addition, those high on trait resilience had more rapid cardiovascular recovery after the stressor, and the effect of trait resilience was completely mediated through higher levels of positive affect (Tugade & Fredrickson, 2004).

In field studies, trait-resilient individuals were more likely to report positive emotions in the context of stress and to experience positive outcomes, such as increased personal resources and greater perceptions of growth in the wake of the stress, compared to low-resilient individuals (Fredrickson, Tugade, Waugh, & Larkin, 2003). In daily diary studies, those who were high on trait resilience recovered more quickly from daily stressful experiences than those low in trait resilience (Ong, Bergeman, Bisconti, & Wallace, 2006). Importantly, daily positive emotions fully mediated the effect of trait resilience on the next day's negative emotion, providing further support that those who are dispositionally resilient may use positive emotions to cope better with stress.

Positive Affect in the Context of Stress

Empirical support for the unique beneficial role of positive affect in the context of stress is accumulating. Much of this work stems from the surprising observation that positive affect can occur with relatively high frequency, even in the most dire stressful context, and can occur at the same time that symptoms of depression and distress are significantly elevated. In our study of caregiver partners of men with AIDS, the depression scores of the caregivers in the study were in the range that would classify them as being at risk for clinical depression, both during caregiving and after the death of the partner (Folkman, Chesney, Collette, Boccellari, & Cooke, 1996). However, with the exception of the time immediately surrounding the death of the partner, when asked to report how often they experienced various positive and negative affects in the previous week, the participants reported experiencing overall positive affect more frequently than they experienced overall negative affect (Folkman, 1997). Three years after the death of the partner, the mean depression score of the bereaved caregivers was still significantly higher than the general population mean (Moskowitz, Folkman, & Acree, 2003). Again, however, positive affect occurred more frequently than negative affect. We have found a similar co-occurrence of positive and negative affect among participants in a study of people newly diagnosed with HIV (Moskowitz, 2008), as have studies of other samples experiencing severe stress (Viney, 1986; Viney, Henry, Walker, & Crooks, 1989; Wortman, 1987).

The fact that positive affect co-occurs with negative affect suggests that positive affect may play a functional role in the context of stress (Folkman, 1997; Folkman & Moskowitz, 2000; Fredrickson & Joiner, 2002; Fredrickson et al., 2003; Tice, Baumeister, Shmueli, & Muraven, 2007; Wichers et al., 2007; Zautra, Smith, Affleck, & Tennen, 2001). Recent work supports this hypothesis. In a 12-week study of women with arthritis or fibromyalgia, the association of positive affect with reduced pain and lowered negative affect was stronger during high-stress weeks compared to low-stress weeks (Zautra, Johnson, & Davis, 2005). Similarly, in a longitudinal study of widows, daily positive affect buffered the effect of stress on negative affect. Compared to periods of low stress, positive affect in periods of high stress predicted lower levels of negative affect (Ong et al., 2006). Furthermore, laboratory studies suggest that positive affect may have beneficial *physiological* effects in the context of stress. Fredrickson and Levenson (1998) induced negative affect in subjects by showing them a film that elicited fear. Subjects were then shown one of four films designed to elicit contentment or amusement (positive affect), sadness (negative affect), or no affect (neutral condition). Measures of cardiovascular reactivity indicated that individuals who were shown the contentment or amusement film had faster recovery to baseline than did subjects shown the sad or neutral film. These studies indicate that positive affect may counteract or "undo" some of the negative physiological and psychological effects associated with stress.

A number of studies have now demonstrated that positive affect is uniquely associated with lower risk of morbidity and mortality in people with chronic conditions (Chida & Steptoe, 2008; Pressman & Cohen, 2005). In a sample of men with AIDS, higher average scores on the positive affect subscale from the Center for Epidemiologic Studies Depression Scale (CES-D) uniquely predicted significantly lower risk of mortality (Moskowitz, 2003). When risk estimates were adjusted for the time-dependent covariates of CD4 cells, antiretroviral use, and the other subscales of the CES-D, positive affect remained significantly predictive of lower risk of AIDS mortality. Positive affect is also associated with lower risk of mortality in samples with other chronic illnesses. We analyzed data from the National Health and Nutrition Examination Survey (NHANES) and NHANES Epidemiologic Follow-up Study (NHEFS) to determine whether positive affect was associated with mortality in a sample of people who reported having diabetes at baseline (Moskowitz, Epel, & Acree, 2008). Again, the Positive Affect subscale of the CES-D was significantly associated with lower risk of mortality, whereas Negative Affect was not. The protective effects of positive affect are not confined to measurement with the CES-D. Danner, Snowdon, and Friesen (2001) analyzed handwritten autobiographies by 180 Catholic nuns just prior to entering the convent. Positive affective content in the autobiographies was strongly inversely associated with risk of mortality over the next 60 years when they controlled for age, education, and measures of linguistic ability. Consistent with the growing literature showing an association between positive affect and beneficial health outcomes (Chida & Steptoe, 2008; Pressman & Cohen, 2005), these findings demonstrate the unique adaptive role of positive affect in coping with chronic illness.

Theoretical Support for the Adaptive Role of Positive Affect in Response to Stress

Early emotion theories, if they addressed positive affect at all, proposed that it served as a safety signal and was likely to lead to decreased vigilance and shallower processing of information compared to negative affect (for reviews, see Aspinwall, 1998; Fredrickson, 1998). If this were the case, positive affect would be detrimental in the context of a stressful medical diagnosis because it would counteract the adaptive attentional and motivational effects of negative affect. However, in the past decade, three theories have emerged that explicitly include positive affect and make a place for it in explaining resilient responses to serious stress: Folkman's (1997, 2008) revised stress and coping

theory; Fredrickson's (1998, 2001) broaden-and-build theory of positive emotion; and the dynamic model of affect proposed by Zautra, Reich, and colleagues (Reich, Zautra, & Davis, 2003; Zautra et al., 2001).

According to the original stress and coping theory (Lazarus & Folkman, 1984), the coping process begins when an event is appraised as threatening, harmful, or challenging. These appraisals are associated with affect (negative affect in response to threat or harm, a mix of positive and negative affect in response to challenge) and prompt coping. If the event is resolved favorably, a positive affective state is the result. If the event is resolved unfavorably, or if it is unresolved, a negative affective state results, and the coping process continues through reappraisal and another round of coping. Folkman (1997) proposed a revision to the stress and coping theory that explicitly posits a role for positive affect in the coping process. The revised model suggests that the negative affect associated with unfavorable resolution motivates meaning-focused coping processes that draw on important goals and values, including goal-directed, problem-focused coping and values-based positive reappraisal. These coping processes result in positive affect, which provides a psychological time-out and sustains ongoing coping efforts (Folkman, 2008; Lazarus, Kanner, & Folkman, 1980).

Fredrickson (1998) proposed a complementary "broaden-and-build" model of the function of positive affect. In contrast to the specific action tendencies and narrowed attention associated with negative affect, Fredrickson reviewed evidence that positive affect broadens the individual's attentional focus and behavioral repertoire, and, as a consequence, builds social, intellectual, and physical resources. Under stressful conditions, such as diagnosis with a serious illness, the functions of positive affect suggested by the model become especially important. The "broadening" function of positive affect would enable the individual to see beyond the immediate stress and possibly come up with creative approaches to coping with the diagnosis. The "building" function would help to rebuild resources (e.g., self-esteem and social support) that can be depleted by enduring stressful conditions but are important for coping with stress. Subsequent work by Fredrickson and colleagues has provided support for both the broadening and building functions of positive affect (e.g., Fredrickson & Branigan, 2005; Fredrickson, Cohn, Coffey, Pek, & Finkel, 2008; Fredrickson & Levenson, 1998).

The dynamic model of affect (DMA) (Reich et al., 2003; Zautra et al., 2001) posits that positive affect has stronger beneficial effects under conditions of stress compared to lower stress situations. The theory is based on the finding that the correlation between positive and negative affect varies depending on the degree to which the situation is stressful. Under normal, lower stress conditions, positive and negative affect are relatively independent, but under higher stress conditions, the association between positive and negative affect becomes more strongly inversely related (e.g., Potter, Zautra, & Reich, 2000). Under normal (low stress) conditions, cognitive demands are comparatively low, and the individual gains maximum information if positive and negative affect are distinct (less correlated), thus providing a wider range of clues about what is going on in the environment. However, under stressful conditions, cognitive capacity is taxed, attention is narrowed, and the complexity of affective information is decreased, leading to a strong inverse correlation between positive and negative affect. For example, among patients with arthritis, positive and negative affect are more highly inversely correlated on high pain days than on low pain days (Zautra et al., 2005). The implications for intervention with people experiencing serious stress are clear: if positive affect is experimentally increased, negative affect should decrease as a result. The DMA has received support from a growing body of studies (e.g., Ong et al., 2006; Zautra et al., 2005).

The revised stress and coping theory, the broaden-and-build theory of positive emotion, and the DMA have different but complementary foci. The revised stress and coping theory emphasizes coping responses that maintain positive affect under conditions of stress, the broaden-and-build theory focuses on the consequences of positive affect under both normal and higher stress conditions, and the DMA emphasizes the association between positive and negative affect, and the contextual determinants of that association. However, the three theories are consistent in their emphasis on the unique importance of positive affect, and all speak to the potential role of positive affect in enhancing resilience in the context of stress.

Development of a Positive Affect Intervention for People Coping with a New HIV Diagnosis

In response to increasing calls for novel, effective interventions to help people adjust to serious life stressors, such as diagnosis with serious illness (e.g., Lyubomirsky, Sheldon, & Schkade, 2005; Mancini & Bonanno, 2006; Ong et al., 2006), and motivated by data indicating that positive affect predicts beneficial psychological, behavioral, and physical outcomes in people newly diagnosed with HIV (Moskowitz, 2008), we developed an intervention to increase positive affect and, ultimately, the likelihood of more resilient psychological and physical adjustment trajectories in people newly diagnosed with HIV.

People newly diagnosed with HIV are in the acute phase of a major stressful life event and face significant challenges, including the need to interact with a complex health care system; constraints on sexual behavior; the need for disclosure of serostatus to friends, family, and sexual partners; stigma; and, in many cases, a struggle to come to terms with a new identity as someone with HIV (Hult, Maurer, & Moskowitz, 2009; Moskowitz, Wrubel, Hult, Maurer, & Stephens, 2007).

As with other serious diagnoses, testing positive for HIV is stressful, and the period immediately following HIV-positive serostatus notification is characterized by increases in depression and anxiety (Ironson, LaPerriere, Antoni, & O'Hearn, 1990; Jacobsen, Perry, & Hirsch, 1990; LaPerriere, Antoni, Schneiderman, & Ironson, 1990; Ostrow, Joseph, Kessler, & Soucy, 1989; Perry, Fishman, Jacobsberg, & Frances, 1992; Rundell, Paolucci, Beatty, & Boswell, 1988). Even years after diagnosis, people living with HIV are at elevated risk of depression (Bing et al., 2001), and depressive mood is associated with a number of undesirable outcomes, including increased risky sexual behavior (Marks, Bingman, & Duval, 1998) and more rapid HIV disease progression (Ickovics et al., 2001; Leserman, 2000; Mayne, Vittinghoff, Chesney, Barrett, & Coates, 1996). Although interventions designed to reduce depression in people living with HIV have met with some moderate success (Antoni, Ironson, & Schneiderman, 2007; Chesney, Chambers, Taylor, Johnson, & Folkman, 2003; Himelhoch, Medoff, & Oyeniyi, 2007), none has targeted newly diagnosed individuals. We designed our present intervention specifically for those who are newly diagnosed with a serious illness such as HIV.

This positive affect intervention, named IRISS (intervention for those recently informed of their seropositive status), comprises five one-on-one sessions in which a facilitator teaches the individual eight different skills for increasing positive affect: (1) noting daily positive events; (2) capitalizing on or savoring positive events; (3) gratitude; (4) mindfulness; (5) positive reappraisal; (6) focusing on personal strengths; (7) goal setting and working toward attainable goals; and (8) small acts of kindness. The content of the intervention was drawn from empirical findings, reviewed below, of predictors of positive affect in the context of stress and previously developed interventions designed explicitly to increase well-being (as opposed to simply decreasing negative affect).

With a few noted exceptions, none of these previous studies were conducted in samples of people with HIV or other serious illness. Although there are some uniquely stressful aspects of HIV (e.g., disclosure to sexual partners, persistent stigma), from a broader perspective, the intervention we developed is applicable in a wide variety of samples experiencing all kinds of serious stress. As we describe below, nothing about the skills taught in the intervention is specific to HIV, and there is no reason to expect that the intervention would only be effective in people coping with HIV. Instead, these skills to increase positive affect in daily life are drawn from a variety of empirical studies that may be applied to everything from the stress of daily living to the stress of a diagnosis of a serious illness, including but not limited to HIV.

Interventions Demonstrating Promise for Positive Affect Skill Building

Although not as widely tested as interventions to decrease depression and negative affect, a handful of multicomponent interventions have been designed explicitly to increase positive affect (Fava, Rafanelli, Cazzaro, Conti, & Grandi, 1998; Fava & Ruini, 2003; Fordyce, 1981, 1983). Thirty years ago, Fordyce reported a program of research testing an intervention that comprised "14 fundamentals" of happiness (e.g., keep busy and be more active; spend more time socializing, become present oriented, stop worrying). Happiness levels in the intervention group were compared to levels in control group members who were given the expectation that participation in a class on psychological adjustment would increase their happiness. In a series of six studies, Fordyce (1981, 1983) demonstrated that students who engaged in the happiness intervention had significant increases in happiness compared to the controls. In a seventh study (Fordyce, 1983), the intervention groups continued to have elevated happiness 9–18 months after the intervention.

More recently, Seligman, Rashid, and Parks (2006) have begun testing a treatment for depression called positive psychotherapy that focuses on increasing positive emotion, engagement, and meaning. In group positive psychotherapy, clients participated in six weekly sessions with home exercises. In an initial study of the intervention, students with mild to moderate depression were randomly assigned to group positive psychotherapy or to a no-treatment control group. Although there were no significant differences between the two groups immediately postintervention, depression scores in the positive psychotherapy group were marginally (p = .06) lower at 3 months and significantly lower at 6 and 12 months postintervention. Similarly, the differences in satisfaction with life were not significant at the posttest but became significant at 3-, 6-, and 12-month follow-up assessments. In a second pilot test of positive psychotherapy (Seligman et al., 2006), in which participants were assigned to individual sessions (vs. group sessions, described earlier), 46 clients seeking treatment for depression at a university health center were randomly assigned to positive psychotherapy or to treatment as usual. Clients seeking treatment for depression and being treated with antidepressants served as a second control condition (they were not randomized but were matched on several characteristics to the positive psychotherapy group). At the postintervention assessment, both the positive psychotherapy and the medication groups improved on depressive symptoms and overall functioning compared to the treatment as usual (no medication) group. Participants in the positive psychotherapy condition had significantly higher scores on happiness than both the treatment as usual and the medication groups.

Positive Events and Capitalizing

A number of studies demonstrate that positive life events are associated with increases in positive affect (Murrell & Norris, 1984;

Reich & Zautra, 1981; Zautra & Reich, 1983), and scheduling "pleasant events" is a central part of some types of therapy for depression (Krause, 1998; Lewinsohn & Amenson, 1978; Lewinsohn, Hoberman, & Clarke, 1989; Lewinsohn, Sullivan, & Grosscup, 1980). Our previous work with caregivers of partners with AIDS demonstrated that even in the midst of severe stress, people experience and note positive events that may help them cope with the stress (Folkman, Moskowitz, Ozer, & Park, 1997). Even seemingly minor things can become positive events to people coping with a new diagnosis of HIV. For example, one participant in our ongoing observational study of people newly diagnosed with HIV said: "I think before I was HIV-positive I wasn't very aware of how much small things make people happy." These findings led us to hypothesize that under enduring stressful conditions, people may consciously seek out or create positive events that can increase their positive affect and, as a result, replenish their psychological resources and help to sustain their coping efforts. *Capitalizing* is an expressive response to positive events and includes telling others about it, marking the occurrence in some way, or even thinking about the event again later on (Langston, 1994). Simply experiencing positive events is associated with increased positive affect, but capitalizing strengthens the association between positive events and positive affect (Langston, 1994). In other words, savoring (Bryant, 1989) or capitalizing on positive events leads to more positive affect. Of note, Langston (1994) found that the effect is not the same for negative events. Whereas expressive responses to positive events amplified the effect on positive affect, expressive responses to negative events were not related to positive affect. Thus, it is not simply that expressing emotion after an event is associated with more of that emotion—the effect is specific to positive events and positive affect. Savoring is one of the components of positive psychotherapy (Seligman et al., 2006).

Gratitude

Gratitude is defined as a feeling of thankfulness and appreciation expressed toward others—other people, nature, God. The association between intentionally noting things for which one is grateful and increased well-being is empirically well supported (Emmons, 2007). Studies on gratitude in student samples and in people with serious illness have demonstrated that keeping a gratitude journal is associated with less negative affect, fewer physical symptoms, better sleep quality, and greater satisfaction with life (Emmons & McCullough, 2003). Kashdan, Uswatte, and Julian (2006) found that gratitude predicted greater daily positive affect in Vietnam War veterans with PTSD. In a study reported by Lyubomirsky and colleagues (2005), students who were asked to "count their blessings" once per week had a significant increase in positive affect over 6 weeks compared to a control group. Gratitude is also one of the components of positive psychotherapy (Seligman et al., 2006).

Mindfulness

Mindfulness is defined as the ability to attend to intentionally and maintain non-judgmental awareness of one's experience (thoughts, feelings, physical sensations) in the present moment (Kabat-Zinn, 2003). Trait and state mindfulness are associated with higher positive affect and lower negative affect (Brown & Ryan, 2003), and interventions to increase mindfulness have been shown to increase positive affect (Grossman, Tiefenthaler-Gilmer, Raysz, & Kesper, 2007; Shapiro, Brown, & Biegel, 2007). Davidson and colleagues (2003) randomized 25 healthy people to mindfulness meditation and 16 to a control group. Measures of brain electrical activation showed significant increases in left-sided anterior activation, a pattern previously associated with positive affect, in the mindfulness group compared to the control group. Fredrickson and colleagues (2008) demonstrated that a 7-week loving kindness meditation intervention increased daily experience of positive affect, compared to a waiting-list control condition. Positive affect, in turn, was associated with increased life satisfaction, decreased levels of depression, and better physical health approximately 3 months after the baseline assessment. Reich and colleagues (2003) suggest that mindfulness training may help to "decouple" positive and negative affect, and allow higher levels of positive affect even in the context of high stress and negative affect.

Positive Reappraisal

According to stress and coping theory (Lazarus & Folkman, 1984), the extent to which an event is experienced as stressful depends on the individual's *appraisal*—the interpretation of the significance of the event for the individual. Positive reappraisal is a form of coping in which the significance of the event is reinterpreted in a more positive way. For example, seeing the silver lining in a stressful event is one form of positive reappraisal. In the coping literature, positive reappraisal is one of the few ways of coping that is consistently associated with increased positive affect (Carver & Scheier, 1994; Folkman, 1997; Sears, Stanton, & Danoff-Burg, 2003). In a study of coping with caregiving and bereavement, positive reappraisal was consistently and significantly associated with positive affect both during bereavement and after the death of the partner (Moskowitz, Folkman, Collette, & Vittinghoff, 1996). In a meta-analysis of coping with HIV (Moskowitz, Hult, Bussolari, & Acree, 2009) positive reappraisal was among the ways of coping most strongly associated with increased positive affect (7 studies, average $r = .22$, $p < .0001$). Forms of positive reappraisal are included in several interventions for people with HIV (e.g., Antoni et al., 2007; Chesney et al., 2003; Chesney, Folkman, & Chambers, 1996), but the reappraisals in these interventions usually concern replacing negative thoughts with more rational ones and do not explicitly focus on possible positive aspects of the situation.

Focusing on Personal Strengths

We hypothesize that reminding participants of their personal strengths and the ways these can help them cope with stressful events will provide self-affirmation and help participants appraise events as less stressful. We chose the personal strengths content based on theory and research on secondary appraisal and self-affirmation. Secondary appraisal is part of the coping process in which the individual evaluates his or her personal, social, and material resources to cope with a stressful event (Lazarus & Folkman, 1984). A secondary appraisal of sufficient resources, such as personal strengths, leads to a less severe stress appraisal. Focusing on one's strengths is a form of self-affirmation that is sometimes used as a positive affect manipulation in laboratory studies. Reed and Aspinwall (1998) found that women who were given the opportunity to affirm a positive aspect of themselves oriented to information regarding their risk of a serious illness more quickly than did those not given the opportunity to affirm another aspect of the self. They also found the information more convincing and recalled more of the risk-confirming information at a 1-week follow-up session. Self-affirmation is also associated with positive affect after failure feedback (Koole, Smeets, van Knippenberg, & Dijksterhuis, 1999). Other social-psychological research demonstrates that *self-enhancing cognitions* (thoughts about one's positive qualities) are associated with better psychological adjustment to illness (Taylor et al., 1992; Taylor & Lobel, 1989) and healthier biological profiles (Taylor, Lerner, Sage, & McDowell, 2003). Focusing on personal strengths is one of the components of positive psychotherapy (Seligman et al., 2006).

Attainable Goals

Goal setting is common in health education and intervention programs (Strecher et al., 1995). It has been used in interventions for people with HIV (e.g., Antoni et al., 2007; Sikkema, Kalichman, Kelly, & Koob, 1995). Observational research on goals indicates that perceptions of goal progress are associated with greater life satisfaction and higher levels of positive affect (Brunstein, Schultheiss, & Grassmann, 1998; Carver & Scheier, 1990; Lent et al., 2005), and pursuit of attainable goals (vs. more global distant goals) is associated with higher subjective well-being (Emmons, 1986, 1992). Sheldon and Houser-Marko (2001) tested an intervention to foster goal attainment in students and found that those in the intervention had greater increases in the ratio of positive to negative affect over the course of several weeks. In her revision of stress and coping theory, Folkman (1997) reviewed data indicating that problem-focused coping is related to positive affect in the context of stress. She hypothesized that this is due to the successes in goal-directed behavior that resulted from problem-focused coping, which was consistently associated with higher levels of positive affect in a number of different samples (Blalock, DeVellis, & Giorgino, 1995; Folkman, 1997; Moskowitz et al., 1996). In our meta-analysis of coping with HIV, problem-focused coping was significantly associated with increased positive affect (seven studies, average $r = .18$, $p < .0001$; Moskowitz et al., 2009).

Altruistic Behaviors/Acts of Kindness

Volunteerism and other altruistic behaviors are associated with lower risk of mortality (Musick & Wilson, 2003; Oman, Thoresen, & McMahon, 1999) and serious illness (Moen, Dempster-McCain, & Williams, 1993) in large representative samples. Ironson and colleagues (2002) found that helping others was associated with long-term survival in people with AIDS. In a study that explicitly compared the effects of giving and receiving support in a sample of older adults, giving support was associated with a significantly lower risk of death, whereas receiving support was associated with an *increased* risk of death, when researchers controlled for self-rated health, interviewer-rated health, health behavior, mental health, socioeconomic status, and personality variables (Brown, Nesse, Vinokur, & Smith, 2003). Altruistic behavior may be associated with positive affect because it distracts the individual from his or her own problems, increases self-esteem, or increases a sense of control or efficacy (Penner, Dovidio, Piliavin, & Schroeder, 2005). Lyubomirsky and colleagues (2005) reported preliminary data that engaging in five acts of kindness per week for 6 weeks increased positive affect in students, especially if they engaged in all five activities on a single day each week (rather than one per day). Recent work by Dunn, Aknin, and Norton (2008) demonstrates that spending money on others is associated with significant increases in happiness, when researchers controlled for income and other relevant predictors. In our qualitative analysis of HIV illness appraisals in a sample of HIV-positive men prior to highly active antiretroviral treatment (HAART), the central characteristic of one of the appraisal groups was their focus on others (Moskowitz & Wrubel, 2005). We labeled this group Outward Focus (other groups were Future Focus, Detached, Stigma, and Aware/Avoid). A significantly higher proportion of participants in the Outward Focus group performed HIV/AIDS-related volunteer service and offered support to others as a way of coping more often than any other appraisal group. At the end of the 2-year longitudinal study, the Outward Focus group did not differ from the others on negative affect but was significantly higher than the other four groups on positive affect. This finding led us to recognize the potential for altruistic behaviors or acts of kindness to others as ways to increase positive affect.

A Pilot Study of the Positive Affect Intervention

We conducted a small pilot study of IRISS to test the feasibility of the intervention and to gather preliminary evidence on whether we could increase positive affect in participants during the first few months after an HIV-positive diagnosis. As noted earlier, the five weekly, individually delivered sessions of the intervention covered eight behavioral and cognitive "skills" for increasing positive affect: (1) noting daily positive events; (2) capitalizing on or savoring positive events; (3) gratitude; (4) mindfulness; (5) positive reappraisal; (6) focusing on personal strengths; (7) setting and working toward attainable goals; and (8) small acts of kindness.

We compared data gathered in the IRISS pilot to data from an ongoing longitudinal observational study of people newly diagnosed with HIV, the CHAI (Coping, HIV, and Affect Interview) study (Hult, Maurer, & Moskowitz, 2009; Moskowitz, 2008), which provided data on a "normative" trajectory of depression in the months after diagnosis with HIV and allowed us to determine whether we altered that course in the IRISS pilot sample to a more resilient trajectory.

For the pilot, we recruited 11 participants who had tested positive for HIV within the past 12 weeks (mean, 8 weeks after diagnosis; range, 3–15 weeks). Nine were men, two were women. One participant dropped out after the first session. Ten participants completed all five weekly sessions; nine of these completed the postintervention evaluation at Week 6, as well as a follow up phone call a month later. We measured positive and negative affect, using a modified version of the Differential Emotions Scale (DES) (Fredrickson et al., 2003; Izard, 1977), and depressive mood, using the CES-D (Radloff, 1977), at seven time points: weekly at the start of each intervention session, and at the two follow-up points 1 week and 4 weeks after completion of the intervention.

The intervention appeared to increase positive affect significantly from week 1 of the intervention to the first postintervention follow-up (Moskowitz et al., 2009). IRISS participants had an average increase of 3.9 (SD = 3.8) points on the DES Positive scale. In comparison, the average scores on the CES-D in CHAI increased 1.2 points over the comparable time period after diagnosis. At the start of the intervention, approximately 8 weeks postdiagnosis, the average DES positive score in IRISS was 17.6 (SD = 5.5; possible range, 0–36). The average preintervention DES Positive score on IRISS was slightly lower than the average DES Positive scores in CHAI at 8 weeks postdiagnosis (mean, 19.27, SD = 7.4). At the first postintervention follow-up (approximately 13 weeks after diagnosis), the average DES Positive score in IRISS was 21.4 (SD = 3.1), compared to an average score at 13 weeks postdiagnosis in CHAI of 20.5 (SD = 7.4).

Comparison between IRISS intervention and CHAI participants provides additional support for the hypothesis that a positive affect intervention in the early postdiagnosis period can lead to a more resilient trajectory of depressive mood (see Figure 22.1). During the intervention, the CES-D scores for the IRISS participants were comparable to those of the CHAI participants. However, whereas the CHAI participants' average CES-D score continued to be elevated up to 17 weeks postdiagnosis, the IRISS participants' average score declined significantly at the two postintervention follow-up points (comparable to CHAI at 13 and 17 weeks postdiagnosis). At the final intervention session, IRISS participants' average CES-D was 15.44 (SD = 8.5), close to the cutoff of 16, which generally is considered "at risk" for clinical depression (Radloff, 1977). By the 1-week postintervention assessment, scores had dropped to 12.3 and continued to drop to 9.0 (SD = 6.4) by the 4-week follow-up assessment, comparable to the average score in the general population (Radloff, 1977).

In the Words of the Participants

In the first postintervention follow-up session, we asked participants for feedback on the intervention. Overall, the feedback was very positive and highlighted the potential for the IRISS intervention to increase positive affect and resilience in people coping with the onset of a serious chronic illness.

"This is a great study to be involved in. Helped me see my life in the larger sense— I'm really doing well."

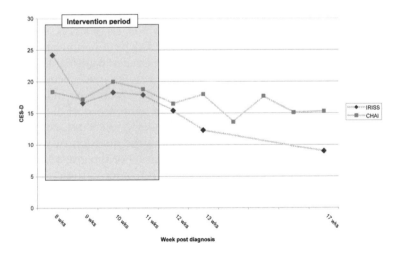

FIGURE 22.1. CES-D scores in IRISS and CHAI participants by week postdiagnosis.

"It's like collecting pennies under your sofa. But then the whole jar fills up and you realize you have a lot more than you thought. This is the same thing. There are many more positive things in my life than I realized."

"The acts of kindness component was really nice. Such a beautiful idea. If I could do it more often, it would make me a happier person. I was amazed."

"This intervention was a life change type of thing for me."

"It's good for people dealing with HIV because there is a lot of shame and doubt. It's a time in your life when you can potentially really cut yourself down so [the intervention] was a really important exercise. It helps you discover yourself—not to be so self-absorbed and drowning in the depression. It draws you out of your slump. Makes you look at yourself from a different angle and validates who you are and the importance of what you are and what you are doing in the world. The HIV, that's in my life, but these positive things are also in my life as well."

Questions and Future Directions

Our IRISS pilot indicates that a positive affect intervention in the period immediately following diagnosis with a serious illness is feasible and potentially effective in altering the short-term course of depressive mood to a more resilient trajectory. Based on theory and research demonstrating that positive affect has unique adaptive effects in the context of stress, these early results are promising and provide a strong foundation for future work to test more thoroughly the intervention in a variety of samples experiencing serious stress.

Results are preliminary, however, and a number of questions arise in response to

them. First, how much does the timing of the intervention matter? Is there a critical window in which a positive affect intervention has a maximal effect? Or is the effect just as powerful later on in the course of the illness? The DMA (Reich et al., 2003; Zautra et al., 2001) would suggest that the acute onset of the stress of a chronic illness is the optimal time because experimentally induced positive affect may serve to decrease negative affective outcomes during this critical period. Similarly, the broaden-and-build model (Fredrickson, 1998) would suggest that a positive affect intervention at this early point serves to "undo" the deleterious effects of negative affect. It may be that such an intervention at a later time would be less effective if the individual is not experiencing sufficient stress for positive affect to have its buffering or undoing effects. In their cognitive-behavioral stress management intervention for women with breast cancer, Antoni, Carver, and Lechner (2008) found that the intervention was particularly beneficial for women with elevated depression. The extent to which the same would be true for interventions that focus solely on positive affect is not clear. Possible ways to test whether the effects are specific to high-stress periods include implementing a positive affect intervention at different points in the course of an illness or testing the effects of the intervention in groups experiencing different levels of stress. Such designs would allow a determination of whether individuals experiencing normative levels of daily life stress reap as much benefit from a positive affect intervention as individuals experiencing the acute stress of diagnosis.

Similarly, there are currently no data to address the question of whether the beneficial effects of the intervention would be the same for other chronic illnesses, or whether HIV is a special case. We are currently conducting a large randomized controlled trial to test more fully the efficacy of the IRISS positive affect intervention in people newly diagnosed with HIV and have plans for testing the intervention in other samples of newly diagnosed people with other serious illnesses, such as cancer or type 2 diabetes. Our hypothesis is that positive affect is beneficial across a range of conditions, but the precise process by which positive affect leads to adaptive outcomes may differ depending on characteristics of the illness. For example, there are multiple pathways through which positive affect is likely to have beneficial health effects—behavioral, autonomic, neuroendocrine, and immune—and it may be that the behavioral pathway is strongest for diseases in which health behaviors have a large impact on outcomes, such as type 2 diabetes. For diseases that are particularly strongly driven by immune factors, such as HIV or perhaps cancer, the immune pathway may be the strongest. Again, answers to these questions await further research.

The IRISS intervention comprises multiple skills and, at this early point, it is not clear that any one of the skills is more effective than the others in increasing positive affect. To some extent, we will be able to test whether specific skills are particularly effective in our larger trial of IRISS. However, we do not anticipate finding one or two skills that work particularly well for all participants. Instead, we agree with Lyubomirsky, King, and Diener (2005), who argue that an important characteristic of successful positive affect interventions is the match of the person to the activity. It is likely that different activities will work for different people, so having several options to choose from may increase the likelihood that the intervention as a whole will have an effect. In addition, having a variety of skills to choose from may help to avoid the "hedonic treadmill" (Diener, Lucas, & Scollon, 2006). If one type of skill starts to lose its impact, the participant can try another one.

A fundamental difference between the IRISS and most other psychosocial interventions is that the focus is on positive affect per se, and not on current life stress or negative affect. Will positive affect interventions such as IRISS prove to be at least as effective in enhancing physical and psychological resilience as interventions aimed at reducing negative affect and stress? Definite answers to this question await further studies that directly compare positive affect interventions to stress reduction interventions. However, a recent study of patients with rheumatoid arthritis (Zautra et al., 2008) compared the effects of an emotion regulation intervention that included some components similar to those in IRISS (e.g., mindfulness; pleasant event scheduling) to a cognitive-behavioral therapy (CBT) condition that included managing daily activities, cognitive coping, and problem solving with respect to pain. For some outcomes (positive affect, negative affect, coping efficacy, catastrophizing, swelling, and tenderness), the emotion regulation condition resulted in significantly greater improvements than the CBT condition, particularly among participants with recurrent depression. These results suggest that interventions with less focus on depression and distress, and more emphasis on positive affect, may ultimately prove to be more effective.

The risk of this positive affect focus is that it may appear to minimize the pain and serious individual and societal consequences associated with major stressful events. We are not advocating a simplistic "don't worry— be happy" approach, nor do we believe that simply increasing positive affect will prove to be a cure-all for the very real and complex issues facing newly diagnosed people with serious illness. However, we argue that an intervention to increase positive affect may set the stage for a cascade of adaptive consequences. Given the high levels of stress, distress, and depression documented in samples of people diagnosed with serious illness, we consider increasing positive affect to be an inherently worthwhile intervention goal. Ultimately, positive affect interventions at the time of diagnosis may serve as the seeds for resilience down the line.

References

Adriaanse, M. C., Snoek, F. J., Dekker, J. M., Spijkerman, A. M., Nijpels, G., Twisk, J. W., et al. (2004). No substantial psychological impact of the diagnosis of type 2 diabetes following targeted population screening: The Hoorn Screening Study. *Diabetic Medicine, 21*(9), 992–998.

Alonzo, A. A. (2000). The experience of chronic illness and post-traumatic stress disorder: The consequences of cumulative adversity. *Social Science and Medicine, 50,* 1475–1484.

American Psychiatric Association. (1994). *Diagnostic and statistical manual of mental disorders* (4th ed.). Washington, DC: Author.

Antoni, M., Carver, C. S., & Lechner, S. C. (2008). Enhancing positive adaptation: Example intervention during treatment for breast cancer. In C. L. Park, S. C. Lechner, M. H. Antoni, & A. L. Stanton (Eds.), *Medical illness and positive life change: Can crisis lead to personal transformation?* Washington, DC: American Psychological Association.

Antoni, M. H., Ironson, G., & Schneiderman, N. (2007). *Cognitive-behavioral stress management for individuals living with HIV.* New York: Oxford University Press.

Aspinwall, L. G. (1998). Rethinking the role of positive affect in self-regulation. *Motivation and Emotion, 22,* 1–32.

Bellizzi, K. M., & Blank, T. O. (2007). Cancer-related identity and positive affect in survivors of prostate cancer. *Journal of Cancer Survivorship, 1,* 44–48.

Bing, E. G., Burnam, M. A., Longshore, D., Fleishman, J. A., Sherbourne, C. D., London, A. S., et al. (2001). Psychiatric disorders and drug use among human immunodeficiency virus-infected adults in the United States. *Archives of General Psychiatry, 58*(8), 721–728.

Blalock, S. J., DeVellis, B. M., & Giorgino, K. B. (1995). The relationship between coping and psychological well-being among people with osteoarthritis: A problem-specific approach. *Annals of Behavioral Medicine, 17,* 107–115.

Block, J., & Kremen, A. M. (1996). IQ and ego-resiliency: Conceptual and empirical connections and separateness. *Journal of Personality and Social Psychology, 70,* 349–361.

Bonanno, G. A., Galea, S., Bucciarelli, A., & Vlahov, D. (2007). What predicts psychological resilience after disaster?: The role of demographics, resources, and life stress. *Journal of Consulting and Clinical Psychology, 75,* 671–682.

Brown, K. W., & Ryan, R. M. (2003). The benefits of being present: Mindfulness and its role in psychological well-being. *Journal of Personality and Social Psychology, 84,* 822–848.

Brown, S. L., Nesse, R. M., Vinokur, A. D., & Smith, D. M. (2003). Providing social support may be more beneficial than receiving it: Results from a prospective study of mortality. *Psychological Science, 14,* 320–327.

Brunstein, J. C., Schultheiss, O. C., & Grassmann, R. (1998). Personal goals and emotional well-being: The moderating role of motive dispositions. *Journal of Personality and Social Psychology, 75*(2), 494–508.

Bryant, F. B. (1989). A four-factor model of perceived control: Avoiding, coping, obtaining, and savoring. *Journal of Personality, 57,* 773–797.

Carver, C. S., & Antoni, M. H. (2004). Finding benefit in breast cancer during the year after diagnosis predicts better adjustment 5 to 8 years after diagnosis. *Health Psychology, 23*(6), 595–598.

Carver, C. S., Pozo, C., Harris, S. D., Noriega, V., Scheier, M. F., Robinson, D. S., et al. (1993). How coping mediates the effect of optimism on distress: A study of women with early stage breast cancer. *Journal of Personality and Social Psychology, 65,* 375–390.

Carver, C. S., & Scheier, M. F. (1990). Origins and functions of positive and negative affect: A control process view. *Psychological Review, 97,* 19–35.

Carver, C. S., & Scheier, M. F. (1994). Situational coping and coping dispositions in a stressful transaction. *Journal of Personality and Social Psychology, 66,* 184–195.

Carver, C. S., Smith, R. G., Antoni, M. H., Petronis, V. M., Weiss, S., & Derhagopian, R. P. (2005). Optimistic personality and psychosocial well-being during treatment predict psychosocial well-being among long-term survivors of breast cancer. *Health Psychology, 24,* 508–516.

Chalfant, A. M., Bryant, R. A., & Fulcher, G. (2004). Posttraumatic stress disorder following diagnosis of multiple sclerosis. *Journal of Traumatic Stress, 17,* 423–428.

Chesney, M., Chambers, D., Taylor, J. M., Johnson, L. M., & Folkman, S. (2003). Coping effectiveness training for men living with HIV: Results from a randomized clinical trial testing a group-based intervention. *Pyschosomatic Medicine, 65*, 1038–1046.

Chesney, M. A., Folkman, S., & Chambers, D. (1996). Coping effectiveness training. *International Journal of STD and AIDS, 7*(Suppl. 2), 75–82.

Chida, Y., & Steptoe, A. (2008). Positive psychological well-being and mortality: A quantitative review of prospective observational studies. *Psychosomatic Medicine, 70*, 741–756.

Danner, D. D., Snowdon, D. A., & Friesen, W. V. (2001). Positive emotions in early life and longevity: Findings from the Nun Study. *Journal of Personality and Social Psychology, 80*, 804–813.

Davidson, R. J., Kabat-Zinn, J., Schumacher, J., Rosenkranz, M., Muller, D., Santorelli, S. F., et al. (2003). Alterations in brain and immune function produced by mindfulness meditation. *Psychosomatic Medicine, 65*(4), 564–570.

Diener, E., Lucas, R. E., & Scollon, C. N. (2006). Beyond the hedonic treadmill: Revising the adaptation theory of well-being. *American Psychologist, 61*, 305–314.

Dunn, E. W., Aknin, L. B., & Norton, M. I. (2008). Spending money on others promotes happiness. *Science, 319*, 1687–1688.

Emmons, R. A. (1986, August). *The dual nature of happiness: Independence of positive and negative moods*. Paper presented at the annual meeting of the American Psychological Association, Washington, DC.

Emmons, R. A. (1992). Abstract versus concrete goals: Personal striving level, physical illness, and psychological well-being. *Journal of Personality and Social Psychology, 62*, 292–300.

Emmons, R. A. (2007). *Thanks!: How the new science of gratitude can make you happier.* New York: Houghton Mifflin.

Emmons, R. A., & McCullough, M. E. (2003). Counting blessings versus burdens: An experimental investigation of gratitude and subjective well-being in daily life. *Journal of Personality and Social Psychology, 84*, 377–389.

Fava, G. A., Rafanelli, C., Cazzaro, M., Conti, S., & Grandi, S. (1998). Well-being therapy: A novel psychotherapeutic approach for residual symptoms of affective disorders. *Psychological Medicine, 28*, 475–480.

Fava, G. A., & Ruini, C. (2003). Development and characteristics of a well-being enhancing psychotherapeutic strategy: Well-being therapy. *Journal of Behavior Therapy and Experimental Psychiatry, 34*, 45–63.

Fife, B. L. (2005). The role of constructed meaning in adaptation to the onset of life-threatening illness. *Social Science and Medicine, 61*, 2132–2143.

Folkman, S. (1997). Positive psychological states and coping with severe stress. *Social Science and Medicine, 45*, 1207–1221.

Folkman, S. (2008). The case for positive emotions in the stress process. *Anxiety, Stress and Coping, 21*, 3–14.

Folkman, S., Chesney, M., Collette, L., Boccellari, A., & Cooke, M. (1996). Postbereavement depressive mood and its prebereavement predictors in HIV+ and HIV– gay men. *Journal of Personality and Social Psychology, 70*, 336–348.

Folkman, S., & Moskowitz, J. T. (2000). Positive affect and the other side of coping. *American Psychologist, 55*, 647–654.

Folkman, S., Moskowitz, J. T., Ozer, E. J., & Park, C. L. (1997). Positive meaningful events and coping in the context of HIV/AIDS. In B. H. Gottlieb (Ed.), *Coping with chronic stress* (pp. 293–314). New York: Plenum Press.

Fordyce, M. W. (1981). *The psychology of happiness: Fourteen fundamentals.* Fort Meyers, FL: Cypress Lake Media.

Fordyce, M. W. (1983). A program to increase happiness: Further studies. *Journal of Counseling Psychology, 30*, 483–498.

Fredrickson, B. L. (1998). What good are positive emotions? *Review of General Psychology, 2*, 300–319.

Fredrickson, B. L. (2001). The role of positive emotions in positive psychology. *American Psychologist, 56*, 218–226.

Fredrickson, B. L., & Branigan, C. (2005). Positive emotions broaden the scope of attention and thought-action repertoire. *Cognition and Emotion, 19*, 313–332.

Fredrickson, B. L., Cohn, M. A., Coffey, K. A., Pek, J., & Finkel, S. M. (2008). Open hearts build lives: Positive emotions, induced through meditation, build consequential personal resources. *Journal of Personality and Social Psychology, 95*, 1045–1062.

Fredrickson, B. L., & Joiner, T. (2002). Positive emotions trigger upward spirals toward emotional well-being. *Psychological Science, 13*(2), 172–175.

Fredrickson, B. L., & Levenson, R. W. (1998). Positive emotions speed recovery from the cardiovascular sequelae of negative emotions. *Cognition and Emotion, 12*, 191–220.

Fredrickson, B. L., Tugade, M. M., Waugh, C. E., & Larkin, G. R. (2003). What good are positive emotions in crises?: A prospective study of resilience and emotions following the terrorist attacks on the United States on September 11th, 2001. *Journal of Personality and Social Psychology, 84*, 365–376.

Groake, A., Curtis, R., Coughlin, R., & Gsel, A. (2005). The impact of illness representations and disease activity on adjustment in women with rheumatoid arthritis: A longitudinal study. *Psychology and Health, 20*, 597–613.

Grossman, P., Tiefenthaler-Gilmer, U., Raysz, A., & Kesper, U. (2007). Mindfulness training as an intervention for fibromyalgia: Evidence of postintervention and 3-year follow-up benefits in well-being. *Psychotherapy and Psychosomatics, 76*, 226–233.

Hack, T. F., & Degner, L. F. (2004). Coping responses following breast cancer diagnosis predict psychological adjustment three years later. *Psychooncology, 13*(4), 235–247.

Himelhoch, S., Medoff, D. R., & Oyeniyi, G. (2007). Efficacy of group psychotherapy to reduce depressive symptoms among HIV-infected individuals: A systematic review and meta-analysis. *AIDS Patient Care and STDs, 21*(10), 732–739.

Hult, J., Maurer, S., & Moskowitz, J. T. (2009). "I'm sorry, you're positive": A qualitative study of individual experiences of testing positive for HIV. *AIDS Care, 21*, 185–188.

Ickovics, J. R., Hamburger, M. E., Vlahov, D., Schoenbaum, E. E., Schuman, P., Boland, R. J., et al. (2001). Mortality, CD4 cell count decline, and depressive symptoms among HIV-seropositive women: Longitudinal analysis from the HIV Epidemiology Research Study. *Journal of the American Medical Association, 285*(11), 1466–1474.

Ironson, G., LaPerriere, A. R., Antoni, M. H., & O'Hearn, P. (1990). Changes in immune and psychological measures as a function of anticipation and reaction to news of HIV-1 antibody status. *Psychosomatic Medicine, 52*(3), 247–270.

Ironson, G., Solomon, G. F., Balbin, E. G., O'Cleirigh, C., George, A., Kumar, M., et al. (2002). The Ironson–Woods Spirituality/Religiousness Index is associated with long survival, health behaviors, less distress, and low cortisol in people with HIV/AIDS. *Annals of Behavioral Medicine, 24*(1), 34–48.

Izard, C. E. (1977). *Human emotions.* New York: Plenum Press.

Jacobsen, P. B., Perry, S. W., & Hirsch, D.-A. (1990). Behavioral and psychological responses to HIV antibody testing. *Journal of Consulting and Clinical Psychology, 58*(1), 31–37.

Jadresic, D., Riccio, M., Hawkins, D. A., Wilson, B. Shanson, D. C., & Thompson, C. (1994). Long-term impact of HIV diagnosis on mood and substance use-St. Stephen's cohort study. *International Journal of STD and AIDS, 5*(4), 248–252.

Kabat-Zinn, J. (2003). Mindfulness-based interventions in context: Past, present, and future. *Clinical Psychology: Science and Practice, 10*, 144–156.

Kashdan, T. B., Uswatte, G., & Julian, T. (2006). Gratitude and hedonic and eudaimonic well-being in Vietnam War veterans. *Behaviour Research and Therapy, 44*, 177–199.

Koole, S. L., Smeets, K., van Knippenberg, A., & Dijksterhuis, A. (1999). The cessation of rumination through self-affirmation. *Journal of Personality and Social Psychology, 77*, 111–125.

Krause, N. (1998). Positive life events and depressive symptoms in older adults. *Behavioral Medicine, 14*, 101–112.

Langston, C. A. (1994). Capitalizing on and coping with daily-life events: Expressive responses to positive events. *Journal of Personality and Social Psychology, 67*, 1112–1125.

LaPerriere, A. R., Antoni, M. H., Schneiderman, N., & Ironson, G. (1990). Exercise intervention attenuates emotional distress and natural killer cell decrements following notification of positive serologic status for HIV-1. *Biofeedback and Self-Regulation, 15*(3), 229–242.

Lazarus, R. S., & Folkman, S. (1984). *Stress, appraisal, and coping.* New York: Springer.

Lazarus, R. S., Kanner, A. D., & Folkman, S. (1980). Emotions: A cognitive-phenomenological analysis. In R. Plutchik & H. Kellerman (Eds.), *Theories of emotion* (pp. 189–217). New York: Academic Press.

Lent, R. W., Singley, D., Sheu, H.-B., Gainor, K. A., Brenner, B. R., Treistman, D., et al. (2005). Social cognitive predictors of domain and life satisfaction: Exploring the theoretical precursors of subjective well-being. *Journal of Consulting and Clinical Psychology, 52,* 429–442.

Leserman, J. (2000). The effects of depression, stressful life events, social support, and coping on the progression of HIV infection. *Current Psychiatry Reports, 2,* 495–502.

Lewinsohn, P. M., & Amenson, C. S. (1978). Some relations between pleasant and unpleasant mood-related events and depression. *Journal of Abnormal Psychology, 87,* 644–654.

Lewinsohn, P. M., Hoberman, H. M., & Clarke, G. N. (1989). The coping with depression course: Review and future directions. *Canadian Journal of Behavioral Science, 21,* 470–493.

Lewinsohn, P. M., Sullivan, M., & Grosscup, S. J. (1980). Changing reinforcing events: An approach to the treatment of depression. *Psychotherapy: Theory, Research, and Practice, 17,* 322–334.

Lyubomirsky, S., King, L., & Diener, E. (2005). The benefits of frequent positive affect: Does happiness lead to success? *Psychological Bulletin, 131,* 803–855.

Lyubomirsky, S., Sheldon, K., & Schkade, D. (2005). Pursuing happiness: The architecture of sustainable change. *Review of General Psychology, 9,* 111–131.

Mancini, A. D., & Bonanno, G. A. (2006). Resilience in the face of potential trauma: Clinical practices and illustrations. *Journal of Clinical Psychology, 62,* 971–985.

Marks, G., Bingman, C. R., & Duval, T. S. (1998). Negative affect and unsafe sex in HIV-positive men. *AIDS and Behavior, 2*(2), 89–99.

Masten, A. S., & Reed, M.-G. J. (2002). Resilience in development. In C. R. Snyder & S. J. Lopez (Eds.), *Handbook of positive psychology* (pp. 74–88). London: Oxford University Press.

Mayne, T. J., Vittinghoff, E., Chesney, M. A., Barrett, D. C., & Coates, T. J. (1996). Depressive affect and survival among gay and bisexual men infected with HIV. *Archives of Internal Medicine, 156*(19), 2233–2238.

Moen, P., Dempster-McCain, D., & Williams, R. M. (1993). Successful aging. *American Journal of Sociology, 97,* 1612–1632.

Moskowitz, J. T. (2003). Positive affect predicts lower risk of AIDS mortality. *Psychosomatic Medicine, 65,* 620–626.

Moskowitz, J. T. (2008, March). *The role of positive affect in adjustment to chronic illness.* Paper presented at the annual meeting of the American Psychosomatic Society, Baltimore.

Moskowitz, J. T., Epel, E. S., & Acree, M. (2008). Positive affect uniquely predicts lower risk of mortality in people with diabetes. *Health Psychology, 27,* S73–S82.

Moskowitz, J. T., Folkman, S., & Acree, M. (2003). Do positive psychological states shed light on recovery from bereavement?: Findings from a 3-year longitudinal study. *Death Studies, 27,* 471–500.

Moskowitz, J. T., Folkman, S., Collette, L., & Vittinghoff, E. (1996). Coping and mood during AIDS-related caregiving and bereavement. *Annals of Behavioral Medicine, 18*(1), 49–57.

Moskowitz, J. T., Hult, J. R., Bussolari, C., & Acree, M. (2009). What works in coping with HIV?: A meta-analysis with implications for coping with serious illness. *Psychological Bulletin, 135,* 121–141.

Moskowitz, J. T., Hult, J. R., Maurer, S., Duncan, L. G., Cohn, M. A., & Bussolari, C. (2009). *A positive affect intervention for people newly diagnosed with serious illness: Development and pilot data.* Manuscript in preparation.

Moskowitz, J. T., & Wrubel, J. (2005). Coping with HIV as a chronic illness: Illness appraisals, coping, and well-being. *Psychology and Health, 20,* 509–531.

Moskowitz, J. T., Wrubel, J., Hult, J., Maurer, M. J., & Stephens, E. (2007, August). *Illness appraisals and coping in people newly diagnosed with HIV.* Paper presented at the annual meeting of the American Psychological Association, San Francisco.

Murrell, S. A., & Norris, F. H. (1984). Resources, life events, and changes in positive affect and depression in older adults. *American Journal of Community Psychology, 12*(4), 445–464.

Musick, M. A., & Wilson, J. (2003). Volunteering and depression: The role of psychological and social resources in different age groups. *Social Science and Medicine, 56,* 259–269.

Oman, D., Thoresen, C. E., & McMahon, K. (1999). Volunteerism and mortality among the community-dwelling elderly. *Journal of Health Psychology, 4,* 301–316.

Ong, A. D., Bergeman, C. S., Bisconti, T. L., & Wallace, K. A. (2006). Psychological resilience, positive emotions, and successful adaptation to stress in later life. *Journal of Personality and Social Psychology, 91,* 730–749.

Ostrow, D. G., Joseph, J. G., Kessler, R., & Soucy, J. (1989). Disclosure of HIV antibody status: Behavioral and mental health correlates. *AIDS Education and Prevention, 1*(1), 1–11.

Ozer, E. J., Best, S. R., Lipsey, T. L., & Weiss, D. S. (2003). Predictors of posttraumatic stress disorder and symptoms in adults: A meta-analysis. *Psychological Bulletin, 129*, 52–73.

Park, C. L., Lechner, S. C., Antoni, M. H., & Stanton, A. L. (Eds.). (2009). *Medical illness and positive life change: Can crisis lead to personal transformation?* Washington, DC: American Psychological Association.

Penner, L. A., Dovidio, J. F., Piliavin, J. A., & Schroeder, D. A. (2005). Prosocial behavior: Multilevel perspectives. *Annual Review of Psychology, 56*, 365–392.

Perry, S. W., Fishman, B., Jacobsberg, L., & Frances, A. J. (1992). Relationships over 1 year between lymphocyte subsets and psychosocial variables among adults with infection by human immunodeficiency virus. *Archives of General Psychiatry, 49*(5), 396–401.

Potter, P. T., Zautra, A. J., & Reich, J. W. (2000). Stressful events and information processing dispositions moderate the relationship between positive and negative affect: Implications for pain patients. *Annals of Behavioral Medicine, 22*(3), 191–198.

Pressman, S. D., & Cohen, S. (2005). Does positive affect influence health? *Psychological Bulletin, 131*, 925–971.

Radloff, L. S. (1977). The CES-D scale: A self-report depression scale for research in the general population. *Applied Psychological Measurement, 1*, 385–401.

Reed, M. B., & Aspinwall, L. G. (1998). Self-affirmation reduces biased processing of health-risk information. *Motivation and Emotion, 22*, 99–132.

Reich, J. W., & Zautra, A. (1981). Life events and personal causation: Some relationship with satisfaction and distress. *Journal of Personality and Social Psychology, 41*, 1002–1012.

Reich, J. W., Zautra, A. J., & Davis, M. (2003). Dimensions of affect relationships: Models and their integrative implications. *Review of General Psychology, 7*, 66–83.

Rundell, J. R., Paolucci, S. L., Beatty, D. C., & Boswell, R. N. (1988). Psychiatric illness at all stages of human immunodeficiency virus infection. *American Journal of Psychiatry, 145*, 652–653.

Sears, S. R., Stanton, A. L., & Danoff-Burg, S. (2003). The yellow brick road and the emerald city: Benefit finding, positive reappraisal coping and posttraumatic growth in women with early-stage breast cancer. *Health Psychology, 22*(5), 487–497.

Seligman, M. E. P., Rashid, T., & Parks, A. C. (2006). Positive psychotherapy. *American Psychologist, 61*, 772–788.

Shapiro, M., Brown, K. W., & Biegel, G. M. (2007). Teaching self-care to caregivers: Effects of mindfulness-based stress reduction on the mental health of therapists in training. *Training and Education in Professional Psychology, 1*, 105–115.

Sheldon, K. M., & Houser-Marko, L. (2001). Self-concordance, goal attainment, and the pursuit of happiness: Can there be an upward spiral? *Journal of Personality and Social Psychology, 80*, 152–165.

Sikkema, K. J., Kalichman, S. C., Kelly, J. A., & Koob, J. J. (1995). Group intervention to improve coping with AIDS-related bereavement: Model development and an illustrative clinical example. *AIDS Care, 7*, 463–475.

Stanton, A. L., & Snider, P. R. (1993). Coping with a breast cancer diagnosis: A prospective study. *Health Psychology, 12*, 16–23.

Stevens, P. E., & Doerr, B. T. (1997). Trauma of discovery: Women's narratives of being informed they are HIV-infected. *AIDS Care, 9*(5), 523–538.

Strecher, V. J., Seijts, G., Kok, G. J., Latham, G. P., Glasgow, R., DeVellis, B. M., et al. (1995). Goal setting as a strategy for health behavior change. *Health Education Quarterly, 22*, 190–200.

Taylor, S. E., Kemeny, M. E., Aspinwall, L. G., Schneider, S. G., Rodriguez, R., & Herbert, M. (1992). Optimism, coping, psychological distress, and high-risk sexual behavior among men at risk for acquired immunodeficiency syndrome (AIDS). *Journal of Personality and Social Psychology, 63*, 460–473.

Taylor, S. E., Lerner, J. S. Sherman, D. K., Sage, R. M., & McDowell, N. K. l. (2003). Are self-enhancing cognitions associated with healthy or unhealthy biological profiles? *Journal of Personality and Social Psychology, 85*, 605–615.

Taylor, S. E., & Lobel, M. (1989). Social comparison activity under threat: Downward evaluation and upward contacts. *Psychological Review*, *96*, 569–575.

Tice, D. M., Baumeister, R. F., Shmueli, D., & Muraven, M. (2007). Restoring the self: Positive affect helps improve self-regulation following ego depletion. *Journal of Experimental Social Psychology*, *43*, 379–384.

Tugade, M. M., & Fredrickson, B. L. (2004). Resilient individuals use positive emotions to bounce back from negative emotional experiences. *Journal of Personality and Social Psychology*, *86*, 320–333.

Urcuyo, K. R., Boyers, A. E., Carver, C. S., & Antoni, M. H. (2005). Finding benefit in breast cancer: Relations with personality, coping, and concurrent well-being. *Psychology and Health*, *20*, 175–192.

Valle, M., & Levy, J. A. (2008). Finding meaning: African American injection drug users' interpretations of testing HIV-positive. *AIDS Care*, *20*, 130–138.

Van't Spijker, A., Trijsburg, R. W., & Duivenvoorden, H. J. (1997). Psychological sequelae of cancer diagnosis: A meta-analytical review of 58 studies after 1980. *Psychosomatic Medicine*, *59*, 280–293.

Viney, L. L. (1986). Expression of positive emotion by people who are physically ill: Is it evidence of defending or coping? *Journal of Psychosomatic Research*, *30*, 27–34.

Viney, L. L., Henry, R., Walker, B. M., & Crooks, L. (1989). The emotional reactions of HIV antibody positive men. *British Journal of Medical Psychology*, *62*(2), 153–161.

Wichers, M. C., Myin-Germeys, I., Jacobs, N., Peeters, F., Kenis, G., Derom, C., et al. (2007). Evidence that moment-to-moment variation in positive emotions buffer genetic risk for depression: A momentary assessment twin study. *Acta Psychiatrica Scandinavica*, *115*, 451–457.

Wortman, C. B. (1987). Coping with irrevocable loss. In G. R. Van den Bos & B. K. Bryant (Eds.), *Cataclysms, crises, and catastropes: Psychology in action* (pp. 189–235). Washington, DC: American Psychological Association.

Zautra, A. J., Davis, M. C., Reich, J. W., Nicassario, P., Tennen, H., Finan, P., et al. (2008). Comparison of cognitive behavioral and mindfulness meditation interventions on adaptation to rheumatoid arthritis for patients with and without history of recurrent depression. *Journal of Consulting and Clinical Psychology*, *76*(3), 408–421.

Zautra, A. J., Johnson, L. M., & Davis, M. C. (2005). Positive affect as a source of resilience for women in chronic pain. *Journal of Consulting and Clinical Psychology*, *73*, 212–220.

Zautra, A. J., & Reich, J. W. (1983). Life events and perceptions of life quality: Developments in a two-factor approach. *Journal of Community Psychology*, *11*, 121–132.

Zautra, A. J., Smith, B., Affleck, G., & Tennen, H. (2001). Examinations of chronic pain and affect relationships: Applications of a dynamic model of affect. *Journal of Consulting and Clinical Psychology*, *69*(5), 786–795.

23

Asset-Based Strategies for Building Resilient Communities

John P. Kretzmann

Many residents of lower-income inner-city neighborhoods face a relentless set of difficult challenges in their daily lives. Not the result of natural disasters, these challenges often reflect decades of economic and political forces that have left devastated communities in their wake. On Chicago's West Side, for example, racial segregation, business disinvestment, failing schools, and indifferent government have characterized a half-dozen neighborhoods and affected thousands of households.

People who not only survive but thrive in such conditions know a lot about resilience. It is instructive to attend to their strategies for revitalizing their communities, which may prove to be applicable in other challenging situations as well.

Beyond simply trying to cope, to survive from one day to the next, people in places like the West Side of Chicago tend to look first to government or other outside resources to prop up what they perceive (rightly) to be very needy people in a very destitute place. To attract the programs and interventions that are available from public, private, and nonprofit sources, local leaders must become highly skilled at communicating the depth and breadth of the economic, social, and institutional disasters they experience daily. They must, in other words, construct a self-portrait emphasizing their problems, challenges, and deficiencies—a kind of "needs map" (Figure 23.1).

This map represents one accurate, partial portrait of the realities of struggling communities, but by no means is it the full picture. In addition, the needs map is usually not the dominant self-portrait drawn by residents themselves, though they know that the problems are very real. Instead this relentless focus on the needs, problems, and deficiencies of neighborhoods often originates outside the community—in the offices of city, state, or federal officials; or in the suites of philanthropic groups; in the research agendas of academics focused on "urban problems," or in the classrooms of clinically

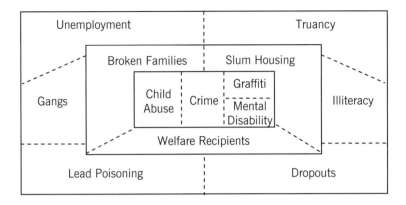

FIGURE 23.1. The neighborhood needs map.

oriented social work courses. Too many people outside struggling communities, usually motivated by an interest in helping, are convinced that communities are defined by their problems and needs—we professionals and our knowledge represent the solutions to their problems. If this needs map is the only, or the most pervasive set of ideas about residents' conditions, the resulting mindset has devastating consequences for the residents themselves.

Among these consequences is a set of both structural and psychological factors that act as powerful barriers to both individual and community resilience. For example:

- Residents of a community that is constantly labeled as needy and deficient may begin to internalize that conception, and begin to think about themselves as incapable of raising thriving children or entering the job market, or working with neighbors to make the area safer.
- Having been convinced that their community's reality is characterized by deficiencies, residents stop turning to each other, or to local religious institutions, block clubs, or businesses to solve problems, and instead look first to resources outside the community—governments, funders, expert helpers—as their rescuers. Critical local relationships, as a result, begin to deteriorate.

- Financial resources from the outside tend to be narrowly defined (categorical funding) and focused on supporting professional helpers, not residents.
- In this funding context appear local leaders whose primary leadership skill involves not motivating and shaping resilient, resident-centered initiatives but instead communicating local deficiencies, "how bad things are here," to outside public, private, and philanthropic sources of funding.
- Because this funding dynamic relies on the agreement that resources will be directed toward the most problematic situations and communities, supplicants are encouraged to fail—as crime increases (or the dropout rate, or teen pregnancy), more resources will flow.
- All of this tends to feed a downward spiral, leading to residents who share a negative self-image and an experience of growing hopelessness.

What, then, is the alternative to this debilitating and dominant focus on the needs, problems, and deficiencies of struggling communities? For many years, the Asset-Based Community Development (ABCD) Institute has explored resilience in struggling urban and rural communities, both within the United States and internationally. Working with and learning from resident leaders fac-

ing very difficult social and economic challenges, the Institute has collected thousands
of "success stories," cases in which significant efforts were initiated and led by local
folks who accomplished important community improvements. For example, locally
driven efforts turned schools around, took
parks back from drug dealers, provided alternatives for young people in trouble, developed political leaders, revived commercial
areas, developed small businesses, and so
forth.

Extensive interviews with the citizen leaders who catalyzed these efforts uncovered a
rich set of lessons for those interested in resilience. The most critical lessons, repeated
in different terms by almost all of the local
leaders who produced significant change,
involved the importance of modifying, or
ignoring, the portrait of their neighbors
and community that emphasized needs and
problems, and substituting instead a focus
on resources and capacities. Interviews revealed that in most of the cases of successful

initiatives, resident leaders utilized combinations of community resources or *assets*.

In effect, they began to create an alternative to the needs map, drawing instead
a mental (and sometimes physical) map of
their community's resources, or assets. Figure 23.2 is an example. As ABCD Institute
researchers interviewed leaders about the
local resources they used to accomplish their
goal, and about the content of their asset
map, six distinct categories of assets began
to emerge. It now appears that every community comprises some unique combination
of these six types of assets:

1. The experiences, skills, gifts, interests,
   and passions of individual residents.
2. The power of local networks and voluntary associations.
3. The resources of local public, private,
   and nonprofit institutions.
4. The physical resources of the community—natural, built, transport, and so
   forth.

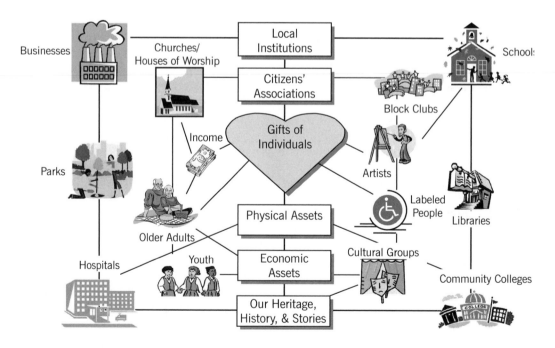

FIGURE 23.2. The neighborhood assets map.

5. The local economy—production, consumption, barter, and so forth.
6. The culture, history, values, and stories that define the community.

Resilient communities, those that establish sustainable development trajectories, appear to employ three asset-focused steps before turning to outside resources. First, they discover their existing assets, or "map" them. This step often involves the use of locally developed tools, such as "capacity inventories" (see below) or association maps. Next, communities that have been made aware of their range of resources begin to connect them for productive purposes (e.g., individuals' skills with local associations or institutions to build relationships or local networks with economic possibilities, or local institutions with the economic development potential of physical assets, such as transit stops). Finally, resilient communities harness their linked assets to a compelling and widely owned vision for the future: What does resilience look like here? What do residents here want their community to be like in 5, 10, or 15 years? What might life for young people be like? What about the economy and living wage jobs? How might the physical environment be enhanced, and so forth?

These three steps—discover the assets, connect them with each other for productive purposes, and harness them to a holistic vision for the future—are not sequential, but continuous. And they form the foundation for proposals that request outside public or philanthropic support. In the words of one successful community builder, "It's not that we don't need help from friends outside our community. But the fact is that we can't know what we need from the outside until what we know what we already have."

What do these strategies look like in real communities? Start with the discovery of individual gifts, skills, and dreams. Figure 23.3 is an interview form developed by volunteers at a soup kitchen who wanted to move beyond feeding folks to providing them with opportunities to reconnect with economic and social opportunities.

These one-on-one personal interviews uncovered musicians, artists, carpenters, plumbers, and dozens of cooks. Findings revolutionized the soup kitchen: Recipients became cooks at the kitchen, provided music during dinner hour, and started carpentry businesses in the neighborhood. Those whose identity was defined by their neediness became valued contributors; clients became useful community citizens.

People whose skills were discovered then were linked to local associations and institutions in the community—choirs and churches, block clubs and parent groups, businesses and community development organizations. For many, these new relationships opened up paths to a fresh set of opportunities. The asset discovery process at the soup kitchen led to a powerful experience of resilience.

Other "capacity inventories," echoing the 4-H Clubs, ask community residents about their gifts of the head (what they know, what they like to discuss, etc.), gifts of the hands (gardening, driving, sports, etc.), and gifts of the heart (do they care most about their children, faith, environment, etc.?). These prompts led interviewees to reconnect with their capacities and open up to new possibilities for their futures. Sometimes, these interviews are designed to uncover skills peculiarly suited to contribute to a predesigned project—improve health in the neighborhood, connect with older adults, or involve young people in improving the neighborhood. At other times, these surveys are aimed at rediscovering the gifts and skills of people who are often thought not to have any gifts and skills (e.g., people with disabilities, young people in trouble, ex-offenders, new immigrants, older adults, and others). Of course, people in all of these groups have so many talents, such a rich set of experiences to contribute, that our communities are impoverished without them.

Beyond discovering and connecting the skills and capacities of individuals, asset-

Introduction

My name is _____, what is your name?

Thank you for coming over. Did someone talk to you about what the "Gift Exchange" is all about? What do you understand it to be?

Basically, we believe that everyone has God-given talents and gifts that can be used to benefit the community. I'd like to spend a few minutes talking to you about your gifts and skills. Before we get started, let me give you a small gift.

Gifts

Gifts are abilities that we are born with. We may develop them, but no one has to give them to us.
1. What positive qualities do people say you have?
2. Who are the people in your life that you give to? How did you give to them?
3. When was the last time you shared with someone else? What was it?
4. What do you give that makes you feel good?

Skills

Sometimes we have talents that we've acquired in everyday life, such as cooking and fixing things.
1. What do you enjoy doing?
2. If you could start a business, what would it be?
3. What do you like to do that people would pay you to do?
4. Have you ever made anything? Have you ever fixed anything?

Dreams

Before you go, I want to take a minute and hear about your dreams—these goals you hope to accomplish.
1. What are your dreams?
2. If you could snap your fingers and be doing anything, what would it be?

Closing

First, I'd like to thank you. We're talking to as many people as we can, and what we'd like to do is begin a Wall of Fame here in the Soup Kitchen highlighting the gifts, skills, and dreams of as many people as possible. The ultimate goal is to find a way to use those gifts in rebuilding the community.

Before you go, can I get your full name? Address? Age?

FIGURE 23.3. New Prospect Baptist Church, Cincinnati, Ohio, survey guidelines.

focused community developers work to discover, connect, and mobilize local voluntary networks and associations. These include a wide range of groups, all of which aggregate the gifts and interests of individuals for more powerful collective expressions. Block clubs and block watches solve local problems and make neighborhoods safer. Religious congregations shape the values of members and organize their community-building involvements. Individual passions connect for the well-being of young people, women, those with disabilities, and others. Local creative energies emerge in murals, reading groups, and community theater productions. All of these efforts connect local residents with ever-stronger bonds and open up possibilities for new community-building initiatives—for stronger efforts to build resilient communities.

Community-building strategies that utilize these first two categories of assets—the gifts and skills of individuals, and the existing local networks and voluntary associations—

are clearly rooted in a long history of studies that emphasize the critical importance of *social capital*, the bonds of interdependence that create trust and reciprocity. Alexis de Tocqueville observed in 1833 that "in no country in the world has the principle of association been more successfully used or applied to a greater multitude of objects than in America. ... In the United States associations are established to promote the public safety, commerce, industry, morality, and religion. There is no end which the human will despairs of attaining through the combined power of individuals united into a society" (de Tocqueville, 1853, pp. 198–199).

In the last decade, the continuing importance of social capital for community resilience has been a central concern for a number of scholars, most prominently Robert Putnam, whose Bowling Alone attempts to document a marked decline in associational life over the last 30 years or so. He argues that diminished social capital has led to a range of negative community outcomes, affecting everything from education to public safety to economic vitality. Our own research in selected lower-income urban communities has indicated, however, that many still contain a surprisingly rich set of local voluntary groups. Strong networks based on communities of origin (e.g., small Southern towns or rural districts for African Americans, common villages for immigrants from Mexico or Central America) spawn new forms of social capital, such as religious groups, block clubs, sports teams, youth groups, and so forth. As in de Tocqueville's day, all of these relationships continue to produce the capacity to respond to individual and community stresses with creativity and resilience.

Another set of critical community assets includes all of the local public and not-for-profit institutions. Schools, libraries, police and fire stations, parks, hospitals, and the enormous range of nonprofit agencies represent resources in two distinct ways. First, of course, they all have a distinctive mission and purpose, and the more successfully they pursue it, the stronger the community. Everyone recognizes the importance of good schools, safe streets, attractive parks, and access to high-quality health care. But less obvious is that each of these institutions represents an array of valuable assets that could be connected to residents and their associations for community-building purposes. A school, for example, is not just a place where students and teachers interact around a curriculum. It can also function as a community and meeting center, and make available to the wider community not only its space but also its materials and equipment. It can try to hire and buy locally, whenever possible. It can facilitate useful community work on the parts of both students and teachers. When the local school, along with all of the other public and nonprofit institutions, begins to think about all of its assets, and opens them up to be utilized by the community, even people in the most struggling neighborhood quickly find themselves to be richer than they thought.

In the last decade or so, leaders in a number of institutional sectors have begun to recognize that more robust partnerships with community residents and associations can contribute to the success of their own missions as well. So, for example, the growth of the "community school" movement seeks not only to make the school a center for human service and health care providers but also to extend its availability for afterschool and evening activities—to reintroduce the school as a valuable community center.

Similarly, law enforcement leaders have increasingly recognized that police can only do so much to ensure safety. Increasing evidence that a well-organized community is also important has led to the nationwide growth of *community policing.* In the criminal justice system, more and more judges and policymakers are looking toward community-based diversion activities as a workable alternative to expensive and ineffective incarceration.

A few more examples of the expansion of these powerful partnerships between professionals and communities are as follows: Doctors and other health professionals increasingly recognize that providing high-quality, affordable, accessible medical care is only part of what it takes to keep people healthy; a community mobilized to enhance healthy behaviors, provide social supports for families and individuals, and open up economic opportunities represents a critical part of the partnership to foster health; finally, a number of the service professions whose practitioners have been trained to "treat" or "fix" people with problems— young people in trouble, people with disabilities, older adults—are now opening up to the possibility that their "clients" have gifts and interests that can be connected to those of other individuals and associations in the community.

It is important to emphasize that all of these partnerships represent "two-way streets": both the professionals and their institutions on the one hand and local communities on the other are beneficiaries.

Each renewed set of relationships is now generating its own descriptive and analytic literature. It is beyond the scope of this chapter to introduce these emerging fields, but they are easily accessed by searching topics such as *community schools, community policy, restorative justice, engaged libraries, service learning,* and so forth.

The fourth category of assets used to build resilient communities is physical in character—the natural and built environments, transportation, infrastructure, and so forth. Urban neighborhoods on the rebound feature residents who construct inviting public spaces, such as markets, parks, and attractive streetscapes; support vibrant meeting or "bumping into" places; calm, control, or eliminate excessive automobile traffic; value high-volume public transportation and the economic development projects it can support; and work to preserve culturally significant and historic buildings. Creative community development groups can see potential even in eyesores—a rubble strewn

empty lot offers a recycling opportunity, the space to create new affordable housing, or a community garden or playground.

Factors contributing to the physical and economic vitality of cities and neighborhoods have been explored by visionary social commentators such as Jane Jacobs and William H. Whyte, whose ideas are embodied today in hundreds of community development corporations and in practically prophetic groups, such as the Project for Public Spaces.

In rural areas, where small family farms are being swallowed up by larger corporate operations, or where the long-standing extraction industries such as mining, forestry, and fishing are shrinking, small towns are reinventing their social and economic futures based largely on a combination of the skills of local residents and the assets represented by the land. Forests, farmland, and coastal areas are magnets for tourists, and when coupled with the craft-producing residents of Appalachia, western Maine, or the Georgia Sea Islands, can produce promising economic futures.

In fact, it is this local economic activity that constitutes the fifth category of assets. In even the lowest-income communities, residents produce, consume, and barter. Small businesses repair, clean, sew, sell, cook, serve, and provide jobs. Investing in these businesses produces significant returns. Powerful strategies such as microlending support expanded entrepreneurial activity. In many communities, both urban and rural, local economies are constantly renewed as new residents arrive. Many small towns now boast more than one Mexican restaurant, and in Minneapolis one can visit the Mercado Central, featuring more than 40 small businesses, then walk down the street to the Somalian equivalent. Concerted efforts by chambers of commerce and community development groups now encourage "buy local" and even "eat local" campaigns. Resilient communities learn to support the businesses and economic activities already in place, at the same time welcoming and nurturing new efforts.

Finally, every community is importantly defined by its unique stories, which reveal a culture, broadly defined, and some measure of a shared history and values. The most creative communities find ways to celebrate their past. One group in Chicago's West Side commissioned young people to conduct scores of oral history interviews with elders, then produced a multimedia presentation they called *Looking Backward to Move Forward*. This same group collected a pair of old shoes from each of 50 "neighborhood heroes" and proudly displayed them, with pictures and biographies, and with the challenge to "walk in their shoes."

To gather a community's stories, many have found the tools of *appreciative inquiry* very useful. Put simply, discussions begin with a question like "When were you proudest of your community?" or "Tell me when you felt most valued here?" or the direct resilience question, "Can you recall a time when your family, or the whole community, bounced back from some very negative event or experience?" After collecting a series of these success stories, residents analyze the circumstances, causes, and lessons to be learned from them. Then, they strategize about how to make more successes happen in the future. The whole process, obviously, is designed to project a positive future that residents feel is realistic and attainable: We've done it before. Why can't we succeed again?

Are asset-based approaches to building stronger, more resilient communities limited to urban North American settings? Recent evidence suggests that building communities from the inside out is working in the developing world as well. The Coady International Institute at St. Francis Xavier University in Nova Scotia has been studying and working with community development groups in the Global South for decades, as well as training nongovernmental organization leaders in strengths-based strategies. Their collection of case studies, *From Clients to Citizens: Communities Changing the Course of Their Own Development*, documents the rich experiences of 13 urban and rural communities, most from developing countries, that have charted a resilient course based on their existing human, social, physical, and cultural assets.

Finally, many communities of indigenous peoples, from North and South America, and Australia, are rediscovering the power of their own cultures, skills, and histories to forge paths to more hopeful futures. In the mountainous Chimborazo region of Ecuador, for example, indigenous women formed the Jambi Kiwa cooperative, which built on traditional knowledge of medicinal and aromatic plants to find a global marketplace. Hundreds of families in remote villages have discovered the power of inherited skills to connect with the 21st-century economy (Cunningham, 2008). Other native villages have conducted "capacity inventories" to identify elders who possess traditional knowledge and skills, and who are willing to pass those down to younger people. One rich example from Alaska's Inuit people is found in Appendix 23.1.

Asset-based community development, then, represents a perspective and a set of strategies for rebuilding towns and neighborhoods from the inside out. Resilient communities are not self-sufficient. They recognize the larger regional, state, and national contexts that interact with their local agendas. They know that some of the resources they need must come from the outside, from public, private, nonprofit, and philanthropic sources. But resilient communities are determined to set the terms for the infusion of those resources. They refuse to allow others to define them as needy and deficient, as worthy recipients of charity. Rather, they look first to the processes of locating, connecting, and mobilizing assets they already have, then inviting the outsiders to invest in their success, to join as partners in producing communities that are increasingly vital and resilient.

APPENDIX 23.1. Releasing Individual Capacities: Big Dipper Community Circle

Hello, I'm with Big Dipper Community Circle. We're talking to everyone in Kotzebue about their skills and interests—what they already know and new things they'd like to do or learn. We want to make it easier for people to find others with similar interests and concerns—also connections for interesting experience trying out new things or working to help each other or to help the community. May I ask you some questions about what you've done, what you might like to learn or do?

Part I: Skills Information

I'm going to read to you a list of skills. It's a long list, so I hope you'll stick with me. I'll read the list and you tell me whether you know it or can do it, can teach it to someone else or, if you don't have that skill, whether you would like to learn it.

We're interested in all your skills and abilities—also in things you're interested in learning or doing. For now, think about what you're learned by experience at home or with your family. Remember what you've learned at church, in the community, from other people—wherever. There may be things you've learned at work, too, either on your own job or watching others. As I read the list, tell me which things you know, which things you would be able to teach others, and which things you would like to learn.

We'll start with some traditional Inupiaq skills and then go on to others.

	Know	Could teach	Want to learn
Inupiaq History and Customs			
Know Inupiaq history			
Know village history			
Identify landmarks near villages			
Know Inupiaq stories			
Understand legends			
Understand short stories			
Understand songs			

Knows customs of celebrating first catch			
Eskimo games			
Eskimo football			
NYO games			
Rules for proper play			
Eskimo dancing			
Drumming			
Songs			
Fishing			
Do you fish?			
Jigging			
Build and use fish trap			
Chop ice hole			
Clear ice hole			
Fish underwater with a net			
Check seining net			
Set net			
Hang net			
Repair net			
Make needed tools			
If yes, which ones?			
Make floats and sinkers			
Make net			
Make knots properly			
Measure net gauge correctly			
Make correct gauge for big and small fish			
Handling Meat			
Skin and butcher a caribou			
Choose organs good for eating			
Use all parts of a caribou			
Nigukkaq			
Makes arts and crafts from skin, hoofs, antlers			
Make fish rack			
Butcher a seal			

Make seal oil			
Make seal oil with black meat			
Butcher an Ugruk			
Butcher a beluga			
Butcher a bowhead whale			
Know how to divide shares			
Store caribou or seal meat in freezer			
Cut meat for drying			
Store frozen fish			
Store fermented frozen fish			
Dry fish			
Cut fish			
Smoke fish			
Pluck ducks			
Run an outboard motor			
Row a boat			
Winterize boat			
Winterize outboard motor			
Repair sled			
Build sled			
Guns			
Teach gun safety			
Choose correct gun for task			
Shoot accurately			
Dog Team			
Hitch up a team			
Use dog team for transportation			
Mush a team			
Care for a team			
Train a dog team			
Make dog posts			
Make harnesses			
Make collars			
Make mushing lines			

Know about dog mushing nutrition			
Arctic Survival			
Understand weather			
Predict weather			
Dress appropriately for travel in different types of weather			
Identify ice conditions			
Recognize dangerous or thin ice			
Choose grass good for insulation			
Pack sled correctly			
Make emergency snow shelter			
Office			
Typing (___ words per minute)			
Operating adding machine/calculator			
Filing alphabetically/ numerically			
Taking phone messages			
Writing business letters (not typing)			
Receiving phone orders			
Operating a switchboard			
Keeping track of supplies			
Shorthand or speedwriting			
Transaction from tape			
Bookkeeping (by hand)			
Inupiaq Language			
Can you speak Inupiaq?			
Understand spoken Inupiaq?			
Read Inupiaq?			
Write Inupiaq?			
(Stop here if no affirmative response by this point; skip to next section.)			

Translate spoken Inupiaq into English?			
Translate spoken English into Inupiaq?			
Translate written Inupiaq into English?			
Translate written English into Inupiaq?			
Transcribe audiotapes into Inupiaq?			
Edit audiotape?			
Edit Inupiaq language videotape?			
Make public service announcements in Inupiaq?			
Teach language?			
Type Inupiaq in computer?			
Trapping			
What tools to use			
Make a rabbit or ptarmigan snare			
Set rabbit/ptarmigan snare			
Identify good snare tapping locations			
Identify fur trapping locations			
Butcher and skin fur bearing animals			
Dry furbearing animals properly			
Food and Medicine			
Locate good berry patches			
Pick berries			
Preserve berries			
Identify edible greens			
Know season to harvest			
Harvest greens			
Preserve greens			
Make doughnuts			
Make Akutuq			

Practice traditional tribal medicine			
Bloodletting (kapi-)			
Massage or manipulation (i.e., savit for health reasons)			
Internal (specialty)			
Bone			
Circulation			
Exercise			
Outdoor Camping Skills			
Cut wood (spruce, alder)			
Chop wood (spruce, elder, driftwood)			
Saw wood			
Operate lantern			
Gas			
Kerosene			
Seal oil			
Operate camp stove			
Pitch up a tent			
Sewing			
Make parkas/*atikluk*			
Fur			
Cloth			
Long, short			
For men, women, children			
Make fancy trim			
Skin Sewing			
Tan skins			
Make *mukluks*			
Make ruffs			
Make slippers			
Make mittens			
Make yo-yos			
Beading			
Wood Carving			
Ivory Carving			
Basket Making			

Make baleen baskets			
Make birch bark baskets			
Make grass baskets			
Make willow baskets			
Ulu Making			
Jigging Stick Making			
Making Skin Scraper			
Make a Log Cabin			
Build a Sod House			
Make Birch Frames			
Make Beaded Frames			
Make Miniature Dolls, Gayaqs, Sleds, etc.			
Crochet			
Knit			
Socks			
Gloves			
Headband			

Selected Bibliography

Cooperrider, D., Whitney, D., & Stavros, J. (2007). *Appreciative inquiry handbook* (2nd ed.). Brunswick, OH: Crown Custom Publishing.

Cunningham, G. (2008). The Jambi Kiwa story: Mobilizing assets for community development in Ecuador. In A. Mathie & G. Cunningham (Eds.), *From clients to citizens: Communities changing the course of their own development*. Warwickshire, UK: Practical Action.

de Tocqueville, A. (1853). *Democracy in America*. New York: Vintage Books.

Green, G., Haines, P., & Haines, A. (2002). *Asset building and community development*. Thousand Oaks, CA: Sage.

Jacobs, J. (1961). *The death and life of great American cities*. New York: Random House/Vintage Books.

Kingsley, G. T., McNeely, J., & Gibson, J. (1997). *Community building coming of age*. Washington, DC: Development Training Institute and the Urban Institute.

Kretzmann, J., & McKnight, J. (1993). *Building communities from the inside out: A path toward finding and mobilizing a community's assets*. Evanston, IL: Institute for Policy Research, Northwestern University.

Mathie, A., & Cunningham, G. (Eds.). (2008). *From clients to citizens: Communities changing the course of their own development*. Rugby, UK: Practical Action.

Putnam, R. D. (2001). *Bowling alone: The collapse and revival of American community*. New York: Simon & Schuster.

Whyte, W. H. (2001). *The social life of small urban spaces*. Naperville, IL: Conservation Foundation, 1980/Reissued in paperback by Project for Public Spaces, Inc.

ABCD Institute Publications

A Guide to Mapping and Mobilizing the Economic Capacities of Local Residents

A Guide to Mapping Local Business Assets and Mobilizing Local Business Capacities

A Guide to Mapping Consumer Expenditures and Mobilizing Consumer Expenditure Capacities

A Guide to Capacity Inventories: Mobilizing the Community Skills of Local Residents

A Guide to Evaluating Asset-Based Community Development: Lessons, Challenges, and Opportunities

A Guide to Creating a Neighborhood Information Exchange: Building Communities by Connecting Local Skills and Knowledge

City-Sponsored Community Building: Savannah's Grants for Blocks Story

Newspapers and Neighborhoods: Strategies for Achieving Responsible Coverage of Local Communities

A Guide to Mapping and Mobilizing the Associations in Local Neighborhoods

Leading by Stepping Back: A Guide for City Officials on Building Neighborhood Capacity

A Guide to Building Sustainable Organizations from the Inside Out: An Organizational Capacity Building Toolbox from the Chicago Foundation for Women

The Organization of Hope: A Workbook for Rural Asset-Based Community Development

Community Transformation: Turning Threats into Opportunities

Asset-Based Strategies for Faith Communities

Building the Mercado Central: Asset-Based Development and Community Entrepreneurship

24

Health in a New Key
Fostering Resilience through Philanthropy

Roger A. Hughes

From colonial America to the dawn of global society in the early 21st century, philanthropy has played a pivotal role in promoting healthy, resilient individuals and communities. It has helped to both define and shape civil society, which in turn has nurtured modern markets and government, and has been instrumental in the development of the economic, cultural, and social capital necessary to build diverse networks characterized by the capacity for learning, adaptation, and self-organization.

As resilience is forged in adversity, so, too, has philanthropy's role in American society been contested for much of the 20th century. Conservatives fault modern philanthropy—in the form of large foundations—for turning to instrumentalist, managerial, and social science "engineering" approaches to "solve" the problems of society and abandoning its civil society roots of promoting voluntary association, charity, free markets, personal responsibility, moral traditions, and the family

(Joyce & Richardson, 1993). Critics on the left paint these same philanthropic organizations as "cooling out agencies" that perpetuate the status quo of ruling class elites and oppress the interests of minorities, the working class, and more fundamental social and economic reform (Arnove, 1980). Still others fault modern philanthropic organizations for not being strategic enough, and for flitting from issue to issue, without focus and long-term commitment to social change (Fleischman, 2007). As a field, philanthropy contains fundamental differences in values and political outlook, the optimum balance between the roles of individuals, civil society, markets, and government; and the very definition of terms such as *philanthropy* and *resilience* themselves.

While there is a remarkable symmetry between the role philanthropy played in the early years of American history and its role today, there is a potential discontinuity on the horizon. The complexity of the world we live in, and our ability to adapt successfully to rapid social, economic, and technological change, calls into question both the scope and scale of philanthropy to "make a difference"—its mantra as judged by the number of times it is chanted by the faithful—compared to its impact in the past. The world is fundamentally changing, and in ways we may not fully comprehend. The issue is whether *philanthropy*—considered as the voluntary contribution of human and financial resources for the benefit of the public good—still has a critical role to play in fostering resilience, and if so, what that role might be.

That question is the subject of this chapter. To set the stage, I briefly trace the historical roots of American philanthropy and community development from the colonial period through the modern era, beginning with the rise of the industrial state at the turn of the 20th century and reaching its aegis at the start of the so-called "postindustrial" period in the 1970s and 1980s. I then argue that as we move from modern culture to the "Hyperculture," those working in organized philanthropy may need to reframe their work in a "new key" if they wish to continue to "make a difference" in fostering resilient individuals and communities.

A Note on Definitions

A brief reference to the terms *philanthropy* and *resilience* helps to set the context.

Philanthropy

I use the term *philanthropy* in its broadest sense as the voluntary contribution of time, talent, and money to promote the public good. This is in contrast to much of the literature on modern philanthropy, which is often focused on grant making alone, and especially the world of big foundations and donors (Fleischman, 2007; Frumpkin, 2006). Indeed, the term *philanthropic sector* is used interchangeably with terms such

as *organized* philanthropy and the *business* of philanthropy, where grants (investments) are made for specific purposes (strategic objectives) over extended periods of time by philanthropists and the professional class of "philanthrocrats" who work for them, or the institutions they create. Much of this language can be traced to the rise of industrialism, science, and social progressivism in the late 19th and early 20th century, when great American philanthropists such as Andrew Carnegie and John D. Rockefeller created foundations to invest in solutions to pressing issues (e.g., poverty and poor health) by providing a "hand up, not a handout." Purpose-driven philanthropy then, as now, was distinguished from *charity*—the direct provision of assistance to those in need—and thought to be superior to it.

I use this broader definition not to detract from the emphasis on organized and strategic giving but to capture the vast undertow of volunteering and giving that has always comprised the bulk of American philanthropy. For example, in 2006, giving by foundations accounted for 12.4% ($36.5 billion) of the amount counted as "charitable giving" ($295 billion). The great majority of giving came from individuals (75.6%), and of that, approximately 33% went to churches and other religious organizations and causes (Giving USA Foundation, 2007). Presumably, millions of Americans support local institutions and causes, with nary a thought as to whether they are "making a difference" or being "strategic." They do it because it feels good, because it is the right thing to do, because someone asked them to, or because they have a relationship with a particular cause or organization. Or perhaps they do it for social status, feelings of guilt or peer pressure, to express their deepest values, and even to "give back" to the community for all of the blessings afforded them, real or imagined. If one adds to this the unpaid hours of 61 million Americans (Bureau of Labor Statistics, 2007) who volunteer in their local communities, the impact is huge. In a direct and tangible way, this voluntary contribution of time, money, and talent to advance the public good in all of its myriad forms is the glue that holds social capital together.

Although much of the later analysis of approaches to increasing resilience in individuals and communities is focused on the more strategic aspects of modern philanthropy, this broader definition underscores the importance of giving and volunteering at all levels of society both to maintain and enhance a common life. This social reciprocity is critical to any understanding of how to foster resilient individuals and communities, and we return to it time and time again.

Resilience

A growing body of research on *resilience* in social–ecological systems defines it as the degree to which the system can absorb change and "still retain the same controls on function and structure; the degree to which the system is capable of self-organization; [and] the ability to build and increase the capacity for learning and adaptation." In social systems, resilience takes on "the added capacity of humans to anticipate and plan for the future," as well as the capacity to deal with complex issues widely dispersed across social networks (Resilience Alliance, 2008).

Here, we are primarily interested in resilience as the ability or process of *adaptation* in response to significant dislocation and turmoil, and not simply as a passive "bouncing back" from adversity to some alleged "stable" state. As a process, resilience emerges from a set of malleable resources at both individual and community levels. Human agency, social capital, economic development, information and communication, and community competence are all networked resources that we draw on to foster resilience (Norris, Stevens, Pfefferbaum, Wyche, Pfefferbaum, 2008). Philanthropy's investment in these resources is what is of interest here.

For individuals, the commonsense notion of resilience as the ability to "snap back" from stress and adversity applies as well as

the process of adaptability. For example, *resilience* in children can be defined as getting "good outcomes in spite of serious threats to development" (Masten, 2000). Resilience in adults, such as those suffering from cancer, is linked to social support, spirituality/faith, and helping others (Pentz, 2005). For individuals with arthritis and other chronic, debilitating diseases, *resilience* is defined in the context of having a sense of control over the disease and a feeling of well-being in the face of adversity (Zautra & Kruszewski, 2008). Resilient people who have lost a spouse, a job, or otherwise experienced significant dislocation are able to "pick themselves up" after a period of time and continue to be hopeful about the future.

Philanthropic organizations that seek to foster resilience in individuals and communities use these general definitions to inform their work. They make grants to promote "strong institutions, dense networks and flexible coping mechanisms" in communities, and feelings of hope, optimism, and social connectedness in individuals (J. W. McConnell Family Foundation, 2006). With a growing awareness of the threat of global warming and the impact of economic and social forces on communities all over the world, philanthropy-sponsored researchers are also investigating characteristics of resilience in the context of sustainability of ecological and social systems, primarily from "complex system" and "transdisciplinary" approaches. Issues such as developing renewable sources of energy, water management, biodiversity, transportation, and the future of "megapolitan" regions, among others, top the agenda (Global Institute of Sustainability, 2007). Whereas the focus of this investigation is primarily on the social aspects of resilience in individuals and communities, and on the ability to adapt and plan for the future in the face of major change, a great deal of the research and philanthropic interest in resilience is directed at biological, mechanical, and economic systems specifically, and the interstices of those domains and social systems more generally.

One issue of interest is whether this *system* definition of resilience can be separated from its *normative* aspects, which are invariably situated within value-laden conceptions of civil society and its political, economic, and sociocultural context. I return to this point later.

The Roots of Philanthropy in Fostering Resilience

In her book *American Creed*, historian Kathleen McCarthy (2003) convincingly demonstrates how philanthropy helped both to define and shape society from the colonial period to the Civil War by creating civic associations, public–private partnerships, social advocacy organizations, and economic development strategies that in turn nurtured the market and government sectors, and established the importance of giving, volunteerism, and participation in civil society to fostering resilient communities and individuals. Key to this process was the ascendancy of an American creed "that held that every citizen had an implicit right to create organizations, lobby for change, and participate in political and economic developments through the voluntary sphere" (p. 202).

Unlike the emphasis in philanthropy today on giving by wealthy individuals and foundations, participation in philanthropy in America's early period was broad and deep, and included both men and women, rich and poor, and black and white. In addition to establishing charities, schools, religious institutions, communal self-help societies, and social reform organizations, philanthropists entered into partnerships with government (the prototype of what we refer to today as public–private partnerships), created savings banks and loan pools (the prototype of today's credit unions and microfinancing mechanisms in developing countries), and helped to foster market values "through associational sales and investments in business development and public works, as well as social causes" (McCarthy, 2003, p. 6). All of this expanded the social, political, and

economic roles of volunteers and trustees, and underscored the fact that "rather than separate spheres, philanthropy, governance and the economy were inherently linked."

McCarthy's account of philanthropy's role in shaping civil society during America's early years contains several important lessons for understanding how to foster resilience in communities and individuals.

1. Social reciprocity and the establishment of trust between individuals is a necessary condition for *asset formation*, whether considered as resources that people use to create a life for themselves and others, or as the capabilities people have to act on those resources (sometimes referred to as human *agency*). In the early years of community building in America, market and government forces were limited, and people came together through voluntary association and developed their own assets. Critical to this was philanthropic investment in human agency. For example, as a young apprentice in the newspaper business in 1727, Benjamin Franklin created the Junto Society, a "volitional community" of fellow apprentices drawn from a variety of trades for purposes of engaging in self-education, public service, and self-help. Members of the Junto, a highly successful alliance that lasted over three decades, were encouraged by Franklin to go out and start similar self-help societies to promote their own businesses, have more influence in public affairs, and "do well by doing good." The Junto was literally "a template for the creation of social capital, the trust that enables individuals to work collaboratively to benefit themselves and the larger society" (McCarthy, 2003, p. 18). As an early proponent of what is referred to today as philanthropic *leverage*, Franklin's entire career demonstrated the effectiveness of an asset-based approach to individual and community development, and the importance of social "bridging" networks of learning and practice to the ability of individuals to adapt and thrive during a period of economic and social turmoil.

2. Another necessary condition for the development of strong, resilient communities is the existence of *social protection*—services, organizations, and policies that protect and promote the well-being of the poor and infirmed, and help them to cope with risks and shocks (Moser, 2006). Early American philanthropists and social activists, such as Isabella Graham, who founded one of the country's first female-controlled charities, the Society for the Relief of Poor Widows with Small Children, were instrumental in knitting together a network of charities, orphanages, hospitals, and similar institutions following the ravages of the Revolutionary War, providing a "safety net" for those who otherwise would never have been able to "bounce back" on their own from adversity. Philanthropists, many of whom were women with social connections, were able to secure charters to establish social protection organizations because they provided vital services for cash-strapped governments. "In effect, they subsidized the state by cutting social service costs through their contributions of money and time" (McCarthy, 2003, p. 38). These associations were early examples of public–private partnerships and laid the ground for the contentious dialogue on the optimal balance between the spheres of civil society, the market, and the state that continues to this day. Then, as now, there were those who scorned charity as unnecessary and degrading for "self-reliant" and "independent" souls, and the accomplishments of these social entrepreneurs were all the more remarkable because of it. Were it not for the development of these early social protection networks, it is likely that early American communities would not have been as resilient as they ultimately proved to be.

3. In addition to promoting individual and social agency in early America, philanthropists invested in *economic agency*. For example, upon his death, Franklin bequeathed an amount of money to be given as low-cost loans to bakers, bricklayers, blacksmiths, hatters, and other tradesmen embarking on their careers—not unlike microloans given

today to people starting businesses in developing countries. The Society for the Prevention of Pauperism, founded in 1817 by prominent New York philanthropists, government officials, and businessmen, received a charter to develop the volunteer-run Savings Bank of New York to provide a means for the poor to save for the future, escape poverty, and promote "habits of economy" and "prudent conduct" (McCarthy, 2003). Similar savings banks began to appear in Philadelphia, Baltimore, Boston, and other American cities. This generated controversy because people were being swept by market forces from an agrarian to a wage economy, and many distrusted the charities that were displacing the so-called "autonomy" of an earlier era, but it illustrates how philanthropy, in partnership with government and business, sought to create avenues of adaptability and social cohesion in the face of major economic and social dislocation. These efforts were complex and contested, and played out much differently in the agrarian South than in the more industrialized North, but in all cases they illustrated the impact of philanthropy in the creation of public–private partnerships to address issues of economic agency and prepare citizens for the future.

4. Philanthropy also fostered resilience in early American society by promoting *social advocacy*. First Amendment guarantees of the right to free speech and petitioning the government for grievances unleashed a torrent of activity by citizens across a broad economic and social spectrum to shape policy agendas and pursue legislative change. These voluntary activities led to the development of a highly charged public sphere, a key dimension of civil society in a democracy, where conflicts between disparate groups could be mediated and diffused before they exploded into physical combat (McCarthy, 2003). In many cases, such as the development of the Free African Society in the North, this social advocacy was conjoined with an emphasis on mutual aid, charity, self-help, and a strict moral code of conduct. Social advocacy grew in tandem with the prominence of

women in public affairs, many of whom established fund-raising auxiliaries, charities, and self-help groups that fueled economic and political activity, as well as a growing emphasis on literacy, which in turn fostered even more social advocacy.

As important as philanthropy was to this process, little of it would have occurred without the federal government's early subsidization of a growing postal network, which by 1828 had twice as many offices as the postal system in Great Britain, and over five times as many offices as the postal system in France. What the French aristocrat Alexis de Tocqueville described in 1831 as the "astonishing circulation of letters and newspapers among these savage woods" knitted together a network of voluntary associations, business enterprises, and political parties that created a distinctive national state (Skocpol, 1996). Philanthropy played a seminal role in this process, but as the economic and governmental structures it helped to create grew in size and impact, its own development began to take a different turn.

Resilience and Modern Philanthropy

Historians of American philanthropy place its modern genesis in the period of social and economic change following the Civil War and into the beginning of the 20th century, when the amassing of great industrial fortunes, rapid advances in scientific and technological progress, and pressing issues of poverty, social dislocation, and economic and cultural upheaval combined to usher in the first "Golden Age" of giving. Early donors such as Andrew Carnegie and John D. Rockefeller felt it was their moral and practical duty to "give a ladder up" to their fellow citizens by stressing self-help and improvement, and not traditional charity and almsgiving. Rather than ameliorate poverty and human suffering, they sought to address the *causes* of poverty through the same

principles of science, organization, and the "systematic application of knowledge" that informed the development of their vast industrial enterprises. This came to be known around the turn of the century as *scientific giving* (Sealander, 2003) and, in its rejection of charity as the dominant philanthropic impulse, defined the reimagination, if not the bulk, of philanthropy during the first part of the 20th century (Frumpkin, 2006).

On the one hand, this was not as radical a break with the past as it might appear. The great majority of people still volunteered their money, time, and talent in promoting human agency, social protection, economic development, and social advocacy. Thousands of self-improvement groups, hospitals, schools, welfare agencies, churches, and social/fraternal organizations continued to take root in local communities across the country, aided by a growing transportation and communication infrastructure of postal, telegraph, rail, telephone, and the automobile. The bulk of giving was still an expression of local community values and concerns, much of it fused with strong religious values and shared norms of moral conduct in response to the effects of industrialism on work and social relationships, and waves of new immigrants entering the country who had to be assimilated and "prepared" for citizenship. Not surprisingly, many people distrusted the rich specifically, and the growing reach of large industrial enterprises and governmental institutions more generally, and were no fans of the emerging "scientific enterprise."

On the other hand, philanthropy, like the country, was becoming more organized, professionalized, and institution-driven. An old order characterized by isolated, independent, self-sufficient, and hierarchical relationships was being replaced by a new order, characterized by efficiency, regularity, control, and bureaucratic relationships (Wiebe, 1967). As the "business" of America became business, so too did large-scale philanthropy become more business-like. The major philanthropists were businessmen first, and they embraced this new order, with its emphasis on self-improvement, social and personal discipline, prudent conduct, and public service. The formal philanthropic institutions they created were based on the same principles and staffed by an ever-increasing cadre of experts in various fields who, through "systematic intervention," sought to bring the material, social, and economic dimensions of life under greater control.

Meanwhile, the welfare activities of the federal government were growing even faster than philanthropy. With the advent of the Great Depression, it became painfully apparent that private, voluntary resources were insufficient to meet basic human needs on a broad scale, calling into question once again the purpose and scope of voluntary giving. Gradually, many of the premier achievements of large-scale philanthropy in the first half of the 20th century—the production of scientific knowledge, the nurturing of great American universities, the eradication of disease, and the development of a network of national social agencies—were superseded by government programs such as Social Security, the GI Bill, the National Institutes of Health, the National Science Foundation, Medicaid, and Medicare. Because most Americans distrusted "Big Government," it became politically expedient to "devolve" many of these social, health, and education functions to state, local, and private sectors, where a rapidly growing array of new "not-for-profit" organizations were funded by the government to provide services. By the 1970s, the federal government was the single largest source of direct and indirect revenue for not-for-profit organizations (Hall, 2003). In 2006, not-for-profit organizations in the United States reported 31% of revenues from government, with as high as 52% for social service nonprofits (Independent Sector, 2006). In fact, what today is characterized as an "independent" sector has been from the colonial period on an *interdependent* sector, where public, private, and market forces intersect in ways that belie the fiction of separate and distinct spheres.

The sheer complexity and diversity of philanthropic activity within this intersection make it difficult to separate its impact in fostering resilience in American life from the impact of larger economic, social, and political forces. Nevertheless, we can trace at least four general trends over the course of the 20th century that link philanthropy and resilience, and set the stage for what some herald as the second "Golden Age" of philanthropy at the beginning of the 21st century.

The Formalization of Human Agency

The ability of people to adapt to a rapidly growing and industrialized society at the turn of the 20th century required ever more formalized programs of education, social amelioration, and control. The investments of philanthropists such as Carnegie in education and libraries, Rockefeller in universities and medical education, Olivia Sage in social service, and Julius Rosenwald in schools for African Americans were "wholesale" transactions in the development of an educational, training, and research infrastructure to enhance individual and community capacity, and not "retail" charitable transactions of goods and services between individuals (Sealander, 2003). Indeed, our growing knowledge of resilience in social-ecological systems comes from the knowledge infrastructure that philanthropy helped to nurture over 100 years ago. Although the magnitude of philanthropic investment in education, training, and research has diminished over the 20th century in comparison to public investment and market-driven activity, voluntary giving continues to be a source of support for innovative programs and projects, some of which are "scaled up" in partnership with business and government. This is the "catalytic" function that many who work in organized philanthropy champion as their pivotal role, as distinct from the role of providing direct human services, which they believe are more properly the province of the public sector.

The Triumph of Technique

The growing industrialization of America in the 20th century spawned an ever more centralized economy and a technological infrastructure characterized by efficiency and control. Whether in the domains of social engineering, the eradication of disease, or increasing agricultural and industrial productivity, a growing cadre of technocratic experts approached all problems as questions of applying optimum techniques, or "the most efficient ensemble of means to achieve a given end" (Ellul, 1967, p. xxv). To cite just one of many examples, the philanthropic foundations of Rockefeller, Ford, and others were instrumental in launching the "Green Revolution" in the 1950s and 1960s, which applied more efficient strains of seeds, fertilizer, and pesticides to increase crop yields dramatically in underdeveloped parts of the world and feed millions of people. Only later did it become apparent that, in the name of efficiency and increased productivity, this approach damaged the environment, favored larger and wealthier agricultural complexes, and drove rural areas deeper into debt. Whatever the pros and cons of the Green Revolution (International Food Policy and Research Institute, 2002), it highlights how the pursuit of efficiency alone can have unintended consequences that may decrease social resilience in the long term by favoring a growth and industrial "monoculture" model over a less efficient but more diverse, adaptable, and sustainable model that can "restore human scale to human enterprise" and "emphasize cooperation over competition, virtue over efficiency and control" (Wolf, 2004). To the degree that efficiency seeks the one "best" solution to achieve a given end, it reduces redundancy, a principal attribute of resilient systems (Resilience Alliance, 2008).

The Changing Nature of Social Capital

The associational aspects of civil society are a primary source of *social capital*, one defi-nition of which is "social networks and the norms of reciprocity and trustworthiness that arise from them" (Putnam, 2000, p. 19). Social support and embeddedness, the presence of strong and weak associational ties, a sense of community, and attachment to place are part of networked adaptive capacities that characterize community resilience (Norris et al., 2008). While mainstream, local philanthropy continued its traditional role of nurturing social capital, funding local institutions and community networks, religious, social, educational, and cultural activities, some of the national "strategic" foundations followed a more formal approach by developing intermediate institutions to "activate community resources behind change" through coordinated, systematic intervention and applied expertise rather than to rely on considerably more messy (and inefficient) grassroots organizing, political mobilization, and local control (O'Connor, 1999). Some of this, such as the Ford Foundation's Gray Area Program in the early 1960s, was considered successful enough to be folded into President Johnson's Great Society antipoverty programs that followed. Critics, however, saw it as one more nail in the coffin of local control and the weakening of indigenous social capital as poor and disenfranchised citizens came to be dependent on outside experts and services for assistance. As we shall see, the issue today is whether the requirements of life in a postindustrial global economy call into question the view that social capital is constructed primarily in shared norms of reciprocity in voluntary civil society—a "Tocquevillian" view of democratic life—and must now factor in a growing technical and "managed" corporate–governmental apparatus that increasingly shapes and regulates our individual and collective capacity to adapt successfully to change.

From Diversity to Pluralism

Resilience in social-ecological systems is characterized by diverse functions, structures, roles, relationships, responses, and activities. Stress in one part of the system can spread out and be absorbed by other parts. This is not the same thing as diversity in the sense of pluralism, a state in which members of diverse ethnic, racial, religious, and social groups are able to maintain their particular interests and cultures within the confines of a larger society. Such a society could, in fact, be remarkably uniform in its central economic and political functions and thus be more, rather than less, susceptible to system shock. An event such as the recent U.S. credit and housing crisis is a case in point. Interestingly, one could make the case that from the height of the civil rights movement in the 1950s and 1960s on, large-scale philanthropy, rather than fostering resiliency through diversity in the first sense, has promoted diversity in the second sense, in the form of support for a rainbow of racial, ethnic, gender, sexual orientation, disability, and interest-specific causes and groups that comprise a new politics of *identity*— of separateness and difference. This in turn has engendered a preoccupation with self-actualization through the identity of one's group rather than the more traditional notion of service in some broader community. Robert Putnam's (2007) recent research on linking immigration and ethnic diversity to lower levels of social solidarity and social capital can be interpreted in this light. To be sure, the turn to identity politics and a focus on self-actualization resulted from a play of economic and cultural forces extending far beyond organized philanthropy, but investments by the Ford Foundation and others in the latter half of the 20th century in issues of social justice and self-determination, while contributing to a more pluralistic and arguably more fair nation, left untouched an increasingly monolithic and less diverse economic and social infrastructure characterized by economic growth and relentless consumerism. Given that these philanthropies themselves were fueled by rapid economic growth, this is not too surprising.

But is a vast global economic and technological monoculture a foregone conclusion? In what ways are the so-called "postmodern" world we are entering different from the modern industrial world that is passing from view, and how might philanthropy adjust to and capitalize on these differences to foster more resilient and healthy individuals and communities?

From Culture to Hyperculture

The recent creation of megafoundations such as the Gates Foundation, the rising tide of billionaire social entrepreneurs, and a projection of more than $40 trillion in transfer of wealth between 2000 and 2055 (Havens & Schervish, 1999) have been cited as evidence that we are entering a second "Golden Age" of philanthropy, in which a new class of philanthropists, steeped in hands-on strategic change and fueled by pragmatic idealism, will work in partnership with market and government forces to create a more sustainable, healthy, and just world. This is stated as a moral imperative: The potential consequences of global warming, economic disparity, the clash of religious and social ideologies, and terrorism/war threaten to destroy human life as we know it unless we act now with boldness, purpose, and direction. Philanthropists everywhere are called upon to step up and play a leadership role.

How much of this is fact, hype, or hope is a question left for another time. Whatever the case, the ability of philanthropy to "make a difference" in the world to the same degree as in the past will be tested by powerful economic, social, psychological, and cultural forces now in play, in varying degrees, in postindustrial society. Here are a few of them.

The Assault on Place

For all of the rhetoric and nostalgia about the importance of community and place in

American life, there is ample evidence that the forces of economic globalism are testing its vitality and survival. The imperatives of increasing productive capacity and efficiency have rent asunder entire industries and the communities that have come to depend on them—a textbook example of what can happen when communities lack economic diversity in the face of social and economic dislocation. In this new economic order, physical place is increasingly contingent on economic criteria as local input and control take a backseat to system decisions made elsewhere. Whether it is a loss of well-paying jobs to outsourcing, displacement of diverse local businesses and social capital by the dominance of "big box" stores like Wal-Mart (Goetz & Rupasingha, 2006), or the loss of civic engagement and local leadership in the face of corporate dislocation (Heying, 2001), communities are increasingly at the mercy of larger forces over which they seemingly have little control. *Place*—physical location—becomes potentially fungible.

Remoteness

The assault on physical place is directly related to the effects of *remoteness*. In a global economic environment, communities may experience the effects of *spatial remoteness*, where decisions are made physically remote from the communities and conditions in which members have a stake. An example is CEOs of companies headquartered elsewhere, who make decisions affecting communities in which they themselves do not live. There is also *consequential remoteness*, where the consequences of decisions impact others but not necessarily those who make them. For example, legislators may decide to cut funding for community mental health services in low-income communities, without the inconvenience of experiencing the effects of the cuts themselves. In another type of remoteness, *temporal remoteness*, decisions we may make today play out in the future and impact others not present. An

example is increasing Medicare benefits, the bill for which will come due in future generations. Finally, there is *virtual remoteness*, where we psychologically "disappear" into a virtual, online world of connections and services that supersedes social connectivity and reciprocity in physical settings: the teenager who feels more connected to her online community of friends than she does to her friends at school; the person who prefers to purchase goods and services online instead of socializing in the local marketplace; and so forth. Whatever the type, remoteness reduces the resilience of communities by masking shared responsibility and conditions of cause and effect. Communities high on the remoteness index—companies with headquarters outside the area, a large number of entitlement programs set by outside regulators or exclusionary age-based communities that have trouble seeing the connection between paying taxes and the education of children not their own—may be less successful than those communities with less remoteness in adapting to the economic, social, and environmental stressors of a rapidly changing world.

A Shrinking Future

Today, many of us live and work in the *Hyperculture*, which is a kind of semantic shorthand that refers to the symbol-mediated presentation of social, political, and economic reality through modern commercial media in all of their myriad forms and venues. It is a culture of hyperbole, or *hype*. It is characterized by exaggeration, speed, short-attention spans, compressed time frames, "fast-breaking" events, fragmented lives and lifestyles, desire for immediacy, and addiction to choice and novelty. It is thought by some to foster purposeless and frantic activity, and to destroy cultural memory and stability of self and society (Bertman, 1998). In the Hyperculture, the future shrinks into the "Long Now." Faith in the future becomes tenuous; philanthropic foundations that once were designed to last "in perpetuity" are increasingly set up to "sunset" after a specified number of years; projects designated as "long term" typically last 5 years or less; the focus shifts to addressing deficits and problems that are at the front door *now*. The issue, of course, is whether the sense of urgency that attends the perception of compressed time and a shrinking future mitigates against fostering individual and community resilience, the characteristics of which literally take a *lifetime* to develop.

The Eclipse of Public Space

Over 80 years ago, philosopher John Dewey (1927) foresaw the eclipse of the public in the rise of a mass-mediated culture of rapid, continuous information, and a growing dependence on experts and a technocratic elite for "solving" problems, instead of people's active participation in a common political life. For Dewey, the distractions of "the movie, cheap reading matter and the motor car" were dominant and drew people's attention away from participation in civic life; today it is cell phones, computers, the Internet, and a mind-boggling, 24/7 industrial "infotainment" complex that comprises the very infrastructure in which public policy is defined, marketed, and "sold" to individual consumers and various "publics" of identifiable interests. In the Hyperculture, everything singular becomes plural: publics, not public; policies, not policy. The promise of technology to enhance a common public life has instead appropriated public space into a breathtaking pluralism of private spaces occupied by these publics. Whether there is traction in technologies, such as the Internet, to create broad-based social networks, public journalism, and a rebirth of active participation in civil discourse remains to be seen; what is beyond dispute is that philanthropy, if it is to direct its resources toward fostering healthy communities, is going to have to learn how to adapt and even shape this new communications arena, the contours of which we do not yet fully comprehend.

The Search for Community

The assault on place, remoteness, a shrinking future, and the eclipse of public space combine to call into question both the definition and experience of *community*, a common definition of which is "a group of people with diverse characteristics who are linked by social ties, shared common perspectives, and engage in joint action in geographical locations or settings" (MacQueen et al., 2001, p. 1929). The experience of community can be fragmented into the experience of "communities," organized both in real-time and virtual settings by interests, ethnicity, religion, age, work, and other dimensions. The experience of community may be very different in more homogeneous, rural communities than in large urban settings, with myriad physical, economic, and sociocultural localities. For example, the resilience of New Orleans in the face of Hurricane Katrina broke down into the attributes and joint action capabilities of quite different subcommunities defined by economics, race, physical location, and function, including the "community" of federal workers and volunteers who assisted with rescue and rebuilding. One of the challenges facing organized philanthropies that seek to foster resilience in communities lies in defining the boundaries of community in the first place.

From Growth to Adaptation

The opportunity before us today is to move from a fixation on increasing productive capacity alone to one of increasing *adaptive* capacity. Clearly, productive capacity is critical to growth and development, but if we are to improve the sustainability of our natural and social environment, we need to turn our attention to encouraging adaptation and learning through a broad diversity of critical functions, economic and social supports, knowledge, institutions, and human opportunities. The concept of resilience, considered both as a metaphor and a process, provides an organizing set of principles and strategies for undertaking this enterprise.

With regard to philanthropy's role, we must consider both the normative and the theoretical and descriptive dimensions of resilience because the goal of philanthropy is to promote the public good, and that leads us to an exercise in moral philosophy, or to investigate norms and ethical principles that comprise what we mean by *the good*. We do not have to pursue that exercise here to appreciate the fact that, in the end, we cannot talk about philanthropy and resilience without also talking about issues such as freedom, autonomy, social justice, democracy, and beneficence, among others. We can give a descriptive account of how to foster resilience through philanthropy, but in the practice of philanthropy in our daily lives, we are compelled to bear witness to ethical principles that imbue our common *public* life and give it its richest meaning. This is why some characterize philanthropy as the "social history of the moral imagination" (Payton, 1987).

Based on one review of the literature, there are four primary sets of *networked adaptive capacities* that foster resilience: economic development, social capital, community competence, and information/communication (Norris et. al., 2008). I take these up in turn, link them back to the role philanthropy has historically played in fostering resilience, and suggest how philanthropists might approach these in light of the selected forces of the Hyperculture, briefly outlined earlier, to continue to be effective in their strategic work. I conclude with some lessons beginning to emerge from the work of one public foundation, St. Luke's Health Initiatives in Phoenix, Arizona, in fostering community resilience.

There are two caveats. The first—and it is an important one—is that there is no single right, or even preferred, way of increasing individual or community resilience through philanthropy. The same diversity of approaches, functions, knowledge, and institutional arrangements that foster resil-

ience must of necessity be present in philanthropy as well. The ideas explored here are thus offered as hypotheses, subject to revision based on experimentation. They are, in short, meant to be *adaptable*. The second caveat restates the qualification previously noted in the definition of *philanthropy*, which historically has included the contribution of time, money, and talent by ordinary citizens from all walks of life to promote the common good, and not simply the distribution of grants from wealthy donors and large foundations to address major problems of the day. The danger is that *philanthropy* in the latter sense will become a spectator sport, as millions of citizens read about and watch the activities of wealthy, celebrity-like philanthropists in the supercharged world of the Hyperculture, and become disengaged from pursuing social change in their own communities. This is already happening: the TV and media personality Oprah has a reality show, *The Big Give*, in which participants "compete" to give away $1 million.

Communities as Adaptive Markets

One way to think of the core adaptive capacities that promote resilience in communities is to characterize communities as potential markets of relationships and opportunities for value, choice, and access (Traynor, 2008). Philanthropy can help to extend these opportunities through networks characterized by a high degree of civic engagement; diversity in economic base, environmental resources, skills, roles, relationships, perspectives and beliefs; redundancy in the sense of overlapping functions and institutions; and robust and stable feedback loops of information, communication, and social connectivity.

Economic Development

I have briefly described how philanthropy has promoted economic development throughout the course of American history in active partnership with private market forces and government. Today, some philanthropic organizations are going back to the "roots" of basic community asset building after 20th-century forays into a more top-down, technocratic, and social engineering approach. One example is the Ford Foundation's Asset Building and Community Development Program, which invests in community economic and material infrastructure (community development corporations, housing and financing intermediaries, basic organizational capacity building, and technical assistance) scaled up in partnership with government and private businesses to develop better public policies, promote the more equitable distribution of power and resources, and create communities of practice and social learning (Ford Foundation, 2004). Others, such as the Skoll Foundation, invest in a burgeoning class of social entrepreneurs such as Martin Fischer, who in 1991 helped to create ApproTec, an nongovernmental organization (NGO) in Kenya that today has created more than 28,000 businesses and 0.5% of Kenya's total gross domestic product (GDP) (Osberg, 2007). In all of this, the challenge is to resist becoming seduced by communities of technocratic elites (some of whom work in large philanthropic organizations) and the exclusivity of specialists who have access to money and tools, and remain open to more inclusive processes and adaptation at the local level of physical and place-bound communities. Another challenge, especially when thinking about how to "scale up" community building through economic development, is to resist the "bigger is better" monoculture of productive efficiency alone, and balance it with a more sustainable, though perhaps less efficient, focus on smaller communities of diverse economic and social supports, networked with each other to disperse the impact of system shocks.

Social Capital

In the communities as adaptive markets model, social capital is best understood as access (networks) plus resources, as distinct from focusing on shared norms of social reciprocity and voluntary association alone (Foley, Edwards, & Diani, 2001). Access to networks of social support, strong organizational linkages and cooperation, diverse sources of capital, and a high degree of civic participation and formal leadership roles are predictors of economic activity, a significant portion of which today rests upon a vast communications, financial, and regulatory infrastructure. Attachment to place and sense of community, as important as they are, are increasingly provisional and temporary; feelings of remoteness and a sense of a shrinking future call into question either the ability or suitability of traditional civil society configurations (unions, community organizations, traditional nonprofits) both to critique the ideology of relying on consumer market forces alone to supply public goods and to present a viable alternative to it.

But what alternatives are there? The growing prevalence of bridging networks based on identity politics, advocacy, professional services/interests, and faith-based activities is a fruitful area to explore. Here, the role of philanthropic organizations as independent conveners and providers of information and technical assistance is as important as supplying funds for organizational and network support. This comes down to "re-creating" social capital at the cellular level. Today, people move in and out of these networks quickly, and their level of commitment to, and interest in, a specific physical place or community of practice is itself influenced by their personal situation (education, income, mobility, etc.). In an increasingly unstable economic and sociocultural environment, these bridging networks—real-time, place-bound, or virtual—have to be as fluid and adaptable as individuals themselves, and provide substantive and timely access to social and economic resources. Furthermore, these networks must exhibit a high measure of redundancy and strong feedback loops of shared information and collaboration. For example, a recent foundation-sponsored study in a large, urban metro area on the pathways people use to access behavioral health services, and to share common interests and conditions, documented an impressive web of interconnected self-help groups, institutions, businesses, churches, government agencies, and informal circles of family and friends (Hughes, 2005). This web of economic and social reciprocity was not necessarily efficient, but it was effective. It was not necessarily stable or permanent, but it was adaptable. It did not arise whole cloth as the result of some top-down "strategic" planning exercise with techniques of formal intervention and control, but it grew organically from the bottom-up, through networks of social reciprocity. In short, it was literally *self-organizing*.

Community Competence

Resilience is rooted in individual and community agency, or the capabilities for meaningful, intentional action. Unless communities have the capacity to acquire information, reflect critically on it, and solve emerging problems, strategic planning becomes an academic exercise at best and is of no practical use at all. Throughout American history, philanthropists from all walks of life have invested in asset building and human agency: providing educational opportunities, building institutions of social support, investing in research and knowledge development, creating economic opportunities, supporting advocacy, extending communication networks across groups of diverse and even divergent interests, and developing leadership. This new Golden Age of philanthropy, if in fact it occurs on the large scale projected, must continue this investment in all of its myriad forms, including building partnerships with the business and government sectors.

The latter is especially important. It is tempting to wax nostalgic about a return to smaller communities, local control, and people coming together to "take care of their own" through community-based (and financed) services, but the fact of the matter

is that local communities are increasingly dependent on, and interdependent with, large-scale global economic forces and a financial/regulatory infrastructure that is relentlessly extending its reach into communities all across the world. If this structure itself is to prove adaptable and resilient, it is imperative that philanthropists look for ways to invest in the open, transparent, intelligent, and responsive government structures we need at all jurisdictional levels, and not reject government involvement for ideological reasons alone. Paradoxically, we will create vital, local communities with a high degree of civic engagement, diversity of opportunities, and supports through the intelligent investment of resources and ideas in governmental and regulatory infrastructure—and vice versa. Interdependency and integration, not separateness and fragmentation, comprise the operable state of all sustainable social-ecological systems.

The other salient point about investing philanthropic resources to increase community competence is to note the sheer amount of "noise" arising in the Hyperculture from adversarial conflict and dissension. The ability of communities to address conflict is enhanced by engaging constructively in group processes, being able to collect and analyze relevant information, to resist undesirable influences, and to participate in a constructive political process that involves all citizens, and not just special interest groups. This community "empowerment" process is enhanced by both investing in the skills necessary to collaborate with others and creating the public space in which such collaboration can occur. This translates into increased philanthropic investment in the activities of citizen engagement, advocacy, grassroots organizing, and leadership development. This can generate even more "noise," of course, but it is only through the process of active and ongoing citizen engagement—not through uncritical and passive acceptance of the manipulated messages of the Hyperculture—that we will increase adaptive capacity and community competence.

Information and Communication

In the face of system stress and shock, having access to a trusted source of information and a robust communications infrastructure is necessary for a community's ability to respond and adapt quickly. According to one private foundation official, the ability of New York City to weather and bounce back from the 9/11 crisis in 2001 was due to both the "official" communications infrastructure of the city to respond to emergencies and the "unofficial" infrastructure of small organizations all over the city that connected with thousands of undocumented and marginalized persons who needed basic humanitarian help and advice (Berresford, 2007). Again, the lesson is that a *diversity* of trusted, reliable information and communication resources, and not just one source, characterizes resilient communities.

I am talking here about more than the necessity of a strong communication and information system for disasters and emergencies. I am also talking about the communications infrastructure that carries *narratives* of shared meaning and purpose in community life. This is increasingly the province of mass media—many of which are in the hands of private corporations—that shape the terms, set the agenda, and referee the debate on the disposition of conflicting values and the allocation of scare resources to address common social and economic issues through public policy. Like it or not, mass media dominate our collective perceptual space. It is impossible to ignore the impact of the Hyperculture on the adaptive capacity of individuals and communities in the face of social and economic dislocation. Indeed, some in philanthropy believe that it is impossible to operate effectively in this "mediated" environment without themselves being "information brokers" and policy players. "A culture of timidity is useless in the Information Age," the president of a major health care foundation told his philanthropic colleagues over a decade ago. "You have to make your voice

heard. It isn't important what your point of view is. Just have one" (Altman, 1996).

In the Hyperculture, even journalists are spectators and consumers first, and participants in civic discourse second. To counter this, some in philanthropy support a burgeoning civic (public, participatory) journalism movement, either through funding various national, regional, and local initiatives (Ford Foundation, among others) or getting into the business of producing independent information and analysis in partnership with public media (Kaiser Family Foundation and Pew Charitable Trusts, among others). Still others are investigating the use of social media on the Internet (Web 2.0) and the use of personal technologies, such as cell phones and portable computers, to provide new information and communication avenues for narratives based on substantive civic engagement. The exploration of this growing movement is outside the scope of this chapter, but it is potentially one of the ways in which philanthropists can reinvigorate the participation of citizens in public life, and away from a passive spectator role of "consuming" orchestrated news and cultural amusements.

Resilience: Health in a New Key

In 2003, St. Luke's Health Initiatives (SLHI) personnel had a series of conversations with the editors of this handbook that resulted in publication of the report *Resilience: Health in a New Key* (Hughes, 2003). In the traditional sense, *health* is viewed as the absence of illness and pathology. This is the principal focus of the formal U.S. health care system: to treat disease and affliction, and to "restore" the patient to health. In a "New Key" definition, however, *health* is defined as the harmonious integration of mind, body, and spirit within a responsive community. This normative definition places equal weight on both physical–psychological–spiritual integration and its interdependency within a responsive social-ecological environment, where *responsive* is directly tied to the networked adaptive capacities of communities. *Resilience*, too, is a normative term in this context, to the degree that it encompasses the values of collaboration and social reciprocity, and encourages active participation in civic life and democratic processes.

Based on its knowledge of the local Phoenix metro area, and the history of philanthropy and community development more generally, SLHI adopted an asset-based—as distinct from the more pervasive deficit-based—approach to community development (Kretzmann & McKnight, 1993) and began to put theory into practice. Space does not allow for a more complete discussion of the principles and strategies of asset-based community development, but they infuse the following "emerging lessons" from one foundation's early experience in fostering resilience through philanthropy at the local level.

1. *Resilience is enhanced by connecting civic and political institutions.* This is hardly a novel lesson in the history of American democracy, but it can be a difficult one for foundations to learn, especially those that wish to avoid the messy world of advocacy. In 1999, SLHI made a grant to the Arizona Interfaith Partnership (AIP), a network of approximately 170 member congregations, unions, schools, and other educational organizations to develop a multicity health care initiative. What foundation staff thought was a "planning" grant resulted in an intense political process, where almost 5,000 people convened in Phoenix at the end of the project period and, in a political rally atmosphere, asked foundation and other local leaders to "take the pledge" to demand health care coverage for all citizens, a livable wage, education, and other conditions of social justice. Some SLHI board members thought the foundation would lose its reputation for independence and being an "honest broker" if it funded organizations that had a "political" agenda; others were sufficiently impressed by the success of AIP to argue that the foundation should support those organizations that could move an agenda consistent with the mission and goals of SLHI. The foundation went on to fund AIP for the next 6 years, focusing on a successful effort to create a special tax district to support the region's public hospital system, and creating education partnerships to train low income persons for entry-level jobs in the health care field. The experience underscored the capacities for social capital embedded in religious institutions, and the power that comes from grassroots organizing at the local level (Warren, 2001). In the face of the alienating aspects of the Hyperculture, many churches remain a "haven in a heartless world," where people physically gather to establish norms of social reciprocity and take social and political action. They are often *anchor stores* in communities, where people who share common values can tap into community strengths and assets in ways that service organizations run by outside professionals cannot. For foundations focused on social change, it is impossible to swim in this water without getting wet. Some are more comfortable with supporting advocacy than others, and it remains a point of vigorous discussion among the SLHI trustees.

2. *Resilience is enhanced by community wells.* At the local level, space- and time-bound communities are enhanced by the presence of accessible and trusted "wells" of information, services, and social connections. This is especially true in communities characterized by high rates of transience and diverse populations, such as the Phoenix metro area, one of the fastest growing regions in the country. Based on SLHI's experience in working with leaders and organizations in specific locations, there is a marked difference between communities that have these wells and those that do not. In one low-income community in North Central Phoe-

nix, for example, with a high transient rate and a multiplicity of languages and cultures, a local hospital system, the John C. Lincoln Health Network, has for many years been a stabilizing, trusted source of social support and connection. Their Desert Mission program, which SLHI has supported with planning and technical assistance grants over the past 8 years, has been the *well*—the hub, the anchor—in a network of organizations that work on neighborhood housing and revitalization issues, family assistance, child care, dental care, community health, and a food bank. There are diverse services and funding sources, and an emphasis on leveraging local assets and leadership in the various ethnic communities.

In contrast, SLHI is beginning to work in a community in South Phoenix that has been decimated by high rates of crime, poverty, and racial tension. A number of governmental and nonprofit agencies provide services in the community, but there is currently no established, trusted source of information and social connections that community members themselves "own." Ironically, programs targeted for specific "populations" (Hispanics, African Americans, people with mental illnesses, etc.) increase social separateness and reinforce identity with a specific group, and not with the larger community. When asked what they "need," residents simply say "more services." Locked in a deficit model, agencies have never asked people in the community what their interests are, what strengths they think they have, and what they can *do* instead of what they *need*. In situations like this, more money for more services is not the answer. Philanthropy can play an important role simply by helping to frame the community conversation from a deficit model to an asset-based perspective and begin patiently to convene both the outside agencies and community leaders to discuss how to move forward in a different way. Based on SLHI's experiences, the leaders are there; they just need to be identified and encouraged to get involved.

3. *Resilience is enhanced by leveraging local culture.* Steven Schroeder (2007), past president of the Robert Wood Johnson Foundation, concluded that in the world of large philanthropic foundations, "execution trumps strategy" (p. 56). SLHI would go one step further and say that "culture trumps execution." If a foundation does not start from where people are rather than where they think they ought to be, it is likely to have little impact. For example, SLHI is learning the importance of balancing its own perception of time and measures of performance (project "periods," funding "cycles," "benchmarks" of success, etc.) with perceptions of time and social cohesiveness among quite distinct communities, such as recently arrived immigrants and Native Americans. As simple as it sounds, the importance of convening people and sharing a meal cannot be overstated. In a culture of virtual encounters and short attention spans, people from all walks of life crave meaningful human contact. SLHI hosts over 300 community meetings a year at its facilities, and most of them revolve around food. At one recent gathering of immigrants being trained as medical interpreters, each person brought a dish from his or her own country, and the group celebrated their shared identity as a "community of learners." It was a powerful moment for all involved. By providing an environment in which people meet and break bread together, SLHI both gains the trust and acceptance of a growing community of local partner organizations and leaders, and nurtures bonds of social reciprocity among participants. This in turn enhances trust and communication in the daily work of community development. All of this takes time and cannot easily be fit into neatly defined beginning and ending points. The current fascination among some in the philanthropic community with adopting the principles and language of venture capitalism, with its emphasis on focus, metrics, and time-driven results, may be out of sync with the considerably slower pace of some local cultures and

communities. Once again, remaining flexible and adaptable to local conditions is key.

4. *Resilience is enhanced through strong feedback loops.* Robust and stable connectivity, both in a biological and a social sense, allows individuals and communities to monitor and adapt to change. One of the ironies of today's hyperconnected world is that the surface communication networks that fill up the perceptual space of mass culture and constitute our "common" commercial life are often not well connected to the more informal, place-bound communication networks of local communities. Philanthropic organizations spend a great deal of time in the former, but the experts and professionals they employ do not necessarily live in the latter or understand fully the opportunities and challenges there. SLHI has focused much of its work on developing social connectivity in targeted Health in a New Key communities through helping to develop strong feedback loops among community leaders, technical assistance consultants, and various programs and agencies that work in these communities. Still, the foundation finds that there is much to learn about how to engage residents themselves in addressing common issues. For example, in a Hispanic community on Phoenix's West Side, a local community center employed *promotoras* (Hispanic health workers) as part of an SLHI-sponsored project to address issues in maternal child health, among other things. In going door to door, however, the *promotoras* discovered that residents were much more concerned with issues of community safety, and especially with the presence of unleashed dogs in the neighborhood that made it unsafe for children to play outside. This led to the residents and the *promotoras* exploring ways to work together with the City of Phoenix to address the problem, potentially giving the residents a sense of accomplishment and empowering them to get more directly involved with community social networks instead of passively waiting for services and "solutions." This does not happen without ongoing, monitored feedback between all the community stakeholders.

Conclusion

Health in a New Key is one of many examples of ways in which philanthropy can foster resilience in individuals and communities. It is not that different from what philanthropy has always sought to do throughout American history: promote the common good through investment in human agency, social support, economic development, and social advocacy. The playing field has changed—civil society, the market, and government are now inextricably intertwined in a global culture of economic interdependency, and characteristics of the emerging Hyperculture have dramatically altered the perceptual field and the ways in which ideas, values, and policy are formed—but philanthropy across a broad spectrum of society continues to support education, research, social services, cultural activities, health, and other dimensions of human life to "make a difference" in communities all over the world. Diversity of species, functions, responses, human opportunity, and economic options is a critical component of resilient communities, and so must it be with philanthropy. The danger is that we will continue to equate a linear conception of human progress with the greater production of goods and services, and apply technology to bring the natural environment under control to serve that narrow conception rather than apply human ingenuity to learn how to live in harmony with the natural world in ways that sustain freedom, choice, justice, and hope in adaptive, responsive communities. This, in the end, is what ties philanthropy at the beginning of the 17th century to philanthropy at the beginning of the 21st century. It was then, and remains today, a profound moral imperative: to serve and to help others, so that we all ultimately may help ourselves. Bound thus together, we will learn to adapt successfully and thrive in the face of ceaseless change.

References

Altman, D. (1996, February 22). Remarks made at the annual conference of Grantmakers in Health, Los Angeles, CA.

Arnove, R. 1980. *Philanthropy and cultural imperialism*. Bloomington: Indiana University Press.

Berresford, S. (2007). Partnerships for foundation effectiveness and regulation. In J. M. Juergens & B. R. Sievers (Eds.), *Stanford conversations in philanthropy*. Stanford, CA: Stanford University Press.

Bertman, S. (1998). *Hyperculture: The human cost of speed*. New York: Praeger.

Bureau of Labor Statistics, United States Department of Labor. (2007). *Volunteering in the United States, 2007*. Retrieved January 26, 2008, from *www.bls.gov/news.release/pdf/volun.pdf*.

Dewey, J. (1927). *The public and its problems*. New York: Holt.

Ellul, J. (1967). *The technological society*. New York: Vintage Books.

Fleischman, J. (2007). *The foundation: A great American secret*. New York: Public Affairs.

Foley, M. W., Edwards, B., & Diani, M. (2001). Social capital reconsidered. In B. Edwards, M. W. Foley, & M. Diani (Eds.), *Beyond Tocqueville: Civil society and the social capital debate in comparative perspective* (pp. 266–280). Hanover, NH: University Press of New England.

Ford Foundation. (2004). *Asset building for social change: Pathways to large scale impact*. Retrieved January 24, 2008, from *www.fordfound.com/pdfs/impact/assets_pathways.pdf*.

Frumpkin, P. (2006). *Strategic giving: The art and science of philanthropy*. Chicago: University of Chicago Press.

Giving USA Foundation. (2007, June 25). Press release on U.S. Charitable Giving. Retrieved January 26, 2008, from *www.aafrc.org/press_releases/gusa/20070625.pdf*.

Global Institute of Sustainability. (2007). Arizona State University. Retrieved November 16, 2007, from *sustainability.asu.edu*.

Goetz, S. J., & Rupasingha, A. (2006). Wal-Mart and social capital. *American Journal of Agricultural Economics*, 88(5), 1304–1310.

Hall, P. D. (2003). The welfare state and the careers of public and private institutions since 1945. In L. Friedman & M. McGarvie (Eds.), *Charity, philanthropy and civility in American history* (pp. 363–383). Cambridge, UK: Cambridge University Press.

Havens, J. J., & Schervish, P. G. (1999). *Millionaires and the millennium: New estimates of the forthcoming wealth transfer and the prospects for a golden age of philanthropy* [Report]. Chestnut Hill, MA: Boston College, Social Welfare Research Institute.

Heying, C. H. (2001). Civic Elites and corporate delocalization: An alternative explanation for declining civic engagement. In B. Edwards, M. W. Foley, & M. Diani (Eds.), *Beyond Tocqueville: Civil society and the social capital debate in comparative perspective* (pp. 101–111). Hanover, NH: University Press of New England.

Hughes, R. (2003). *Resilience: Health in a new key*. Phoenix, AZ: St. Luke's Health Initiatives.

Hughes, R. (2005). *Mind, mood and message: Community pathways in behavioral health*. Phoenix, AZ: St. Luke's Health Initiatives.

Independent Sector. (2006). *Charitable fact sheet*. Retrieved March 19, 2008, from *www.independentsector.org/programs/research/charitable_fact_sheet.pdf*.

International Food Policy and Research Institute. (2002). *Green revolution: Curse or blessing?* Retrieved March 28, 2008, from *ifpri.org/pubs/ib/ib11.pdf*.

Joyce, M., & Richardson, H. (1993). *What is conservative philanthropy?* [Heritage Foundation research paper]. Retrieved March 13, 2008, from *www.heritage.org/research/politicalphilosophy/upload/92068_1.pdf*.

J. W. McConnell Family Foundation. (2006). *Resilient communities*. Retrieved December 19, 2007, from *mcconnellfoundation.ca//default.aspx?page=100&lang=en-us*.

Kretzmann, J., & McKnight, J L. (1993). *Building communities from the inside out: A path toward finding and mobilizing a community's assets*. Chicago: ACTA Publications.

Masten, A. S. (2000). *Children who overcome adversity to succeed in life* [University of Minnesota Extension]. Retrieved December 19, 2007, from *www.extension.umn.edu*.

MacQueen, K., McLellan, E., Metsger, D., Kegeles, S., Strauss, R., Scotti, R., et al. (2001) What is community?: An evidence-based definition for participatory public health. *American Journal of Public Health*, 91(12), 1929–1937.

McCarthy, K. (2003). *American creed: Philanthropy and the rise of civil society, 1700–1865*. Chicago: University of Chicago Press.

Moser, C. (2006). *Asset-based approaches to poverty reduction in a globalized context* [Brookings Institution]. Retrieved January 5, 2008, from *www.brookings.edu/papers/2006/11sustainabledevelopment_moser.aspx*.

Norris, F. H., Stevens, S. P., Pfefferbaum, B., Wyche, K. F., & Pfefferbaum, R. L. (2008). Community resilience as a metaphor, theory, set of capacities, and strategy for disaster readiness. *American Journal of Community Psychology*, 41, 127–150.

O'Connor, A. (1999). The Ford Foundation and philanthropic activism in the 1960s. In E. Lagemann (Ed.), *Philanthropic foundations: New scholarship, new possibilities* (pp. 169–194). Bloomington: Indiana University Press.

Osberg, S. (2007). Time present, time future: Choosing to last. In J. M. Juergens & B. R. Sievers (Eds.), *Stanford conversations in philanthropy* (pp. 97–110). Stanford, CA: Stanford University Press.

Payton, R. (1987). *Philanthropy as a concept*. Retrieved April 18, 2008, from *www.payton-papers.org/output/pdf/0081.pdf*.

Pentz, M. (2005). Resilience among older adults with cancer and the importance of social support and spirituality–faith: "I don't have time to die." *Journal of Gerontological Social Work*, 44(3–4), 3–22.

Putnam, R. D. (2000). *Bowling alone: The collapse and revival of American community*. New York: Simon & Schuster.

Putnam, R. D. (2007). *E pluribus unum*: Diversi-

ty and community in the twenty-first century: The 2006 Johan Skytte Prize Lecture. *Scandinavian Political Studies*, 30(2), 137–174.

Resilience Alliance. (2008). *Key concepts*. Retrieved February 2, 2008, from *www.resalliance.org/576.php*.

Schroeder, S. (2007). Lessons learned: Twelve-and-a-half-years at the Robert Wood Johnson Foundation. In J. M. Juergens & B. R. Sievers (Eds.), *Stanford conversations in philanthropy* (pp. 53–60). Stanford, CA: Stanford University Press.

Sealander, J. (2003). Curing evils at their source: The arrival of scientific giving. In L. Friedman & M. McGarvie (Eds.), *Charity, philanthropy and civility in American history* (pp. 217–239). Cambridge, UK: Cambridge University Press.

Skocpol, T. (1996). What Tocqueville missed. *Slate Magazine*. Retrieved March 3, 2008, from *www.slate.com/id/2081*.

Traynor, B. (2008, Spring). The bright future of community building. *Nonprofit Quarterly*, pp. 24–29.

Warren, M. R. (2001). Power and conflict in social capital. In B. Edwards, M. W. Foley, & M. Diani (Eds.), *Beyond Tocqueville: Civil society and the social capital debate in comparative perspective* (pp. 169–182). Hanover, NH: University Press of New England.

Wiebe, R. (1967). *The search for order, 1877–1920*. New York: Hill & Wang.

Wolf, R. (2004). *The triumph of technique*. Halls, TN: Ruskin Press.

Zautra, A., & Kruszewski, D. (2008). Psychosocial factors in arthritis. In J. H. Klippel, J. H. Stone, L. J. Crofford, & P. H. White (Eds.), *Primer on rheumatic diseases* (13th ed., pp. 609–613). New York: Springer.

Author Index

Subject Index

Page numbers followed by *f* indicate figure; *n*, note; *t*, table.